W9-BHY-299

BASIC TECHNIQUES IN CLINICAL LABORATORY SCIENCE

Third Edition

Basic Techniques in Clinical Laboratory Science

Third Edition

Jean Jorgenson Linné, B.S., M.T.(ASCP)

Assistant Professor
Department of Laboratory Medicine and
*   Pathology*
University of Minnesota Medical School
Minneapolis, Minnesota

Karen Munson Ringsrud, B.S., M.T.(ASCP)

Assistant Professor
Department of Laboratory Medicine and
*   Pathology*
University of Minnesota Medical School
Minneapolis, Minnesota

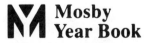

Mosby
Year Book

St. Louis   Baltimore   Boston   Chicago   London   Philadelphia   Sydney   Toronto

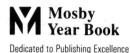
Mosby Year Book

Dedicated to Publishing Excellence

Sponsoring Editor: Stephanie Manning
Assistant Editor: Jane Petrash
Assistant Director, Manuscript Services: Frances M. Perveiler
Production Manager: Nancy C. Baker
Proofroom Manager: Barbara Kelly

Copyright 1992 by Mosby–Year Book, Inc.
A C. V. Mosby Company imprint of Mosby–Year Book, Inc.

Mosby–Year Book, Inc.
11830 Westline Industrial Drive
St. Louis, MO 63146

All rights reserved. No part of this publication may be reproduced, stored in a retrieval system, or transmitted, in any form or by any means, electronic, mechanical, photocopying, recording, or otherwise, without prior written permission from the publisher. Printed in the United States of America.

Permission to photocopy or reproduce solely for internal or personal use is permitted for libraries or other users registered with the Copyright Clearance Center, provided that the base fee of $4.00 per chapter plus $.10 per page is paid directly to the Copyright Clearance Center, 21 Congress Street, Salem, MA 01970. This consent does not extend to other kinds of copying, such as copying for general distribution, for advertising or promotional purposes, for creating new collected works, or for resale.

1 2 3 4 5 6 7 8 9 0 CL/MV 96 95 94 93 92

Library of Congress Cagaloging-in-Publication Data
Linné, Jean Jorgenson.
    Basic techniques in clinical laboratory science / Jean Jorgenson
Linné, Karen Munson Ringsrud.
        p.   cm.
    Rev. ed. of: Basic techniques for the medical laboratory. 2nd ed.
c1979.
    Includes bibliographical references and index.
    ISBN 0-8016-2864-4
    1. Diagnosis, Laboratory—Laboratory manuals. I. Ringsrud, Karen
Munson. II. Linné, Jean Jorgenson. Basic techniques for the
medical laboratory. III. Title.
    [DNLM: 1. Technology, Medical. QY 25 L758ba]
    RB37.L68 1991   91-28014
    616.07′5—dc20   CIP
    DNLM/DLC
    for Library of Congress

To David, David and Jonathan
Peter and Erik

PREFACE TO THE THIRD EDITION

More than 20 years have passed since the publication of the first edition of this textbook, and there have been significant changes in the practice of clinical laboratory science during those years. The response to editions one and two has been encouraging and we have been asked to prepare this third edition. To keep abreast of these many changes, even the title has changed with each subsequent revision. The third edition has been titled *Basic Techniques in Clinical Laboratory Science,* to present the material using vocabulary currently in use. The reader will find many of the same basic concepts and much of the same general background material that was originally included in the 1970 edition because basic information remains constant throughout the years. What has evolved in the clinical laboratory is the introduction of more technology, more automation, more consideration of safe work habits and generally more emphasis on efficacy of doing the various laboratory tests.

An extensive effort has been made to completely revise this third edition to allow for the significant advances in the field of clinical laboratory science since the second edition. The primary aim of the book remains unchanged: it is a source of general information for performing the many types of routine tests done in clinical laboratories of various sizes and locations—hospital laboratories, clinic laboratories, and laboratories in physicians' offices. We have sought to maintain the topics pertinent to routine assays performed in clinical laboratories. The original intent of the first edition—to present material in a very basic, thorough manner—difficult to find in any other single textbook—has been retained. We hope that we also have retained the style, organization, and level of presentation so the material can be used by students and laboratorians of many levels.

We have thoroughly revised the material for the third edition. Several new concepts are discussed, with consideration of the innovations in technology available—the use of immunoassays, for example. Outdated information has been removed that is no longer of any general value. We make no pretense of including all laboratory assays performed in a routine clinical laboratory because of the variation between sites and situations. With these limitations in mind, we hope that the reader will find the following material useful in their role as a clinical laboratorian.

We acknowledge Dr. G. Mary Bradley at the University of Minnesota Medical School for her constant support in encouraging us in this endeavor. As an author herself, she knows what goes into such a production. She was always available for advice, information, and encouragement.

No authors can write a book without the support and involvement of their families. It takes over all of their lives. We are thankful for the patience and support of our husbands, David Linné and Peter Ringsrud, and our children, who have gone from infants to young adults in the process of these three editions.

Jean Jorgenson Linné, B.S., M.T.(ASCP)
Karen Munson Ringsrud, B.S., M.T.(ASCP)

CONTENTS

PART *I*

FUNDAMENTALS OF THE CLINICAL LABORATORY

1 Safety in the Clinical Laboratory

Key Terms

Aerosols	Hepatitis C virus (HCV)
Barrier precautions	Human immunodeficiency virus (HIV)
Basic first aid	Infection control
Biohazard	Material Safety Data Sheet (MSDS)
Biohazard containers	National Committee for Clinical Laboratory Standards (NCCLS)
Bloodborne pathogens	
Carcinogens	Occupational Safety and Health Administration (OSHA)
Decontamination	
Etiologic agent	Safety manual
Hazard indentification system	Sharps containers
Hepatitis B virus (HBV)	Universal precautions

The importance of laboratory safety and correct first-aid procedures cannot be overemphasized to anyone working in the clinical laboratory. Students as well as laboratory personnel should be constantly reminded of safety precautions. Most accidents do not just happen—they are caused by carelessness or lack of proper communication. For this reason, safety should be foremost in the mind of anyone involved in doing laboratory work of any kind.

Most laboratory accidents are preventable by the exercise of good technique and by the use of common sense. There are many potential hazards in the laboratory, but they can be controlled by taking simple precautions. In every medical institution, the administration supplies the laboratory with safety devices for equipment and personal use, but it is up to the individual to make use of them. Safety is personal, and its practice must be a matter of individual desire and accomplishment. Real appreciation for safety requires a built-in concern for the other person, for an unsafe act may harm the bystander without harming the person who performs the act.

SAFETY MANUAL

Each laboratory should have a **safety manual** readily available which covers all safety practices and precautions. It should be updated frequently with additional or new information as it becomes available. This manual should also include regulations covering the proper use of laboratory equipment and the handling of all hazardous or infectious materials. Anything which poses a potential safety hazard for persons in the laboratory should be described in the safety manual. All persons in the laboratory setting should be familiar with the contents of this manual.

EMERGENCY PRECAUTIONS

A posted plan for evacuation of the laboratory in the event of an emergency must be readily available. Routes for exiting the room and building must be made known to all persons working in that setting, as well as familiarity with the location of the various safety devices—fire extinguishers, emergency showers, eye washers, fire blankets, and other equipment such as respirators or goggles. Implementation of periodic unannounced safety drills may motivate the laboratory personnel to acquire familiarity with current safety practices.

SAFETY STANDARDS AND GOVERNING AGENCIES

Standards for clinical laboratories are initiated, governed, and reviewed by several agencies or committees—the US Department of Labor's **Occupational Safety and Health Administration (OSHA)**; the **National Committee for Clinical Laboratory Standards (NCCLS)**, a nonprofit educational organization providing a forum for development, promotion, and use of national and international standards; the Centers for Disease Control (CDC), a part of the US Department of Health and Human Services' Public Health Service; and the College of American Pathologists (CAP), to name a few.

To ensure that workers have safe and healthful working conditions, the United States government created a system of safeguards and regulations under the Occupational Safety and Health Act of 1970. This system touches almost every person working in the United States today. It is especially relevant to discuss the meaning of the act in any presentation concerning safety in the clinical laboratory. In this setting there are special problems with respect to potential safety hazards, and diseases or accidents associated with preventable causes cannot be tolerated.

The Occupational Safety and Health regulations apply to all businesses with one or more employees and are administered by the US Department of Labor through OSHA. The program deals with many aspects of safety and health protection, including compliance arrangements, inspection procedures, penalties for noncompliance, complaint procedures, duties and responsibilities for administration and operation of the system, and how the many standards are set. Responsibility for compliance is placed on both the administration of the institution and the employee.

The OSHA standards, where appropriate, include provisions for warning labels or other appropriate forms of warning to alert all workers of potential hazards, suitable protective equipment available, exposure control procedures, and implementation of training and education programs—all for the primary purpose of assuring safe and healthful working conditions for every American worker.

A person who understands the potential hazards in a laboratory and knows the basic safety precautions can prevent accidents. The Occupational Safety and Health Act requires a safety program in every clinical laboratory. Identification of potential hazards is an important part of any such program. In each department in the laboratory, the type of hazard is slightly different. However, many hazards are commonly found throughout the laboratory.

LABORATORY HAZARDS

Biological Hazards and Infection Control

Because many hazards of the clinical laboratory are unique, a special term, **biohazard,** was devised. This word is posted throughout the laboratory to denote infectious materials or agents that present a risk or even a potential risk to the health of humans or animals in the laboratory. The potential risk can be either through direct infection or through the environment. Biological infections are frequently caused by accidental aspiration of infectious material, accidental inoculation with contaminated needles or syringes, animal bites, sprays from syringes, **aerosols** from uncapping specimen tubes, and centrifuge accidents. Some other sources of laboratory infections are cuts or scratches from contaminated glassware, cuts from instruments used during animal surgery or autopsy, and spilling or spattering of pathogenic samples on the work desks or floors. Persons working in laboratories on animal research or other research involving biologically hazardous materials are also susceptible to the problems of biohazards. The symbol shown in Figure 1–1 is used to denote the presence of biohazards.

One safeguard that can be taken is to see that all containers are properly labeled. Labeling may be the simplest, single important step in the proper handling of any hazardous substance. A label for a container should include a date and the contents of the container. When the contents of one container are transferred to another container, this information should also be transferred to the new container. Proper labeling of containers is discussed further *later in this chapter*.

Laboratories must exert every effort to implement a program for infection control. This can start with prevention of contamination while the specimens are collected

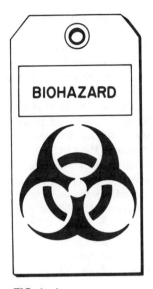

FIG 1–1.
Biohazard symbol.

and delivered to the laboratory. A large percentage of the specimens sent to the laboratory contain blood, and their safe collection and transportation must take top priority in any discussion of safety in the laboratory (see Chapter 2).

Infection Control Programs

Since the clinical laboratory functions to test the various biological specimens from the patient, one of the most important OSHA regulations covers exposure to biological hazards. Protection from **bloodborne pathogens** is of major importance. Clinical specimens received from patients pose a potential hazard to laboratory personnel because of infectious agents they may contain. The CDC recommend safety precautions concerning the handling of all patient specimens. These are known as **universal precautions** (or universal blood and body fluid precautions) and are published in the *Morbidity and Mortality Weekly Report (MMWR),* a series of recommendations from the CDC to protect health care workers and others from acquiring infection with bloodborne pathogens.

Recommendations from OSHA include an infection control plan, engineering and work practice controls, personal protective clothing and equipment, sufficient education and training, signs and labels, provision of **hepatitis B virus (HBV)** vaccination, and medical follow-up for exposure incidents.

The NCCLS has also issued guidelines for the laboratory worker in regard to protection from bloodborne diseases spread via contact with patient specimens.

Together, these agencies are working to lessen the risk of exposure for health care workers to bloodborne pathogens. An infectious disease program must be in place in any health care facility to ensure the safety of the people working there. The US Department of Labor (under OSHA) has developed standards of practice for health care institutions. The CDC have issued guidelines for implementation of these standards. The College of American Pathologists offers a voluntary accreditation program for clinical laboratories. The requirements include safe work practices which, in turn, include biosafety measures.

Universal Precautions

The term *universal precautions* refers to a system of infectious disease control which assumes that every direct contact with body fluids is infectious. These controls include personal protective devices, good work practices, and the proper implementation of engineering controls. It requires that every employee exposed to direct contact with body fluids be protected as though such body fluids were infected with HBV or **human immunodeficiency virus (HIV).** Since not all patients carrying bloodborne pathogens are identified prior to the handling of their specimens, all persons who handle patient specimens or who come in contact with patients in a health care setting should exercise certain consistent precautions on a routine basis. These universal precautions recognize the infectious potential of any patient specimen. The CDC recommendations also recognize that while all patients are potentially infectious, not all types of specimens pose the same degree of risk for the health care personnel.

Blood and certain body fluids pose the greatest risk for those persons whose activities involve contact with them. Body fluids which are included in this classification are semen and vaginal secretions, tissues, cerebrospinal fluid, synovial fluid, peritoneal fluid, and amniotic fluid. For the purposes of prudent laboratory practice, however, adherence to universal precautions for the handling of all biological patient specimens is recommended. In following these precautions, both the prevention of cross-transmission of infectious disease to patients as well as protection to laboratory personnel from infected patients will be addressed. In most health care institutions, all patient specimens and body substances encountered during patient care are regarded as infectious and are handled using the universal precautions policy.

The essence of any universal precaution policy is the avoidance of direct contact with patient specimens in general. When contact with any patient specimen is anticipated, health care workers should use the appropriate barrier precautions to prevent cross-transmission and exposure of their own skin and mucous membranes.

Protection from Specimen-borne Pathogens

Precautions for exposure to possible specimen-borne infection focus mainly on HBV, HIV, and human T cell lymphotropic viruses (HTLV). Focus on HBV and HIV transmission is emphasized owing to the severity of hepatitis B and acquired immunodeficiency syndrome (AIDS)—risks to health care workers that have grave consequences. There are other viruses of concern to laboratory workers, hepatitis non-A, non-B virus **(hepatitis C),** for example, but it is felt that the precautions recommended for HBV and HIV are sufficient for these also.

Virus Transmission.—The major infectious pathogens, HBV and HIV, may be transmitted in the laboratory directly by three main routes:

1. *Percutaneous:* parenteral inoculation of blood, plasma, serum, or body fluids which can occur by accidental needle sticks, scalpel cuts, etc., and by transfusion of infected blood or blood products.
2. *Nonintact skin:* transfer of infected blood, plasma, serum, or body fluids in the absence of overt punctures of the skin, through the contamination of pre-existing minute cuts, scratches, abrasions, burns, weeping or exudative skin lesions, etc.
3. *Mucous membranes:* contamination of mucosal surfaces with infected blood, plasma, serum, or body fluids as may occur with mouth pipetting, splashes, spattering, or other means of oral or nasal mucosal or conjunctival contact.

HBV can be transmitted indirectly from such common surfaces as telephones, test tubes, laboratory instruments, and work surfaces. HIV *may* be similarly transmitted, but no environmentally mediated transmission of HIV has been documented. HIV has been isolated from blood, semen, vaginal excretions, saliva, tears, breast milk, cerebrospinal fluid, amniotic fluid, alveolar fluid, and urine. However, only blood, semen, vaginal excretions, and breast milk have been implicated in the transmission of HIV to date. Hepatitis B is of special concern in laboratories of hospitals where organ transplants are done, necessitating large volumes of blood and blood products being used. Those most heavily exposed to blood from renal transplant patients—for example, through accidental inoculation, ingestion of blood, or inhalation of blood aerosols while doing laboratory work on these samples—are at the greatest risk of infection from HBV.

Hepatitis B and C viruses transmit the most frequent laboratory-associated infections. As a precautionary measure against potential exposure to HBV, a licensed inactivated vaccine (HB) is available. The CDC's Advisory Committee on Immunization Practices (ACIP) recommends the use of this vaccine as a precautionary step for those persons who are at a substantially greater risk for HBV infection—medical technologists, phlebotomists, and pathologists.

Hepatitis B Virus Exposure.—After skin or mucosal exposure to blood that is known to contain or might contain hepatitis B antigen, ACIP recommends immunoprophylaxis, dependent on several factors. If the worker has not been vaccinated against HBV, a single dose of hepatitis B immune globulin should be given as soon as possible, within 24 hours if practical, along with doses of HB vaccine at a later date. Specific protocol for these measures will rest with the institution's infection control division.

Hepatitis C Virus Exposure.—After exposure to blood of a patient infected or suspected to be infected with HCV, immune globulin should be given as soon as possible.

Human Immunodeficiency Virus Exposure.—The antibody status of the patient or specimen source should be determined, if it is not already known. If the source is a patient, voluntary consent should be obtained, if possible, for testing for HIV antibodies as soon as possible. One possible prophylaxis after exposure to blood or body fluids potentially infectious for HIV by percutaneous, permucosal, or nonintact skin routes, is the use of AZT (zidovudine).

If HIV antibodies are not detected in the blood source, it is probably desirable to test for HIV antigen using a polymerase chain reaction (PCR). If the source patient is seronegative, the exposed worker should be

tested at 3 and 6 months. If the source patient is at high risk for HIV infection, more extensive follow-up of both the worker and blood source patient may be needed.

If the source specimen is HIV-positive (HIV antibodies, HIV antigen, or HIV DNA by PCR), the blood of the exposed worker should be tested for HIV antibodies within 48 hours, if possible. Exposed workers who are initially seronegative for the HIV antibody should be tested again 6 weeks after exposure. If this test is negative, the worker should be tested again at 12 weeks and 6 months after exposure. Most reported seroconversions have occurred between 6 and 12 weeks after exposure.

During the early follow-up period after exposure (especially the first 6–12 weeks), the worker should follow the recommendations of the CDC regarding the transmission of AIDS, including:

1. Refraining from donating blood or plasma.
2. Informing potential sex partners of the exposure.
3. Avoiding pregnancy.
4. Informing health care providers of their potential exposure, so necessary precautions can be taken by them.
5. Not sharing razors, toothbrushes, or other items which could become contaminated with blood.
6. Cleaning and disinfecting surfaces on which blood or body fluids have spilled.

The exposed worker should be advised of and alerted to the risks of infection and evaluated medically for any history, signs, or symptoms consistent with HIV infection. Serologic testing for HIV antibodies should be made available to health care workers who are concerned that they have been infected with HIV.

Procedure 1–1. First Aid for Skin Puncture or Mucosal Contamination

1. For skin puncture or surface skin contamination, wash skin site with soap and water while encouraging bleeding. If appropriate, bandage the site. Report incident to supervisor.
2. For contaminated mucosal or conjunctival sites, wash with large amounts of water for an extended period of time. Report incident to supervisor.

Safe Work Practices

To eliminate the risk of transmitting infectious pathogens, those working in the laboratory with blood specimens must take several precautions. Washing the hands frequently is one of the most important ways of preventing contamination. At least one sink in the laboratory should be equipped with a foot pedal for operating the faucets, and it should also have a foot pedal dispenser with a detergent solution for the hands.

Handwashing.—Handwashing is the most important means of interrupting transmission of infectious pathogens. Immediately after any accidental skin contact with blood, body fluids, or tissues, hands or other skin areas must be thoroughly washed. If the contact occurs through breaks in gloves, the gloves must be removed immediately and the hands thoroughly washed according to established procedure for the laboratory. It is also good practice to wash the hands any time there is visible contamination with blood or any body fluid, after completion of laboratory work and before leaving the laboratory, after removing gloves, and before any activities which involve contact with mucous membranes, eyes, or breaks in the skin.

Handwashing Procedure (Procedure 1–2).— Washing with soap and water is recommended, although any standard detergent product acceptable to the personnel may be used. Unless in a unique situation, the use of hand towelettes and cleansing foams is not recommended because they do not provide the necessary dilution and detergent action with the proper rinsing action to follow.

Procedure 1–2. Handwashing

1. Wet both hands and wrists with warm water only; do not use very hot or very cold water.
2. Apply soap from a dispenser to the palms first (about one teaspoonful).
3. Lather well and wash hands and wrists, fingernails, and between the fingers. Do this for a minimum of 5 seconds.
4. Rinse well with warm water and dry completely.
5. If the sink being used is not equipped with foot- or knee-operated controls, turn off the hand faucets using a paper towel to avoid recontamination of clean hands.

No additional benefit has been established for washing with antiseptic soaps or solutions. Any product which disrupts the integrity of the skin should be avoided. Moisturizing hand creams or lotions may reduce skin irritation caused by the frequency of handwashing which is so necessary.

Food and Drink Restrictions.—Since the safety of the laboratory personnel is the reason for such scrutiny in the handling of specimens, etc., previously discussed, it is only prudent that there be no eating, drinking, smoking, and application of cosmetics in the laboratory. Hands may be contaminated with infectious organisms which can easily be spread to the mouth during the above-mentioned activities.

Personal Protective Equipment

Protective equipment, including that for eyes, face, head, and extremities; protective clothing; respiratory devices; and protective shields and barriers are to be provided to laboratory personnel whenever necessary by reason of the potential hazards of processes or environment. This equipment should not only be provided but be maintained in a sanitary and reliable condition. OSHA requires that institutions provide their personnel with personal protective equipment.

Barrier Precautions

As discussed previously, precautions for exposure to possible specimen-borne infection focus mainly on HBV and HIV. Protective devices and **barrier precautions** will prevent transmission of most infectious disease if compliance is strictly maintained.

In the laboratory, the skin (especially when scratches, abrasions, dermatitis conditions, or lesions are present) and the mucous membranes of the eye, mouth, nose, and possibly the respiratory tract can be considered potential pathways for entry of the infectious pathogen. Puncture with needles, sharp instruments, broken glass, and other sharp objects must be avoided. The careful handling and discard of these objects must be done in a consistent manner. Constant vigil and care must be exercised in the handling of infected cell-culture liquid or other virus-containing materials. Barrier precautions are implemented to prevent exposure to infectious pathogens.

Gloves.—Protective gloves must be worn by all persons who engage in procedures which involve direct contact of skin with biological specimens. The implementation of universal precautionary practices is recommended for handling clinical specimens, body fluids, and tissues from humans or from infected or inoculated laboratory animals.

Gloves must be manufactured from the appropriate material, usually intact latex or intact vinyl, of the appropriate quality for the procedures required, and of the appropriate size for each health care worker. Gloves should be thrown away and not washed and used again. Since barrier protection is the ultimate goal, gloves must be discarded if they are peeling, cracking, or discolored (indications of deterioration), or if they have tears or punctures. Proper discard of used gloves is necessary.

Gloves are worn when doing phlebotomies and processing body fluid and blood specimens in the laboratory. After the gloves are removed, the hands must be washed immediately.

Gowns.—All laboratory workers should wear a long-sleeved laboratory coat or gown with a closed front. Gowns and coats worn in the laboratory should be removed when the worker leaves. If personnel desire to wear a laboratory coat out of the laboratory, it is recommended to have coats of different colors—one color to be worn while in the laboratory (considered to be contaminated) and a different color to be worn outside of the laboratory (considered to be noncontaminated).

When splashes to the skin or clothing are likely to occur, a special protective gown, apron, or laboratory coat must be worn. This protective clothing should be manufactured of fluid-proof or fluid-resistant material and should protect all areas of exposed skin.

Masks and Eye Protectors.—When contamination of mucosal membranes (mouth, eyes, or nose) is likely to occur, the use of masks and protective eyewear or face shields is required. Such contamination can occur with body fluid splashes or aerosolization. Protective eyewear should be worn when transferring blood from a collection syringe into the specimen container, for example. Potential splashes can also occur when using chemicals. Certain laboratory reagents are known to be especially caustic to the mucosa. Broken glassware projectiles and vapors from some chemicals can also cause serious eye injuries. The eyes should always be protected with goggles when cleaning glassware with analytic cleaners and when preparing laboratory reagents using strong acids and bases or any other hazardous material.

Protection From Aerosols

Biohazards are generally treated with great respect in the clinical laboratory. The adverse effects of pathogenic substances on the body are well documented. The presence of pathogenic organisms is not limited to the culture plates in the microbiology laboratory. Aerosols can be found in all areas of the laboratory where human specimens are used.

Biosafety Cabinets.—These are protective devices used to control the presence of infectious agents in the air. Microbiology laboratories selectively utilize biological safety cabinets for doing those procedures which generate infectious aerosols. Several common procedures in processing specimens for culture—grinding, mincing, vortexing, centrifuging, and preparation of direct smears—are known to produce aerosol droplets. Air containing the infectious agent is sterilized, either by heat, ultraviolet light, or, most commonly, by passage through a high-efficiency particulate air (HEPA) filter. They not only remove air contaminants through a local exhaust system but provide an added safety measure by confining the aerosol contaminant within an enclosed cabinet, thereby isolating it from the worker.

Specimen Processing Protection.—Specimens should be transported to the laboratory in plastic leak-proof bags. Protective gloves should always be worn when handling biological specimens of all kinds.

Substances can become airborne when the stopper (cap) is popped off a blood-collecting container, a serum sample is poured from one tube to another, or a serum tube is centrifuged. When removing the cap from a specimen tube or blood collection tube, the top should be covered with a disposable gauze pad or special protective pad. Gauze pads with an impermeable plastic coating on one side can reduce contamination of the gloves. The tube should be held away from the body and the cap gently twisted to remove it. Snapping off the cap or top can cause some of the contents to aerosolize. When not in place on the tube, the cap should still be kept in the gauze and not placed directly on the work surface or counter top.

Specially constructed plastic splash shields are used in many laboratories for the processing of blood specimens. The tube caps are removed behind or under the shield, which acts as a barrier between the person and the specimen tube. This is designed to prevent aerosols from entering the nose, eyes, or mouth. Laboratory safety boxes are commercially available and can be used for unstoppering tubes or doing other procedures which might cause spattering. Splash shields and safety boxes should be periodically decontaminated.

When centrifuging specimens, the tube caps should always be kept on the tubes. Centrifuge covers must be used and left on until the centrifuge stops. The centrifuge should be allowed to stop by itself and not be manually stopped by the worker.

Another step that should be taken to lessen the hazard from aerosols is to exercise caution in handling pipettes and other equipment used to transfer human specimens, especially pathogenic materials. These materials should be discarded properly and carefully.

Seven Rules for Biosafety in the Laboratory

1. Never mouth-pipette.
2. Treat infectious fluids carefully to avoid spills and to minimize aerosolization.
3. Restrict use of needles and syringes to procedures where there is no alternative; use needles, lancets, and other "sharps" carefully to avoid self-inoculation; dispose of sharps in leak- and puncture-resistant containers.
4. Use protective laboratory coats and gloves.
5. Wash hands frequently: following all laboratory activities, after removing gloves, and immediately following contact with infectious materials.
6. Decontaminate work surfaces before and after use; wipe up any spills immediately.
7. Never eat, drink, store food, or smoke in the laboratory.

Other Hazards

The fact that clinical laboratories present many potential hazards simply because of the nature of the work done there cannot be overemphasized. In addition to biological hazards, open flames, electrical equipment, glassware, chemicals of varying reactivity, flammable solvents, and toxic fumes are but a few of the other hazards present in the clinical laboratory.

Flammable Substances

One serious hazard in laboratory work is the potential for fire and explosion when flammable solvents such

as ether and acetone are used. These materials should always be stored in special safety cans or other appropriate storage receptacles. Even with proper storage of these materials, there is always some release of flammable vapors in a working laboratory. A good ventilation system in the room and vent sites for the storage area will help to eliminate some of the potential hazard. When using flammable materials, proper precautions must be taken; for instance, flammable liquids should be poured from one container to another slowly, they should never be used when there is an open flame in the room, and they should be kept in closed containers when they are not being used.

Chemical Hazards

Other sources of injury in the laboratory are poisonous, volatile, caustic, or corrosive reagents such as strong acids or bases. Chemicals and reagents can present different types of hazards. Some are dangerous when inhaled (sulfuric acid), some are corrosive to the skin (phenol), some are caustic (acetic acid), some are volatile (many solvents), and some combine these hazards. Acids and bases should be stored separately in well-ventilated storage units. When not in use, all chemicals and reagents should be returned to their storage units. Bottles of particularly volatile substances should not be left open for extended periods.

OSHA is also involved in setting standards directed at minimizing occupational exposures to hazardous chemicals in laboratories. The OSHA hazard communication standard (the employee "right-to-know" rule) is designed to ensure that laboratory workers are fully aware of the hazards associated with chemicals in their workplace. This necessitates the development of comprehensive plans at each work site to implement the practice of safety measures throughout the laboratory insofar as the use of laboratory chemicals is concerned. A chemical hygiene plan for each laboratory must outline the specific work practices and procedures that are necessary to protect workers from any health hazards associated with hazardous chemicals. Information and training regarding hazardous chemicals must be provided to all workers in the laboratory setting. The individual states have also enacted "right-to-know" laws to ensure that available information is disseminated at the local level.

Information about signs and symptoms associated with exposures to hazardous chemicals used in the laboratory must be communicated to all. Reference materials for this information are included in the **material safety**

data sheets (MSDS) provided by all chemical manufacturers and suppliers. This information concerns hazards, safe handling, storage, and disposal of hazardous chemicals used in the laboratory.

Material Safety Data Sheets (MSDS).—Information is provided by chemical manufacturers and suppliers about each chemical. This information is to accompany the shipment of all chemicals and should be available for anyone to review. Each laboratory must have on file all MSDSs for the hazardous chemicals used in that laboratory. Use of MSDSs is a common way that potential product hazard information is made available and OSHA requires this provision by all chemical manufacturers. The health care facility is, in turn, required to provide this information to its workers in the laboratory.

Each MSDS contains basic information about the specific chemical or product. Trade name, chemical name and synonyms, chemical family, manufacturer's name and address, emergency telephone number for further information about the chemical, hazardous ingredients, physical data, fire and explosion data, and health hazard and protection information are included for each chemical.

Protection.—When using any potentially hazardous solution or chemical, protective equipment for the eyes, face, head, and extremities, as well as protective clothing or barriers, should be used. Volatile or fuming solutions should be used under a fume hood. In case of accidental contact with a hazardous solution or a contaminated substance, quick action is essential. The laboratory should have a safety shower where quick, all-over decontamination can take place immediately. Another safety device that is essential in all laboratories is a face or eye washer that streams aerated water directly onto the face and eyes to prevent burns and loss of eyesight. Any action of this sort must be undertaken immediately, so these safety devices must be present in the laboratory area.

Measures to limit exposure to hazardous chemicals must be implemented. Appropriate work practices, emergency procedures, and use of personal protective equipment are to be employed by all. Many of the measures taken are also those needed for protection from biological hazards, as discussed previously (see under Personal Protective Equipment). This includes the use of gloves, keeping the work area clean and uncluttered, the proper and complete labeling of all chemicals, the use of proper

eye protection, fume hood, respiratory equipment, and any other emergency or protective equipment as necessary.

Chemical waste must be deposited in appropriately labeled receptacles for eventual disposal.

Specific Hazardous Chemicals.—Some specific chemicals that must be handled with care and some potential hazards in their use are:

- *Sulfuric acid:* at a concentration above 65% may cause blindness; may produce burns on the skin; if taken orally may cause severe burns, depending on the concentration.
- *Nitric acid:* gives off yellow fumes that are extremely toxic and damaging to tissues; overexposure to vapor can cause death, loss of eyesight, extreme irritation, smarting, itching, and yellow discoloration of the skin; if taken orally can cause extreme burns, may perforate the stomach wall, or cause death.
- *Acetic acid:* severely caustic; continuous exposure to vapor can lead to chronic bronchitis.
- *Hydrochloric acid:* inhalation of vapors should be avoided; any acid on the skin should be washed away immediately to prevent a burn.
- *Sodium hydroxide:* extremely hazardous in contact with the skin, eyes, and mucous membranes (mouth), causing caustic burns; dangerous even at very low concentrations; any contact necessitates immediate care.
- *Phenol (a disinfectant):* can cause caustic burns or contact dermatitis even in dilute solutions; wash off skin with water or alcohol.
- *Carbon tetrachloride:* damaging to the liver even at an exposure level where there is no discernible odor.
- *Trichloroacetic acid:* very severely caustic; respiratory tract irritant.
- *Ethers:* cause depression of central nervous system.

Select Carcinogens.—These are substances regulated by OSHA as **carcinogens.** Carcinogens are any substance that causes the development of cancerous growths in living tissue and are considered hazardous to people working with them in laboratories. When possible, substances which are potentially carcinogenic have been replaced by those which are less hazardous. If necessary, with the proper safeguards in place, potentially carcinogenic substances can be used in the laboratory. Lists of potential carcinogens used in a particular laboratory must be available to all who work there. These lists can be long.

Hazard Warning.—A **hazard identification system** was developed by the National Fire Protection Association. This system provides at a glance, in words, symbols, and pictures, information on the presence of potential health, flammability, and chemical reactivity hazards of materials used in the laboratory. This information is provided on the labels for all containers for hazardous chemicals.

The hazard identification system consists of four small, diamond-shaped symbols grouped into a larger diamond shape (Fig 1–2). The top diamond is red and indicates a flammability hazard. The diamond on the right is yellow and indicates a reactivity-stability hazard. These materials are capable of explosion or violent chemical reactions. The diamond on the left is blue and indicates a possible health hazard. The diamond on the bottom is white and indicates special hazard information. It can indicate information about radioactivity, special biohazards, and other dangerous elements. The system also indicates the severity of the hazard using numerical designations from 4 to 0. Using this designation, 4 is extremely hazardous and 0 is no hazard.

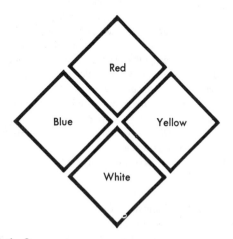

FIG 1–2.
Identification system of the National Fire Protection Association. (From Kaplan LA, Pesce AJ: *Clinical Chemistry: Theory, Analysis, and Correlation*, ed 2. St Louis, Mosby–Year Book, Inc, 1989, p 24. Used by permission.)

Electrical Hazards

Shocks from electrical apparatus in the clinical laboratory are a common source of injury if one is not aware of the potential hazard. This may be one of the most serious hazards in the laboratory. The important thing to understand with respect to danger to the human body is the effect of an electrical current. Current flows when there is a difference in potential between two points, and this knowledge is used in determining the approach to safety in the use of electrical equipment. Grounding of all electrical equipment is essential. If there is no path to ground, such a path might be established through the human in contact with the apparatus, resulting in serious injury. Attempts to repair or inspect a disabled electrical device should be left to someone who is trained to do this work.

Hazards With Glassware

The use of many kinds of glassware is basic to anyone working in the clinical laboratory. Caution must be used to prevent unnecessary or accidental breakage. Some types of glassware can be repaired, but most glassware used today is discarded when it is broken. Any broken or cracked glassware should be discarded in a special container for broken glass, and not thrown into the regular waste container. Common sense should be used in storing glassware, with heavy pieces placed on the lower shelves and tall pieces placed behind smaller pieces. Shelves should be placed at reasonable heights; glassware should not be stored out of reach. Broken or cracked glassware is the cause of many lacerations, and care should be taken to avoid this laboratory hazard.

Fire Hazards

In case of fire hazards, various types of fire-extinguishing agents must be available and their use must be understood. Fire in clothing should be smothered with a fire blanket or heavy toweling or the flame should be beaten out; it should not be flooded with water. Everyone in the laboratory should know the correct use of the fire alarm and the procedure to follow in the event of a fire (see under Emergency Precautions).

Pipetting Safeguards: Automatic Pipetting Devices

It is a generally accepted rule that all pipetting must be done by mechanical means. For pipetting use either mechanical suction or aspirator bulbs. This procedure safeguards against burning the mouth with caustic reagents and against contamination by pathogenic organisms in samples. All specimens of human origin that are used in the laboratory (blood, urine, spinal fluid, stools, etc.) should be considered potentially infectious.

To eliminate the use of aspirator bulbs and to give increased pipetting accuracy, a form of automatic pipetting device is frequently used. These devices offer fast, accurate means for dispensing repetitive volumes. They can be set to deliver volumes in different ranges depending on the device used. In general, a syringe reservoir is filled with the reagent to be measured, the volume to be delivered is determined by setting the dispenser dial, and the dispensing button is depressed to deliver the amount selected. The syringe mechanisms are usually autoclavable and the pipette tips are disposable.

Another device, a bottle top dispenser, can be used to deliver repetitive aliquots of reagents. These are designed as bottle-mounted systems which can dispense repetitive selected volumes in an easy, precise manner. They are usually trouble-free and require a minimum of maintenance.

DECONTAMINATION

It is important to keep the laboratory workplace in a clean and sanitary condition. Cleaning and disinfecting the working surfaces after contact with blood or other potentially infectious materials are of prime importance. Most disinfectants are less active in the presence of high concentrations of protein. Blood and other body fluids contain high concentrations of protein and for this reason, these specimens, if spilled, should first be absorbed as completely as possible with disposable towels or gauze pads prior to disinfection. After absorption of the liquid, all contaminated materials (paper towels, etc.) should be discarded as biohazard waste. After absorption, clean the spill site with an aqueous detergent solution, then disinfect with a high-level hospital disinfectant such as a dilution of household bleach.

Use of Bleach

Sodium hypochlorite, liquid household bleach, is often used as an intermediate-level disinfectant. Dilutions of bleach—a 1% solution made from a 5% solution (one part 5% sodium hypochlorite and four parts wa-

ter)—should be made up fresh weekly to prevent the loss of germicidal action during prolonged storage.

To clean up the laboratory work area, a strong bleach solution can be used for any spills of biological materials. Desk tops can be cleaned daily with a dilute solution of bleach. Any contaminated laboratory ware that must be reused cannot be cleaned with bleach because it corrodes stainless steel containers and coagulates proteins. A strong detergent solution such as 3% phenolic detergent can be used before autoclaving. Contaminated pipettes should be placed in long horizontal covered trays deep enough to minimize the chance of spilling when they are transported to the autoclave.

Autoclaves

Material which is to be autoclaved should be loosely packed so the steam can circulate freely around it. Autoclaving depends on humidity, temperature, and time. Under pressure, steam becomes hotter than boiling water and kills bacteria much more quickly. Autoclaves must be used with caution.

Autoclaves should be monitored regularly for their performance in adequately sterilizing the materials to be decontaminated. This monitoring procedure should be part of the ongoing quality assurance program for the laboratory.

LABORATORY WASTE DISPOSAL

OSHA standards provide for the implementation of a waste disposal program. Receptacles used for the disposal of medical wastes should be manufactured from leakproof materials and be maintained in a sanitary condition. The purpose of waste disposal control is to confine or isolate any possible hazardous material from all workers—laboratory personnel as well as custodial and housekeeping personnel.

Infectious Waste

OSHA has defined *infectious waste* as blood and blood products, contaminated sharps, pathologic wastes, and microbiological wastes. Infectious waste is to be packaged for disposal in color-coded containers and should be labeled as such with the universal symbol for biohazards. Final disposal is by incineration or autoclaving.

Containers for Waste

Containers must be easily accessible to personnel needing them and located in the laboratory areas where they are commonly used. They should be constructed in such a manner that their contents will not be spilled if the container is tipped over accidentally.

Sharps Container

After use, disposable syringes and needles, scalpel blades, and other sharp items should be placed in puncture-resistant **Sharps containers** for disposal. The most widespread control measure required by OSHA and NCCLS is the use of puncture-resistant sharps containers. The primary purpose of using these containers is to eliminate the need for anyone to transport needles and other sharps while looking for a place to discard them. Sharps containers are to be located in the patient areas as well as conveniently placed in the laboratory. Use of the special sharps container permits quick disposal without recapping the needle. This supports the recommendation against recapping, bending, breaking, or otherwise manipulating any sharp needle or lancet device by hand. Most needle-stick accidents have occurred when recapping a needle after doing a phlebotomy. If a needle must be recapped, it should be done in a one-handed fashion with one hand held behind the back. Injuries also can occur to housekeeping personnel when contaminated sharps are left on a bed, concealed in linen, or disposed of improperly in a waste receptacle. Most accidental disposal-related exposures can be eliminated by the use of sharps containers.

Biohazard Containers

Body fluid specimens, including blood, must be placed in well-constructed **biohazard containers** with secure lids to prevent leakage during transport and for future disposal. Contaminated specimens and other materials used in laboratory tests should be decontaminated before reprocessing for disposal or be placed in special impervious bags for disposal in accordance with established waste removal policies. If outside contamination of the bag is likely, a second bag should be used.

Hazardous specimens and potentially hazardous substances should be tagged and identified as such. The tag should read "biohazard" or the biological hazard symbol should be used. All persons working in the laboratory area must be informed as to the meaning of the tags used and what precautions should be taken for each.

Contaminated equipment must be placed in a designated area for storage, washing, decontamination, or disposal. With the increased use of disposable protective clothing and gloves, etc., the volume of waste for discard will be on the increase.

Biohazard Bags

Plastic bags are appropriate for disposal of most infectious waste materials, but rigid, impermeable containers should be used for disposal of sharps and broken glassware. Red or orange plastic bags with the biohazard symbols and lettering in black prominently visible should be used in secondary metal or plastic cans. These cans can be decontaminated on a regular basis or immediately when visibly contaminated. These biohazard containers should be used for all blood, body fluids, tissues, and other disposable materials contaminated with infectious agents and should be handled wearing gloves.

Final Decontamination of Waste in Containers

Final decontamination of materials in bags or containers is done by either incineration or autoclaving, either off or on site.

Disposal of medical waste should be done by licensed organizations which will ensure that no environmental contamination or anything aesthetically displeasing occurs. Congress has passed various acts and regulations regarding the proper handling of medical waste to assist the Environmental Pollution Agency to carry out this process in the most prudent fashion.

SAFETY REFERENCE LIBRARY

Every clinical laboratory should have at its disposal a safety reference library. This library should be available at all times to all technical personnel, students, and employees. It should include books and manuals that will be helpful in preventing unsafe conditions and that provide a guide to safe procedures to be employed in the event of an accident in the laboratory. The following publications are recommended for a safety reference library:

1. Committee on Hazardous Biological Substances in the Laboratory, Board on Chemical Sciences and Technology, Commission on Physical Sciences, Mathematics, and Resources National Research

Council: *Biosafety in the Laboratory*. Washington, DC, National Academy Press, 1989.

2. *Hazardous Materials, Storage and Handling Pocketbook*. Alexandria, Va, Defense Logistics Agency, 1984.

3. Miller B (ed): *Laboratory Safety: Principles and Practices*. Washington DC, American Society for Microbiology, 1986.

4. Occupational exposure to bloodborne pathogens: Proposed rule and notice of hearing. *Federal Register* 1989; 54(May 30):23042–23139.

5. Occupational exposures to hazardous chemicals in laboratories, final rule. *Federal Register* 1990; 55(Jan 31):3327–3335.

6. *Protection of Laboratory Workers From Infectious Disease Transmitted by Blood, Body Fluids, and Tissue*. Villanova, Pa, National Committee for Clinical Laboratory Standards. 1989; 9(January):MT29-T.

7. Richardson J, Barkley WE (eds): *Biosafety in Microbiological and Biomedical Laboratories*, ed 2. Washington, DC, US Department of Health and Human Services, Public Health Service, Centers for Disease Control, and National Institutes of Health, 1988.

8. Rose S: *Clinical Laboratory Safety*. Philadelphia, JB Lippincott Co, 1984.

9. *Safety in Academic Chemistry Laboratories*, ed 4. Washington, DC, American Chemical Society, Committee on Safety, 1985.

BASIC FIRST-AID PROCEDURES

Since there are so many potential hazards in a clinical laboratory, it is easy to understand why a knowledge of **basic first aid** should be an integral part of any educational program in clinical laboratory medicine. The first emphasis should be on removal of the accident victim from further injury; the next involves definitive action or first aid to the victim. By definition, *first aid* is "the immediate care given to a person who has been injured or suddenly taken ill." Any person who attempts to perform first aid before professional treatment by a physician can be arranged should remember that such assistance is only a stopgap—an emergency treatment to be followed until the physician arrives. Stop bleeding, prevent shock, then treat the wound—in that order.

A rule to remember in dealing with emergencies in the laboratory is to keep calm. This is not always easy to do, but it is very important to the well-being of the victim. Keep crowds of people away and give the victim plenty of fresh air.

Because so many of the possible injuries are of such an extreme nature and because in the event of such an injury immediate care is most critical, application of the proper first-aid procedures must be thoroughly understood by every person in the medical laboratory. A few of the more common emergencies and the appropriate first-aid procedures are listed below. These should be learned by every student or person working in the laboratory.

1. *Alkali or acid burns on the skin or in the mouth:* Rinse thoroughly with large amounts of running tap water. If the burns are serious, consult a physician.

2. *Alkali or acid burns in the eye:* Wash out thoroughly with running water for a minimum of 15 minutes. Help the victim by holding the eyelid open so that the water can make contact with the eye. An eye fountain is recommended for this purpose, but any running water will suffice. Use of an eyecup is discouraged. A physician should be notified immediately, while the eye is being washed.

3. *Heat burns:* Apply cold running water (or ice in water) to relieve the pain and to stop further tissue damage. Use a wet dressing of 2 tablespoons of sodium bicarbonate in 1 quart of warm water. Bandage securely but not tightly. If it is a third-degree burn (the skin is burned off), do not use ointments or grease, and consult a physician immediately.

4. *Minor cuts:* Wash carefully and thoroughly with soap and water. Remove all foreign material, such as glass, that projects from the wound, but do not gouge for embedded material. Removal is best accomplished by careful washing. Apply a clean bandage if necessary.

5. *Serious cuts:* Direct pressure should be applied to the cut area to control the bleeding, using the hand over a clean compress covering the wound. Call for a physician immediately.

In cases of serious laboratory accidents, such as burns, medical assistance should be summoned while first aid is being administered. For general accidents, competent medical help should be sought as soon as possible after the first-aid treatment has been completed. In cases of chemical burns, especially where the eyes are involved, speed in treatment is most essential. Remem-

General Rules for Safety in the Clinical Laboratory

1. Know where the fire extinguishers are located, the different types for specific types of fires, and how to use them properly.
2. Pipette *all* solutions by using mechanical suction or an aspirator bulb. Never use mouth suction.
3. Handle all flammable solvents and fuming reagents under a fume hood. Store in a well-ventilated cabinet.
4. Use an explosion-proof refrigerator to store ether. Never use ether near an open flame. It is highly flammable.
5. Do not use *any* flammable substance near an open flame.
6. Wear gloves when handling infectious substances or toxic substances such as bromine or cyanide.
7. Mercury is poisonous. Clean up spilled mercury immediately.
8. If glass tubing is to be cut, hold the tubing with a towel to prevent cuts of the hands. This precaution also applies to putting a piece of glass tubing through a rubber stopper.
9. Use extreme caution when handling laboratory glassware. Broken glass is probably the greatest source of injury in the laboratory. Immediately discard cracked or broken glassware in a separate container, not with other waste.
10. If strong acids or bases are spilled, wipe them up immediately, using copious amounts of water and great care. Keep sodium bicarbonate on hand to assist in neutralizing acid spillage.
11. Plainly label all laboratory bottles, specimens, and other materials. When a reagent bottle is no longer being used, store it away in its proper place.
12. Put away safely or cover any equipment that is not being used.
13. Replace covers, tops, or corks on all reagent bottles as soon as they are no longer being used. Never use a reagent from a bottle that is not properly labeled.
14. If water is spilled on the floor, wipe it up immediately. Serious injuries can result from falls caused by slipping on a wet floor.
15. Never taste any chemical. Smell chemicals only when necessary and then only by fanning the vapor of the chemical toward the nose.
16. When handling blades or needles, use extreme caution to avoid cuts and infections. Dispose of all blades and needles in Sharps container.
17. Always pour acid into water for dilution. Never pour water into acid. Pour strong acids or bases slowly down the side of the receiving vessel to prevent splashing.
18. Use universal precautions when obtaining any specimen from a patient. Handle blood, serum, plasma, cerebrospinal fluid, urine, or any other patient specimen carefully, as if it was infectious. Severe infections and illnesses can result from handling specimens carelessly.
19. Wear gloves when handling any biological specimen.
20. Wash hands frequently while working in the laboratory, especially after handling patient specimens or reagents. *Always* wash hands before leaving the laboratory.
21. Wear safety goggles when preparing reagents with strong chemicals (such as the dichromate acid cleaning solution used to clean laboratory glassware, or aqua regia, another cleaning solution). Some states (e.g., Minnesota) have enacted laws that require students, teachers, and visitors in educational institutions who are participating in or observing activities in eye-protection areas (areas where work is performed that is potentially hazardous to the eyes) to wear devices to protect their eyes.
22. In case of severe fire or burns, know where the safety shower is located and how to operate it.
23. Know the location of a fire blanket, which is used to smother flames in case of fire.
24. Most hospitals and teaching institutions have some type of warning signal and a procedure to follow in the event of a fire. This procedure should be understood thoroughly by anyone working in that institution, whether as a student or an employee. Such institutions also have disaster plans, with which every worker must be thoroughly familiar.

Continued.

25. When using burners and other heating devices, keep them far enough away from the working area that there is no possibility that anything will catch on fire.
26. Never lean over an open flame. Extinguish flames when not in use.
27. Learn the procedure used in the laboratory for discarding hazardous substances such as strong acids and bases.
28. Never pour volatile liquids down a sink.
29. To free a frozen glass stopper, run hot water over it, tap it lightly with a towel wrapped around it, or grasp it with a rubber glove or tourniquet.
30. Wear gloves when cleaning glassware in case there is broken glass in the sink or soaking bucket.
31. Handle all hot objects with tongs, not hands. Extremely hot objects are to be handled with asbestos gloves.
32. If contaminated materials such as human specimens or bacterial agents are spilled on the work area, discard the contaminated material properly and wipe off the work area with bleach solution or other laboratory disinfectant.
33. Cover all centrifuges to avoid flying broken glass and aerosols. Do not open centrifuges before they have stopped. Do not stop the centrifuge head by hand.
34. Be familiar with the OSHA rules and regulations and be ready for an inspection by OSHA.

ber that first aid is useful not only in your working environment, but at home and in your community. It deserves your earnest attention and study.

BIBLIOGRAPHY

Henry JB (ed): *Clinical Diagnosis and Management by Laboratory Methods,* ed 18. Philadelphia, WB Saunders Co, 1991.

National Fire Protection Association: *Hazardous Chemical Data.* Boston, Mass, National Fire Protection Association, 1975, No. 49.

Occupational exposure to bloodborne pathogens: Proposed rule and notice of hearings. *Federal Register,* 1989; 54(May 30):23134–23139.

Occupational exposure to hazardous chemicals in laboratories, final rule. *Federal Register* 1990; 55(Jan 31):3327–3335.

Occupational safety and health standards. *Federal Register* 1978; 43(Oct 24, Nov 17).

Protection of Laboratory Workers from Infectious Disease Transmitted by Blood, Body Fluids, and Tissue, Tentative Guidelines. Villanova, Pa, National Committee for Clinical Laboratory Standards, 1989; 9 (January):M29-T.

Recommendations for prevention of HIV transmission in health-care setting. *MMWR* 1987; 36 (suppl):3s.

Standards for the tracking and management of medical waste, interim final rule and request for comments. *Federal Register* 1989; 40 (March 24):12326.

Update, universal precautions for prevention of transmission of human immunodeficiency virus, hepatitis B virus, and other bloodborne pathogens in health-care settings. *MMWR* 1988; 37:377.

2 Collecting and Processing Laboratory Specimens

Key Terms

Additives, anticoagulants	Patient's bill of rights
Bedside testing	Phlebotomist
Body cavity fluids	Protective isolation
Capillary blood collections	Serum separator gels
Fasting blood	Syringe and needle collection system
First morning urine specimen	Timed urine collection
Hematomas	Tourniquet
Hemolysis	Vacuum tube and needle collection system
Heparin-locks	Vascular access device (VAD)
Indwelling lines	Venipuncture
Infusion set (butterfly)	Voided midstream urine specimen
Quality assurance	

QUALITY ASSURANCE

The term **quality assurance** is used to describe management of the treatment of the whole patient. As it applies to the clinical laboratory, quality assurance requires establishing policies that maintain and control, as much as possible, the many processes that involve the patient and any laboratory results for that patient. It includes properly preparing the patient for any specimens to be collected, collecting valid samples, correctly performing the laboratory analyses needed, validating the test results, correctly recording and reporting the test results, and getting those results into the patient's record. Another very important aspect of quality assurance is the policy regarding how records describing quality assurance practices and quality control measures used for laboratory analyses are documented, maintained, and made available, if needed, for review.

The purpose of a quality assurance policy is to make certain that over a long period of time, the laboratory provides reliable data that accurately reflect the status of the patient. Since physicians use laboratory test data to make diagnoses and to determine a course for therapy, it is essential that the results be reliable. As stated previously, the accuracy of the test result begins with the quality of the specimens received by the laboratory. The quality of the specimen depends on how it was collected, transported, and processed. The person drawing the blood specimen or collecting any patient specimen has the responsibility of ensuring that the specimen is collected in the best manner possible. By following established policy and with training and experience, specimens can be collected which will yield valid results, thus promoting good-quality patient care.

The laboratory test can be no better than the specimen on which it is performed. If the specimen is improperly collected, is not stored correctly, or is generally mishandled in some way, the most quantitatively perfect determination is of no use because the results are invalid and cannot be used by the physician in diagnosis or treatment.

GENERAL SPECIMEN REQUIREMENTS

All samples sent to the laboratory must be processed according to certain established policies. Each division of the laboratory will have unique requirements for specimens used in that division, but there are several general considerations that apply to all specimens. Special requirements for the collection, preservation, and processing of laboratory specimens are discussed where appropriate in subsequent chapters.

Patient Identification

Initial identification of the patient is extremely important. It is essential that a specimen from a particular patient is placed in the appropriate container and labeled for that patient. The patient's name, hospital identification number and room number, date and time of collection are commonly found on the label. All specimens sent to the laboratory must be properly labeled. For some tests, labels *must* include the time of collection of the specimen and the type of specimen. A properly completed request slip should accompany all specimens sent to the laboratory.

Labels

Quality assurance policies are implemented in the clinical laboratory to protect the patient from any adverse consequences of errors due to an improperly handled specimen—beginning with the collection of that specimen. Laboratory quality assurance and accreditation require that specimens be properly labeled at the time of collection.

An unlabeled container or one labeled improperly should not be accepted by the laboratory. Specimens are considered improperly labeled when there is no patient identification on the tube or container holding the specimen. Many specimen containers are transported in leakproof plastic bags. It is not acceptable that the bags be labeled without also labeling the container in the bag. If the identification is illegible, the specimen is also unacceptable. In laboratories where computers are used, labels are generated which assist in making certain that the proper identification information is included for each patient. A specimen is unacceptable if the specimen container identification does not match exactly the identification on the request form for that specimen. Each laboratory will have a specific protocol for the handling of mislabeled or "unacceptable" specimens.

All specimen containers must be labeled by the person doing the collection to ensure that the specimen is indeed collected from the patient whose identification is on the label.

ISOLATION TECHNIQUES

With the adoption of universal precautions, the need for using the isolation category called "blood and body fluid isolation," (formerly referred to as "strict isolation") has been for the most part eliminated. The Centers for Disease Control (CDC) previously recommended several disease-specific isolation policies for patients known to be or suspected of being infected with bloodborne pathogens. With strict adherence to universal precautions, no diagnosis or suspicion of a transmissible disease is necessary as all sources of specimens (patients) are considered potentially pathogenic or infectious, i.e., all specimens are treated in the same way. The use of proper collection techniques and barriers to prevent transmission of infectious agents is discussed in Chapter 1.

For known airborne pathogens (such as tuberculosis) or other highly communicable diseases that are spread by airborne or contact routes, specific additional precautions should be taken for blood collection, e.g., masks should be worn to enter the room. A "stop sign alert" should be placed on the door of a room occupied by a patient with an airborne disease to indicate that disease-specific precautions should be taken. The individual health care facility will initiate these specific precautions. Always follow the procedure of the hospital or patient care unit regarding isolation policies.

Additional *contact precautions* must be used for patients with volumes of drainage, skin infections, lice, scabies, cytomegalovirus infections, etc., when giving direct care.

Protective Isolation

Protective isolation is used to protect the patient from infectious agents. For example, a burn patient is very susceptible to infection, so that anyone entering the room of a burn patient must use protective isolation procedures. When collecting specimens from patients with leukemia, severe burns, or those receiving organ or bone marrow transplants, body radiation therapy, and plastic surgery, who must be protected from exposure to pathogens and other bacteria, a sterile gown, cap, gloves, and mask should be worn. Shoe coverings may also be required. With a patient having a kidney transplant or dialysis, protective isolation technique should be used for the sake of the patient and extremely careful collecting technique for the sake of the laboratory.

TYPES OF SPECIMENS COLLECTED

Several different kinds of specimens are analyzed routinely in the clinical laboratory. The specimen most often tested in the clinical laboratory is blood. It is true that blood represents a large percentage of the specimens sent to the laboratory, but urine specimens are also sent in great numbers. Blood and urine specimens are discussed throughout this book under the various laboratory departments covered.

Many pathologic conditions may be associated with the fluid that accumulates in the various cavities of the body. Laboratory examination of body cavity fluid may yield useful information regarding its formation and constituents. The physician can also be alerted to the type of disease process present by the information obtained from the laboratory analysis of a patient's various body cavity fluids. Some of the body cavity fluids examined in the laboratory are pleural, pericardial, peritoneal, synovial, amniotic, and cerebrospinal.

Fecal specimens and many kinds of specimens for microbiological tests, such as throat cultures and abscesses from wounds, are also sent to the laboratory.

Blood

Blood represents a large percentage of the total specimens used in laboratory determinations. Blood specimens are obtained by several different types of health care personnel, depending on the facility. In some institutions, this work is done by the clinical laboratory scientists, medical technologists, or medical technicians. In other institutions, there are specially trained individuals who do the blood collecting. The person who practices this specialty is called a **phlebotomist.**

The Phlebotomist

A professional phlebotomist has specific training in the technical skills of drawing blood. The phlebotomist is an important connection between the patient and the clinical laboratory. In addition to becoming skilled in obtaining blood by venipuncture, he or she is also trained to do **capillary blood collections** and perform special skin punctures used, e.g., when taking specimens from infants in neonatal care units. Drawing specimens from **indwelling lines** is another technique to be learned when specializing in the drawing of blood.

Related areas of specimen receiving and processing must also be fully understood by the phlebotomist and by anyone who collects blood specimens. It is important therefore, to understand the proper means for collecting, preserving, and processing blood samples.

Approaching the Patient

Because it is relatively easy to obtain a blood sample, numerous studies are done on blood in diseased and normal states. Much valuable information is readily available at relatively low cost and with little discomfort to the patient. Certain routine blood studies are part of new hospital admissions. Many of these studies are carried out in the hematology and chemistry departments (see Chapters 10 and 11). Blood is also cultured in the microbiology department.

Anyone who plans to assume a duty or occupation where contact with patients is required must consider several factors. These persons are providing a service to the patient. Adequate performance of this service involves not only technical knowledge but sincere and concerned interest in people. This is a quality that, unfortunately, cannot be taught readily. It is a quality that each one must learn as a part of reaching maturity. Those in the medical laboratory field must be not only academically capable but also psychologically and socially responsible.

Patient's Bill of Rights.—When collecting blood specimens, it is important that the rights of patients be kept in mind at all times. Being considerate of these rights is consistent with good patient care. Phlebotomy involves direct patient contact and it is essential that all people engaged in this aspect of laboratory work remember to serve the patient well.

Many hospitals have adopted a patient's bill of rights as declared by the Joint Commission on Accreditation of Healthcare Organizations (JCAHO). In some states, laws have been passed making the patients' rights mandatory (California and Minnesota have done this). This law could become the basis of litigation if a patient

---

Patient's Bill of Rights

The patient has a right to:
1. Impartial access to treatment or accommodations that are available or medically indicated, regardless of race, creed, sex, national origin, or sources of payment for care.
2. Respectful, considerate care and treatment.
3. Confidentiality of all communications and other records and data which pertain to the care received by the patient.
4. Expect that any discussion or consultation involving the patient's case will be conducted discreetly and respectfully and that persons not directly involved in the case will not be present without the permission of the patient or guardian.
5. Expect reasonable personal safety in accord with the hospital practices and environment.
6. Know the identity and professional status of individuals providing service and to know which physician or other practitioner is primarily responsible for his or her care.
7. Obtain from the practitioner complete and current information about diagnosis, treatment, and any known prognosis, in terms which can reasonably be understood by the patient.
8. Reasonable and informed participation in decisions involving his or her health care. The patient shall be informed if the hospital proposes to engage in or perform human experimentation or other research or educational projects affecting his or her care or treatment. The patient has the right to refuse participation in such activity.
9. Consult a specialist at the patient's own request and expense.
10. Refuse treatment to the extent permitted by law.
11. Request and receive an itemized and detailed explanation of the total bill for services rendered in the hospital regardless of the source of payment.
12. Be informed of the hospital rules and regulations.

feels that his or her rights have been violated. As endorsed by JCAHO, the box on page 21 is a summary of basic patient rights:

Patient Considerations.—A patient in the hospital experiences several emotions, including anxiety and fear. The patient, separated from familiar surroundings, is also probably not feeling well, is concerned about his or her physical condition, and may be afraid of what is going to happen next. For these and other reasons, the patient's mental state is probably at its worst during hospitalization. It is extremely important that the patient be shown kindness and understanding. The collection of blood specimens is one area where laboratory personnel have an opportunity to meet patients. It is essential, therefore, that those doing the blood collecting strive for a real understanding of what the patient is feeling. Try to imagine what it would be like if you were the patient, and act accordingly. Try to talk to patients the way you would like someone to talk to you—be friendly, pleasant, and outgoing.

When approaching a patient for the first time, there are certain procedures to remember. First, make certain that the patient on whom the test is being done is actually the right patient. Checking the hospital number of the patient is essential. Check the wrist tag of the patient to make certain it is the right patient. Ask the patient's name—this is also a good way to start conversation. A mix-up in labeling tubes or drawing blood from the wrong patient can be disastrous. Always label the tubes of blood at the bedside of the patient, as well as any slides, pipettes, or other materials used for taking specimens. Proper and immediate labeling is essential.

Pediatric Patients.—When working with a pediatric patient, you must first gain the patient's confidence. This may be the first time a child has had blood drawn. If this first experience is a bad one, it will be remembered and feared for years to come. It is therefore important to take some extra time to gain the child's confidence before going ahead with the collection procedure. Get acquainted with the child by using a book or a toy, for example. Keep your equipment tray as inconspicuous as possible. Be frank with the child. Sometimes you may be able to tell a story about what you are doing. It is important in working with pediatric patients to bolster their morale as much as possible. Ask for help in restraining a very small or uncooperative child.

Older children may be more responsive when permitted to "help," by holding the gauze, for example. If your technique is efficient and you talk to the patients convincingly, you will be able to "take a picture from their finger" before they realize what has happened. Handling a child often involves handling the parents also. This is best accomplished by allowing the parents to know, by your attitude, that you are kind but very definitely in charge of the situation. This attitude, which is so basic for laboratory personnel, can be developed only with practice.

In the nursery, each hospital will have its own rules, but a few general precautions apply. After working with an infant in a crib, be sure to put up the crib sides. If an infant is in an incubator, keep the portholes closed. When oxygen is in use, do not forget to close the openings when you have finished with the infant. Dispose of all waste materials properly.

Adult Patients.—Adult patients must be told briefly what is expected of them and what the test involves. With adults and especially when dealing with children, complete honesty is important. It is unwise to say that a finger puncture will not hurt, when it really will. However, if possible, avoid saying that the puncture will hurt.

Greet the patient in a friendly and tactful manner. Do not become overly familiar; carry on conversation in a pleasant and calm manner. Tell the patient why you are there and what you are going to do. Speak quietly at all times. Discuss personal information the patient relates to you softly; this is being told to you in confidence. Respect the religious beliefs of the patient. Keep all laboratory reports confidential, and also keep any personal information about the patient confidential. Firmly refuse information about other patients or physicians. If you see the same patient frequently, become familiar with his or her interests, hobbies, or family and use these as topics of conversation. Many patients in the hospital are lonely and need a friend. Occasionally you will find, especially with the extremely ill, that patients do not wish to talk at all; in this case, respect their wishes. Do not irritate the patient. It is important to be honest, but boost the patient's morale as much as possible. Smile, be cordial, and leave the room in a friendly fashion.

Even if the patient is disagreeable (and many are), remain pleasant. It is important to repeat at this point that it is helpful if you enter the patient's room wearing a pleasant expression; a smile will often work miracles. Be firm when the patient is unpleasant, remain cheerful, and express confidence in the work to be done. Young children who do not understand words seem pacified by the sound of a confident voice. Talking pleasantly to every patient is essential.

In a hospital setting, check before leaving the patient's room to see that you have returned everything to your laboratory tray. Keep the tray holding your supplies and equipment out of reach of the patient. This is especially important when working with children, but it applies to all patients.

Collection Procedures

Any discussion concerning blood specimens must include collection procedures for blood. There are two general sources of blood for clinical laboratory tests: peripheral, or capillary, blood and venous blood. This applies to all areas of the clinical laboratory. For small quantities of blood for some hematologic or microchemical determinations, capillary blood is suitable. This is obtained from the capillary bed by puncture of the skin. The tip of the finger is the site most commonly punctured. For larger quantities of blood, a puncture is made directly into a vein (phlebotomy), using a sterile **syringe and needle collection system** or **vacuum tube and needle collection system**. A vein in the upper forearm (or antecubital fossa) area is most often chosen for venipuncture as these veins are easily palpable and fairly well fixed.

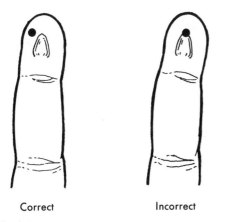

Correct   Incorrect

FIG 2–1.
Sites for capillary puncture: finger stick. (From Powers LW: *Diagnostic Hematology.* St Louis, Mosby–Year Book, Inc, 1989, p 433. Used by permission.)

Gloves.—Before any contact with the patient is made, the phlebotomist must put on protective gloves to implement the necessary barrier protection required by the universal precaution policy.

Peripheral or Capillary Blood

For the small quantities of blood required for most hematologic procedures and for microchemical techniques requiring serum or plasma, an adequate blood sample may be obtained from the capillary bed by puncture of the skin. From certain patients, such as babies, burned patients, or amputees, it may be necessary or desirable to draw only a very small amount of blood. This can be accomplished quite easily by means of capillary puncture. This blood is collected into suitable capillary tubes or pipettes or used directly to prepare blood films.

Capillary blood is often used for **bedside testing** for glucose using one of several available meter devices and the accompanying reagent strips. This same procedure is done by countless diabetics on their own blood to ascertain the level of their blood glucose.

In adults and older children, the tip of the finger is punctured (Fig 2–1); in infants, the plantar surface of the heel or the large toe is punctured (Fig 2–2). In general, the ear lobe should be avoided for puncture because there is a slower flow of blood there and the concentration of cells and hemoglobin will be greater. Blood obtained by puncturing the earlobe has been found to contain a higher concentration of hemoglobin than fingertip or venous blood and also is not reliable for white blood cell counts. The ear lobe is sometimes the desirable source of blood for the preparation of blood films used to study leukocyte abnormalities, since larger cells are frequently trapped in the capillary bed because of the slow circulation. Blood obtained by skin puncture of these types is generally called *capillary blood,* but it is closer to arteriolar blood in its composition. The results of tests from venous and capillary (fingertip) blood compare well if the capillary blood is free-flowing. To ensure free flow of capillary blood, the finger must be warm.

Various types of disposable lancets or blades are used for skin puncture. Use of nondisposable blades is not recommended because of the risk of infectious pathogens. Some blades require the operator to gauge the depth of the puncture, while others have a safety gauge on them.

Precautions to Note When Obtaining Capillary Blood.—If the patient's fingers are cold, slight rubbing

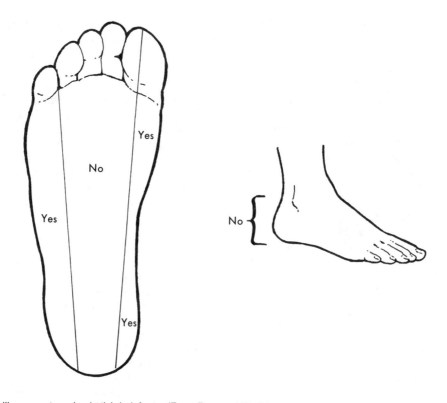

FIG 2–2.
Sites for capillary puncture: heel stick in infants. (From Powers LW: *Diagnostic Hematology.* St Louis, Mosby–Year Book, Inc, 1989, p 435. Used by permission.)

may help to warm them. The finger or heel must not be squeezed excessively, because tissue fluid may dilute the blood sample or cause the blood to clot faster than it normally would. The first drop of blood is usually removed because it contains tissue fluid, alcohol, or perspiration, which will dilute the blood. Immediately after surgery, patients with low blood pressure and those in surgical shock may require more than one puncture. Only one sterile blade is used at a time. The tip of the blade should not touch anything until it punctures the skin of the patient. Contaminated blades are discarded properly and new ones used. After the puncture is made, the blade is discarded immediately. Clean hands are essential when working with patients.

Skin Puncture Devices (Procedure 2–1).—A variety of automatic, spring-activated puncturing devices are commercially available. Clean, rapid incisions can be made of a consistent depth with the use of one of these devices. Devices such as the Autolet (Ulster Scientific,

Inc., Highland, NY 12528) have a lancet held in place by a cocking lever (Fig 2–3). When released, the blade penetrates the skin to a depth of 2 to 3 mm, depending on the choice of platform used. The platform regulates the depth of the puncture. Disposable blades and platforms or guards are used with these devices. The device itself can be cleaned with a bleach or disinfectant solution.

It is important that all used blades and platforms be discarded in a container for sharps. Transmission of bloodborne infections must be prevented (see under Universal Precautions in Chapter 1).

Procedure for Heel Puncture.—For infants under 3 months of age, the heel is the most commonly used site for obtaining a blood sample. Any wound-inflicting device can result in serious injury when excessive pressure and skin indentation accidentally allow the wound depth to reach the heel bone.

The foot must be held securely in place for the

Procedure 2–1. Finger Puncture

1. Assemble the necessary equipment: lancet device, alcohol pad, dry gauze, slides, and capillary tubes or other supplies necessary to receive the blood.
2. Be sure that the patient is seated comfortably.
3. Put on gloves.
4. Choose an area for the puncture that is free from calluses, edema, or cyanosis. Warm the puncture site if it is cold by immersing it in warm water or by rubbing it.
5. Clean the skin of the puncture site on the third or fourth finger vigorously with a pad soaked in an alcohol solution. This will remove dirt and epithelial debris, increase the circulation, and leave the area relatively sterile. Allow the area to air-dry.
6. Grasp the finger firmly and make a quick, firm puncture about 2 to 3 mm deep with a sterile disposable lancet or automated lancet device (Fig 2–4). This puncture should be made at right angles to the fingerprint striations on the patient's finger midway between the edge and midpoint of the fingertip (see Fig 2–1). The puncture should not be made too far down on the finger and should not be too close to the fingernail. A deep puncture hurts no more than a superficial one and it gives a much more satisfactory flow of blood.
7. Discard the lancet in the sharps disposal container. Used lancets should never be left lying on the work area. They should be discarded immediately after use and should not be touched again.
8. Wipe away the first drop of blood, using a clean piece of dry gauze or tissue. This drop is contaminated with tissue fluid and will interfere with some laboratory results if used. The succeeding drops are used for tests.
9. If a good puncture has been made, the blood will flow freely. If it does not, use gentle pressure to make the blood form a round drop. Excessive squeezing will cause dilution of the blood with tissue fluid.
10. Collect the specimens by holding a capillary tube to the blood drop or by touching the drop to a glass slide. Rapid collection is necessary to prevent coagulation, especially when several tests are to be done using blood from the same puncture site.
11. When the blood samples have been collected, have the patient hold a sterile, dry piece of gauze or cotton over the puncture site until the bleeding has stopped.
12. Remove gloves and wash hands.

---

puncture (Fig 2–5). The lateral or medial plantar surface of the foot should be used for the skin puncture (see Fig 2–2). The site and depth of the puncture is of critical importance. The depth should not exceed 2.4 mm. The central portion and posterior curvature of the heel are not used because the bone lies too close to the surface. Puncture of the heel bone (calcaneous) can result in osteochondritis or osteomyelitis. The National Committee for Clinical Laboratory Standards has established recommendations for heel punctures in neonates (Procedure 2–2).

A semiautomatic device for performing heel punctures is called Tenderfoot™ (International Technidyne Corporation, Edison, NJ) and makes an incision that is 1 mm deep and 2.5 mm wide, allowing free-flowing collection of up to 3 mL of blood. The blade of the device

---

Procedure 2–2. Heel Puncture

1. Perform the puncture on the most medial or most lateral portion of the plantar surface (see Fig 2–2).
2. Puncture no deeper than 2.4 mm.
3. Do not perform punctures on the posterior curvature of the heel.
4. Do not puncture through previous sites which may be infected.

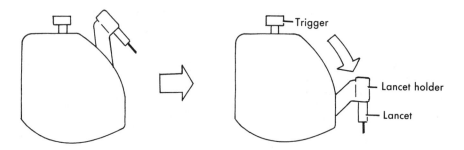

FIG 2–3.
Automated lancet, spring-driven and trigger-activated (Autolet, Ulster Scientific, Inc, Highland, NY). (From Powers LW: *Diagnostic Hematology.* St Louis, Mosby–Year Book, Inc, 1989, p 430. Used by permission.)

automatically retracts following the skin incision, ensuring that neither the blood collector nor the infant is accidentally punctured. When compared with other puncturing devices, Tenderfoot causes less hemolysis of the sample, requires fewer punctures to obtain the desired sample, and produces less physical trauma to the heel of the infant. It is a sterile, completely disposable device, reducing the possibilities of introducing infection in the infant. The depth and width of the incision are controlled, thus eliminating the possibility of calcaneal puncture and osteomyelitis. The amount of sample collected and the free-flowing nature of the blood following the puncture makes squeezing the foot unnecessary. It reduces the number of heel punctures needed. The detailed procedure for using this device accompanies the product.

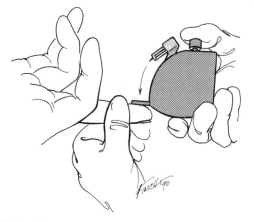

FIG 2–4.
Finger puncture technique using automated lancet device. (Courtesy of Autolet, Ulster Scientific, Inc, Highland, NY.)

Glucose Testing on Capillary Blood at the Bedside.—Capillary blood samples for glucose testing are used frequently in many health care facilities. Quantitative determinations for glucose are made available within 1 or 2 minutes, depending on the system employed. This test is also done by many outpatient diabetics using their own blood and one of several glucose measuring devices. It is important for patients with diabetes, especially those with insulin-dependent diabetes mellitus, to monitor their own blood glucose several times a day and to be able to adjust their dosage of insulin accordingly.

For the inpatient diabetes patient, bedside glucose testing is a valuable tool for management of the disease. The blood glucose is often quite unstable in these patients and may require frequent adjustments of insulin dosage. Ordering and collecting venous blood specimens for glucose tests with the necessary frequency and rapidity of reporting required is often impractical. Whole blood samples should be collected by puncture from the heel (for infants only), finger, or flushed heparinized line using policies for universal precautions to protect against the transmission of bloodborne pathogens. Arterial or other venous blood should not be used, unless the manufacturer's directions so specify. The instrument should be calibrated and the test performed according to the manufacturer's directions. Results should be recorded permanently in the patient's medical record in a manner which distinguishes between bedside test results and laboratory test results.

It is critical to understand the limitations of each detection system so that reliable results are obtained. The specific limitations described by each manufacturer must be considered. The use of a quality assurance program is

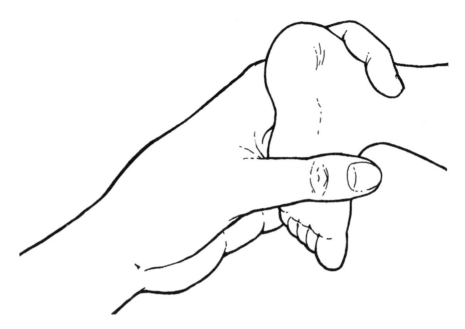

FIG 2–5.
Holding an infant's heel for capillary puncture. (From Powers LW: *Diagnostic Hematology.* St Louis, Mosby–Year Book, Inc, 1989, p 436. Used by permission.)

mandatory to ensure reliable performance of these procedures. The use of bedside testing or self-testing for glucose is intended for management of diabetes patients and not for initial diagnosis. It is not used to replace the standard laboratory tests for glucose, but only as a supplement.

Several commercial instruments are available, the Glucometer 3 (Miles Inc., Diagnostics Division, Elkhart, IN) and Accu-Chek II (Boehringer Mannheim Diagnostics, Indianapolis, IN) are examples. With each product, a meter provides quantitative determination of glucose present when used with a reagent strip which is designed to accompany the meter (GlucoFilm for the Glucometer 3 and ChemStrip bG for the Accu-Chek II). A drop of capillary blood is touched to the reagent strip pad and, following the specific procedure, read in the meter. The instrument provides an accurate and standardized reading when used according to the manufacturer's directions. The reagent strips must be handled with care and used within their proper shelf life. The strips are specific only for glucose. The meters are packaged in convenient carrying cases and are small enough to be placed in a pocket or briefcase.

Capillary Blood Specimen Containers.—Once the skin has been punctured and the blood is flowing, the capillary sample can be collected in a variety of containers. For general purposes, glass tubes with or without heparin can be used and the blood allowed to flow into the tube by capillary action. For example, a heparinized capillary tube is used to collect blood for doing the microhematocrit test in the hematology laboratory.

Another capillary sampling device is called the Unopette (Becton, Dickinson & Co., Rutherford, N.J.) (Fig 2–6). It consists of a disposable capillary pipette which measures a fixed volume and a reservoir of diluent appropriate to the test being performed. This pipette and diluent system can be used with either capillary or venous blood and the general system has been adapted for several chemical and hematologic determinations. Unopettes are described further in Chapter 11 in their use for measuring hemoglobin and for doing manual white cell and platelet counts.

Another microcontainer consists of a small plastic tube with a blood drop collector as part of the lid (see Fig 2–6). One such commercially available system is the Microtainer (Becton, Dickinson & Co., Rutherford, NJ).

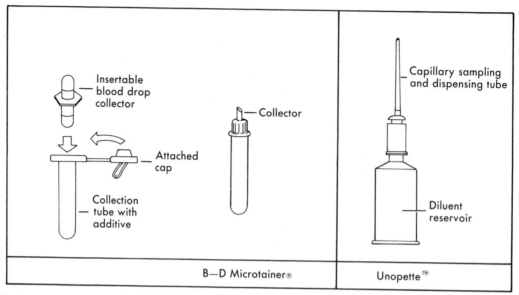

FIG 2–6.
Types of microcontainer tubes and collecting devices. (From Powers LW: *Diagnostic Hematology.* St Louis, Mosby–Year Book, Inc, 1989, p 431. Used by permission.)

This allows the specimen to be collected by capillary action and results in a relatively large amount of specimen in a single container. When the collection is finished, the lid with the capillary tube is removed and discarded. The remaining container can be capped and processed by centrifugation, if serum is to be obtained. These microcontainers are available with various additives, including **serum separator gels.**

Venous Blood

The veins that are generally used for venipuncture are those in the forearm, wrist, or ankle. The first choice for a venipuncture site is a vein in the forearm. They are larger and fuller than those in the wrist, hand, or ankle regions. The wrist, hand, and ankle veins are used only if the forearm site is not available. Venipuncture must be performed with great care and technical skill. The veins of the patient are the main source of blood for testing, and the entry point for medications, intravenous solutions, and blood transfusions. A patient has only a limited number of accessible veins, and it is important that everything possible be done to preserve their good condition and availability. Part of this responsibility lies with the person doing the blood drawing.

Blood may be obtained directly from a vein (phle-

botomy) by using a sterile syringe and needle or a vacuum tube and needle system. The use of the evacuated (vacuum) tube system allows the blood to pass directly from the vein into the collection tube. Veins in the forearm are most commonly used. The three main veins in the forearm are the cephalic, median cubital, and median basilic (Fig 2–7). The median cubital vein is usually chosen for **venipuncture.** The median basilic might roll or move, and the skin over the cephalic might be tougher to penetrate. Other sites may be used when necessary.

The phlebotomy may be made by either the syringe method or the vacuum tube method (Fig 2–8). In the syringe method, a needle is attached to a syringe and inserted into the vein. The plunger of the syringe is drawn back, which creates suction, drawing the blood into the syringe. In the vacuum tube method, one end of a two-way needle is partially attached to the rubber stopper of a specially purchased vacuum tube. The other end of the two-way needle is inserted into the vein. Once in the vein, the needle in the rubber stopper is pushed through the stopper to make a direct connection to the vacuum tube. (Fig 2–9). The vacuum tube creates suction, which draws the blood into the tube. One commercially available vacuum tube system is called Vacutainer (Becton, Dickinson & Co.).

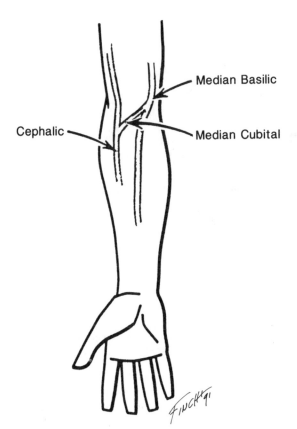

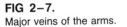

FIG 2–7.
Major veins of the arms.

When doing a venipuncture, the phlebotomist should remain in a standing position, which gives the greatest freedom of movement. The patient should assume a comfortable position. Bed patients should remain lying down, and ambulatory patients should be seated comfortably. The seated patient should put an arm on a table or other firm support and extend it for the pheboto-mist.

Blood Collection Variables.—The majority of clinical laboratory determinations are done on whole blood, plasma, or serum. Many of these are done in the hematology or chemistry laboratories, but many other areas of the laboratory require venous blood for testing.

Most venous blood specimens are drawn from fasting patients. Most **fasting blood** is drawn in the morning before breakfast. This means that the food from the previous meals has been completely digested and absorbed

and any excess has been stored. Food intake, medication, activity, and time of day can all influence the laboratory results for blood specimens. Some of these facts are rarely taken into account by the persons interpreting the laboratory results. The fasting state is one fact that is carefully noted, however, especially for glucose and phosphorus determinations. Through numerous studies it has been found that the average meal has no significant effect on the concentration of most blood constituents, with certain exceptions, such as tests for glucose, phosphorus, and triglycerides. Eating significantly affects blood glucose and triglycerides, giving a falsely high result, and phosphorus, giving a falsely low result. Because it is the most efficient time of day to draw specimens for the laboratory, most of the blood collecting is done early in the morning, and for this reason most of the patients are in the fasting state. Fasting specimens, however, are not necessary for many laboratory determinations. Blood should not be collected while intravenous solutions are being administered, if possible.

Other controllable biological variations in blood include posture (whether the patient is lying in bed or standing up), immobilization (resulting from prolonged bed rest, for example), exercise, circadian variations (cyclical variations throughout the day), recent food ingestion (caffeine effect, for example), smoking (nicotine effect), alcohol ingestion, and administration of drugs. The concentration of certain plasma constituents is affected by some of these factors, and for some laboratory tests it is important to take into consideration the time of day, posture of the patient, dietary intake, and so forth, prior to collection of the blood specimen. Standardization of collection policies can minimize the effect of these variables on test values, but in most health care facilities, this is difficult to do.

Application of the Tourniquet.—The use of a **tourniquet** is desirable to enlarge the veins, so that they become more prominent. A strip of flat tubing (about 1 in. wide) can serve as a tourniquet. It is applied around the arm just above the bend in the elbow and should be just tight enough to stop the blood flow (Fig 2–10). The patient should also be instructed to clench the fist, to aid in building up the blood pressure in the area of the puncture. The proper way to apply an elastic tubing tourniquet is as follows:

1. Place the tourniquet under the patient's arm just above the bend in the elbow.

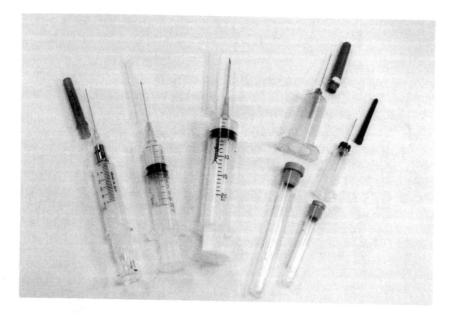

FIG 2–8.
Phlebotomy equipment: syringe, needles, and evacuation system. *Left* to *right:* glass syringe with Luer-Lok needle, disposable plastic syringes and needles, Vacutainer evacuation systems. (From Powers LW: *Diagnostic Hematology.* St Louis, Mosby–Year Book, Inc, 1989, p 418. Used by permission.)

2. Grasping the ends of the tourniquet, pull up so that tension is applied to the tourniquet. This tension must be maintained throughout the procedure.

3. With the proper tension, tuck a loop in the tourniquet from the top down. Do not tie a bow or a knot.

The loop must be made in such a way that it can easily be released when the tourniquet is to be removed (see Fig 2–10).

4. Do not leave the tourniquet on for long periods of time because this will cause stoppage of the circulation (stasis). Prolonged stasis results in gross alterations

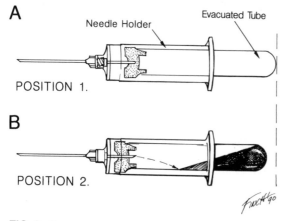

FIG 2–9.
Standard double-ended blood collecting needle with holder using vacuum tube system. **A,** preparation for venipuncture. **B,** collection of specimen.

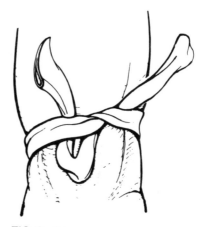

FIG 2–10.
Application of a tourniquet.

in the blood constituents. Stasis should be allowed for a minimum time only.

General Venipuncture Considerations.—The most prominent vein is usually chosen for venipuncture. If the veins are difficult to find, have the patient open and close the fist a few times; this will build up more pressure. Veins may be made more prominent by allowing the arm to hang down for 2 to 3 minutes, by massaging the vein toward the trunk of the body, or by lightly slapping the site of the puncture. Veins may be hardened or rubbery in elderly persons or in those who have had repeated venipuncture. Rolling veins may be held in place by putting the thumb and index finger on the vein so that 2 to 5 cm of vein lies between them. As soon as the vein is entered, the thumb and finger are removed. The veins can be felt by touching or palpating with the index finger. They reveal themselves as elastic tubes under the surface of the skin. By pressing up and down on the vein gently several times, the path of the vein can be felt.

Once the site for venipuncture has been chosen and the vein observed or palpated, the area is cleaned with an antiseptic solution. One suitable antiseptic is a solution of medicated alcohol (or isopropyl alcohol). The area of puncture is rubbed thoroughly with the antiseptic. After application of the antiseptic, the area must not be touched until after the actual puncture is made.

To insert the needle properly into the vein, the gloved index finger is placed alongside the hub of the needle with the bevel of the needle facing up. The vein is fixed by grasping the patient's arm with the other hand and pulling the skin taut. This can be accomplished by placing the thumb about 1 or 2 in. below the puncture site (Fig 2–11). The needle should be pointing in the same direction as the vein. The syringe or vacuum tube apparatus should be held so that it makes a 30- to 40-degree angle with the patient's arm. The tip of the needle is then placed on the vein and pushed deliberately forward. When the vein has been punctured and a suitable amount of blood removed into the tube or syringe, the patient releases the clenched fist, the tourniquet is released, dry gauze is placed over the puncture site, and the needle is withdrawn slowly. After removing the needle, pressure may be applied on the puncture site, using dry gauze.

If difficulty is experienced in entering the vein (no blood appears in the tube or syringe) and especially if a **hematoma** (collection of blood under the skin) starts to form, release the tourniquet and promptly withdraw the

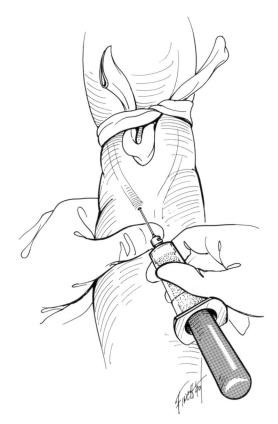

FIG 2–11.
Venipuncture technique using vacuum tube system.

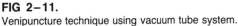

needle, applying pressure to the wound. It is best to select an alternate site for repeated venipunctures on the same patient.

It is most important that the tourniquet be released *before* the needle is removed from the skin. If this is not done, excessive bleeding will occur. If the venipuncture is poorly done (if there is trauma to the tissues), a hematoma may result. This should be avoided, if at all possible.

General Considerations for Problem Venipunctures Using the Vacuum Tube System

1. If a tube begins to fill and then stops, change the position of the needle, first in a forward direction, then slightly backward, or rotate the needle half a turn. Loosen the tourniquet.

2. If a tube is not filling with blood but the needle

Procedure 2–3. Venipuncture Using the Vacuum Tube System

1. Wash hands and put on gloves to comply with policies for universal precautions for blood.
2. *Identify* and reassure the patient. Ask the patient to state his or her full name. Always check the wrist identification to confirm the identity of the patient. This is especially important when drawing blood specimens from unconscious or mentally impaired patients.
3. *Assemble necessary equipment and supplies* (Fig 2–12).
   a. Thread the short end of the double-pointed needle (called the hub of the needle) into the plastic holder and tighten securely using the needle sheath as a wrench (see Fig 2–9).
   b. Assemble sterile evacuated blood collection tubes as needed for the tests desired, ascertaining the proper order for collection.
   c. Place the vacuum tube in the holder and push the stopper of the blood collection tube into the shorter shielded needle (within the holder) up to the recessed guideline on the needle holder. The needle will thus be embedded in the stopper without puncturing it and losing vacuum in the tube (see Fig 2–9,A). *Do not push the tube beyond the guideline* as a premature loss of vacuum may result. Because of this potential problem, some phlebotomists prefer not to attach the tube at this stage.
   d. Remove the needle shield and inspect the tip of the longer needle visually to see if it is free of hooks at the end of the point and the opening is clear. Leave the needle covered loosely until the actual venipuncture can be performed. Do not contaminate it.
4. *Position the patient.* For ambulatory patients, a chair with side supports is used to prevent accidental falling. The patient should be seated comfortably in the chair with the arm extended to form a straight line from the shoulder to the wrist and inclined in a downward position. The arm should rest across a narrow table or on a slanting armrest which can be part of the chair. The arm and elbow should be supported firmly and not be bent at the elbow. Add more support if needed.

   For patients in bed, make certain they are in a comfortable supine position. If additional support is needed, a pillow may be placed under the arm on which the venipuncture is to be done. The patient should extend the arm to form a straight line from the shoulder to the wrist.
5. *Close the patient's hand* (unnecessary if veins are prominent).
6. *Select the vein site to be used.* If possible, the site is selected without the tourniquet. However, on many patients the tourniquet is used at this point. Observe both arms. Select the median cubital vein that appears fullest. These veins are usually easily palpable, fairly well anchored in place, and bruise less. If necessary, use the cephalic vein in preference to the basilic vein. The cephalic vein does not roll and bruise as easily as does the basilic although the blood usually flows more slowly. Palpate and trace the vein several times with the tip of the index finger. Feel the "bounce" of a full vein. A vein feels much like an elastic tube and gives under pressure. Even if you can see the vein, palpate until you can be certain of its location and direction.

   Unlike veins, arteries pulsate and have a thick wall. Thrombosed veins feel cordlike and roll. Muscle tendons are usually apparent.

   Blood can be forced into the vein by gently massaging the arm from wrist to elbow. Several sharp taps at the vein site with the index and second finger may cause the vein to dilate. Application of heat to the site may have the same result. Lowering the arm over the chair will allow the veins to fill to capacity. If a vein is not readily apparent, use a tourniquet temporarily.

   The best location to perform the venipuncture is at the bend of the elbow, but if these sites are not usable, the flexor surfaces of the forearm, the wrist area above the thumb, the volar area of the wrist, or the back of the hand can be used. Use of the foot or ankle is rarely necessary.

   Collection of blood from a site on which the tourniquet has been used for more than 2 minutes can

Continued

result in some inaccurate laboratory analyses. A tourniquet prevents the blood from flowing freely and the balance of fluid and blood elements may be disrupted.

Do not use areas of obvious **hematomas,** where blood has been collected before, as some laboratory results may be erroneous. If no other veins are available, collect below (distal to) the hematoma.

Do not collect blood from scarred areas or from an arm where intravenous fluids are being given. USE THE OTHER ARM. Special procedures must be followed if blood is collected from an arm where an intravenous solution is being administered.

Only experienced phlebotomists should draw blood specimens from a cannula, fistula, vascular graft, or heparin-locked catheter.

7. *Apply the tourniquet so it can be easily released.* The tourniquet increases venous filling with blood and makes the veins more prominent and easier to enter. *Do not leave the tourniquet on for longer than 1 minute if possible; apply just before venipuncture is to be performed.* Never apply a tourniquet above an intravenous site, a fistula, shunt, cannula, or a heparin-locked catheter. Avoid pinching the skin. (A Velcro-type band tourniquet avoids this.) The tourniquet should remain "flat" around the patient's arm.

8. *Clean the skin at the venipuncture site.* Usually the vein site is cleaned with an isopropyl alcohol solution or medicated alcohol on a gauze pad using a circular motion starting from the actual site of entry to the periphery. This is done to prevent any chemical or microbiological contamination of either patient or specimen. Allow the area to air-dry in order to prevent hemolysis of the blood sample and alcohol seepage into the puncture. For blood culture collection, a triple application of iodine solution is required.

If the area is touched before the puncture, it should be recleaned.

9. *Place the selected collection tubes and needle assembly within easy reach.*

10. *Grasp the patient's arm and anchor the vein.* The patient's arm should be grasped firmly with the palm of the hand under the elbow. The patient's arm should be fully extended. Use the thumb, placed 1 or 2 in. below the puncture site, to anchor the vein by drawing the skin taut. Ask the patient to open and close the fist.

11. *Perform the venipuncture:*
    a. Keep the patient's arm in a downward position and maintain the tube below the site throughout the procedure to prevent backflow from the tube into the patient's vein.
    b. Turn the needle so that the bevel side is up.
    c. Line up the needle with the vein.
    d. Puncture the vein. The puncture of the skin and vein should be done in two steps, if possible, the skin first and then the vein, at approximately a 30-degree angle and in a direct line with the vein. A sensation of resistance will be felt followed by ease of penetration as the vein is entered.
    e. Being sure the needle is positioned sufficiently in the vein, insert the vacuum tube into the needle holder as far as it will go so that blood can flow into the vacuum tube (see Fig 2–9,B). Do this by grasping the flange of the needle holder from the top between the index and third fingers and triggering the tube forward by pushing with the thumb until the hub end of the needle punctures the stopper. This will activate the vacuum action to draw the blood into the collection tube.
    f. Allow the tube to fill until the vacuum is exhausted and blood flow ceases in order to ensure the correct ratio of anticoagulant to blood. The tube normally will not be filled completely. As the blood flow ceases, remove the tube from the needle holder, being careful not to change the position of the needle in the vein. If multiple samples are to be drawn, remove the tube as soon as the blood flow stops and insert the next tube into the holder. The shut-off valve on the hub of the needle covers the point at which the tube is removed and stops the blood from flowing until the next tube is inserted. Adhere to the proper order for the draw: first, sterile tubes for culture, then nonadditive tubes, tubes for coagulation studies, and finally the tubes with additives.

Continued.

g. As the tube containing an additive is removed, *mix immediately by gently inverting the tube five to ten times*. To avoid hemolysis, do not mix vigorously.

h. To collect multiple samples, carefully insert the next tube into the holder taking care not to change the position of the needle in the vein. Collect as many tubes as needed, using the same technique.

12. *Open the patient's hand*. Ask the patient to open his or her hand; this reduces the amount of venous pressure.

13. *Release the tourniquet* (preferably at 1 minute). Remove the tourniquet as soon as blood flow is established in the last tube to be drawn. If the tourniquet has been left on too long before blood is acquired, some test results are altered owing to stasis of cells and movement of fluid out of the vein into the tissue. The arm will become cyanotic.

THE TOURNIQUET MUST ALWAYS BE RELEASED BEFORE THE NEEDLE IS REMOVED FROM THE VEIN.

14. *Position a dry gauze pad*. Lightly place a gauze pad over (covering) the venipuncture site.

15. *Quickly, but gently, remove the needle. Then apply pressure on the gauze pad*. Hold the dry gauze pad over the needle and puncture site. Quickly remove the needle while keeping the bevel in an upward position, exercising care not to scratch the patient's arm. Apply mild pressure to the site as soon as the needle is withdrawn. Continue to apply pressure on the gauze pad until bleeding is stopped. Special attention should be given to patients with prolonged bleeding.

16. *Bandage the arm, if needed*. If the patient continues to bleed, apply a pressure bandage over the venipuncture site. Tell the patient to leave the bandage on for 15 to 30 minutes. It is recommended that adhesive bandages not be placed on small children; they may remove, chew, or swallow them.

17. *Dispose of the puncturing unit*. AVOID PUNCTURING YOUR OWN SKIN. Do not attempt to reshield the needle. Special sharps biohazard disposal systems are available which allow for direct disposal of the needle. DISPOSE OF ALL WASTE SUPPLIES IMMEDIATELY IN THE PROPER DISPOSAL CONTAINERS.

18. *Label tubes*. Be sure to properly label all tubes with the patient's name, identification number, date of collection, and other necessary patient information and mix the tubes adequately with their additive or anticoagulant. In the clinical laboratory, blood tube labels must exactly match the patient data on the test request forms.

19. *Remove gloves and wash hands*.

20. *Leave the patient only after all signs of bleeding have stopped*.

---

is in the vein, try another vacuum tube; sometimes the vacuum tubes are defective.

3. Do not probe with the needle. It is painful for the patient.

4. If another venipuncture attempt is necessary, try the other arm in the cubital fossa, or another puncture in the same arm in a site below the first puncture.

5. Never attempt a venipuncture more than twice. Request that another phlebotomist or physician attempt to draw the specimen.

6. Sometimes a capillary puncture may be used in place of the venipuncture.

7. Clothing may be too tight above the site of the venipuncture. This can slow the flow of blood and may cause a hematoma.

8. If the tourniquet is too tight (the radial pulse should be felt at all times), arterial flow of blood will stop and this may cause the vein to disappear before the puncture is done. A tight tourniquet may cause pinching of skin (an unnecessary discomfort), cyanosis, fluid shifts, and possible erroneous laboratory results.

9. Needle placement and angle of entry are important. The angle of the needle with the skin should be about 30 degrees. If the angle is greater than 45 degrees, the needle can pass straight through the vein. If skin and vein are penetrated at one time, blood may spurt from the puncture hole. The needle bevel should be well covered by skin before the vacuum tube is fully attached or the vacuum will be lost. With small veins, the bevel may be rotated down to help increase blood flow.

10. If the vein disappears at puncture (some veins collapse when touched), try increasing the tourniquet pressure slightly.

11. If the vacuum collapses the vein (the size and

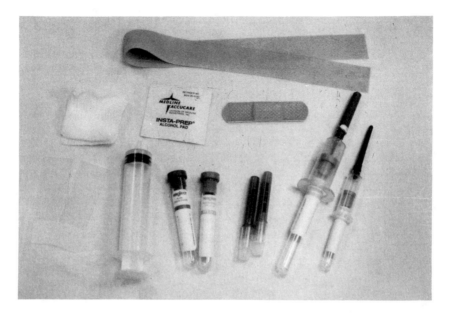

FIG 2–12.
Assembled phlebotomy supplies. (From Powers LW: *Diagnostic Hematology.* St Louis, Mosby–Year Book, Inc, 1989, p 423. Used by permission.)

softness of veins vary), tighten the tourniquet, press the needle down gently, or rotate it so that the vein wall is not occluding the bevel.

12. Undue bleeding and hematoma formation can be prevented if the puncture is made only in the upper-most wall of the vein and by making certain that it is fully penetrated; by removing the tourniquet before re-moving the needle; by immediately applying pressure to the venipuncture site after removing the needle; by ap-plying pressure on the gauze pad over the venipuncture site for several minutes until bleeding stops; or by cover-ing the site with an adhesive dressing, except with small children. If bleeding appears to be excessive, a roll of gauze under an adhesive bandage may be effective. Pa-tients with bleeding must be observed again at 5 minutes.

13. To prevent hemolysis in the blood specimen, avoid drawing blood from an area where there is a hema-toma and, in general, do not mix blood in nonadditive tubes (except for serum separator tubes which must be tipped two or three times to activate the clotting pro-cess). Allow blood to clot at room temperature for 15 minutes before centrifuging for serum separation. Mix anticoagulated specimens thoroughly but by *gentle* inver-sion five to ten times.

Hemolysis, when destruction of red cells has oc-curred, causes erroneous results in some chemistry mea-surements using serum. Hemolytic serum will appear pink.

Venipuncture Using Syringe and Needle.—A sy-ringe and needle are often used to collect blood from pa-tients with difficult veins. Using the same preparation procedures as for use of the vacuum tube system, the sy-ringe and needle system is assembled and the vein en-tered (see Fig 2–12). When making preparations for do-ing the venipuncture, remove the syringe from its protec-tive wrapper and the needle from the sterile package and assemble them, allowing the covering to remain over the needle when not in use. Attach the needle so that the bevel faces in the same direction as the graduation marks on the syringe. Check to make sure the needle is sharp, the syringe moves smoothly, and there is no air left in the syringe.

Blood will enter the syringe spontaneously if a clean entry into the vein has been made. In persons with low venous pressure, the plunger of the syringe is withdrawn slightly to make certain the needle has entered the vein. Withdraw the blood by using the left hand to pull back the plunger while steadying the syringe with the right hand.

When sufficient blood has been withdrawn, release the tourniquet and remove the needle and syringe from the vein. Place a dry gauze pad over the site of the venipuncture and maintain gentle pressure for a few minutes. Do not leave the patient until the bleeding stops.

Remove the needle from the syringe and gently expel the blood into a collection tube. Avoid foaming or rupture of the cells by using gentle pressure on the plunger of the syringe. Stopper the tube and invert gently to mix blood with additive, if one is used.

If a Vacutainer collection tube is used to hold the blood, push the needle through the stopper and allow the blood to collect in the tube using the vacuum in the tube.

A syringe and needle or **infusion set (butterfly)** is often used for coagulation studies, for babies and small children with small veins, for very obese patients whose veins are hard to find, for patients receiving intravenous chemotherapy for cancer (whose veins have become scarred), for patients who have frequent venipunctures (leukemia patients), and for veins other than those in the cubital fossa.

Venipuncture Using the Infusion Set (Butterfly).— The infusion set, or butterfly, is generally used when drawing a blood specimen from a patient with small, fragile, "rolly" veins or when drawing from veins in the wrist area, back of the hand, ankle, foot, or scalp veins. The infusion set is *often* used when drawing blood specimens from pediatric patients.

An infusion set is used with an additional collection method—either by attaching it to a sterile syringe and manually filling the syringe or by attaching it to an adapter which is in turn attached to an evacuated tube holder. The specimen is eventually transferred to or collected directly into an evacuated tube.

Obtaining Blood From Indwelling Lines.—When vascular access is needed over an extended period of time, for administration of therapeutic blood products, for infusion of fluids, medications, or parenteral nutrition solutions, the use of a **vascular access device (VAD)** is used. This device is also called an *indwelling line*. It is also possible, with skill and experience, to collect a venous or arterial blood sample from these devices.

Because infection and septicemia are serious consequences, especially in immunosuppressed patients, adherence to a strict infection control protocol for collec-

tion from VADs is imperative. The VAD specimen drawing procedure should maintain rigid sterile technique and use a consistent protocol to prevent complications from infection. For this reason, a special training program for VAD phlebotomists is necessary.

The VAD consists of a silicon catheter and a self-sealing silicon septum encased in a metal or plastic port. It is surgically implanted using local or general anesthesia. The catheter is tunneled through the subcutaneous tissue to a major blood vessel and the portal is secured to the fascia under the skin. The device is accessed by needle puncture through the skin into the port. For venous ports, catheters are placed in a vein. There are several different manufacturers of VADs.

The decision to use the VAD for obtaining a blood specimen is made by the attending physician.

Obtaining Blood With Heparin Locks.—This system consists of an indwelling winged butterfly needle and can be used in a vein for 36- to 48-hour periods to administer medication intravenously or as a source for venous blood samples. This device is used to "save" veins for patients and to lessen trauma to the veins. Repeated venipunctures can be painful to patients and can, after time, result in scarring of the vein lining which makes the vein unusable.

The butterfly system is carefully placed in the vein and must be maintained using careful infection control procedures, since the needle is a foreign body being injected directly into the patient's vein. This includes the use of antibiotic ointments and careful monitoring for signs of inflammation.

A dilute heparin solution is used in the line to keep the blood in it from clotting. This heparin flush is injected through the tubing and a plug at the end of the butterfly line holds the solution in place. Before any blood is used for analysis, a waste specimen of 2 to 3 mL must be withdrawn and discarded to free the specimen of the heparin solution. There must be a special period of training and education before a phlebotomist draws specimens from a heparin lock.

Blood Collection for Culture.—To ensure that the blood collected for culture is free from contamination (from the patient, phlebotomist, personnel), extra precautions are taken for cleaning the skin and collection tube prior to the actual collection. The skin is cleaned three times with a povidone-iodine solution or a chlorhexidine gluconate preparation. Using a scrub applicator, the povidone-iodine solution must be applied to the puncture site in a concentric outward-moving circle, beginning at the site. This step is repeated three times. After the triple cleaning, the povidone-iodine may be removed with an alcohol pad if the color of the solution makes it difficult to locate the vein. If for any reason the vein must be touched prior to the actual venipuncture, the phlebotomist's gloved finger must be triple-cleaned with povidone-iodine. Perform the venipuncture using a sterile syringe and needle.

Each culture bottle top must be cleaned with an alcohol pad prior to injecting the required amount of blood sample into the bottle. Culture bottles are labeled and brought to the laboratory.

General Considerations for Venipunctures.—The vacuum tube system is an ideal means of collecting multiple samples with ease. A multiple-sample needle is used. After blood has filled the first tube, remove the tube from the needle holder, leaving the needle in the vein, and insert a second tube. Blood will fill the second tube just as it did the first. Remember to thoroughly mix any anticoagulated blood immediately to ensure proper mixing of the additive and blood. The multiple-sample needle has a special adaptation that prevents blood from leaking out during the exchange of tubes. Some vacuum tube collection systems can be purchased with an added guard closure which helps to shield the laboratorian against exposure to blood specimens. Be certain to label all the tubes collected in this manner.

If blood must be drawn from a patient who has intravenous equipment attached to one arm, the blood sample should be drawn from a vein in the other arm. If neither arm is free, an ankle vein is the site of choice for the venipuncture.

In weak or elderly patients, the venous pressure may be so low that the pressure of the needle or the negative pressure of the vacuum tube may collapse the vein. In these cases it is advisable to use a syringe, for then the negative pressure can be controlled.

If the patient's clothing is too tight above the venipuncture site, it will slow down the flow of blood and may cause a hematoma. If the tourniquet is too tight it will cause the arterial flow to stop. The radial pulse should be felt with the tourniquet in place correctly. A tight tourniquet can cause cyanosis, and it pinches the skin, causing unnecessary discomfort to the patient. It may also cause the vein to disappear before the puncture is made. When this happens the vein has collapsed, and

the tourniquet should be released for a few minutes and the procedure repeated.

The placement of the needle—the angle of entry and the entry itself—is important. The angle of entry with the skin should be 30 to 45 degrees. If the skin and vein are penetrated at one time, the needle may go straight through the vein. It is best to make the penetration in two steps: the skin first and then the vein. The bevel of the needle must always be covered by skin before the vacuum tube is fully engaged, otherwise the vacuum in the tube is lost. If there is a poor flow of blood, the needle may be half into the vein or the bevel may be partly occluded. To correct this problem, gently turn the needle, push in, or press down to keep the vein wall off the bevel. The needle must be in line with the vein to have a good flow of blood.

Circulation of Blood

Blood, although a liquid, can also be called a tissue. It circulates throughout the body, acting as a transportation system. As it circulates through the system of blood vessels (the vascular system), oxygen is transported from the lungs to the tissues of the body, products of digestion are absorbed in the intestine and carried to the various body tissues, and substances produced in various organs are transferred to other tissues for use. Cellular elements of the blood may also be transported to fight infection or aid in the coagulation of the blood. At the same time, waste products from the body tissues are picked up by the blood, and these end products of metabolism are then excreted through the skin, kidneys, and lungs.

The heart is the pump that forces the blood, under pressure, out through the arteries to all parts of the body. If an artery is cut, blood spurts out in small bursts each time the heart contracts. Near organs and muscles, the arteries branch out into smaller and smaller blood vessels called arterioles. Still smaller branches from the arterioles are called capillaries. In the tiny capillaries, the blood cells give up the oxygen they have been carrying and exchange it for the waste product from the body tissues, carbon dioxide. The capillary blood carrying carbon dioxide flows into larger vessels called venules, and then into still larger vessels called veins. The veins carry the blood back to the heart. As the blood flows through the capillaries, it gradually loses pressure. In the veins it has still less pressure. Therefore, if a vein is cut the blood oozes out; it does not spurt out. After the veins have carried the blood back to the heart, the blood is pumped into the alveoli, or air sacs of the lung. In the alveoli the carbon dioxide is removed from the red blood cells, which take up oxygen in its place. The blood then returns to the heart to be pumped out to the body once again through the arteries. It is important to understand the basics of the blood circulation so that the proper sites for blood collection are used.

The chemical compound in the red blood cells that actually picks up the oxygen and exchanges it for carbon dioxide is hemoglobin. When hemoglobin is saturated with oxygen, it is bright red in color. When oxygen is replaced by carbon dioxide, the hemoglobin becomes darker red. When blood from an artery is compared with blood from a vein, the arterial blood is a visibly brighter red because of the nature of the hemoglobin compound.

Additives and Anticoagulants

Blood is a combination of formed elements (red cells, white cells, and platelets) in a liquid portion called plasma. In vivo (in the body) the blood is in a liquid form, but in vitro (outside the body) it will clot in a few minutes. Blood that is freshly drawn into a glass tube appears as a translucent, dark red fluid. In a matter of minutes it will start to clot, or coagulate, forming a semisolid jellylike mass. If left undisturbed in the tube, this mass will begin to shrink, or retract, in about 1 hour. Complete retraction normally takes place within 24 hours. When coagulation occurs, a pale yellow fluid called serum separates from the clot and appears in the upper portion of the tube. During the process of coagulation certain factors present in the original blood sample are depleted or used up (See also Coagulation and Hemostasis, Chapter 12.) Fibrinogen is one important substance found in the circulating blood (in the plasma portion) that is necessary for coagulation to occur. Fibrinogen is converted to fibrin when clotting occurs, and the fibrin lends structure to the clot in the form of fine threads in which the red cells (erythrocytes) and white cells (leukocytes) are embedded. To assist in obtaining serum, the use of collection tubes with a separator gel additive in them is commonly used (Fig 2–13). Serum is used extensively for chemical, serologic, and other laboratory testing, and can be obtained from the tube by centrifuging.

If coagulation is prevented by the addition of an anticoagulant, the formed elements of the blood—the red cells, white cells, and platelets—can be separated from the plasma. If the anticoagulated blood is centrifuged, it

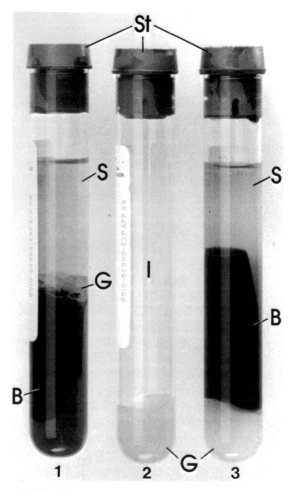

FIG 2–13.
Vacutainer phlebotomy tubes containing barrier gel (red-gray tops). *(1)* Tube filled with blood and centrifuged. *(2)* Unfilled tube. *(3)* Tube filled with blood and not centrifuged. Note positions of gel before *(3)* and after centrifugation *(1)*. B = clotted blood; St = red-gray stoppers; G = barrier gel; S = serum. (From Kaplan LA, Pesce AJ: *Clinical Chemistry, Theory, Analysis, and Correlation,* ed 2. St Louis, Mosby–Year Book, Inc, 1989, p 43. Used by permission.)

separates into three main layers: the red cells, the buffy coat (consisting of white cells and platelets), and the plasma. Hematologic studies are done primarily on whole anticoagulated venous blood or on capillary blood. It is important that everyone involved in collecting blood specimens thoroughly understands the reason for using an anticoagulant. Use of the appropriate additive is essential, and to do this the type of determination to be done by the laboratory must be indicated on the request slip.

Several anticoagulants are available for various purposes in the clinical laboratory. Some of the more commonly used anticoagulants are:

1. *Sodium fluoride:* This is a dry additive, a weak anticoagulant, used primarily for blood glucose specimens since it is also an enzyme poison (preventing glycolysis, or destruction of glucose). More information on the use of this anticoagulant may be found under Glucose in Chapter 10.

2. *Oxalates:* These dry additives are available as sodium, potassium, ammonium, or lithium oxalates. The oxalate in the anticoagulant forms an insoluble complex with the calcium in the blood, inhibiting the clotting mechanism. When calcium ions are combined with oxalate and are therefore not available to participate in clotting, the blood does not clot.

3. *Ammonium and potassium oxalate.* Also called balanced oxalate, or double oxalate, this combination is a dry additive. It is used for some hematology work. It is not used in chemistry, as a rule, because the presence of ammonium in the anticoagulant interferes with some of the chemistry determinations. This anticoagulant has become obsolete in most laboratories since the advent of EDTA.

4. *EDTA (ethylenediaminetetraacetic acid, Versene, Sequestrene).* EDTA is used as a disodium or dipotassium salt. It prevents coagulation by chelating (binding) calcium in the plasma. It is a dry additive used primarily in the hematology laboratory. It is the anticoagulant of choice for blood to be used in cell counts, hematocrit, hemoglobin, and cell differentials on stained blood films, to name but a few tests, because it preserves the morphologic structure of the blood cell elements.

5. *Sodium citrate.* This additive is widely used for coagulation procedures, including prothrombin times and partial thromboplastin tests. It prevents coagulation by inactivating calcium ions. The citrate helps to prevent the rapid deterioration of labile coagulation factors such as factor V and factor VII.

6. *Heparin.* This additive is theoretically the best anticoagulant, because it is a normal constituent of blood and introduces no foreign contaminants in the blood specimen. Heparin is available as sodium, lithium, potassium, and ammonium salts. It is, however, expensive, and has only a temporary effect as an anticoagulant. It prevents coagulation for approximately 24 hours by neutralizing thrombin, thus preventing the formation of fibrin from fibrinogen. Only a small amount of heparin is needed, so that simply coating the insides of tubes or syringes is often enough to give a good anticoagulant effect. Heparin is used for blood gas determinations and pH assays.

Color Coding for Vacuum Tubes.—Stopper color codes for additives have been generally accepted by manufacturers of vacuum (evacuated) tubes for blood collection. The codes in Table 2–1 apply.

TABLE 2–1.

Color Coding for Vacuum Tubes

Stopper Color	Use	Additive
Gray	Plasma or whole blood	Oxalate
Gray	Glycolysis inhibition	Fluoride
Yellow	Sterile interior of tube	SPS (sodium polyanetholesulfonate)
Green	Plasma or whole blood	Lithium, ammonium, or sodium heparin
Red	Serum	None
Red and black	Serum	Inert serum separator gel
Light blue	Plasma or whole blood	Sodium citrate
Royal blue	Plasma or whole blood	Sodium heparin
Lavender	Plasma or whole blood	EDTA

Order for Drawing Blood Into Collection Tubes.—To avoid any possible cross-contamination of additives between tubes, blood collection tubes must be drawn in a specific order. Each health care facility will implement its specific policy for the order of drawing tubes for laboratory analyses. Policies vary from place to place on coagulation studies and blood cultures, for example. In general, however, it is important to draw any sterile blood culture specimens first, then specimens that require no additives (plain tubes), followed by tubes needed for coagulation studies (usually sodium citrate or heparin), if drawn at the same time. Lastly, tubes with the various other additives are drawn, with EDTA first, then oxalates and fluorides. It is possible that there can be additive contamination from tube to tube, especially if the blood drawing is slow and difficult. If, for example, the EDTA tube is collected prior to the heparin tube for electrolyte analysis, the potassium salt of EDTA may falsely elevate the potassium determination.

Adverse Effects of Additives.—The additives chosen for specific determinations must be such that they do not alter the blood components and do not affect the laboratory tests to be done. The following are some adverse effects of using an improper additive or using the wrong amount of additive.

1. The additive may contain a substance that is the same, or reacts in the same way, as the substance being determined. An example would be the use of sodium oxalate as the anticoagulant for a determination of sodium.

2. The additive may remove the constituent to be measured. An example would be the use of an oxalate anticoagulant for a calcium determination; oxalate removes calcium from the blood by forming an insoluble salt, calcium oxalate.

3. The additive may affect enzyme reactions. An example would be the use of sodium fluoride as an anticoagulant in an enzyme determination. Fluoride destroys many enzymes.

4. The additive may alter cellular constituents. An example would be the use of oxalate in cell morphology studies in hematology. Oxalate distorts the cell morphology; red cells become crenated, vacuoles appear in the granulocytes, and bizarre forms of lymphocytes and monocytes appear rapidly when oxalate is used as the anticoagulant. Another example is the use of heparin as an anticoagulant for blood to be used in the preparation of blood films that will be stained with Wright's stain. Unless stained within 2 hours, heparin gives a blue background with Wright's stain.

5. If too little additive is used, partial clotting will occur. This interferes with cell counts.

6. If too much liquid anticoagulant is used, it dilutes the blood sample and thus interferes with certain quantitative measurements.

Laboratory Processing of Blood Specimens

As discussed previously, if no anticoagulant is used, blood clots and serum is obtained. After being placed in a plain tube, the blood is allowed to clot. The serum is then removed from the clot by centrifugation and is placed in a clean, dry storage tube or vial.

Serum Separator Devices.—To assist in the processing of clotted whole blood to obtain the serum, special serum separator collection tubes are available. An evacuated glass tube serves as the single system for both collection and processing of the blood. Serum separator tubes are of two major types, those used during centrifugation and those used after centrifugation.

The tubes used during centrifugation may either be integrated gel tube systems or devices inserted into the collection tube just before centrifugation. The integrated gel tubes contain a special silicon gel layer, which, because of its viscosity and density, moves to form a barrier between cells and serum during centrifugation (see Fig 2–13). Blood is forced into the gel layer during centrifugation causing a temporary change in viscosity. The gel starts out at the bottom of the collection tube. Blood is added to the tube and the clot allowed to form. After clot formation, the tubes are centrifuged. The gel rises and lodges between the packed red cells and the top layer of serum. The gel hardens and forms an inert barrier. These tubes do not have to be unstoppered before centrifugation, thus eliminating aerosol production and possible evaporation. The serum separator tubes also give a higher yield of serum as well as a shorter processing time because only a single centrifugation step is needed.

Processing Blood for Serum.—Serum can be used in the chemistry laboratory for tests for sodium, potassium, calcium, phosphorus, acid and alkaline phosphatase, cholesterol, uric acid, and liver function, to mention but a few. Serum is also used for serology testing.

It is important to remove the plasma or serum from the remaining blood cells, or clot, as soon as possible.

Since biological specimens are being handled, the need for certain safety precautions is stressed. Using the universal precautions policy, all blood specimens represent a potential contamination problem (see Chapter 1). Blood specimens should be handled while wearing protective gloves. The outsides of the tubes may be bloody, and initial laboratory handling of all specimens necessitates direct contact with the tubes. The stoppers on the tubes must be removed carefully and not popped off, as this could cause infection by inhalation or by contact of the infectious aerosol with mucous membranes. Stoppers should be twisted gently while covering them with protective gauze to minimize the risk from aerosol. This processing step can be done using a protective plastic shield so no direct splashes can take place. To separate the serum and plasma from the remaining blood cells, the tube must be centrifuged. It is generally best to remove the serum and plasma as quickly as possible to prevent alterations from taking place in the sample to be tested. It is especially important to remove the plasma quickly from the cell layer when potassium oxalate has been used as the anticoagulant, because the salt (potassium oxalate) shrinks the red blood cells and the intracellular water diffuses into the plasma (fluid inside the red cell leaves the cell and thus causes shrinkage). Centrifuge covers should be in place during centrifugation to protect the worker from the specimens, and the centrifuge should be placed as far from laboratory personnel as possible. The safest procedure for separating the centrifuged serum or plasma from the cell mass left in the tube is by pipetting instead of pouring. Pipette the serum or plasma by using mechanical suction and a disposable pipette. All serum and plasma tubes, as well as the original blood tubes, should be discarded properly in biohazard containers when they are no longer needed for the determination.

Appearance of Processed Specimens.—Those working with specimens in the laboratory must be able to recognize the appearance of normal as opposed to abnormal plasma or serum. Normally, serum or plasma is straw-colored, but various shades of yellow are also normally seen. Abnormal-appearing serum and plasma can be clinical indications of serious disorders. Also, the use of such abnormal specimens can interfere with determinations, especially chemistry tests.

Hemolysis in specimens is perhaps the most common cause of the abnormal appearances to be considered in this section. A specimen that is hemolyzed appears red, usually clear red, because the red blood cells have been lysed and the hemoglobin has been released into the liquid portion of the blood. Often the cause of hemolysis in specimens is the technique used for venipuncture. A poor venipuncture, with excessive trauma to the blood vessel, can result in a hemolyzed specimen. Collecting the blood in dirty tubes or tubes that are not entirely dry can also result in hemolysis. In these cases, carefully repeating the venipuncture and using clean, dry equipment will produce a normal-appearing specimen that can be used for chemical determinations. Hemolysis of blood can also be caused by freezing, prolonged exposure to warmth, unnecessarily forceful spraying of blood from the needle of a syringe when transferring it to a specimen tube, or allowing the serum or plasma to remain too long on the cells before removing it to another tube. Hemolyzed serum or plasma is unsuitable for several chemistry determinations. The procedure to be done should always be checked first to see if abnormal-appearing specimens can be used.

Jaundiced serum or plasma is another specimen with an abnormal-looking appearance. When serum or plasma takes on a brownish-yellow color, there has most likely been an increase in bile pigments, namely bilirubin. Excessive intravascular destruction of red blood cells, obstruction of the bile duct, or impairment of the liver leads to an accumulation of bile pigments in the blood, and the skin becomes yellow. When this occurs, the skin of the patient is said to be *jaundiced*. The serum or plasma can also be jaundiced, or yellow. Those performing clinical laboratory determinations should note any abnormal appearance of serum or plasma and record it on the report slip. Another term for jaundiced is *icteric*. Jaundiced serum or plasma is seen in patients with hepatitis. Once again, we stress the importance of being observant in all areas of laboratory work—noticing things like jaundiced specimens can assist the physician in making a diagnosis.

When the blood, serum, or plasma takes on a milky appearance, the specimen is said to be *lipemic*. The presence of lipids, or fats, in the serum causes this abnormal appearance. A blood specimen drawn from a patient soon after a meal may often appear lipemic. Lipemic specimens, for the most part, do not interfere with chemical determinations.

The processing of individual serum or plasma tubes will depend on the analysis to be done and the time that will elapse before it. Serum or plasma may be kept at room temperature, refrigerated, frozen, or protected from light, depending on the circumstances and the determination to be done. Some specimens must be analyzed immediately after they reach the laboratory, such as specimens for blood gas and pH analyses. Blood specimens for hematology studies can be stored in the refrigerator for 2 hours before being used in testing. After storage, anticoagulated blood, serum, or plasma must be thoroughly mixed after it has reached room temperature.

Plasma and serum often can be frozen and preserved satisfactorily until the determination can be done. Whole blood cannot be frozen because red blood cells rupture on freezing. Freezing preserves most chemical constituents in serum and plasma and provides a method of sample preservation for the laboratory. In general, refrigerating specimens retards alterations of many constituents. With all biological specimens, however, preservation should be the exception rather than the rule. A laboratory determination is best done on a fresh specimen.

Urine

The urine specimen has been referred to as a liquid tissue biopsy of the urinary tract that is painlessly and easily obtained. Urine yields a great amount of valuable information quickly and economically but, as for all other human specimens used in the laboratory, the specimen must be carefully collected, preserved, and processed for the information to be regarded as reliable. A routine urine analysis (urinalysis) is included with most hospital admissions.

Types of Urine Collections

The composition of urine in random samples collected at different times during the day is likely to vary considerably, because the work of the kidney is so variable. It is not practical to collect an entire day's specimen (24-hour specimen), as it would take too long for any results to be ready for the physician; also, as urine stands, many of the more important constituents found in it disappear or are altered. A 24-hour specimen is required only when it is necessary to know the entire day's volume of urine output, or for quantitative tests in which the exact amount of urine must be known so that the exact amount of substance present may be reported.

Since a 24-hour collection is not necessary for a routine urinalysis, any random specimen that is passed during the day may be used. A **voided midstream urine specimen** is suitable for most routine urine tests. The

first urine voided in the morning is usually recommended. This is true primarily because the **first morning urine specimen** is the most concentrated one passed during the day. It is more concentrated because less fluid (or water) is excreted during the night, while the same amount of solid or dissolved substance must be excreted for the kidney to perform its function of maintaining the composition of the extracellular fluid. When testing for the presence of urine sugar, the best specimen to use is one voided 2 to 3 hours after a meal. This is the one exception to the recommended use of the first morning specimen.

Containers for Urine Collection

It is of prime importance that the containers used to collect the urine specimen be clean and dry. Several types of containers are suitable for this purpose. Disposable, inert, plastic containers and plastic bags or jars are most often used. These are available in several sizes and are preferred for routine screening urinalysis. Conical containers are less likely to tip over. Containers for routine urine tests should have a capacity of 50 to 100 mL with a round opening at least 2 in. in diameter and should have screw caps. Sterile containers with lids for collecting urine for microbiological studies (cultures) are available. There are also special pediatric urine-collecting bags made of clear polyethylene. If a 24-hour pediatric specimen is required, a special tube can be attached to the bag, which is in turn connected to a collection bottle.

Large plastic containers with wide mouths and screw caps are used to collect timed specimens (24-hour collections) from adults, usually with added preservatives. The collection bottles should be refrigerated between voidings. Any bedpans that are used to collect voided urine must be scrupulously clean. Any collection containers used must be labeled with complete patient identification.

Preservation of Urine Specimens

If a fresh specimen of urine is left at room temperature for a period of time, the urine rapidly undergoes changes. It is for this reason that a good routine urinalysis should include the use of a *fresh specimen*. Decomposition of urine begins within 30 minutes after collection. Specimens left at room temperature will soon begin to decompose, mainly owing to the action of bacteria in the urine. Urea-splitting bacteria produce ammonia, which on combination with hydrogen ions forms ammonium. This causes an increase in urine pH. The increase in pH will result in decomposition of casts, if present in the urine. The various laboratory tests to be done on a specimen of urine should be done within 30 minutes after collection, if possible; no longer than 1 or 2 hours should elapse before the tests are done unless the urine is preserved in some way.

If it is impossible to examine the urine specimen when fresh or if a **timed urine collection** (2-, 12-, or 24-hour) is required, the *urine must be preserved*. Various methods of preserving urine are available, most of which inhibit the growth of bacteria, thus preventing many of the alterations from occurring. The best method is immediate refrigeration during and after collection. The specimen may be kept 6 to 8 hours under refrigeration with no gross alterations with no chemical preservative added. There are several chemical preservatives which are available as additives for routine urine specimens. Most of them interfere in some way with the testing procedures, however, and it is best if no chemical preservative is added.

Toluene is one chemical preservative which can be used. It is a liquid that works by preventing the growth of bacteria. A thin layer of toluene is added, just enough to cover the surface of the urine. The toluene should be skimmed off or the urine pipetted from beneath it when the urine is examined. Toluene (toluol) is the best all-around preservative, because it does not interfere with the various tests done in the routine urinalysis. Other common preservatives for urine specimens are formaldehyde (formalin), thymol, and boric acid. Thymol, a crystalline substance, works to prevent the growth of bacteria. However, thymol may interfere with tests for urine protein and bilirubin. Formalin, a liquid preservative, acts by fixing the formed elements in the urinary sediment. It may, however, interfere with the reduction tests for urine sugar and may form a precipitate with urea that interferes with the microscopic examination of the sediment. Preservative tablets that produce formaldehyde are commercially available. The tablets are more convenient to use than the liquid formalin and do not interfere with the usual chemical and microscopic examination.

Various disposable collecting systems are available commercially for collecting, storing, transporting, and testing urine specimens. New systems are continually introduced to the market.

In general, it should be remembered that a fresh urine specimen is best for urinalysis tests. It is usually easy to collect and will give the most satisfactory results.

Collecting Urine Specimens

As stated previously, the specimen for urinalysis should be collected in a clean, dry container, and the specimen should be fresh (Procedure 2–4). For routine screening and for most bacteriologic examinations, a fresh, midstream (freely flowing) voided urine specimen is usually suitable (see also Chapter 16). For most routine urinalysis, including protein content and urinary sediment constituents, the concentrated first morning specimen is the most satisfactory one to use.

Occasionally it may be necessary to obtain a catheterized urine specimen, but this procedure is not encouraged because of the risk of patient infection. These urine specimens are obtained by introducing a catheter into the bladder, through the urethra, for the withdrawal of urine. This procedure should be avoided whenever possible, as there is always a risk of introducing bacteria into an otherwise sterile bladder. This could initiate a urinary tract infection. Catheterized specimens are necessary when contamination by vaginal contents in female patients may alter the examination (especially during menstruation). It may also be necessary for obtaining urine specimens for bacteriologic examination when a sterile sample is needed. Under many conditions, however, a freely flowing voided specimen is satisfactory for bacteriologic cultures. Urine obtained by means of catheterization should be *handled very carefully* in the laboratory. Remember that it is an unpleasant procedure for the patient and it does involve some degree of risk.

When both a bacteriologic culture and a routine urinalysis are needed on the same specimen, the culture should always be done first and then the routine tests.

Since many urine specimens are usually sent to the laboratory on a single day, it is especially important that each container be properly labeled when it is collected from the patient. Each specimen must be accompanied by a request slip.

When a 24-hour urine specimen is sent to the laboratory, it must be ascertained first that it has been properly collected. A preservative must have been added at the beginning of the collection time, and the correct collection time must have been used (24 hours total time, for example). In the laboratory, the total volume of specimen is measured and recorded, the urine is thoroughly mixed, and an aliquot is withdrawn for analysis.

Procedure 2–4. Voided Midstream Urine Specimen

Males

1. Instruct the patient who is uncircumcized to retract his foreskin.
2. The patient should pass the first portion of the urination into the toilet, the midportion into the appropriate container, and the last portion into the toilet.
3. If the patient is weak, ill, or otherwise unable to perform the collection without assistance, help him.

Females

1. Ask the patient to sit on the toilet and then to manually separate the labia minora with one hand and keep them separated while voiding the first portion of the urination into the toilet.
2. Tell the patient to catch the midportion of the urination in the appropriate container without contaminating the lip or inside of the container with her hand.
3. Ask the patient to finish voiding into the toilet.
4. If the patient is ill, weak, or otherwise unable to collect her urine unassisted, help her.

Collection of Timed Urine Specimens.—The patient is carefully instructed about details of the collection process, if the collection will be done on an outpatient basis. The bladder is emptied at the starting time (8 A.M., for example) and this time is noted on the collection container. This urine is discarded and *not* put into the container. All subsequent voidings are collected and put into the container up to and including that at 8 A.M. the following morning. This urine specimen will complete the 24-hour collection. For timed collections of other than 24 hours, the sample collection principle applies. The first urine voided at the beginning of the collection is always discarded. These timed collection specimens are preserved by refrigeration in between collections with the appropriate chemical preservative being added to the container prior to beginning the collection process.

The total volume of the timed collection sample is measured, recorded, and the sample well mixed before a measured aliquot is withdrawn for analysis.

Collection of Urine for Culture.—A clean, voided midstream urine specimen is desirable for culture. It is important that the glans penis in the male and the urethral orifice in the female be thoroughly cleaned with a mild antiseptic solution using sterile gauze or cotton balls. In the female, each side of the urinary orifice should also be cleaned and then rinsed twice with sterile water-soaked gauze or cotton balls. The patient should be instructed to urinate forcibly, and to allow the initial stream of urine to pass into the toilet or bedpan. Throughout the urination process for the female, the labia should be separated so no contamination results. The midstream specimen should be collected in a sterile container and no portion of the perineum (female) should come in contact with the collection container. After the specimen has been collected, the rest of the urine is passed into the toilet or bedpan.

Body Cavity Fluids (Extravascular)

When fluids normally found in small amounts in various cavities or spaces in the body increase in amount and mechanically inhibit the action of certain key organs such as the heart or lungs, or when such a fluid is needed for diagnostic purposes, the fluid is aspirated. The procedure is done under sterile conditions by a physician. Fluids aspirated from the chest, abdomen, joints, cysts, or abscesses are often brought to the laboratory for various types of tests. The origin of the fluid and the tests to be done should be noted on the container and request slip along with the usual label information required (patient name, hospital number, etc.). Many different tests can be ordered on body cavity fluids, including chemistry determinations, cultures, cell counts and differentials, and examination for tumor cells.

The various types of extravascular fluids, or body cavity fluids, are examined in various departments of the clinical laboratory, depending on what test is to be done and what type of fluid is to be examined. Cell counts are done on most body fluid specimens. For this reason, in many hospitals, body cavity fluid specimens are brought first to the hematology laboratory, and are either examined there or sent on from there to a specific department.

Most normal body cavity fluids are pale and straw-colored. As the cell count and any abnormal debris and constituents increase, the fluid becomes more turbid.

Since cell counts are done on many body cavity fluid specimens, the specimen must be a fresh one. If it is not fresh, cell disintegration will occur. No cell counts may be done on a clotted specimen; anticoagulants must be used to prevent coagulation of the specimen when a cell count is needed. Specific-gravity tests must also be done on a clot-free specimen. Tests for mucin and protein, however, can be done on clotted specimens. When a glucose determination is ordered, the specimen must be immediately preserved with sodium fluoride to prevent glycolysis. Generally, a blood glucose test is done simultaneously for comparison purposes. Body cavity fluid specimens to be cultured should be sent to the microbiology laboratory. Specimens to be tested for a chemical constituent should be sent to the chemistry laboratory as soon as possible. Sometimes only one specimen is sent to the laboratory, and several tests are required; except for culture, cell counts should always be done before other tests. For cell counts, the anticoagulant of choice is heparin or EDTA. For examination for tumor cells, the fluid may be collected in EDTA or heparin. If the fluid is collected without any anticoagulant, clotting may be observed. The presence of clotting indicates a substantial inflammatory reaction. Sometimes so much fluid is aspirated that it must be collected in a gallon container instead of the usual tube. It is important to remember that the suitable anticoagulant must be placed in this large container just as in the tube. Most laboratory tests cannot be done on a clotted specimen of body fluid. With the universal precautions policy, all body cavity fluids should be considered contaminated, and all equipment must be decontaminated or discarded after being used.

All body cavity fluids are either *transudates* or *exudates*. Transudates are ultrafiltrates of plasma resulting from a difference in osmotic pressure across a membrane. Exudates are fluids that occur as a result of an inflammatory condition that leads to an increase in the permeability of a membrane. Generally, a transudate has a specific gravity below 1.018, a protein value of less than 2.5 g/dL, and very few cells. An exudate has a specific gravity above 1.018, a protein value greater than 2.5 g/dL, and many cells. These values often overlap in certain inflammatory states and can cause confusion about whether the fluid is a transudate or an exudate.

Cerebrospinal Fluid

Cerebrospinal fluid is the most frequently tested body cavity fluid other than blood or urine. It fills the ventricles of the brain, the central canal of the spinal cord, and the subarachnoid spaces of the brain and spinal cord. It is formed in the ventricles and has many of the same characteristics as plasma, since most of its components are derived from the blood plasma. The only known function of the cerebrospinal fluid is mechanical—providing protection for the brain and spinal cord. Examination of the spinal fluid is important in the diagnosis of neurologic disorders, inflammatory diseases, and hemorrhage in the meninges.

The cerebrospinal fluid, or spinal fluid, is obtained by puncturing one of the spaces between the lumbar vertebrae with a needle. It is collected by lumbar puncture into the L3-4 lumbar interspace to avoid damaging the spinal cord. This procedure is done by a physician. The spinal fluid is usually collected into three or four sterile containers (numbered according to the order of collection), each containing between 1 and 3 mL of fluid. It is essential that the containers be properly labeled and handled with extreme care as the procedure of collection cannot be easily repeated. There is a certain risk to the patient in this procedure and for this reason the specimen is extremely precious and must be treated with the utmost care. Cerebrospinal fluid is considered infectious, and universal precautions must be used in connection with the specimen. A 5% phenol, concentrated bleach solution, alcohol solution, or other disinfectant solution can be used for decontamination of equipment that is not disposable. Specific decontamination protocol varies according to the laboratory facility. There is always the danger of spreading infectious pathogens if cerebrospinal fluids are not handled properly. Cell counts on a spinal fluid specimen must be done as soon as possible after the spinal tap has been completed, since the cells present will disintegrate within a short time. Tests for glucose in spinal fluid must also be performed immediately to prevent glycolysis. The use of sodium fluoride will slow down the glycolytic process. A blood specimen for a glucose assay should accompany a request for spinal fluid glucose for comparison purposes. For the chemical tests ordered, the specimen should be sent to the chemistry laboratory.

Normal cerebrospinal fluid appears clear and colorless. If the fluid is grossly bloody or blood-tinged, the patient may have a serious brain or spinal injury. Sometimes, however, a drop of blood gets into the sample from the puncture needle. It is important for this reason to observe the collected tubes and to note the order in which they were collected. If blood has gotten into the tube from a traumatic tap (blood from the needle, skin, or muscle) the tubes will progressively clear. That is, the first tube collected will have more blood in it and the succeeding tubes will have less. This is one reason why it is important to observe *all* the tubes collected, not just one. If all the tubes are bloody to the same degree, a hemorrhage in the brain or spinal cord is more likely. If the spinal fluid in the tubes appears cloudy, there is good reason to suspect an infection in the central nervous system. Most conditions for which spinal fluid testing is requested are very serious and require immediate diagnosis and treatment. This is why the laboratory tests are so important and speed is essential.

Synovial Fluid

Synovial fluid is the fluid that lines the joints. Normal synovial fluid resembles uncooked egg white and is straw-colored, viscous, and does not clot. Examination of this fluid from the joints provides information about joint diseases such as infections, gout, and rheumatoid arthritis.

Synovial fluid differs from other body cavity fluids because of the importance of finding crystals in the specimen and because it is normally very viscous. The specimen should be collected into two tubes: one should be in a tube with anticoagulant, preferably heparin, for culture, cell counts, crystal identification, and prepared smears; the other should be in a plain tube without anticoagulant to observe fibrinogen clots and for chemistry tests. Heparin is the additive of choice because other anticoagulants are likely to have undissolved crystals present when the amount of specimen aspirated is small. Normal joints have very little synovial fluid. The additive crystals can cause confusion when the specimen is being examined for the presence of crystals. To test for clot formation, the fluid must be collected in a plain tube without anticoagulant. Glucose determination requires collection in sodium fluoride.

Pericardial, Pleural, and Peritoneal Fluid

These fluids are called *serous fluids* and are fluids of the pericardial, pleural, and peritoneal cavities. They normally are formed continuously in the body cavities and are reabsorbed leaving only a very small volume. The normal appearance of these fluids is pale and straw-colored. The fluid becomes more turbid as the cell count rises, an indication of inflammation.

An increase in the amount of these body cavity fluids formed is seen in inflammation and when the serum protein level falls. Serous fluids are aspirated because

they are mechanically inhibiting the function of the associated organs or for diagnostic purposes. These aspirations are done by the physician. The specimen is collected into various containers, depending on the laboratory testing to be done. An EDTA tube is used for cell counts and smear evaluation, sterile tubes for cultures, and oxalate or fluoride tubes for protein, glucose, or other chemistry tests. If a large volume of fluid is aspirated, it is collected in a gallon jar with an appropriate additive to prevent clotting. If the fluid clots, it is useless for many analyses.

Swabs for Culture

Swabs with samples of specimens from wounds, abscesses, throats, and so forth are brought to the laboratory in a sterile transport tube for culture. These swabs are potentially from infectious areas and should be treated very carefully in the laboratory. Again, the container with the swab in it must be properly labeled and the culture done immediately (see Chapter 16). Most bacteria will die if stored on a dry swab, so if the culture

---

Procedure 2–5. Throat Culture

1. Ask the patient to open his or her mouth.
2. Using a sterile tongue blade to hold the tongue down, and a sterile swab to collect the specimen, take the specimen directly from the back of the throat, being careful not to touch the teeth, cheeks, gums, or tongue when inserting or removing the swab (Fig 2–14).
3. The tonsillar fauces and rear pharyngeal wall should be swabbed, not just gently touched, in order to remove organisms adhering to the membranes. White patches of exudate in the tonsillar area are especially productive for isolating the streptococcal organisms.
4. The swab containing the specimen can be placed in a special container with transport media. Commercial collection sets containing both swabs and transport media are available. Streptococci survive on dry swabs for up to 2 to 3 hours and on swabs in transport (holding) media at 4° C for 24 to 48 hours.
5. The specimen container must be labeled with the necessary patient identification.

cannot be done immediately some means to keep the swab moist and cool must be used. Most organisms can live for many hours if stored properly. Immediate culture is still best, however. Proper technique for disposal of contaminated material must be used.

Throat Culture Collection (Procedure 2–5)

Throat swab specimens are used for detection of group A β-hemolytic streptococci. The specimen collected can be used for the classic culture on sheep blood media or for one of the rapid direct tests utilizing extraction of the cell wall polysaccharide antigen and its recognition by antibody. These rapid tests have gained popularity, especially in physician's offices, because results are available within minutes instead of hours (see Chapter 16).

Feces

Feces, or stool specimens, should be collected in a clean plastic container. The specimen should be collected and covered without being contaminated with urine. The amount collected depends on the test to be done. Most testing is done on a random specimen. The container should be labeled properly, including the time of collection (for a timed specimen) and the laboratory tests desired.

Small amounts of fecal material are frequently analyzed for the presence of occult, or hidden, blood. Occult blood is recognized as a most important sign of the presence of a bleeding ulcer or malignant disease in the gastrointestinal tract. The specimen is applied to commercially prepared filter paper slides which have been impregnated with reagent. These slides are then sent to the laboratory for analysis. Outpatients are often asked to recover small amounts of their own feces that have been excreted into the toilet and apply them directly to the slides which have been supplied by the physician. These slides are then mailed back to the physician or laboratory for testing.

Feces from infants is usually recovered from the child's diaper for trypsin activity screening tests to detect cystic fibrosis. In adults, for certain metabolic balance studies and for measurement of fecal nitrogen and fat, 3-day (72-hour) fecal collections are needed.

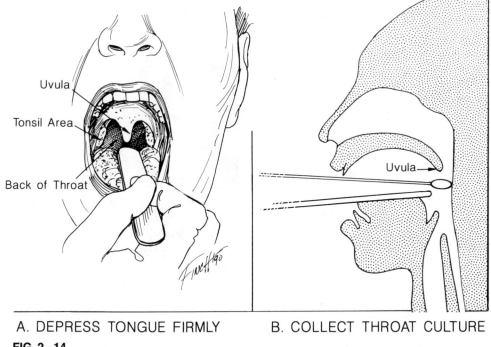

A. DEPRESS TONGUE FIRMLY   B. COLLECT THROAT CULTURE

FIG 2–14.
Obtaining a throat culture.

Other Specimens

Other types of specimens such as gallstones, kidney stones, sputum, seminal fluid, or tissue samples may be sent to the laboratory for analysis. Each requires special collection and processing.

CHAIN-OF-CUSTODY SPECIMEN INFORMATION

When specimens are involved in possible medicolegal situations, certain specimen handling policies are required. Medicolegal, or forensic, implications require that any data pertaining to the specimen in question will be recognized by a court of law. Processing steps for such specimens, including the initial collection, transportation, storage, and analytic testing, must be documented by careful record-keeping. Documentation ensures that there has been no tampering with the specimen by any interested parties, that the specimen has been collected from the appropriate person, and that the results reported are accurate. This document is called the *chain of custody*.

The chain-of-custody document must be signed by every person who has handled the specimens involved in the case in question. The actual process may vary in different health care facilities, but the general purpose of this process is to make certain that any data obtained by the clinical laboratory will be admissible in a court of law and that all steps have been taken to ensure the integrity of the information produced.

SPECIMEN TRANSPORTATION

Once the specimen has been collected and properly labeled, it must be transported to the laboratory for processing and analysis. Placing the specimen container in a leakproof plastic bag is used in many institutions as a further protective measure to prevent pathogen transmission—the implementation of the universal precaution policy and the use of barriers. The request form must be placed on the *outside of this bag*. Many of these transport bags have a special pouch provided on the outside of the bag into which the request slip is placed.

Since some laboratory analyses require special handling of the specimens to be tested, beginning with the transport of the specimen to the laboratory, specific requirements for specimens should be noted for each particular test to be done. For example, some tests require that the specimen be protected from light to prevent a change in the constituent to be measured. These specimens should be covered as soon as possible with a light-protective foil wrap and then transported to the laboratory for processing and testing. Some tests must be done on the specimen as soon after collection as possible. For other tests, the specimen can be processed and stored until testing is done at a later time. It is always the best rule to transport the specimen to the laboratory as quickly as possible, however, using the transport system implemented by the health care institution.

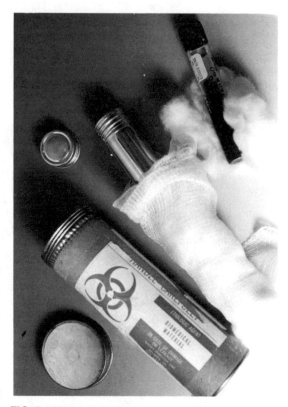

FIG 2–15.
Proper containers for shipping biological specimens. (From Baron EJ, Finegold SM: *Bailey and Scott's Diagnostic Microbiology,* ed 8. St Louis, Mosby–Year Book, Inc, 1990, p 15. Used by permission.)

Shipping Specimens to Reference Laboratories

Sometimes it is necessary to ship a specimen to another laboratory, a large reference laboratory, for example, for testing. Tests infrequently performed, or those needing specialized technology, are sometimes more cost-effective if done in a central laboratory setting where these special tests are performed.

Since biological specimens are potentially infectious, care must be taken to ship them safely following the requirements established by the receiving laboratory. Leakproof and crushproof primary containers and mailing containers should be used (Fig 2–15).

All specimen containers to be shipped must be labeled with the necessary patient identification information and the mailing package must include the properly completed request form for the tests to be done.

BIBLIOGRAPHY

Ancillary (Bedside) Blood Glucose Testing in Acute and Chronic Care Facilities, Proposed Guidelines. Villanova, Pa, National Committee for Clinical Laboratory Standards, 1989; 9(Aug):C30-P.

Henry JB (ed.): *Clinical Diagnosis and Management by Laboratory Methods,* ed 18. Philadelphia, WB Saunders Co, 1991.

Physician's Office Laboratory Guidelines, Tentative Guidelines. Villanova, Pa, National Committee for Clinical Laboratory Standards, Vol 9. 1989. POL1-T.

Procedures for the Collection of Diagnostic Blood Specimens by Skin Puncture, Approved Standard, ed 3 Villanova, Pa, National Committee for Clinical Laboratory Standards, 1991; 11(July), H4–A3.

Procedures for the Collection of Diagnostic Blood Specimens by Venipuncture, Approved Standard, ed 3. Villanova, PA, National Committee for Clinical Laboratory Standards, 1991; 11(July), H3–A3.

Protection of Laboratory Workers From Infectious Disease Transmitted by Blood, Body Fluids and Tissue, Tentative Guidelines. Villanova, Pa, National Committee for Clinical Laboratory Standards, 1989; 9(January) M29-T.

Slockbower JM, Blumenfeld TA: *Collection and Handling of Laboratory Specimens.* Philadelphia, JB Lippincott Co, 1983.

Tietz NW (ed): *Fundamentals of Clinical Chemistry,* ed 3. Philadelphia, WB Saunders Co, 1987.

Tietz NW (ed.): *Textbook of Clinical Chemistry.* Philadelphia, WB Saunders Co, 1986.

3   Use of the Microscope

Description
Parts of the Microscope
General Description, Brightfield Microscope
  Illumination System
    Light source
    Condenser
    Iris Diaphragm
  Magnification System
    Low-Power Objective
    High-Power Objective
    Oil-Immersion Objective
  Adjusting System

Care and Cleaning
Use of the Microscope
  Alignment
  Light Adjustment
  Focusing
Other Types of Microscopes (Illumination Systems)
  Darkfield Microscope
  Fluorescence Microscope
  Polarizing Microscope
  Phase-Contrast Microscope
  Interference Contrast Microscope

Key Terms	
Alignment	Low-power objective
Birefringence	Numerical aperture (NA)
Brightfield microscope	Objectives
Condenser	Oil-immersion objective
Compensated polarized light	Phase-contrast microscope
Eyepiece (ocular)	Polarizing microscope
High-power objective	Resolution
Iris diaphragm	Rheostat

The microscope is probably the piece of equipment that receives the most use (and, unfortunately, misuse) in the clinical laboratory. Microscopy is a basic part of the work in many areas of the laboratory—hematology, urinalysis, microbiology, to name a few. Because the microscope is such an important piece of equipment and is a precision instrument, it must be kept in excellent condition, optically and mechanically. It must be kept clean, and it must be kept aligned.

DESCRIPTION

In simple terms, a microscope is a magnifying glass. The compound light, or **brightfield, microscope** (the type used in most clinical laboratories) consists of two magnifying lenses, the objective and the **eyepiece (ocular).** It is used to magnify an object to a point where it can be seen with the human eye. Here we must introduce the term **resolution,** which is basic in microscopy. Resolution tells how small and how close individual ob-

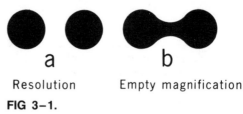

a — Resolution   b — Empty magnification

FIG 3–1.
Resolution vs. empty magnification.

jects (dots) can be and still be recognizable. Practically, the resolving power is the limit of usable magnification. Further magnification of two dots that are no longer resolvable would be "empty magnification" and would result in a dumbbell appearance, as shown in Figure 3–1.

In general terms, the human eye can separate (or resolve) dots that are 0.25 mm (0.25×10^{-3} m or 0.00025 m) apart; the light microscope can separate dots that are 0.25 μm (0.25×10^{-6} m or 0.00000025 m) apart; and the electron microscope can separate dots that are 0.5 nm (0.5×10^{-9} m or 0.0000000005 m) apart.

As mentioned above, the compound light microscope consists of two magnifying lenses, the objective

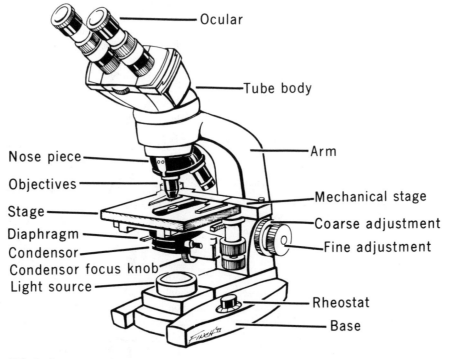

Ocular

Tube body

Nose piece

Objectives

Stage

Diaphragm

Condensor

Condensor focus knob

Light source

Arm

Mechanical stage

Coarse adjustment

Fine adjustment

Rheostat

Base

FIG 3–2.
Parts of the binocular microscope.

and the eyepiece or ocular. The total magnification observed is the product of the magnifications of these two lenses. In other words, the magnification of the objective times the magnification of the ocular equals the total magnification. The magnitude of magnification is inscribed on each lens as a number. These magnification units are in terms of diameters; thus, $\times 10$ means that the diameter of an object is magnified to ten times its original size. (The object itself or its area is not magnified ten times—only the diameter of the object is magnified.)

Because of the manner in which light travels through the compound microscope, the image that is seen is upside down and reversed. The right side appears as the left, the top as the bottom, and vice versa. This should be kept in mind when moving the slide (or object) being observed.

Another term encountered in microscopy is **numerical aperture (NA).** The NA of a lens can be thought of as an index or measurement of the resolving power. As the numerical aperture increases, the resolution (or distance from each other at which objects can be distinguished) decreases. The numerical aperture can also be thought of as an index of the light-gathering power of a lens—a means of describing the amount of light entering the objective. Any particular lens has a constant numerical aperture, and this value is dependent on the radius of the lens and its focal length (the distance from the object being viewed to the lens or the objective). The numerical aperture is also inscribed on each objective lens. It follows that decreasing the amount of light passing through a lens will decrease the numerical aperture. The importance of this value will become apparent when we discuss proper light adjustments with the microscope.

The structures basic to all types of compound microscopes fall in four main categories: (1) the framework, (2) the illumination system, (3) the magnification system, and (4) the adjustment system (Fig 3–2).

PARTS OF THE MICROSCOPE

The framework of the microscope consists of several units. The *base* is a firm, horseshoe-shaped foot on which the microscope rests. The *arm* is the structure that supports the magnifying and adjusting systems. It is also the handle by which the microscope can be carried without damaging the delicate parts. The *stage* is the horizontal platform, or shelf, on which the object being observed is placed. Most microscopes have a *mechanical stage,* which makes it much easier to manipulate the object being observed.

Good microscope work cannot be accomplished without proper illumination. The illumination system is therefore an important part of the compound light microscope. Actually, there are six different illumination techniques or systems that are useful in the clinical laboratory: (1) brightfield, (2) darkfield, (3) fluorescence (using transmitted light), (4) polarizing, (5) phase-contrast, and (6) interference contrast.

GENERAL DESCRIPTION, BRIGHTFIELD MICROSCOPE

The brightfield illumination system is the microscope most commonly employed in the clinical laboratory.

Illumination System

Light Source

The illumination system begins with a *source of light.* The microscope most often has a built-in light source (or bulb). This illumination system also has a control to regulate the light intensity, ensuring both adequate illumination and comfort for the microscopist. The light source is located at the base of the microscope, and the light is directed up through the condenser system. It is important that the bulb be positioned correctly for proper alignment of the microscope. (Proper alignment means that the light path from the source of light throughout the microscope and the ocular is physically correct.) Modern microscopes are designed so that the light bulb filament will be centered if the bulb is installed properly. Many styles or types of bulbs are available, and it is important that the bulb designed for a particular microscope be used.

Some microscopes have an external rather than a built-in illumination system. These tend to be older, less commonly used microscopes. A mirror is part of the illumination system when a microscope has an external light source. It is located at the base of the microscope, approximately where the light bulb is in microscopes with built-in light sources. The mirror reflects the beam of light directed at it upward. It has two sides, one flat and the other concave. The concave side should be used for clinical microscopy work. To be certain that the mirror is at the correct angle, an ocular is removed and the light is centered while looking through the body tube.

Condenser

Another part of the illumination system is the **condenser.** Microscopes generally use a substage Abbé-type condenser. The condenser directs and focuses the beam of light from the bulb or mirror onto the material under examination. The Abbé condenser is a conical lens system (actually consisting of two lenses) with the point planed off. The condenser position is adjustable; it can be raised and lowered beneath the stage by means of an adjustment knob. It must be correctly positioned to correctly focus the light on the material being viewed. When it is correctly positioned, the image field is evenly lighted. The condenser must be positioned because, being a lens, it has a fixed NA. When the microscope is properly used, the NA of the condenser should be equal to or slightly less than the NA of the objective being used. The NA of the condenser can be varied by changing its position; thus the condenser position must be adjusted with each objective used in order to maximize the light focus and the resolving power of the microscope. When the NA of the condenser is decreased below that of the objective, contrast is gained and resolution is lost. This manipulation is often necessary in the clinical laboratory when observing wet, unstained preparations such as urinary sediment. In this case, when scanning a specimen, in order to gain contrast, the condenser is lowered (or the iris diaphragm closed), thus reducing the NA. Preferably, the condenser should be left in a generally uppermost position, at most only 1 or 2 mm below the specimen, and the light adjusted primarily by opening or closing the condenser iris diaphragm. The old procedure of "racking down" the condenser when looking at wet preparations is not acceptable.

Some microscopes are equipped with a top condenser element, which is used in place for low-power work and swings out for high-power. This changes the NA of the condenser, matching it with that of the objective.

Iris Diaphragm

The third and last unit of the illumination systems to be discussed in this section is the **iris diaphragm.** The iris diaphragm also controls the amount of light passing through the material under observation. It is located at the bottom of the Abbé condenser, under the lenses but

within the condenser body. This diaphragm consists of a series of horizontally arranged interlocking plates with a central aperture. It can be opened or closed as necessary to adjust the intensity of the light by means of a lever. The size of the aperture, and consequently the amount of light permitted to pass, is regulated by the microscopist. Such regulation of the light affects the NA of the condenser; decreasing the size of the field under observation with the iris diaphragm decreases the NA of the condenser. Thus, proper illumination techniques involve a combination of proper light intensity regulation, light source position, condenser position, and field size regulation.

Magnification System

The magnification system contains several important parts. This system, too, plays an extremely important role in the use of the microscope. The *ocular,* or *eyepiece,* is a lens that magnifies the image formed by the objective. The usual magnification of the ocular is 10 ($\times 10$); however, $\times 5$ and $\times 20$ oculars are also generally available. Most microscopes have two oculars and are called *binocular* microscopes. Some microscopes have only one ocular, and these are called *monocular microscopes.* The magnification produced by the ocular, when multiplied by the magnification produced by the objective, gives the total magnification of the object being viewed.

The **objectives** are the major part of the magnification system. There are usually three objectives on each microscope, with magnifying powers of $\times 10$, $\times 40$, and $\times 100$. The objectives are mounted on the *nosepiece,* which is a pivot that enables a quick change of objectives. Objectives are also described or rated according to *focal length,* which is inscribed on the outside of the objective. Microscopes used in the clinical laboratory most commonly have 16-, 4-, and 1.8-mm objectives. The focal length is the distance from the object being examined to the center of the lens. Practically speaking, the focal length of a lens is very close in value to the *working distance*—the distance from the bottom of the objective to the material being studied. The greater the magnifying power of a lens, the smaller the focal length and hence the working distance. This becomes very important when using the microscope, as the working distance is very short for the $\times 40$ (4-mm) and $\times 100$ (1.8-mm) objectives. For this reason, correct focusing habits are necessary to prevent damaging the objectives against the slide on the stage. We have now described the objectives in terms of their focal length and magnifying power. The actual magnifying power will vary with different lenses; however, the actual focal length and magnifying power are inscribed directly on the outside of the objective along with the NA and type of lens.

Other terms that are commonly used to describe microscope objectives are *low power, high power* (also *high dry*), and *oil immersion.*

Low-Power Objective

The **low-power objective** is usually a ×10 magnification 16-mm objective. This objective is used for the initial scanning and observation in most microscope work. For example, blood films and urinary sediment are routinely examined by using the low-power objective first. This is also the lens employed for the initial focusing and light adjustment of the microscope. Some routine microscopes also have a very low power ×4 magnification lens. This is used in the initial scanning in the morphologic examination of histologic sections. Often the term *parfocal* is used in speaking about a microscope. It means that if one objective is in focus and a switch is made to another objective, the focus will not be lost. Thus the microscope can be focused under low power and then switched to the high-power or oil-immersion objective and it will still be in focus except for fine adjustment. The NA of the low-power objective is significantly less than that of the condenser on most microscopes (for the ×10 objective the NA is approximately 0.25; for the condenser it is approximately 0.9). Therefore, to achieve focus, the NAs must be more closely matched by reducing the light to the specimen; this is done by lowering the condenser 1 or 2 mm below the specimen and then reducing the size of the field with the iris diaphragm.

High-Power Objective

The **high-power objective** or high-dry objective is usually a ×40 magnification lens with a 4-mm working distance. This objective is used for more detailed study, as the total magnification with a ×10 eyepiece is ×400 rather than the ×100 magnification of the low-power system. The high-power objective is used to study histologic sections, and to study wet preparations such as urinary sediment in more detail. The working distance of the 4-mm lens is quite short; therefore, care must be taken in focusing. The NA of the high power lens is

fairly close to (although slightly less than) that of most commonly used condensers (for most high-power objectives, NA = 0.85; for the condenser, NA = 0.9). Therefore, the condenser should generally be all the way up and the field slightly closed with the iris diaphragm for maximum focus.

Oil-Immersion Objective

The **oil-immersion objective** is generally a ×100 lens with a 1.8-mm working distance. This is a very short focal length and working distance. In fact, the objective lens almost rests on the microscope slide when in use. An oil-immersion lens requires that a special grade of oil, called *immersion oil,* be placed between the objective and the slide or coverglass. Oil is used to increase the NA and thus the resolving power of the objective. Since the focal length of this lens is so small, there is a problem in getting enough light from the microscope field to the objective. Light travels through air at a greater speed than through glass, and it travels through immersion oil at the same speed as through glass. Thus, to increase the effective NA of the objective, oil is used to slow down the speed at which light travels, increasing the gathering power of the lens.* Since the NA of the oil-immersion objective is greater than that of the condenser in most systems (for the ×100 objective, NA = 1.2; for the condenser, NA = 0.9), the condenser should be used in the uppermost position and the iris diaphragm should generally be open; practically speaking, however, partial closing of the iris may be necessary. The oil-immersion lens, with a total magnification of ×1,000 when used with a ×10 eyepiece, is generally the limit of magnification with the light microscope. The oil-immersion lens is routinely used for morphologic examination of blood films and microbes. The short working distance requires dry films, so wet preparations such as urinary sediment cannot be examined under an oil-immersion lens. The high-power lens is also referred to as a high-dry lens because it does not require the use of immersion oil. Other objectives that might be present on a microscope in the clinical laboratory are a lower-power ×4 scanning lens or a ×50 low oil-immersion lens.

*The speed at which light travels through a substance is measured in terms of the *refractive index.* The refractive index is calculated as the speed at which light travels through air divided by the speed at which it travels through the substance. The refractive index of air is therefore 1.00. The refractive index of glass is 1.515; immersion oil, 1.515; and water, 1.33.

Adjusting System

The *body tube* is the part of the microscope through which the light passes to the ocular. The tube length from the eyepiece to the objective lens is generally 160 mm. This is the tube that actually conducts the image. The adjustment system enables the body tube to move up or down for focusing the objectives. This system usually consists of two adjustments, one coarse and the other fine. The coarse adjustment gives rapid movement over a wide range and is used to obtain an approximate focus. The fine adjustment gives very slow movement over a limited range and is used to obtain exact focus after prior coarse adjustment.

A more detailed description of the optics of a microscope can be found in standard physics textbooks.

CARE AND CLEANING OF THE MICROSCOPE

The microscope is a precision instrument and must be handled with great care. When it is necessary to transport the microscope, it should always be carried with both hands; it should be carried by the arm and supported under the base with the other hand. When not in use, the microscope should be covered and put away in a microscope case, or in a desk or cupboard. It should be left with the low power ($\times10$) objective in place, and the body tube barrel adjusted to the lowest possible position.

The surface of most microscopes is finished with a black or gray enamel and metal plating that is resistant to most laboratory chemicals. It may be kept clean by washing with a neutral soap and water. To clean the metal and enamel, a gauze or soft cloth should be moistened with the cleaning agent and rubbed over the surface with a circular motion. The surface should be dried immediately with a clean, dry piece of gauze or cloth. Gauze should *never* be used to clean any of the optical parts of the microscope.

The glass surfaces of the ocular, the objectives, and the condenser are hand-ground optical lenses. These lenses must be kept meticulously clean. Optical glass is softer than ordinary glass and should never be cleaned with paper tissue or gauze. These materials will scratch the lens. To clean the lenses of the microscope, use lens paper. Before polishing with lens paper, care must be

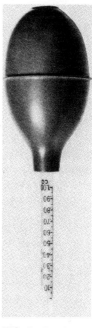

FIG 3–3.
Air syringe.

taken that nothing is present that will scratch the optical glass in the polishing process. Such potentially abrasive dirt, dust, or lint can easily be blown away before polishing. Cans of compressed air are commercially available, or an air syringe can be made simply by fitting a plastic eyedropper or a 1-mL plastic tuberculin syringe with the tip cut off into a rubber bulb of the type used for pipetting (Fig 3–3). This air syringe is used to blow away dust or lint that might otherwise scratch the optical glass in the polishing process.

Oil must be removed from the oil-immersion ($\times100$) objective immediately after use by wiping with clean lens paper. If not removed, oil may seep inside the lens, or dry on the outside surface of the objective. The high-dry ($\times40$) objective should never be used with oil; however, if this or any other objective comes into contact with oil it should be cleaned immediately. If a lens is especially dirty, it may be cleaned with a small amount of xylene or commercial lens cleaner applied to the lens paper. Xylene should be used sparingly, because it can damage the lens mounting if it is allowed to get beyond the front seal. Commercial lens cleaner has the advantage of being less harmful to the mounting medium. To properly clean the oil-immersion lens, first lower the stage, then rotate the objective to the front and wipe gently with clean lens paper. Then clean off the immersion oil with lens paper dampened with special lens cleaner or methanol. In certain cases a small amount of xylene may be used. Alternatively the cleaning agent may be applied to a wooden applicator stick wrapped with cotton or lens paper and moistened with the cleaning agent. *Do not use a plastic applicator stick,* as it will be dissolved by the solvent, ruining the objective. Apply the cleaning agent by blotting and in a circular motion, beginning at the center and moving outward. Repeat with new dampened lens paper as necessary. Finally, blot dry with clean lens paper. Do not rub, as this may scratch the surface of the lens.

Lenses should never be touched with the fingers. Objectives must not be taken apart as even a slight alteration of the lens setting may ruin the objective. Merely clean the outer surface of the lens as described. An especially dirty objective may be removed (unscrewed) from the nosepiece, then held upside down and checked for cleanliness by using the ocular (removed from the body tube) as a magnifying glass. Dust or lint can also be removed from the rear lens of the objective by blowing it away with an air syringe. Such removal of the objective from the nosepiece is *not* a routine cleaning procedure. The final step when using the microscope should always be to wipe off all objectives with clean lens paper.

The ocular or eyepiece is especially vulnerable to dirt because of its location on the microscope and contact with the observer's eye. Mascara presents a constant cleaning problem. Dust can be removed from the lens of the ocular with an air syringe (or camel's hair brush). Air is probably easier to use and more efficient. The lens should then be polished with lens paper. At regular intervals the ocular can be taken apart and cleaned on the inside, by first blowing away dust and lint and then polishing. The ocular can be checked for additional dirt by holding it up to a light and looking through it. When one is looking into the microscope, dirt on any part of the ocular will rotate with the ocular when it is turned. The ocular should not be removed for more than a few minutes, as dust can collect in the body tube and settle on the rear lens of an objective.

The light source (or mirror) and condenser should also be free of dust, lint, and dirt. First blow away the dust with an air syringe or camel's hair brush, then polish the light source and condenser with lens paper. It may be necessary to clean them further with lens paper

moistened with a commercial lens cleaner or methanol before polishing them with lens paper.

The stage of the microscope should be cleaned after each use by wiping with gauze or a tissue. After it has been cleaned thoroughly, the stage should be wiped dry.

The coarse and fine adjustments occasionally need attention, as does the mechanical stage adjustment mechanism. When there is unusual resistance to any manipulation of these knobs, force must not be used to overcome the resistance. Such force might damage the screw or rack-and-pinion mechanism. Instead, the cause of the problem must be found. A small drop of oil may be needed. It is best to call in a specialist to repair the microscope when a serious problem occurs.

USE OF THE MICROSCOPE

Before using a microscope, two conditions must first be met: (1) the microscope must be clean, and (2) it must be aligned. The cleaning procedure was described above; **alignment** is discussed here.

Alignment

When properly aligned, the microscope is adjusted in such a way that the light path through the microscope, from the light source to the eye of the observer, is correct according to the rules of physics. If a microscope is misaligned, the field of view will seem to swing—a very uncomfortable situation, often described as making the observer feel seasick. This can be corrected by properly aligning or adjusting the light path through the microscope. To check the alignment, with the low-power objective in place and the condenser up, remove the eyepiece and look down the body tube. Now close the iris field diaphragm enough to see a constricted (or partially closed) field. Center this field in the body tube by adjusting the centering screws on the condenser. (This alignment operation may be omitted by the new student; the alignment can be adjusted by the instructor or supervisor.) Many microscopes that are produced for student use are aligned by the manufacturer and realignment requires special knowledge and experience, as the field diaphragm, condenser centering adjustment screws, and removable eyepieces are not present.

If the microscope has a field diaphragm it is utilized

in the alignment procedure. A field diaphragm is an iris diaphragm which is part of the built-in illuminator, and is found just over the light source. Using the low-power objective, close down the field diaphragm to a minimum. Then adjust the condenser height until the image of the field diaphragm is visible sharply in the field of view. Next bring the image of the field diaphragm into the center of the field by means of the centering screws located on the condenser. Now open the field diaphragm until it is just contained within the field of view. At this point, it may be necessary to repeat the centering procedure. Finally, open the diaphragm until the leaves are just out of view.

Looking down the microscope body tube with the eyepiece removed, one can also check for the presence of dust, lint, or dirt, which would be readily observed at this point. Besides centering the condenser, one must center the light source to give the correct light path. In microscopes that have a built-in illumination system, the light bulb filament will be correctly centered if the correct bulb is used and is installed properly. For microscopes with an external light source and mirror, use the concave side of the mirror and adjust the mirror angle and light position by centering the light while looking through the body tube with the ocular removed.

Light Adjustment

With the low-power objective in position, the object to be examined, usually on a glass microscope slide, is placed on the stage and secured. Care must be taken to avoid damaging the objective when placing the specimen on the stage. The slide is then positioned so that the specimen is in the light path.

The biggest concern in learning how to use a microscope for the first time is the lighting and fine adjustment maneuvers. One must be certain that the light source, condenser, and iris diaphragm are in correct adjustment. Light adjustment is made before any focusing is done. The power supply is turned on and the light intensity adjusted to a comfortable level. Light adjustment is further accomplished by raising and lowering the condenser and opening and closing the iris diaphragm. At the start of this initial light adjustment, the consenser should be 1 to 2 mm below the slide and the condenser iris diaphragm all the way open, with the low-power ($\times$10) objective in place. While looking through the ocular, the diaphragm can be closed until the light just begins to be reduced.

Or, if possible, the eyepiece is removed and one-fourth of the light darkened out by closing the iris diaphragm while looking down the body tube. Further closing of the iris diaphragm (or lowering of the condenser), while it may increase contrast and depth of focus, will reduce resolution.

Focusing

Focusing is the next technique to be mastered. If using a binocular microscope, the interpupillary distance between the oculars is adjusted so that the left and right fields merge into one.

With the object to be examined on the stage, and while watching from the side, the low-power ($\times$10) objective is brought down as far as it will go, so that it almost meets the top of the specimen. The coarse adjustment is used for this procedure. The objective must not be in direct contact with the specimen. The observer must watch from the side to avoid damaging the objective. Once the objective is just at the top of the specimen, the object is slowly focused upward, using the coarse adjustment knob and looking through the ocular while this is being done. When the object is nearly in focus, it is brought into clear focus by use of the fine adjustment knob. This procedure is done with the right eye. The ocular diopter is then set to the left eye, so that the object will be in focus with both eyes.

Further light adjustment should now be made to ensure maximum focus and resolution. The light intensity is adjusted with the brightness control (**rheostat**) so that the background light is sufficiently bright (white) but comfortable. Next the iris diaphragm is adjusted by opening completely and then slowly closing until the light intensity just begins to be reduced. Alternatively, the eyepiece may be removed and the iris diaphragm closed until three-fourths of the body tube is filled with light.

When changing to another objective, the barrel distance need not be changed. As stated previously, most microscopes are parfocal. The only adjustment necessary should be made with the fine adjustment knob. It is essential to remember that fine adjustment is used continuously during microscopic examination.

When greater magnification is needed, more light is necessary. It is obtained by repositioning the condenser and iris diaphragm in the manner previously described. In general, the condenser will be raised and the iris diaphragm opened as the objective magnification increases. When the oil immersion lens is used, the condenser should be raised to its maximum position.

Additional light is provided by the use of immersion oil which is placed on the viewing slide when the oil-immersion ($\times 100$) objective is used. The oil directs the light rays to a finer point. When the oil-immersion lens is to be used, the desired area on the slide is first found by using the low-power ($\times 10$) objective. Once this area is located, the objective is pivoted out of position, a drop of immersion oil is placed on the slide, and the oil-immersion lens is pivoted into the oil while observing it from the side. The objective is then moved from side to side to avoid the presence of air bubbles. The noisepiece, rather than the objective itself, should be grasped when changing lenses to prevent damage to the objective. The ocular should not be looked through during this adjustment procedure. When the initial adjustment has been made, the fine adjustment is made while looking through the ocular. The oil remaining on the lens of the objective after the study has been completed must be cleaned off with lens paper as described above.

OTHER TYPES OF MICROSCOPES (ILLUMINATION SYSTEMS)

Until recently, brightfield illumination has, with few exceptions, been the primary type of microscope illumination system used in the routine clinical laboratory. Now other illumination systems are becoming increasingly popular as refinements in microscope design have made them more reliable and easier to use in a clinical situation. These other types of illumination systems— darkfield, transmitted light fluorescence, polarizing, phase-contrast, and interference contrast—will now be briefly described. The basic principles of microscopy and rules for usage apply with all of these variations; the primary difference is the character of light delivered to the specimen and illuminating the microscope.

Darkfield Microscope

First we consider *darkfield* illumination. In this system, a special substage condenser is used that causes light waves to cross *on* the specimen rather than pass in parallel waves through the specimen. Thus, when one looks through the microscope, the field in view will be black, or dark, as no light passes from the condenser to the objective. However, when an object is present on the stage, light will be deflected as it hits the object and will pass through the objective and be seen by the viewer. As a result, the object under study appears light against a dark background. Any compound microscope may be converted to a darkfield microscope by use of a special darkfield condenser in place of the usual condenser. The darkfield microscope has long been used in the routine clinical laboratory to observe spirochetes in the exudates from leptospiral or syphilitic infections. A more recent use, facilitated by newer microscope design technology, is as a low-power scanner for urinary sediment.

Fluorescence Microscope

The transmitted light *fluorescence* microscope is a further refinement of the darkfield microscope. It is basically a darkfield microscope with wavelength selection. Certain objects have the ability to fluoresce. This means that they absorb light of certain very short (ultraviolet) wavelengths and emit light of longer (visible) wavelengths. In fluorescence microscopy with transmitted light and a compound microscope, the darkfield condenser is preceded by a special *exciter filter,* which allows only shorter-wavelength blue light to pass and cross on the specimen plane. If the specimen contains an object that fluoresces (either naturally or because of staining or labeling with certain fluorescent dyes) it will absorb the blue light and emit light of a longer yellow or green wavelength. A special barrier filter is placed in the microscope tube or eyepiece. This barrier filter will pass only the desired wavelength of emitted light for the particular fluorescent system. Thus, the fluorescence technique shows only the presence or absence of the fluorescing object. The barrier filter used must be carefully chosen so that only light of the desired wavelength will be passed through the microscope to the observer. Other objects in the specimen that do not fluoresce will not emit light of that wavelength and will not be seen. Fluorescence techniques, in particular fluorescent antibody (FA) techniques, are especially useful in the clinical laboratory. They are used particularly in the clinical microbiology laboratory and for various immunologic studies. Different fluorescent antibody techniques may be used in the primary identification of microorganisms, or in the final identification of bacteria (such as group A streptococci), replacing older serologic methods. Such techniques have the advantage of saving time, which results in earlier diagnosis for the patient, and they are often more sensitive than other techniques. They may also be useful in the identification of organisms that cannot be cultured, such as *Treponema pallidum.*

Polarizing Microscope

Another increasingly popular illumination system is represented by the **polarizing microscope.** A polarizer (or polarizing filter) may be thought of as a sieve that takes ordinary light waves, which vibrate in all orientations (or directions), and allows only light waves of one orientation (say north-south or east-west) to pass through the filter. In a polarizing microscope, a polarizing filter is placed between the light source (bulb) and the specimen. A second *analyzer* (or polarizer) is placed above the specimen, between the objective and the eyepiece (either at some point in the microscope tube or in the eyepiece). One of the polarizers is then rotated until the two are at right angles to each other. This will be seen as the extinction of light through the microscope (one sees a dark field) since both north-south and east-west light waves are cancelled when they are at right angles to each other. However, certain objects have a property termed **birefringence,** which means that they rotate (or polarize) light. An object that polarizes, bends light, and can be seen in such a system. Objects that do not bend light will not be observed in the microscope. An object that polarizes light (or is birefringent) will appear light against a dark background. The polarizing microscope is useful clinically in the study of synovial fluid and urinary sediment, and in some histologic work. This technique is commonly used in geology for particle analysis, and clinically in forensic medicine. With the polarizing microscope the optical properties of an object can be determined.

A further modification of the polarizing microscope involves the addition of a first-order red plate (filter) or full-wave retardation plate placed between the two polarizing filters. With this addition the field background appears red or magenta, while the object that polarizes appears yellow or blue in relation to its orientation to the red filter and its optical properties. This is especially useful clinically for differentiating between sodium acid urate and calcium pyrophosphate dihydrate in synovial fluid. It is also becoming useful in the routine study of urinary sediment.

Phase-Contrast Microscope

Another extremely useful illumination system is the **phase-contrast microscope.** A disadvantage of brightfield illumination is that it is necessary to stain (or dye) many objects to give sufficient contrast and detail. Phase-contrast facilitates the study of unstained structures, which can even be alive, since wet preparations of cells or organisms can be observed without prior dehydration and staining. As the name of the technique implies, the structures observed with this system show added contrast compared with the brightfield microscope. The phase-contrast microscope is basically a brightfield microscope with changes in the objective and the condenser. An annular diaphragm, which is a black ring with a black center, is put into (or below) the condenser. This results in a hollow cone or "doughnut" of light passing through the specimen. A corresponding absorption ring is fitted into the objective. Each phase objective must have a corresponding absorption ring. In microscopes with multiple phase objectives, the annular diaphragms are usually placed in a rotating condenser arrangement. Use of each phase objective requires an adjustment of the condenser to "match" the annular diaphragm and phase ring. The phase microscope may also be used as a brightfield microscope by setting the condenser annulus to the brightfield position. However, since the phase objective blocks out a ring of light, the resolution or detail that can be achieved when using phase objectives for brightfield examination is compromised. For more exact work, an additional brightfield objective should be employed in the microscope.

The annulus and absorption ring must be perfectly aligned or adjusted so that they are concentric and superimposed. Therefore, a problem with the phase-contrast microscope is the necessity for perfect alignment. The net effect is to slow down the speed of light by one-fourth of a wavelength. This diminution of the speed of light makes the system very sensitive to differences in refractive index.

Objects with differences in refractive index, shape, and absorption characteristics show added differences in the intensity and shade of light passing through them. The end result is that one can observe unstained wet preparations with good resolution and detail. In the clinical laboratory, phase contrast is especially useful for counting platelets by using a direct method, and for observing structures in wet preparations of urinary sediment and vaginal smears. Owing to its superior visualization and ease of operation, the phase-contrast microscope has become a common tool in routine urinalysis.

Interference Contrast Microscope

The last illumination technique gaining in clinical use is *interference contrast* illumination. This technique gives the viewer a three-dimensional image of the object under study. Like phase contrast, it is especially useful for wet preparations such as urinary sediment, showing finer details without the need for special staining techniques. The brightfield microscope is modified by the addition of a special beam-splitting (Wollaston) prism to the condenser. The two split beams are then polarized; one passes through the specimen, which alters the amplitude (or height) of the light wave, and the other (which serves as a reference) does not pass through the specimen. The two dissimilar light beams then pass separately through the objective and are recombined by a second Wollaston (beam-combining) prism. This recombination of light waves gives the three-dimensional image to the additive or subtractive effects of the light waves as they are combined.

BIBLIOGRAPHY

Brown BA: *Hematology: Principles and Procedures,* ed 5. Philadelphia, Lea & Febiger, 1988.

Freeman JA, Beeler MF: *Laboratory Medicine/ Urinalysis and Medical Microscopy,* ed 2. Philadelphia, Lea & Febiger, 1983.

Physician's Office Laboratory Procedure Manual, Tentative Guidelines, Villanova, Pa, National Committee for Clinical Laboratory Standards, 1989; 9:POL2-T.

4 Laboratory Measurements: Apparatus and Principles

Key Terms

Analytical balance	Metric system
Automatic pipettes	National Bureau of Standards
Buret	Quantitative transfer
Calibration	Relative centrifugal force (RCF)
Capillary pipette	Standard solution
Centrifugation	Titration
Deionized water	To-contain pipettes
Distilled water	To-deliver pipettes
Grades of chemicals	Tolerance
Graduated pipette	Torsion balance
Gravimetric analysis	Triple-beam balance
International System of Units (SI units)	Volumetric glassware
Material Safety Data Sheet (MSDS)	Volumetric pipette
Measurement of mass	

INTRODUCTION TO LABORATORY MEASUREMENTS: APPARATUS AND PRINCIPLES

If the results of laboratory analyses are to be useful to the physician in diagnosing and treating patients, the tests must be performed as accurately as possible. Many factors constitute the final laboratory result for a single determination. The use of high-quality analytic methods and instrumentation is of prime importance, but other basic principles and procedures also play a role.

In order to unify physical measurements worldwide, the **International System of Units (SI units)** has been adopted. Many of these units also relate to the metric system. A coherent system of measurement units is vital to precise clinical laboratory analyses. The pertinent SI units of measurement are discussed in this chapter.

A general discussion of laboratory glassware and plasticware, including types used for measuring volume, is included. The importance of knowing the correct usage of these various pieces of glassware must be thoroughly appreciated. The four basic pieces of volumetric glassware—volumetric flasks, graduated measuring cylinders, burets, and pipettes—are specialized, each having its own particular use in the laboratory.

The accuracy of laboratory analyses depends to a great extent on the accuracy of the reagents used. Traditional preparation of reagents makes use of balances and volumetric measuring devices such as pipettes and volumetric flasks—examples of fundamental laboratory apparatus. When reagents and standard solutions are being prepared, it is imperative that only the purest water supply be used in the procedure. For this reason, the various types of water are discussed. Discussion about the careful preparation of reagents and standards, along with the necessary knowledge about the chemicals used for these preparations, is basic to any analytic procedure in the clinical laboratory and is included.

Many and varied pieces of laboratory apparatus are used in performing clinical determinations, and knowledge of the proper use and handling of this equipment is an important part of any laboratory work. Measurements of mass, using balances, and measurement of volume, using pipettes and burets, are important basic analytic tools used in the clinical laboratory. Centrifuges are also used in various ways in the laboratory. The use of photometry, and spectrophotometers in particular, is covered in Chapter 5. Autoclaves and incubators are discussed in Chapter 16.

Units of Measurement

SYSTEMS OF MEASUREMENT

The ability to measure accurately is the keystone of the scientific method and anyone engaged in performing clinical laboratory analyses must have a working knowledge of measurement systems and units of measurement. It is also necessary to understand how to convert units measured in one system to units expressed in another system. Systems of measurement included are the English, metric, and SI systems, with emphasis on the last-named.

Metric System

Traditionally, units of measurement in the clinical laboratory have been made in metric units. The **metric system** is based on a decimal system of divisions and multiples of tens. It has not been widely used in the United States, except in the scientific community. The meter (m) is the metric standard unit for measurement of length, the gram (g) is the unit of mass, and the liter (L) is the unit of volume. Multiples or divisions of these reference units constitute the various other metric units.

International System

Another system of measurement, the International System of Units (from le Système International d'Unités, or SI) has been adopted by the worldwide scientific community as a coherent, standardized system based on seven base units. There are also derived units and supplemental units, in addition to the base units, which make up the SI system. The SI base units describe each of seven fundamental, but independent, physical quantities. The derived units are calculated mathematically from two or more base units.

The SI system was established in 1960 by international agreement and is now the standard international language of measurement. The International Bureau of Weights and Measures is responsible for maintaining the standards on which the SI system of measurement is based.

The term *metric system* generally refers to the SI system and, for informational purposes, metric terms that remain in common usage are described where needed.

Since the English system is common in everyday use, English system equivalents are also given in the discussion of units.

The National Committee for Clinical Laboratory Standards (NCCLS) recommends that an extensive educational effort be put forth to implement the SI system in clinical laboratories in the United States. Any changes in units used to report laboratory findings should be done with great care, to avoid misunderstanding and confusion in interpretation of laboratory results.

Base Units for the SI System

In the SI system the base units of measurement are the metre (meter), kilogram, second, mole, ampere, kelvin, and candela. These seven base units of the SI system and accepted symbols are listed in Table 4–1.

All units in the SI system can be qualified by standard prefixes that serve to convert values to more convenient forms, depending on the size of the object being measured. These prefixes are listed in Table 4–2.

Various rules should be kept in mind when combining these prefixes with their basic units and using the SI system; some of these rules follow. An *s* should not be added to form the plural of the abbreviation for a unit or for a prefix with a unit. For example, 25 millimeters should be abbreviated as 25 mm, not 25 mms. Do not use periods after abbreviations (use mm, not mm.). Do not use compound prefixes; instead, use the closest accepted prefix. For example, 24×10^{-9} gram (g) should be expressed as 24 nanograms (24 ng) rather than 24 millimicrograms (25 mμg). In the SI system, commas are not used as spacers in recording large numbers since they

TABLE 4–1.

Base Units of the SI System

Measurement	Unit Name	Symbol
Length	Metre*	m
Mass	Kilogram	kg
Time	Second	s
Amount of substance	Mole	mol
Electric current	Ampere	A
Temperature	Kelvin†	K
Luminous intensity	Candela	cd

*The spelling *meter* is more commonly used in the United States and is used in this book.
†Although the basic unit of temperature is the kelvin, the degree Celsius is regarded as an acceptable unit, since kelvins may be impractical in many instances. Celsius is more commonly used in the clinical laboratory.

TABLE 4–2.

Prefixes of the SI System

Prefix Name	Symbol	Factor	Decimal
Tera	T	10^{12}	1 000 000 000 000
Giga	G	10^{9}	1 000 000 000
Mega	M	10^{6}	1 000 000
Kilo	k	10^{3}	1 000
Hecto	h	10^{2}	100
Deka	da	10^{1}	10
Deci	d	10^{-1}	0.1
Centi	c	10^{-2}	0.01
Milli	m	10^{-3}	0.001
Micro	μ	10^{-6}	0.000 001
Nano	n	10^{-9}	0.000 000 001
Pico	p	10^{-12}	0.000 000 000 001
Femto	f	10^{-15}	0.000 000 000 000 001
Atto	a	10^{-18}	0.000 000 000 000 000 001

are used in place of decimal points in some countries. Instead, groups of three digits are separated by spaces. When recording temperature on the Kelvin scale, omit the degree sign. Therefore, 295 kelvins should be recorded as 295 K, not 295° K. However, the symbol for degree Celsius is ° C, and 22 degrees Celsius should be recorded as 22° C. Multiples and submultiples should be used in steps of 10^{3} or 10^{-3}. Only one solidus or slash (/) is used when indicating *per* or a denominator: thus meters per second squared (m/s^2), not meters per second per second (m/s/s), or millimoles per liter-hour (mmol/L · hour), not millimoles per liter per hour (mmol/L/hour). Finally, although the preferred SI spellings are *metre* and *litre*, the spellings *meter* and *liter* remain in common usage in the United States and are used in this book.

The base units of measurement that are used most often in the clinical laboratory are length, mass, and volume.

Length.—The standard unit for the measurement of length or distance is the meter (m). The meter is standardized as 1,650,763.73 wavelengths of a certain orange light in the spectrum of krypton 86. One meter equals 39.37 inches (in.), slightly more than a yard in the English system. There are 2.54 centimeters (cm) in 1 in.

Further common divisions and multiples of the meter, using the system of prefixes previously discussed, follow. One-tenth of a meter is a decimeter (dm), one-hundredth of a meter is a centimeter (cm), and one-thousandth of a meter is a millimeter (mm). One thousand meters equals 1 kilometer (km). The following examples show equivalent measurements of length:

$$25 \text{ mm} = 0.025 \text{ m}$$

$$10 \text{ cm} = 100 \text{ mm}$$

$$1 \text{ m} = 100 \text{ cm}$$

$$0.1 \text{ m} = 100 \text{ mm}$$

Other units of length that were in common usage in the metric system but are no longer recommended in the SI system are the angstrom and the micron. The angstrom (Å) is equal to 10^{-10} m or 10^{-1} nanometer (nm). This unit is permitted but not encouraged. The micron (μ), which is equal to 10^{-6} m, is replaced by the micrometer (μm).

Mass (and Weight).—Mass denotes the quantity of matter, while weight takes into account the force of gravity and should not be used in the same sense as mass. However, they are commonly used interchangeably and may be so used in this book. The standard unit for the **measurement of mass** in the SI system is the kilogram (kg). This is the basis for all other mass measurements in the system. The standard kilogram is determined by the mass of a block of platinum-iridium kept at the International Bureau of Weights and Measures. One kilogram weighs approximately 2.2 pounds (lb) in the English system. Conversely, 1 lb equals approximately 0.5 kg.

The kilogram is further divided into thousandths, called grams (g). One thousand grams equals 1 kg. The gram is used much more often than the kilogram in the clinical laboratory. The gram is divided into thousandths, called milligrams (mg). Grams and milligrams are units commonly used in weighing substances in the clinical laboratory. One-millionth of a gram, a microgram (μg), may also be encountered. Some examples of weight measurement equivalents follow:

$$10 \text{ mg} = 0.01 \text{ g}$$

$$0.055 \text{ g} = 55 \text{ mg}$$

$$25 \text{ g} = 25{,}000 \text{ mg}$$

$$1.5 \text{ kg} = 1{,}500 \text{ g}$$

Units that were once used to describe mass and that may still be encountered are the gamma and parts per million. The term *gamma* (γ) should not be used; instead, use microgram (μg). The term *parts per million* (ppm) should be replaced by micrograms per gram (μg/g).

Volume.—In the clinical laboratory the standard unit of volume is the liter (L). You may have noticed that it was not included in the list of base units of the SI system. The liter is a derived unit. The standard unit of volume in the SI system is the cubic meter (m^3). However, this unit is quite large and the cubic decimeter (dm^3) is a more convenient size for use in the clinical laboratory. Thus in 1964 the Conférence Générale des Poids et Mésures (CGPM) accepted the litre (liter) as a special name for the cubic decimeter. Previously, the standard liter was the volume occupied by 1 kg of pure water at 4° C (the temperature at which a volume of water weighs the most) and at normal atmospheric pressure. On this basis, 1 L equals 1,000.027 cubic centimeters (cm^3), and the units milliliters and cubic centimeters were used interchangeably, although there is a slight difference between them. One liter is slightly more than 1 qt in the English system (1 L = 1.06 qt).

The liter is further divided into thousandths, called milliliters (mL); millionths, called microliters (μL); and billionths, called nanoliters (nL). Some examples of volume equivalents are:

$$500 \text{ mL} = 0.5 \text{ L}$$

$$0.25 \text{ L} = 250 \text{ mL}$$

$$2 \text{ L} = 2{,}000 \text{ mL}$$

Since the liter is derived from the meter (1 L = 1 dm^3), it follows that 1 cm^3 is equal to 1 mL and that 1 millimeter cubed (mm^3) is equal to 1 μL. The former abbreviation for cubic centimeter (cc) is replaced by cm^3. Although this is a common means of expressing volume in the clinical laboratory, milliliter (mL) is preferred.

Amount of Substance.—The standard unit of measurement for the amount of a (chemical) substance in the SI system is the mole (mol). The mole is defined as the quantity of a chemical equal to that present in 0.0120 kg of pure carbon 12. A mole of a chemical substance is the *relative atomic* or *molecular mass unit* of that substance. Formerly, the terms *atomic* and *molecular weight* were used to describe the mole. These are further defined and discussed below.

Temperature.—Three scales are commonly used to measure temperature, namely, the Kelvin, Celsius, and Fahrenheit scales. The Celsius scale is sometimes referred to as the centigrade scale, which is an outdated term.

The basic unit of temperature in the SI system is the kelvin (K). However, as mentioned previously, the degree Celsius is regarded as an acceptable unit, since the kelvin may be impractical in many instances. The Celsius scale is the one used most often in the clinical laboratory. The Kelvin and Celsius scales are closely related, and conversion between them is simple since the units (degrees) are equal in magnitude. The difference between the Kelvin and Celsius scales is the zero point. The zero point on the Kelvin scale is the theoretical temperature of no further heat loss, which is absolute zero. The zero point on the Celsius scale is the freezing point of pure water. Remember, however, that the magnitude of the degree is equal on both scales. Therefore, since water freezes at 273 kelvins (273 K), it follows that 0 degrees Celsius (0° C) equals 273 kelvins (273 K) and that 0 kelvin (0 K) equals minus 273 degrees Celsius (−273° C). Thus, to convert from kelvins to degrees Celsius, add 273; to convert from degrees Celsius to kelvins, subtract 273.

$$K = {}^\circ C + 273$$

$$^\circ C = K - 273$$

Since the Celsius scale was devised so that 100° C is the boiling point of pure water, the boiling point on the Kelvin scale is 373 K.

Converting from Celsius to Fahrenheit is not as simple, since the degree is not equal in magnitude on these two scales. The Fahrenheit scale was originally devised with the zero point at the lowest temperature attainable from a mixture of table salt and ice, while the body temperature of a small animal was used to set 100° F. Thus, on the Fahrenheit scale the freezing point of pure water is 32°, while the temperature at which pure water boils is 212°. It is rare that readings on one of these scales must be converted to the other, as almost without exception readings taken and used in the clinical laboratory will be on the Celsius scale.

Examples of comparative readings of the three scales with common reference points are given in Table 4–3.

It is possible, however, to convert from one scale to the other. The basic conversion formulas are:

1. $$1^\circ \text{C} = \frac{9}{5}{}^\circ \text{F}$$

   $$1^\circ \text{F} = \frac{5}{9}{}^\circ \text{C}$$

2. To convert Fahrenheit to Celsius:
   Method A: Add 40, multiply by $\frac{5}{9}$, and subtract 40 from the result.
   Method B: $^\circ \text{C} = \frac{5}{9}(^\circ \text{F} - 32)$.
3. To convert Celsius to Fahrenheit:
   Method A: Add 40, multiply by $\frac{9}{5}$, and subtract 40 from the result.
   Method B: $^\circ \text{F} = \frac{9}{5}{}^\circ \text{C} + 32$.

Non-SI Units

There are several non-SI units which are relevant to clinical laboratory analyses. One of these is time, expressed in minutes (min), hours (hr), or days. These units have such historical use in everyday life that it is unlikely that new SI units derived from the second (the base unit in the SI system for time) will be implemented.

TABLE 4–3.

Common Reference Points on the Three Temperature Scales

	Kelvin	Degrees Celsius	Degrees Fahrenheit
Boiling point of water	373	100	212
Body temperature	310	37	98.6
Room temperature	293	20	68
Freezing point of water	273	0	32
Absolute zero (coldest possible temperature)	0	−273	−459.4

Another non-SI unit is volume expressed as liters (L). This has already been discussed under the base SI units of volume. Pressure is expressed as millimeters of mercury (mmHg) and enzyme activity as the International Unit (U) (defined as the amount of enzyme that will catalyze the transformation of 1 mol/sec of substrate in an assay system).

Reporting Results in SI Units

It is important to always report laboratory results with both the numbers and the units by which the result is measured in order to give a meaningful result. The unit expresses or defines the dimension of the measured substance—concentration, mass, or volume—and it is an important part of any laboratory result.

As SI units are adopted in the clinical laboratory, certain previously reported units will change. Whenever the molecular weight of the measured analyte is known, its concentration is to be expressed in moles per liter (mol/L) or a subunit, rather than in mass per liter. If the molecular weight is not known, as in specific proteins, mixtures of proteins, or other complex molecules, the concentration should be expressed in mass per liter.

Conversion to the molar (mol/L) unit from a mass concentration unit (g/dL) first involves multiplication by 10 for volume conversion and then division by the molecular weight of the substance. If any conversion is made, no greater precision should be given than was present in the original measurement.

Laboratory Glassware and Plasticware

The general laboratory supplies, or laboratory ware, described are those used for storage, measurement, and containment for the necessary reactions or analyses needed. Laboratory glassware and plasticware, as well as automatic pipetting and diluting devices are included.

Most laboratory glassware and other laboratory ware can be divided into two main categories according to the use to which they are put: *containers* and *receivers* and *volumetric measurement*. Examples of containers and receivers are beakers, test tubes, Erlenmeyer flasks, and reagent bottles. Examples of volumetric ware are pipettes, automatic and manual; volumetric flasks; graduated cylinders; and burets.

GLASSWARE

Clinical laboratories still use glassware for the greater part of the analytic work done, even with the advent of plasticware. Glassware is used in all departments of the laboratory, and special types of glass apparatus have been devised for special uses. These special types of glassware are discussed where applicable. The chemistry department probably has the greatest variety and amount of glassware. Certain types of glass can be attacked by reagents to such an extent that the determinations done in them are not valid. It is therefore important to use the correct type of glass for the determinations being done.

Types of Glass

Clinical laboratory glassware can be divided into several types: glass with high thermal resistance, high-silica glass, glass with a high resistance to alkali, low-actinic glass, and standard flint glass.

Thermal-Resistant (Borosilicate) Glass

High-thermal-resistant glass is usually a borosilicate glass with a low alkali content. This type of glassware is resistant to heat, corrosion, and thermal shock and should be used whenever heating or sterilization by heat is employed. Borosilicate glass, known by the commercial name of Pyrex (Corning Glass works, Corning, N.Y.) or Kimax (Kimble Glass Co., Vineland, N.J.), is used widely in the laboratory because of its high qualities of resistance. Laboratory apparatus such as beakers, flasks, and pipettes are usually made from borosilicate glass. Other brands of glassware are made from lower-grade borosilicate glass and may be used when a high-quality borosilicate glass is not necessary. If the various pieces of glassware found in the laboratory are examined, it will be seen that one or more of these brand names will be found on many different kinds of glassware. It is essential to choose glassware that has a reliable composition and that will be resistant to laboratory chemicals and conditions. In borosilicate glassware, mechanical strength and thermal and chemical resistance are well balanced. Two other brands of high-thermal-resistant glass are Corex (Corning) and Vycor (Corning). Corex glassware is made from a special alumina-silicate glass that is six times stronger than borosilicate glass.

Vycor glassware can withstand drastic thermal and chemical treatment.

High-Silica Glass

High-silica glass has a silica content of more than 96%, which makes it comparable to fused quartz in its heat resistance, chemical stability, and electrical characteristics. High-silica glass is made from borosilicate glass by removing almost all the elements except silica. This type of glassware is used for high-precision analytic work, is radiation-resistant, and can also be used for optical reflectors and mirrors. It is not used for the type of glassware generally found in the laboratory.

Alkali-Resistant Glass

Glass with high resistance to alkali was developed particularly for use with strong alkaline solutions. It is boron-free. It is often referred to as soft glass, as its thermal resistance is much less than that of borosilicate glass and it must be heated and cooled very carefully. Its use should be limited to times when solutions of, or digestions with strong alkalis are made.

Low-actinic Glass

Low-actinic glassware contains materials that usually impart an amber or red color to the glass and reduce the amount of light transmitted through to the substance in the glassware. It is used for substances that are particularly sensitive to light, such as bilirubin or vitamin A.

Standard Flint Glass

Standard flint glass, or soda-lime glass, is composed of a mixture of the oxides of silicon, calcium, and sodium. It is the most inexpensive glass and is readily made into a variety of types of glassware. This type of glass is much less resistant to high temperatures and sudden changes of temperature, and its resistance to chemical attack is only fair. Glassware made from soda-lime glass can release alkali into solutions and can therefore cause considerable errors in certain laboratory determinations. For example, manual pipettes made from soda-lime glass may release alkali into the pipetted liquid.

Disposable Glassware

The widespread use of relatively inexpensive disposable glassware has greatly reduced the need to clean glassware. This disposable glassware is made to be used and discarded, and no cleaning is necessary either before or after use, in most cases. Disposable glass and plastic is used to manufacture test tubes of all sizes, pipettes, slides, Petri dishes for microbiology, and specimen containers, to mention but a few. Considering the public awareness of the need to conserve resources and raw materials, reusable glassware should still be used when economically feasible.

Containers and Receivers

This category of glassware includes many of the most frequently used and most common pieces of glassware used in the laboratory. Containers and receivers must be made of good-quality glass. They are not calibrated to hold a particular or exact volume, but rather are available for various volumes, depending on the use desired. Beakers, Erlenmeyer flasks, test tubes, and reagent bottles are made in many different sizes (Fig 4–1). This glassware, like the volumetric glassware, has certain information indicated directly on the vessel. The volume and the brand name, or trademark, are two pieces of information found on items such as beakers and test tubes. Containers and receivers are not as expensive as volumetric glassware, because the process of exact volume calibration is not necessary.

Beakers

Beakers are wide, straight-sided cylindrical vessels and are available in many sizes and in several forms. The most common form used in the clinical laboratory is known as the *Griffin low form*. Beakers should be made of glass that is resistant to the many chemicals used in them and also resistant to heat. Beakers are used along with flasks for general mixing and for reagent preparation.

Erlenmeyer Flasks

Erlenmeyer flasks are used commonly in the laboratory for preparing reagents and for titration procedures. They, too, come in various sizes and must be made from a resistant form of glass.

Test Tubes

Test tubes come in many sizes, depending on the use for which they are intended. Test tubes without lips are the most satisfactory, because there is less chance of chipping and eventual breakage. Disposable test tubes are used for most laboratory purposes. Since chemical

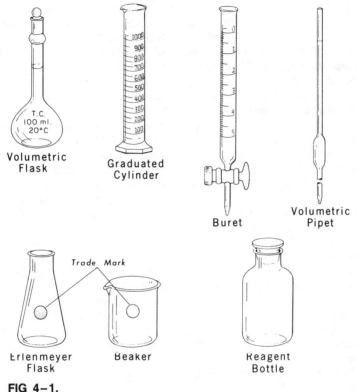

FIG 4-1.
Laboratory glassware. *T.C.* = to contain.

reactions occur in test tubes used in the chemistry laboratory, test tubes intended for such use should be made of borosilicate glass, which is resistant to thermal shock.

Reagent Bottles

All reagents should be stored in a reagent bottle of some type. These can be made of glass or some other material; some of the more commonly purchased ones now are made of plastic. Reagent bottles come in various sizes; the size used should meet the needs for the particular situation.

Photometry Cuvettes

The special tubes used for photometry are called *cuvettes* or *absorption cells*. They may be round, square, or rectangular and may be made of glass, silica (quartz), or plastic. For most routine use in the clinical laboratory, a round cuvette made of good-quality glass is used. The amount of light transmitted by the cuvette varies signifi-

cantly with the material used to make it. To be able to use cuvettes interchangeably, they must be of uniform inside diameters so that the absorbance of a solution will be within a specified tolerance when measured in different cuvettes. To ensure this uniformity, the cuvettes must be calibrated (see under Calibration of Cuvettes for the Spectrophotometer, in Chapter 5).

Volumetric Glassware

Volumetric glassware must go through a rigorous process of volume calibration to ensure the accuracy of the measurements required for laboratory determinations. In very precise work it is never safe to assume that the volume contained or delivered by any piece of equipment is exactly that indicated on the equipment. The calibration process is lengthy and time-consuming; therefore the cost of volumetric glassware is relatively high compared with the cost of noncalibrated glassware (beakers, test tubes, etc.).

Volumetric Flasks

Volumetric flasks are flasks with a round bulb at the bottom. This tapers to a long neck, on which the calibration mark is found. The specifications set up by the **National Bureau of Standards** apply to all volumetric glassware and therefore to volumetric flasks (see Fig 4–1). Volumetric flasks are calibrated to contain a specific amount or volume of liquid, and therefore the letters TC are inscribed somewhere on the neck of the flask. There are many different sizes of volumetric flasks, for the different volumes of liquid that are used. The following are some of the sizes in which volumetric flasks can be purchased: 10, 25, 50, 100, and 500 mL, and 1 and 2 L.

Volumetric flasks have been calibrated individually to contain the specified volume at a specified temperature. They are *not* calibrated to *deliver* this volume. For each size of volumetric flask there are certain allowable limits within which its volume must lie. This is called the tolerance of the flask. All volumetric glassware has a specific tolerance, the capacity tolerance, which is dependent on the size of the glassware. For example, if a 100-mL volumetric flask has a tolerance of ±0.08 mL, conditions are controlled during the calibration of a 100-mL volumetric flask to guarantee these limits. A tolerance of ±0.08 mL indicates that the allowable limits for the volume of a 100-mL volumetric flask are from 99.92 to 100.08 mL. A tolerance of ±0.05 mL for a 50-mL volumetric flask indicates allowable limits ranging from 49.95 to 50.05 mL for the volume of the flask. Volumetric flasks are used in the preparation of specific volumes of reagents or laboratory solutions. They should be used with reagents or solutions at room temperature. Solutions diluted in volumetric flasks should be repeatedly mixed during the dilution so that the contents are homogeneous before they are made up to volume. In this way, errors due to the expansion or contraction of liquids during mixing are made negligible. An important factor in the use of any volumetric apparatus is an accurate reading of the meniscus level. For more information on reading a meniscus, see under General Considerations in Pipetting With Manual Pipettes.

Graduated Measuring Cylinders

A graduated measuring cylinder is a long straight-sided cylindrical piece of glassware with calibrated markings on it. Graduated cylinders are used to measure volumes of liquids when a high degree of accuracy is not essential. They can be made from plastic or polyethylene as well as from glass (see Fig 4–1). Graduated cylinders come in various sizes according to the volumes they measure: 10, 25, 50, 100, 500, and 1000 mL. A 100-mL graduated cylinder can measure 100 mL or a fraction thereof, depending on the calibration, or graduation, marks on it. Most graduated cylinders are calibrated to deliver. This will be indicated directly on the glassware by the inscription TD. The letters TD can be found on many kinds of volumetric glassware, especially on the numerous kinds of pipettes used in the laboratory (see under Pipettes).

Graduated cylinders can be used to measure a specified volume of a liquid, such as water, in the preparation of laboratory reagents. The calibration marks on the cylinder indicate its capacity at different points. If 450 mL of water is to be measured, the most satisfactory cylinder to use would be one with a capacity of 500 mL. Graduated cylinders are not calibrated as accurately as volumetric flasks. Therefore, the capacity tolerance for graduated cylinders allows a greater variation in volume. The capacity tolerance is greater for the larger graduated cylinders. A 100-mL graduated cylinder (TD) has a tolerance of ±0.40 mL, meaning that the allowable limits are from 99.60 to 100.40 mL.

Pipettes

Pipettes are another type of volumetric glassware used extensively in the laboratory. Many types of these pipettes are available. It is important, however, to use only pipettes manufactured by reputable companies. Care and discretion should be used in selecting pipettes for clinical laboratory use, since their accuracy is one of the determining factors in the accuracy of the procedures carried out. A pipette is a cylindrical glass tube used in measuring fluids. It is calibrated to deliver, or transfer, a specified volume from one vessel to another (see Fig 4–1).

Each manual pipette has at least one calibration or graduation mark on it, as does all volumetric glassware. A pipette is filled by using mechanical suction or an aspirator bulb. Mouth suction is never used. Strong acids, bases, solvents, or human specimens are much too potent or contaminated to risk pipetting them by mouth. Caustic liquids and some solvents are very dangerous; some destroy tissue immediately on contact. Some solvents have harmful vapors (see Chapter 1).

For most general laboratory use, there are two main types of manual pipettes: the volumetric (or transfer) pipette and the graduated (or measuring) pipette. They are classified according to whether they contain or deliver a specified amount. For this reason, they may be called **to-contain pipettes** or **to-deliver pipettes.** A to-contain pipette is identified by the inscribed letters TC and a to-deliver one by the letters TD. The TD pipette is filled properly and allowed to drain completely into a receiving vessel. Portions of nonviscous samples, such as filtrates, serum, and standard solutions, are accurately measured by allowing the volumetric pipette to drain while it is held in the vertical position and by using only the force of gravity (see under Pipetting Technique Using Manual Pipettes). For most volumetric glassware the temperature of calibration is usually 20° C, and this is inscribed on the pipette (see under Calibration of Volumetric Glassware).

The opening (orifice) at the delivery tip of the pipette is of a certain size to give a specified length of time for drainage when the pipette is held vertically. A pipette must be held vertically to ensure proper drainage. It will not drain as fast when held at a 45-degree angle. The actual procedure is discussed further under Measurement of Volume: Pipetting and Titration.

The use of diluting pipettes is discussed in Chapter 11.

Volumetric Pipettes.—A pipette that has been calibrated to deliver a fixed volume of liquid by drainage is known as a **volumetric pipette,** or *transfer* pipette. These pipettes consist of a cylindrical bulb joined at both ends to narrow glass tubing. A calibration mark is etched around the upper suction tube, and the lower delivery tube is drawn out to a fine tip. Some important considerations concerning volumetric pipettes are that the calibration mark should not be too close to the top of the suction tube, the bulb should merge gradually into the lower delivery tube, and the delivery tip should have a gradual taper. To reduce drainage errors, the orifice should be of such a size that the flow out of the pipette is not too rapid. These pipettes should be made from a good-quality glass, such as Kimax or Pyrex (Fig 4–2).

Volumetric pipettes are suitable for all accurate measurements of volumes of 1 mL or more. They are calibrated to deliver the amount inscribed on them. This volume is measured from the calibration mark to the tip. A 5-mL volumetric pipette will deliver a single measured volume of 5 mL, and a 2-mL volumetric pipette will deliver 2 mL. The tolerance of volumetric pipettes increases with the capacity of the pipette. A 10-mL volumetric pipette will have a greater tolerance than a 2-mL one. The tolerance for a 5-mL volumetric pipette is ±0.01 mL. When volumes of liquids are to be delivered with great accuracy, a volumetric pipette is used. Volumetric pipettes are used to measure standard solutions, unknown blood and plasma filtrates, serum, plasma, urine, spinal fluid, and some reagents.

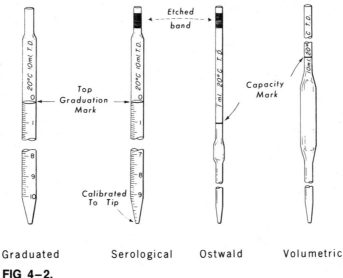

Graduated   Serological   Ostwald   Volumetric

FIG 4–2.
Types of manual pipettes.

Measurements with volumetric pipettes are done individually, and the volumes can only be whole milliliters, determined by the pipette selected (e.g., 1, 2, 5, and 10 mL). To transfer 1 mL of a standard solution into a test tube volumetrically, a 1-mL volumetric pipette is used. To transfer 5 mL of the same solution, a 5-mL volumetric pipette is used. After a volumetric pipette drains, a drop remains inside the delivery tip. This drop is *not* to be blown out: the specific volume the pipette is calibrated to deliver is dependent on the fact that the drop is left in the tip of the pipette. Information inscribed on the pipette includes the temperature of calibration (usually 20° C), capacity, manufacturer, and use (TD). The technique involved in using volumetric pipettes correctly is very important, and a certain amount of skill is required (see under Pipetting Technique Using Manual Pipettes).

Graduated Pipettes.—Another way to deliver a particular amount of liquid is to deliver that amount of liquid contained between two calibration marks on a cylindrical tube, or pipette. Such a pipette is called a **graduated pipette,** or *measuring* pipette. It has several graduation, or calibration, marks (see Fig 4–2). Many measurements in the laboratory do not require the precision of the volumetric pipette. Graduated pipettes are used when great accuracy is not required. This does not mean that these pipettes may be used with less care than the volumetric pipettes. Graduated pipettes are used primarily in measuring reagents, but they are not calibrated with sufficient tolerance to use in measuring standard or control solutions, unknown specimens, or filtrates.

A graduated pipette is a straight piece of glass tubing with a tapered end and graduation marks on the stem separating it into parts. Depending on the size used, graduated pipettes can be used to measure parts of a milliliter or many milliliters. These pipettes come in various sizes or capacities, including 0.1, 0.2, 1.0, 2.0, 5.0, 10, and 25 mL. If 4 mL of **deionized water** is to be measured into a test tube, a 5-mL graduated pipette would be the best choice. Since graduated pipettes require draining between two marks, they introduce one more source of error, compared with the volumetric pipettes with only one calibration mark. This makes measurements with the graduated pipette less precise. Because of this relatively poor precision, the graduated pipette is used where speed is more important than precision. It is used for measurements of reagents and is generally not considered accurate enough for measuring samples and standard solutions.

Two types of graduated pipettes are calibrated for delivery (see Fig 4–2). One (called a *Mohr pipette*) is calibrated between two marks on the stem, and the other (a serologic pipette) has graduation marks down to the delivery tip. The serologic pipette has a larger orifice and therefore drains faster than the Mohr pipette (see under Serologic Pipettes).

The volume of the space between the last calibration mark and the delivery tip is not known in the Mohr pipette. In Mohr graduated pipettes, this space cannot be used for measuring fluids. Graduated pipettes are calibrated in much the same manner as volumetric pipettes; however, they are not constructed to as strict specifications and they have larger-capacity tolerances. The allowable tolerance for a 5-mL graduated pipette is ±0.02 mL.

Micropipettes (to-contain pipettes).—The micropipette, or to-contain pipette, when used properly, is one of the more precise pipettes used in the clinical laboratory. This type of pipette is calibrated to *contain* a specified amount of liquid. If a pipette contains only 10 μL (0.1 mL), and 10 μL of blood is needed for a chemistry determination, then none of the blood can be left inside the pipette. The entire contents of the pipette must be emptied. If this pipette is *rinsed well* with a diluting solution, then all the blood or similar specimen will be removed from it. The correct way to use a to-contain pipette is to rinse it with a suitable diluent. Thus, a to-contain pipette cannot be used properly unless the receiving vessel contains a diluent; that is, a to-contain pipette should not be used to deliver a specimen into an empty receiving vessel. Since all the liquid in a to-contain pipette is rinsed out and used, there is only one graduation mark.

Micropipettes are used when small amounts of blood or specimen are needed. Many procedures require only a small amount of blood, and a micropipette is used for this measurement. Because even a minute volume remaining in the pipette can cause a significant error in micro work, most micropipettes are calibrated to contain the stated volume rather than to deliver it. They are generally available in small sizes, from 1 to 500 μL.

Unopette.—A special disposable micropipette used in the hematology laboratory is a self-filling pipette accompanied by a polyethylene reagent reservoir (see Chapter 11). This unit is called a Unopette (Becton, Dickinson & Co., Rutherford, N.J.) and is used by many laboratories. A glass capillary pipette is fitted in a plastic holder and fills automatically with blood by means of capillary action. The plastic reagent bottle (called the *reservoir*) is squeezed slightly while the pipette is inserted. On release of pressure, the sample is drawn into the diluent in the reservoir. Intermittent squeezing fills and empties the pipette to rinse out the contents. This type of unit has been adapted for several chemical and hematologic determinations.

Capillary Pipettes.—An inexpensive, disposable micropipette is one made of capillary tubing with a calibration line marking a specified volume. These are filled to the line by capillary action and the measured liquid is delivered by positive pressure, as with a medicine dropper. These pipettes are usually calibrated TC and require rinsing to obtain the stated accuracy.

Automatic Micropipettors.—The most common type of micropipette used in many laboratories is one that is automatic or semiautomatic. These are piston-operated devices which allow repeated, accurate, reproducible delivery of specimens, reagents, and other liquids needing measurement in small amounts (see Fig 4–3). Many pipettors are continuously adjustable so that variable volumes of liquids can be dispensed with the same device. Delivery volume is selected by adjusting the settings on the pipette device. Different types or models are available which allow volume delivery ranging from 0.5 µL to 5,000 µL, for example.

The piston, usually in the form of a thumb plunger, is depressed to a stop position on the pipetting device, the tip placed in the liquid to be measured, and then slowly the plunger is allowed to rise back to the original position (see Fig 4–3). This will fill the tip with the desired volume of liquid. The tips are usually drawn along the inside wall of the vessel from which the measured volume is drawn so that any adhering liquid is removed from the end of the tip. These pipette tips are not usually wiped as is done with the manual pipettes because the plastic surface is considered nonwettable. The tip of the pipette device is then placed against the inside wall of the receiving vessel and the plunger is depressed. When following the manufacturer's directions for the device being used, sample delivery volume is judged to be extremely accurate.

The pipette tips are usually made of disposable plastic so no cleaning is necessary. There are various types of tips available. Some pipetting devices are available which automatically eject the tip after use. These will also allow the user to insert a new tip as well as remove the used tip without touching it, minimizing infectious biohazard exposures. (See also Automatic Measurement Devices in this chapter.)

Ostwald Pipettes.—A special type of pipette designed for use in measuring viscous fluids such as whole blood is known as the *Ostwald* pipette (or the *Ostwald-Folin* pipette). When whole blood is to be measured in the chemistry laboratory, the Ostwald pipette can be used, although rarely used anymore. This pipette is similar in appearance to the volumetric pipette, except that the bulb is closer to the delivery tip (see Fig 4–2). Ostwald pipettes are usually calibrated to be blown out, and therefore an etched ring or band will be seen near the suction hole. To minimize the effects of viscosity, the Ostwald pipette is designed with a large oval bulb and a short delivery tip.

Ostwald pipettes come in several sizes; the most common ones are 0.5, 1.0 and 2.0 mL. When using an Ostwald pipette to measure blood, the blood should be allowed to drain as slowly as possible so that no residual film is left on the sides of the pipette. Contrary to the usual practice of reading the bottom of the meniscus for liquids being measured by pipette, when blood is pipetted in the Ostwald pipette, the top of the meniscus is read (blood is not transparent and the bottom of the meniscus cannot be seen clearly).

Serologic Pipettes.—Another pipette used in the laboratory, but not often in the chemistry laboratory, is called a *serologic* pipette. It is much like the graduated pipette in appearance (see Fig 4–2). The orifice, or tip opening, is larger in the serologic pipette than in other pipettes. The rate of fall of liquid is much too fast for great accuracy or precision. For use in chemistry it would be necessary to retard the flow of liquid from the delivery tip of the serologic pipette. The serologic pipette is graduated to the end of the delivery tip and has an etched band on the suction piece. It is therefore designed to be blown out. The serologic pipette is less precise than any of the pipettes discussed above. It is designed for use in serology, where relative values are sought. It is best not to use the serologic pipette for chemistry.

Stopcock Pipettes.—The *stopcock* pipette is designed for delivering blood into a Van Slyke machine, which can be used for the determination and analysis of gases such as oxygen and carbon dioxide. The stopcock pipette can be used to deliver anything that is not to be exposed to the air. It resembles a small volumetric pi-

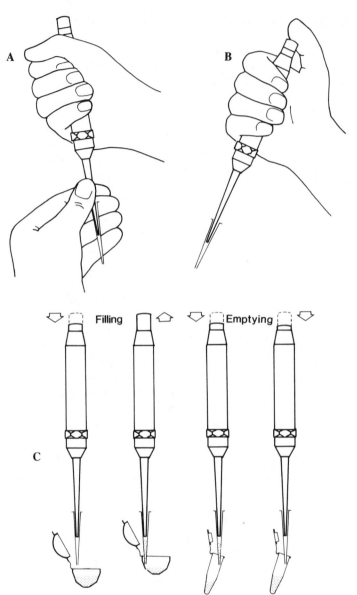

FIG 4–3.
Steps in using piston-type automatic micropipette. **A,** attaching proper tip size for range of pipette volume and twisting tip as it is pushed onto pipette to give an airtight, continuous seal. **B,** Holding pipette before use. **C,** detailed instructions for filling and emptying pipette tip. (From Kaplan LA, Pesce A: *Clinical Chemistry, Theory, Analysis, and Correlation,* ed 2, St Louis, Mosby–Year Book, Inc, 1989, p 15. Used by permission.)

pette with a stopcock attached near the delivery tip; this is used for better control of the delivery of the sample into the machine. Stopcock pipettes have two calibration marks, one on either side of the bulb.

Burets

A **buret** is a long cylindrical tube of glassware with graduation divisions on it and a stopcock closing at one end (see Fig 4–1). The stopcock on the delivery tip of the buret serves to control the flow of liquid. A buret is used to deliver measured quantities of fluids or solutions. Like all other volumetric glassware, burets are carefully calibrated according to the specifications set up by the National Bureau of Standards.

Burets also have a specific capacity tolerance depending on their size. Smaller burets are more accurate than larger ones (they have smaller tolerances). Burets with a maximum capacity of 2 mL or less are called *microburets.* They are usually calibrated with 0.01-mL or smaller divisions. Some common capacities for burets are 5, 10, and 25 mL. The capacity tolerances for burets are similar to those for graduated pipettes, which burets resemble very closely. For a 5-mL buret, the tolerance is ±0.02 mL. This means that the allowable limits for the volume of this particular buret range from 4.98 to 5.02 mL. The chief difference between the buret and the graduated pipette is that the buret has a stopcock. The stopcock is made from either glass or Teflon. A glass stopcock requires the use of a lubricant, but a Teflon stopcock does not. Burets are used in titration, a means of quantitative measurement (see under Titration for more information on the use of the buret).

Calibration of Volumetric Glassware

Calibration is the means by which glassware or other apparatus used in quantitative measurements is checked to determine its exact volume. To calibrate is to divide the glassware or mark it with graduations (or other indices of quantity) for the purpose of measurement. Calibration marks will be seen on every piece of volumetric glassware used in the laboratory. Specifications for the calibration of glassware are established by the National Bureau of Standards.

Each piece of volumetric glassware must be checked and must comply with these specifications before it can be accurately used in the clinical laboratory. Pipettes, burets, volumetric flasks, and other volumetric glassware are supposed to hold, deliver, or contain a specific amount of liquid. This specified amount, or volume, is known as the *units of capacity* and is indicated by the manufacturer directly on each piece of glassware.

Volumetric glassware is usually calibrated by weight, using **distilled water.** Water is commonly used as the liquid for calibration because it is readily available and because it is similar in viscosity and speed of drainage to the solutions and reagents ordinarily used in the clinical laboratory. The units of capacity determined will therefore be the volume of water contained in, or delivered by, the glassware at a particular temperature. The manufacturer knows what the weights of various amounts of distilled water are at specific temperatures. This information is used in the manual calibration of volumetric glassware. If a manufacturer wants a volumetric flask to contain 100 mL, a sensitive balance such as an analytical balance is used. Weights corresponding to what 100 mL of distilled water weighs at a specific tem-

perature are placed on one side of the balance. The flask to be calibrated is placed on the other side of the balance, and distilled water is gradually added to it until equilibrium is achieved. The manufacturer then makes a permanent calibration mark on the neck of the flask at the bottom of the water meniscus level. This flask is then calibrated to contain 100 mL. Other sizes and types of volumetric glassware are similarly calibrated.

The volume of a particular piece of glassware varies with the *temperature.* For this reason it is necessary to specify the temperature at which the glassware was calibrated. Glass will swell or shrink with changes in temperature, and the volume of the glassware will therefore vary with changes in temperature. Most volumetric glassware for routine clinical use is calibrated at 20° C. This means that the calibration process and checking took place at a controlled temperature of 20° C. On all volumetric glassware the inscription 20° C will be seen. Although 20° C is almost universally adopted as the standard temperature for calibration of volumetric glassware, each piece of glassware will have the temperature of calibration inscribed on it. The volume of a volumetric flask is less at a low temperature than at a higher temperature. A 50-mL volumetric flask that was calibrated at 20° C would contain less than 50 mL at 10° C.

Since the laboratory depends to such a great extent on the quality of its glassware to produce reliable results, it is necessary to be certain that the glassware is of the *very best quality.* The glass used for volumetric glassware must meet certain standards of quality. It must be transparent and free from striations and other surface irregularities. It should have no defects that would distort the appearance of the liquid surface or portion of the calibration line seen through the glass.

The *design* and *workmanship* for volumetric glassware is also specified by the National Bureau of Standards. The shape of the glassware must permit complete emptying and thorough cleaning, and it must stand solidly on a level surface.

PLASTICWARE

The clinical laboratory has benefited greatly from the introduction of plasticware. In many cases, plasticware designed for laboratory use has replaced glassware. Much of the laboratory ware in general use, such as beakers, graduated cylinders, reagent bottles, capillary tubing for pipettes, and test tubes, can be manufactured from plastic as well as from glass. Plasticware is cheaper and more durable, but glassware is frequently preferred because of its chemical stability and clarity. Plastic is unbreakable, which is its greatest advantage. Plastic is preferred for certain analyses in which glass can be damaged by chemicals used in the testing. Alkaline solutions must be stored in plastic.

The disadvantages of plasticware are that there is some leaching of surface-bound constituents into solutions, some permeability to water vapor, some evaporation through breathing of the plastic, and some absorption of dyes, stains, or proteins. Because evaporation is a significant factor in using plasticware, small volumes of reagent should never be stored in oversized plastic bottles for long periods of time.

Polymerized organic monomers are used to manufacture plastics for laboratory use. The most commonly used plastics include the polyolefins (polyethylene, polypropylene), polytetrafluoroethylene (Teflon, a fluorinated hydrocarbon), polystyrene, polycarbonate, and polyvinylchloride. These plastics are chemically relatively inert and as a group are unaffected by acids, alkalis, salt solutions, and most aqueous solutions. Most disposable plasticware is made from polyethylene; it is very resistant to high temperatures, but can absorb some pigments and become discolored. Polyvinylchlorides are soft and flexible and are used to manufacture tubing. Some of the plastics can be autoclaved—Teflon, polycarbonate, and some of the polyolefin plastics. Polycarbonate plasticware is clear and is ideal for graduated cylinders. Teflon is useful because it is almost totally chemically inert and is also resistant to a wide range of temperatures. Polyolefins are useful, in general, for their strength and resistance to high temperatures. Specific physical properties for each type of plasticware can be obtained from the manufacturer of the product. Materials used should be tested under the conditions present in the individual laboratory setting.

AUTOMATIC MEASURING DEVICES

Automatic Pipettes

Automatic and semiautomatic pipettes are useful in many areas of laboratory work. Several different types are available and each must be carefully calibrated before use. The problems encountered with automatic pipetting depend to a large degree on the nature of the solution to be pipetted. Some reagents cause more bubbles than others and some are more viscous. The presence of bubbles and viscous solutions can cause problems with measurement and delivery of samples and solutions.

Automatic pipetting devices permit rapid, repetitive measurement and delivery of predefined volumes of reagent or sample. With the use of these devices, efficient delivery of equal volumes of specific liquids is assured. Specimens can be measured efficiently, followed by the addition of the necessary reagents or diluents. Some devices can measure the sample and then follow with a diluting reagent dispensed with the same apparatus. Other devices have tip-ejector capabilities, variable digital settings, or repetitive-dispensing capabilities for added convenience. The capillary tips into which the sample is drawn can be made from glass or plastic. These are usually disposable. This eliminates cleaning and promotes proper discard techniques for infection control. Proper care, calibration, and maintenance are necessary to ensure precise, accurate sampling when using these automatic pipetting devices. It is important to read and follow the manufacturer's instructions for each device used (see also under Automatic Micropipettors in this chapter).

Automatic Dispensers or Syringes

Many types of automatic dispensers or syringes are used in the laboratory for repetitive adding of multiple doses of the same reagent or diluent. These devices are used for measuring serial amounts of relatively small volumes of the same liquid. The volume to be dispensed is determined by the pipettor setting. Dispensers are available with varieties of volume settings. Some are available as syringes and others as bottle top devices. Most of these dispensers can be cleaned by autoclaving.

Diluter-dispensers

In automated instruments, diluter-dispensers are used to prepare a number of different samples for analysis. These devices pipette a selected aliquot of sample and diluent into the instrument or receiving vessel. These devices are mostly of the dual-piston type, one being used for the sample and the other for the diluent or reagent.

CLEANING LABORATORY GLASSWARE AND PLASTICWARE

Among the many factors that ensure accurate results in laboratory determinations is the use of *clean,* unbroken glassware. There is no point in exercising care in obtaining specimens, handling the specimens, and making the laboratory determination if the laboratory ware used is not extremely clean. Plasticware must also be clean.

There are various methods of cleaning glassware, the one chosen depending on the glassware's use. In all cases, glassware for the clinical laboratory must be physically clean, in most cases it must be chemically clean, and in some cases it must be bacteriologically clean, or sterile.

Laboratory ware that cannot be cleaned immediately after use should be rinsed with tap water and left to soak in a basin or pail of water to which a small amount of detergent has been added. Never allow dirty glassware or plasticware to dry out. Once dried out on the surface, it is difficult to remove most soil by ordinary means. For this reason it is important to have a soaking bucket available in the working area. Glassware that is new is often slightly alkaline and should be soaked for several hours in a dilute hydrochloric acid or nitric acid solution (about 1 mL/dL is satisfactory). This glassware should then be washed in the usual manner.

Glassware that is contaminated, as by use with patient specimens, must be decontaminated before it is washed. This can be done by presoaking in 5% bleach, or by boiling, autoclaving, or some similar procedure.

General cleaning methods involve the use of a soap, detergent, or cleaning powder. In most laboratories, detergents are used. If the dirty glassware has been soaking in a solution of the detergent water, the cleaning job will be much easier.

Procedure 4–1. Cleaning Glassware

1. Put the specified amount of detergent into a dishpan or washing bucket containing moderately hot water. Allow the detergent to dissolve thoroughly.

2. Rinse glassware (or other items that can be washed) in tap water before placing it in the detergent solution. Never allow dirty glassware to dry out; always place it in a soaking bucket. Glassware should be completely submerged in the bucket or pan. Fill large pieces with detergent water and set aside to soak. Soaking glassware for at least 1 hour before washing makes the washing procedure much more efficient.

3. Using a cleaning brush, thoroughly scrub the glassware, being certain to clean all parts. Brushes of various sizes should be available to fit the different-sized test tubes, flasks, funnels, and bottles. Excessive brushing and improper use of brushes may cause scratching of the glassware. Avoid the use of abrasive cleaners on glassware.

4. Rinse glassware under running tap water; allow the water to run into each piece of glassware, pour it out, and repeat several times (seven to ten times is sufficient). Rinse the outside of the glassware too. It is especially important to *remove all the detergent from the glassware before use;* if detergent remains, the alkali in it may interfere with laboratory determinations.

5. After thoroughly rinsing the glassware with tap water, rinse it with deionized water (type I or II) three to five times. Certain glassware used for microbiological studies requires even longer rinsing with deionized water. Use deionized (or distilled water in some instances) in the final rinsing of all laboratory glassware.

6. Glassware may be dried in a hot oven (no hotter than 100° C) or at room temperature. If a higher temperature is used, the glassware can become distorted. Always dry glassware or other equipment in an inverted position to ensure complete drainage of water as it dries. Never dry laboratory ware with a towel. Do not dry plasticware or rubber items in an oven.

7. Check the glassware for cleanliness by observing the water drainage. Chemically clean glassware will drain uniformly; dirty glassware will drain leaving water droplets adhering to the walls of the glass.

General Cleaning Procedure

There are various methods of cleaning laboratory ware. Most glassware and plasticware (with the exception of pipettes) can be cleaned as described in Procedure 4–1.

Cleaning Plasticware

Most plasticware can be cleaned in the same manner as glassware and using ordinary glassware washing machines, but the use of any abrasive cleaning materials should be avoided.

Plasticware should be well cleaned and rinsed with deionized water prior to any necessary autoclaving, since some chemical reactions can occur during autoclaving temperatures which do not occur when the plastics are at room temperature. These reactions can cause deterioration of the plastic.

Some of the transparent plastics, such as polystyrene or polycarbonate, may absorb small quantities of water vapor during autoclaving and appear cloudy. This clouding effect will disappear as the plastic dries and the plastic becomes transparent again. Drying the plasticware in a 110° C oven can enhance the clearing effect.

Cleaning Nondisposable Pipettes

Nondisposable pipettes used in the laboratory are cleaned in a special way. Immediately after use, the pipettes should be placed in a special pipette container or cylinder containing water; the water should be high enough to completely cover the pipettes. Pipettes should be placed in the container carefully to avoid breakage. When the pipettes are to be cleaned, they are removed from the cylinder and placed in another cylinder containing a cleaning solution. This cleaning solution can be a detergent or a commercial analytical cleaning product. An acid cleaning solution can be used for pipettes for some analyses where scrupulously clean glassware is needed.

Acid cleaning solution is usually a combination of sulfuric acid and either potassium or sodium dichromate (called acid-dichromate solution). Acid-dichromate cleaning solution may be purchased commercially, or it may be prepared by dissolving 100 g of sodium or potassium dichromate in 100 mL of water and slowly adding, while stirring, the contents of one 9-lb bottle of technical grade sulfuric acid. For safe handling during the preparation, the container of acid solution should be placed in a pan or sink of cold water because of the great amount of heat generated on mixing the acid and water. Safety goggles should always be worn during the preparation of this solution, as should rubber gloves and a protective apron. It is extremely potent and must be handled cautiously or serious burns will result (see Chapter 1). The pipettes are allowed to soak in the cleaning solution for 30 minutes.

The next step involves thorough rinsing of the pipettes. This can be accomplished by hand, but more often it is done with the aid of an automatic pipette washer. The pipettes are rinsed with tap water, using the automatic pipette washer, for 1 to 2 hours. They are then rinsed in deionized or distilled water two or three times and dried in a hot oven.

Cleaning Nondisposable Diluting Pipettes

If nondisposable diluting pipettes are used (as in the hematology laboratory), they are cleaned in a special way. They should always be rinsed immediately after use, preferably by being placed in a tumbler or beaker of water until they are cleaned. There are several ways to clean these pipettes, but in general they are first cleaned with tap water, then with distilled water, and finally rinsed with either alcohol or acetone. Acetone assists in drying the inside of the pipette. Usually the cleaning is done with suction, using a special pipette holder that fits onto the suction apparatus. The pipettes are also dried with suction. Periodically, the pipettes should be cleaned with a detergent solution, rinsed well, and dried.

Cleaning Nondisposable Photometry Cuvettes

Cuvettes must be scrupulously clean and free from grease smudges or scratches. As soon as possible after use, cuvettes should be rinsed with tap water, filled with a mild detergent solution, and placed in a rubberized test tube rack. It is best not to put them into a regular dishwashing bucket where they would rub against one another and be scratched. After standing with the detergent solution, the cuvettes are rinsed several times with tap water and two or three times with distilled or deionized water. When drying cuvettes, high temperatures and unclean air should be avoided. A low to medium oven (not above 100° C) can be used for rapid drying. In some laboratories, there are special dishwashing machines that can adequately handle cuvettes.

GLASS BREAKAGE AND REPLACEMENT

It is important in the clinical laboratory to check all glassware periodically to determine its condition. No broken or chipped glassware should be used. Many laboratory accidents are caused by the use of broken glassware. Serious cuts may result, and infections may set in.

Each time a laboratory procedure is carried out, the glassware used should be checked; equipment such as beakers, pipettes, test tubes, and flasks should not have broken edges or cracks. To prevent breakage, glassware should be handled carefully; carrying too much glassware at one time from one place to another in the laboratory is to be avoided.

When glassware is broken, it must be replaced with another like piece. Breakage should be reported to an instructor or department head, so that replacement can be arranged. Several laboratory equipment catalogs are available from which the required items may be ordered. These catalogs are distributed by supply companies that handle laboratory equipment. They describe the quality, capacity, tolerance, and cost of the available items. To purchase equipment at the most reasonable price it is advisable to compare specific items in several different catalogs.

Laboratory Reagent Water

The quality of water used in the laboratory is very important. Its use in reagent and solution preparation, reconstitution of lyophilized materials, and dilutions of samples demands specific requirements for its level of purity. All water used in the clinical laboratory should be free from substances that could interfere with the tests being performed. It is important that the persons involved in doing the analyses understand the reasons for the special emphasis placed on the kinds of water used and the difficulties involved in obtaining and maintaining a pure reagent water supply. Significant error can be introduced into a laboratory assay if inorganic or organic impurities in the water supply have not been removed prior to analysis.

LEVELS OF WATER PURITY

Three levels of laboratory water quality have been recommended by the National Committee for Clinical Laboratory Standards and the College of American Pathologists: type I, type II, and type III:

Type I Reagent Water

This type of reagent water is the most pure and should be used for procedures which require maximum water purity. For preparation of standard solutions, buffers, controls, in quantitative analytic procedures (especially where nanograms or subnanogram measurements are required), in electrophoresis, in toxicology screening tests, and in high-performance liquid chromatography, type I reagent water must be used.

Type II Reagent Water

When doing qualitative chemistry procedures and for most procedures carried out in hematology, immunology, microbiology, and other clinical test areas, type II water is suitable for use. Type II water can be used when the presence of bacteria can be tolerated.

Type III Reagent Water

This type of water can be used for some qualitative laboratory tests, such as those used in general urinalysis. Type III water can be used as a water source for preparation of type I and type II water and for washing and rinsing laboratory glassware. Any glassware should be given a final rinse with either a type I or II water, depending on the intended use for the glassware.

CRITERIA FOR WATER PURITY

The presence of ionizable contaminants in distilled or deionized water is most easily determined by measuring the conductance, or electrical resistance, of the water. This is the basis for having *purity meters* or conductivity warning lights on distillation and deionization apparatus.

There are several ways to test for water purity. With regard to the presence of inorganic ionized materials, as the purity of the water increases, the amount of dissolved ionized substances decreases and the ability of the water to conduct an electrical current decreases. This principle is used in commercially available resistance test analyzers for water purity. As the ability of the water to conduct an electrical current decreases, the resistance increases.

Water of the highest purity will vary with the actual method of preparation and may be referred to as nitrogen-free water, double-distilled water, or conductivity water, depending on the actual method used. However, a measure of conductance does not consider the presence of nonionized substances (organic contaminants) such as dissolved gases. Especially important in the clinical laboratory is dissolved carbon dioxide. Water free of such dissolved gases may be obtained by boiling it immediately before use and is often referred to as gas-free, or carbon dioxide–free, water. Such water may be necessary for the preparation of strongly alkaline solutions. Another contaminant of water may be the presence of substances dissolved from the storage container.

Accreditation or certification requirements for clinical laboratories set up by state and federal agencies have resulted in specific well-defined criteria for water purity. The classification and specifications for water purity are designed to enable laboratory personnel to specify the quality of the water needed for particular laboratory analyses and reagent preparation, for example. Each test performed in the laboratory must be evaluated as to the type of water needed to avoid potential interference with specificity, accuracy, and precision. It is well known, for example, that water contaminated with metal, when used in analyses of enzymes, can have a dramatic effect on the value obtained.

STORAGE OF REAGENT WATER

It is important to store the reagent water appropriately. Type I water must be used immediately after its production to prevent carbon dioxide from being absorbed into it. There are no specified storage guidelines for type I water, because it is not possible to maintain its high level of purity for any length of time. Types II and III water can be stored in borosilicate glass or polyethylene bottles but should be used as soon as possible to pre-

vent contamination with airborne microbes. Containers should be tightly stoppered to prevent absorption of gases. It is also important to keep the delivery system for the water protected from chemical or microbiological contamination.

METHODS OF PURIFYING WATER

The original source for water varies greatly with the health care facility. Water originating from rivers, lakes, springs, or wells contains a variety of inorganic, organic, and microbiological contaminants. No single purification system can remove all the contaminants. For this reason, a variety of methods, in differing combinations, are used to obtain the particular types of water used in a single laboratory facility. Two general methods are employed to prepare water for laboratory use: deionization and distillation. Sometimes it is necessary to further treat distilled water with a deionization process to obtain water with the acceptable degree of purity needed.

Deionized Water

In the process of deionization, water is passed through a resin column containing positively (+) and negatively (−) charged particles. These particles combine with ions present in the water to remove them. Therefore, only substances that can ionize will be removed in the process of deionization; organic substances and other substances that do not ionize are not removed. Further treatment with membrane filtration and activated charcoal is necessary to remove organic impurities, particulate matter, and microorganisms to produce type I water from deionized water.

Distilled Water

In the process of distillation, water is boiled, and the resulting steam is cooled; condensed steam is distilled water. Many minerals are found in natural water. Among those commonly found in water are iron, magnesium, and calcium. Water from which these minerals and others have been removed by distillation is known as *distilled water*. The process of distillation also removes microbiological organisms, but volatile impurities such as carbon dioxide, chlorine, and ammonia are not removed.

Water which has been distilled meets the specifications for type II and type III water.

Double-Distilled Water

Distilled or deionized water is not necessarily pure water. There may be contamination by dissolved gases, by nonvolatile substances carried over by steam in the distillation process, or by dissolved substances from storage containers. For example, in tests for nitrogen compounds (such as urea nitrogen, a common clinical chemistry determination) it is important to use ammonia-free (nitrogen-free) water. This may be specially purchased by the laboratory for such determinations or prepared in the laboratory by a specific method, double distillation, to remove the contaminating ammonia.

Combinations of Deionization and Distillation

Water of higher purity is also produced by special distillation units in which the water is first deionized and then distilled; this eliminates the need for double distillation. Other systems may first distill the water, then deionize it.

Reverse Osmosis

The process of reverse osmosis passes water under pressure through a semipermeable membrane made of cellulose acetate, or other materials. This treatment removes approximately 90% of dissolved solids, 98% of organic impurities, insoluble matter, and microbiological organisms. It does not remove dissolved gases and only about 10% of ionized particles.

Other Processes of Purification

Filtration of water through semipermeable membranes will remove insoluble matter, pyrogens, and microorganisms if the pore size of the membrane is small enough. Adsorption by activated charcoal, clays, silicates, or metal oxides can remove organic matter. Type I water can be processed through a combination of deionization, filtration, and adsorption.

Tap Water

Rarely is tap water used in the clinical laboratory, the exception being for the initial cleaning of laboratory glassware. Plain tap water is not used in any laboratory analyses or in the preparation of any reagents.

Reagents Used in Laboratory Assays

The validity of the laboratory data obtained by analysis of patient specimens is dependent on the use of specific laboratory measuring apparatus and also on the use of specific reagents and materials or products devised for that apparatus. Analytic procedures require the use of properly prepared solutions or reagents. It is important to understand fully just how valuable reagents are in the total clinical laboratory analyses. The accuracy of the determinations depends to a large extent on the accuracy of the reagents used.

A *reagent* is defined as any substance employed to produce a chemical reaction. In preparing reagents, instructions should be followed exactly. Often certain reagents will be purchased in a fully prepared state; in this case it is important that the reagents be obtained only from reputable chemical companies. To repeat a most important precept, *instructions must be followed*; this is a strict rule in the laboratory. One should never rely on memory in preparing a reagent, but rather follow the set of instructions or directions provided for the preparation of each reagent needed.

REAGENT PREPARATION

Instructions for preparing a reagent resemble a cooking recipe in that they tell what quantities of ingredients to mix together. They tell the names of the chemicals needed, the number of grams or milligrams needed, and the total volume to which the particular reagent should be diluted. The solvent most commonly used for dilution is deionized or distilled water.

Measurement of Mass and Volume

To prepare reagents, either measurement of mass by use of a balance for weighing, or reconstitution of a freeze-dried or otherwise concentrated reagent product is necessary.

Preparation of reagents in the traditional way involves the use of a balance (the analytical, triple-beam, or torsion balance, for example) and other special volumetric measuring devices (such as volumetric flasks and graduated cylinders). The types of volumetric glassware available are discussed under Laboratory Glassware and Plasticware.

Since chemicals are used in the preparation of reagents and the accuracy of laboratory determinations depends on the quality of the reagents employed, it is essential that only chemicals from reliable manufacturers be used.

Concentration of Solutions

Using solutions of the correct concentration is of the greatest importance in attaining good results in the laboratory. Quantitative transfer, along with accurate initial measurement of the chemical, helps to ensure that the solution will be of the correct concentration.

The concentration of a solution may be expressed in different ways. With the use of SI units, traditional expression of concentration in terms of mass of solute per volume of solution has been replaced by the use of moles of solute per volume of solution for analyte analyses whenever possible, and the use of the liter as the reference value.

In the clinical chemistry laboratory, where the vast majority of the total laboratory analyses are performed, most measurements are concerned with the concentration of substances in solutions. The solution is usually blood, serum, urine, spinal fluid, or other body fluid and the substance to be measured is dissolved in the solution. This substance is known as the *solute*. Therefore, the substances being measured in the analyses (whether they are organic or inorganic, or of high or low molecular weight) are solutes. The substance in which the solute is dissolved is known as the solvent.

When a reagent is being prepared, and the solution is being diluted with water, its volume is increased and its concentration decreased, but the amount of solute remains unchanged.

Laboratory Chemicals

A chemical is a substance that occurs naturally or is obtained through a chemical process; it is used to produce a chemical effect or reaction. Chemicals are produced in various purities or grades.

Standards of Purity

There are many grades of chemicals available and it is essential to understand which grade or type should be used for which reagent.

When quantitative determinations are to be performed and accurate standard solutions prepared, it is necessary to use pure chemicals. In such cases, the more costly *reagent-grade* chemicals are necessary for accuracy. Different companies have their own descriptions for the various degrees of purity, and there is no official designation. The label on the bottle and the supplier's catalog may give important information such as the maximum limits of impurities or an actual analysis of the chemical. Directions for reagent preparation usually specify the grade, and in many instances state the particular brand of chemical. These directions must be followed to ensure reliable results.

The purity of organic chemicals is generally inferior to that of inorganic chemicals. This is due both to the manner in which they are prepared or synthesized and to changes that occur as they stand or are stored.

Grades of Chemicals

The following is a general description of the various **grades of chemicals** available for the clinical laboratory.

1. *Reagent grade or analytic reagent (AR) grade.* These chemicals are of a high degree of purity and are used often in the preparation of reagents in the clinical laboratory. The American Chemical Society has developed specifications for many reagent grade or AR chemicals, and those that meet their standards are designated by the letters ACS.

2. *Chemically pure (CP) grade.* These chemicals are sufficiently pure to be used in many analyses in the clinical laboratory. However, the designation does not reveal the limits of impurities that are tolerated, and so they may not be acceptable for research and various clinical laboratory techniques unless they have been specifically analyzed for the desired procedure. It may be necessary to use this grade when higher-purity biochemicals are not available.

3. *USP and NF grade.* These reagents meet the specifications stated in the *United States Pharmacopeia (USP)* or the *National Formulary (NF)*. They are generally less pure than CP grade, as the tolerances are specified such that they are not injurious to health rather than chemically pure.

4. *Purified, practical, or pure grade.* These chemi-

cals may be used as starting materials for synthesis of other chemicals of greater purity but generally should not be used in the clinical laboratory.

5. *Technical or commercial grade.* These chemicals are used only for industrial purposes and are generally not used in the preparation of reagents for the clinical laboratory.

6. *National Bureau of Standards, the College of American Pathologists (CAP), and the National Committee for Clinical Laboratory Standards (NCCLS).* These agencies or bureaus all supply certified clinical laboratory standards. The highest grade or purest chemicals are available from the National Bureau of Standards. However, very few such compounds are available to the clinical laboratory and they are known as *standards, clinical type.*

Physical Forms of Chemicals

Chemicals used in the laboratory have various physical forms. Persons using these chemicals must know the various forms and which form should be used in the preparation of a specific reagent. Some of the common forms are lumps, sticks, pellets, granules, fine granules, crystalline powder, crystals, fine crystals, powder, and liquid. There are some special forms such as chips, scales, and flakes, but these are not frequently used in reagent preparation.

Hazardous Chemicals Communication Policies

Information and training regarding hazardous chemicals must be provided to all persons working with them in the clinical laboratory. The Occupational Safety and Health Administration (OSHA) regulations ensure that all sites where hazardous chemicals are used comply with the necessary safety precautions. Any information about signs and symptoms associated with exposures to hazardous chemicals used in the laboratory must be communicated to all persons. Reference materials about the individual chemicals are provided by all chemical manufacturers and suppliers by means of the **Material Safety Data Sheet (MSDS).** This information accompanies the shipment of all hazardous chemicals and should be available in the laboratory for anyone to review. The MSDS contains information about possible hazards, safe handling, storage, and disposal of the particular chemical it accompanies (see Chemical Hazards in Chapter 1).

Storage of Chemicals

It is important that chemicals kept in the laboratory be stored properly, as described in Chapter 1. Chemicals that require refrigeration should be refrigerated immediately. Solids should be kept in a cool, dry place. Acids and bases should be stored separately and in well-ventilated storage units. Flammable solvents (e.g., alcohol, chloroform) should be stored in specially constructed well-ventilated storage units with appropriate labeling in accordance with OSHA regulations. Flammable solvents such as acetone and ether should always be stored in special safety cans or other appropriate storage devices in appropriate storage units. Fuming and volatile chemicals, such as solvents, strong acids, and strong bases, should be opened and reagent preparation resulting in fumes should be done only under a fume hood so that the vapors will not escape into the room. Chemicals that absorb water should be weighed only after desiccation or drying in a hot oven; otherwise the weights will not be accurate.

It is very important that the label on the chemical be read for instructions about storage details. Most chemicals are stable at room temperature without desiccation. Some must be stored at refrigeration temperature, some frozen, and some that are light-sensitive must be stored in brown bottles.

Chemicals Used to Prepare Standard Solutions

Standards are the most highly purified types of chemicals available. The group includes *primary, reference,* and *certified* standards. Primary standards meet specifications set by the Committee on Analytical Reagents of the American Chemical Society. Each lot of these chemicals is assayed and the chemicals must be stable substances of definite composition. Reference standards are chemicals whose purity has been ensured by the National Bureau of Standards list of standard reference materials (SRM). Certified standards are also available. For example, the CAP certifies bilirubin and cyanmethemoglobin standards, and the NCCLS certifies a standardized protein solution.

Quantitative Transfer and Dilution of Chemical for Reagent

In preparing any solution in the clinical laboratory, it is necessary to utilize the practice known as **quantita-**

tive transfer (Procedure 4–2). It is essential that the *entire* amount of the weighed or measured substance be used in preparing the solution. In quantitative transfer, the entire amount of the measured substance is transferred from one vessel to another for dilution. The usual practice in preparing most laboratory reagents is to weigh the chemical in a beaker (or other suitable vessel, such as a disposable weighing boat) and quantitatively transfer the chemical to a volumetric flask for dilution with deionized or distilled water. The volumetric flask chosen

must be of the correct size; that is, it must hold the amount of solution that is desired for the total volume of the reagent being prepared.

The most common amount of solution prepared at one time is 1 L. If 1 L of reagent is needed, the measured chemical must be transferred quantitatively to a 1-L volumetric flask and diluted to the calibration mark with deionized water or the required solvent. The method of quantitative transfer requires a great deal of care and accuracy.

Dissolving the Chemical in the Solution

There are several methods by which the dissolution of solid materials can be hastened. Heating usually increases the solubility of a chemical, and heat also causes the fluid to move (the currents help in dissolving). Even mild heat, however, will decompose some chemicals, and therefore heat must be used with caution. Agitation by using a stirring rod or swirling by means of a mechanical shaker increases solubility by removing the saturated solution from contact with the chemical. Rapid addition of the solvent is another means of hastening the solution of solid materials. Some chemicals tend to cake and form aggregates as soon as the solvent is added. By adding the solvent quickly and keeping the solids in motion, aggregation may be prevented.

Labeling the Reagent Container

Containers for storage of reagents (usually reagent bottles) should be labeled before the material is added. A reagent should never be placed in an unlabeled bottle or container. If an unlabeled container is found, the reagent in it must be discarded. Proper labeling of reagent bottles is of the greatest importance. All labels should include the name and concentration of the reagent, the date on which the reagent was prepared, and the initials of the person who made the reagent (Fig 4–4).

Checking the Reagent Before Use

After the prepared reagent is in the reagent bottle, it must be checked by some means before it is put into actual use in any procedure. This can be done in one of several ways, depending on the reagent itself. After the reagent has been checked, this is noted on the label, and the solution can then be put into active use in the laboratory.

Procedure 4–2. Quantitative Transfer.

1. Place a clean, dry funnel in the mouth of the volumetric flask.
2. Carefully transfer the chemical in the measuring vessel into the funnel.
3. Wash the chemical into the flask with small amounts of deionized water or the required solvent for the reagent.
4. Rinse the measuring vessel (beaker) three to five times with small portions of deionized water or the required solvent until *all* of the chemical has been transferred from the vessel into the volumetric flask (add each rinsing to the flask).
5. Rinse the funnel with deionized water or the required solvent, and remove the funnel from the volumetric flask.
6. Dissolve the chemical in the flask by shaking it. Some chemicals are more difficult to dissolve than others. On occasion, more special attention must be given to the problem of dissolving the chemical.
7. Add deionized water or the required solvent to about 0.5 in. below the calibration line on the flask, allow a few seconds for drainage of fluid above the calibration line, and then carefully add deionized water or the required solvent to the calibration line (the *bottom* of the meniscus must be exactly on the calibration mark).
8. Stopper the flask with a ground-glass stopper, and mix well by inverting at least 20 times.
9. Rinse a properly labeled reagent bottle with a small amount of the mixed reagent in the volumetric flask. Transfer the prepared reagent to the labeled reagent bottle for storage.

```
┌─────────────────────────────────────────┐
│  Test Used For              ✔O. K.       │
│                                          │
│           Name of Reagent                │
│                                          │
│  Date Prepared          Initial of Maker │
└─────────────────────────────────────────┘
```

FIG 4–4.
Sample label.

READY-MADE REAGENTS

In many laboratories, ready-made reagents are used, especially where large automated instruments are utilized. The manufacturers of these instruments usually provide the necessary specific reagents for use with their instrument. These reagents must be handled with extreme care and always must be used according to the manufacturer's directions.

Immunoreagents

Special commercial reagent kits are commonly used for clinical immunology and radioimmunoassay tests. A typical test kit will contain all necessary reagents, including standards, labeled antigen, and antibody, plus any other associated reagents needed. The laboratory must maintain strict evaluation policies for these kits to ensure their reliability. The disadvantage of these kits is that the laboratory is dependent on the supplier to produce and maintain components which must meet the necessary standards. Each new kit must be evaluated by the laboratory according to a strict protocol and then a periodic monitoring program must be maintained to ensure the reliability of the results produced.

Measurement of Mass: Weighing and the Use of Balances

GENERAL USE OF BALANCES

Probably some of the most important measurement devices are the various types of balances used to measure weight or mass (gravimetric analysis) in preparing the reagents and standard solutions used in the laboratory. This is one method of quantitative analysis in the clinical laboratory. Almost every procedure performed in the laboratory depends to some extent on the use of a balance. Laboratory balances function by either mechanical or electronic means.

In the traditional clinical laboratory, **gravimetric analysis** (analysis by measurement of mass or weight) is used extensively in the preparation of reagents and standard solutions. Most procedures depend on the use of an accurately prepared **standard solution.** In many laboratories today, however, reagents, standard solutions, and control solutions are purchased ready to use and the actual laboratory preparation of these reagents and solutions is not done. Therefore, the use of the various balances is not needed as often. Since measurement of mass remains fundamental to all analyses, the technique of weighing should continue to be fundamental to the base of knowledge for all persons working in a clinical laboratory. Even with the use of purchased laboratory solutions, it is likely that a balance will be needed for preparing reagents or standards for doing certain laboratory determinations. Because of the added cost of purchasing prepared standards, some laboratories routinely prepare their own standard solutions. Another use for weighing is the calibration of volumetric equipment. The measurement of mass continues to be the quantitative means by which this equipment is calibrated.

Balances are used to weigh the chemicals used to prepare the many chemical solutions needed in the laboratory. Some solutions require more accurately weighed chemicals than others. The accuracy needed depends on what the solution is to be used for. One must decide what type of balance (or scale) is most appropriate for the precision or reproducibility required in weighing the chemicals to be used for a particular solution. The different kinds of balances are suited to particular needs. A balance that sacrifices precision for speed should not be used when precision is needed.

TYPES OF BALANCES USED IN THE LABORATORY

The balance considered to be the backbone of the clinical laboratory, especially clinical chemistry, is the **analytical balance.** This balance and other types—

namely the **triple-beam balance,** Cent-O-Gram, and **torsion balance**—are discussed in this section. A single laboratory is likely to have all of these types, and for this reason persons working in a laboratory should understand how the various balances work. Every laboratory should have some type of analytical balance and at least one other less sensitive type of balance. These are the minimum requirements for weighing devices.

Analytical Balance

Many different types of analytical balances are made by different companies and they have various degrees of automatic operation. In this discussion, analytical balances are divided into two types: manually operated (mechanical) analytical (Fig 4–5) and automatic or electronic analytical (Fig 4–6) balances. Each company that manufactures analytical balances has its own trade name for each of the analytical balances produced. Some of the fine analytical balances manufactured for use in the clinical laboratory are the Ainsworth, Voland, Christian-Becker, Mettler, Ohaus, and Sartorius balances. Others are also available. It is important to investigate carefully several different analytical balances before deciding on one for use in a particular laboratory.

General Principles of Analytical Balances

The basic principle in the quantitative measurement of mass is to balance an unknown mass (the substance being weighed) with a known mass. The analytical balance uses the basic concept of a simple lever or beam which pivots on a knife-edge fulcrum which is placed at the center of gravity of the lever. Using this principle, balances are designed in different ways.

In the traditional mechanical analytical balance, two pans of equal mass are suspended from the ends of the lever or beam and calibrated weights are placed on one pan to counterbalance an object of unknown mass on the other pan. A rider or chain weight device is utilized for fractional weights.

The electronic analytical balance is a single-pan balance that uses an electromagnetic force to counterbalance the load placed on the pan. This pan is mechanically connected to a coil which is suspended in the field of a permanent cylindrical electromagnet. When a load is placed on the pan, a force is produced which displaces the coil within the magnetic field. A photoelectric cell scanning device changes position and generates a current just sufficient in amount to return the coil to its original position; this is called *electromagnetic force compensation.* This current is proportional to the weight of the load on the pan and is displayed for the person using the

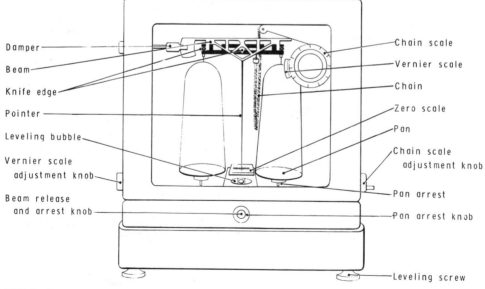

FIG 4–5.
Manual (mechanical) analytical balance.

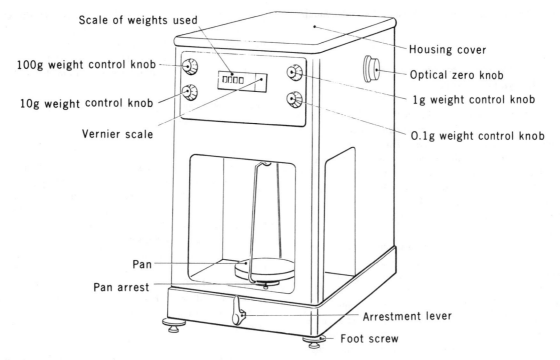

FIG 4–6.
Electronic analytical balance.

balance to see visually or it can be interfaced with a data output device. The greater the mass placed on the pan, the greater the deflecting force and the stronger the compensating current required to return the coil to its original position. There is a direct linear relationship between the compensation current and the force produced by the load placed on the pan. Electronic balances permit fast, accurate weighings with a high degree of resolution. They are easy to use and have replaced the traditional mechanically operated analytical balance in most clinical laboratories.

Uses for the Analytical Balance

All analytical balances are used to weigh very small amounts of substances with a high degree of accuracy, but how this is accomplished differs slightly from one balance to another. Some require little or no manual operation, and some are more time-consuming and require much more manipulation on the part of the operator.

Almost every procedure performed in the traditional clinical laboratory depends on the use of balances, the most important one being the analytical balance. Before any procedure is started, reagents and standard solutions are prepared. Standard solutions are always very accurately prepared, and the analytical balance is used to weigh the chemicals for these solutions. The analytical balance might be called the starting point of each method used in the laboratory. Its accuracy determines the accuracy of many clinical determinations. An instrument that is so sensitive and so essential must be made with great skill and treated very carefully by those using it.

The analytical balance should be cleaned and adjusted at least once a year to ensure its continued accuracy and sensitivity. Its accuracy is what makes this instrument so essential in the clinical laboratory. The accuracy to which most analytical balances used in the clinical laboratory should weigh chemicals is commonly 0.1 mg, or 0.0001 g. Whenever this accuracy is needed, the analytical balance must be used. Differences between electronic and manual analytical balances lie mainly in the manner in which the weights are added in the weighing procedure. In the manual balance the weights are actually placed on one of the balance pans by hand. In the electronic balance the weights are added by manipulating a series of dials.

General Rules for Weighing With an Analytical Balance

Weighing errors will occur if the balance is not properly positioned. It is therefore very important that the balance be located and mounted in an optimal position. The balance must be level. This is usually accomplished by adjusting the movable screws on the legs of the balance. The firmness of support is also important. The bench or table on which the balance rests must be rigid and free from vibrations. Preferably the room in which the balance is set up should have constant temperature and humidity. Ideally, the analytical balance should be in an air-conditioned room. The temperature factor is most important. The balance should not be placed near hot objects such as radiators, flames, stills, or electric ovens. Likewise, it should not be placed near cold objects, especially not near an open window. Sunlight or illumination from high-power lamps should be avoided in choosing a good location for the analytical balance.

The analytical balance is a delicate precision instrument, which will not function properly if abused. When learning to use an analytical balance, one should be responsible for knowing and adhering to the rules for the use of the particular balance being used. The following general rules apply:

1. Set up the balance where it will be free from vibration.
2. Load and unload the balance only when the pans are arrested; if the pans are not arrested, the delicate knife-edges can be damaged.
3. Close the balance case before observing the reading; any air currents present will affect the weighing process.
4. Never weigh any chemical directly on the pan; a container of some type must be used for the chemical.
5. Never place a hot object on the balance pan. If an object is warm, the weight determined will be too light because of convection currents set up by the rising heated air.
6. Whenever the shape of the object to be weighed permits, handle it with tongs or forceps. Round objects such as weighing bottles may be handled with the fingers, but take care to prevent weight changes caused by moisture from the hand. Do not hold any object longer than necessary.

7. On completion of weighing, remove all objects and clean up any chemical spilled on the pans or within the balance area. Close the balance case.
8. Weighed materials should be transferred to labeled containers or made into solutions immediately.

Speed in weighing is obtained only through practice. (Procedures 4–3 and 4–4).

Basic Parts of the Analytical Balance

It is essential that the parts of the analytical balance be thoroughly understood, so that the weighing process can be carried out to the degree of accuracy necessary. Once the correct use of an analytical balance has been mastered, one should be able to use any of the available types, as they all have the same basic parts. Each manufacturer supplies a complete manual of operating directions, as well as information on the general use and care of the balance, with each balance purchased. These directions should be followed. The following are parts common to most analytical balances, electronic or mechanical (manually operated):

1. *Glass enclosure*. The analytical balance is enclosed in glass to prevent currents of air and collection of dust from disturbing the process of weighing.
2. *Balancing screws*. Before doing any weighing on the balance, it must be properly leveled. This is done by observing the leveling bubbles, or spirit level, located near the bottom of the balance. If necessary, adjust the balancing screws located on the bottom of the balance case (usually found on each leg of the balance).
3. *Beam*. This is the structure from which the pans are suspended.
4. *Knife-edges*. These support the beam at the fulcrum during weighing and give sensitivity to the balance. Knife-edges are vital parts and are constructed of hard metals to give a minimum amount of friction.
5. *Pans for weighing*. In the manually operated analytical balance, there are two pans: the weights are placed on the right-hand pan and the object to be weighed is placed on the left-hand pan. In the electronic analytical balance, there is only one pan. The object to be weighed is placed on this pan. The pans are suspended from the ends of the beam.
6. *Weights*. In the manual balance, the weights are found in a separate weight box. These weights are never handled with the fingers but are removed from the box and placed on the balance pan by using ivory-tipped forceps. Mishandling of weights, either by using the fingers

---

Procedure 4–3. Weighing With a Manual (Mechanical) Analytical Balance

1. Sitting directly in front of the center of the balance, dust off the pans and the inside of the balance with a soft brush.
2. Check to see that the balance is level by observing the leveling bubbles. Make any necessary adjustment by means of the leveling screws on the legs of the balance.
3. To adjust the balance to a beginning reading of zero, lower the beam and release the pan arrests, making certain that the chain reading scale and the vernier scale are both set at zero. Note where the pointer comes to rest, and slowly move the chain until the pointer rests exactly at zero. Arrest the pans and raise and lock the beam. Recheck by repeating these same steps once again. The pointer should still rest exactly at zero. By use of the vernier scale adjustment knob, adjust the zero of the vernier scale to match the zero of the chain reading scale.
4. With the beam raised and locked and the pans arrested, place the weighing vessel on the left-hand pan, using tongs if possible.
5. From the box of weights provided with the balance, transfer the first weight to the right-hand pan, using the special forceps. Choose a rather large weight as the first weight: a 20-g weight would be satisfactory for most purposes. Lower the beam and release the pan arrests. Note where the pointer swings in relation to the zero point. If the pointer swings to the left, the weight is heavier than the vessel. If the pointer swings to the right, the weight is lighter than the vessel. Arrest the pans, and raise and lock the beam.
6. Depending on the direction of the pointer's swing in the previous step, either add another weight from the box of weights, or remove the 20-g weight and replace it with a lighter one (10 g). Repeat this process by adding and removing weights (being certain to raise and lock the beam and arrest the pans before each change of weights) until the addition of the smallest weight in the box (100 mg) causes the pointer to swing to the left. Close the balance window.
7. At this point add weight from the chain. The chain has a total weight of 100 mg and is used when no further weights from the box can be used. With the beam locked and the pans arrested, add 50 mg from the chain by moving the chain scale adjustment knob. Lower the beam and release the pans. Observe the pointer. Again, if the pointer swings to the left the chain weight is too light, and more weight must be added. Raise the beam and arrest the pans. Depending on the swing of the pointer, either add weight by moving the chain by 20-mg steps until the addition of 20 mg causes the pointer to swing to the left, or remove weight by 20-mg steps until the pointer swings to the right. When the chain weight has been narrowed down to within 10 mg of true balance, leave the beam lowered and the pans released, and gradually add or remove weight until balance is obtained. The weighing vessel has now been weighed, and the actual weighing of the desired chemical can commence. Record the weights used to obtain balance with the weighing vessel. To obtain the reading to the nearest 0.1 mg, the vernier scale (Fig 4–7) must be used in conjunction with the chain scale. Raise the beam and arrest the pans.
8. To the weight of the weighing vessel add the amount of chemical to be weighed. For example, if the weighing vessel weighs 35.5646 g and the amount of chemical to be weighed is 10.5555 g, the total weight is 46.1201 g. This total weight should be on the right-hand pan. To accomplish this, add the necessary weights from the box of weights and the chain scale to make up the difference.
9. Add the chemical in small amounts, using a clean spatula until balance is achieved. Before each addition of chemical raise the beam and arrest the pans. When balance is obtained, the amount of chemical has been weighed in the weighing vessel. Then transfer it quantitatively to a flask for dilution (see under Quantitative Transfer and Dilution of Chemicals for Reagent).
10. Return all weights to the box, return the chain to zero, and clean up any spilled chemical from the balance area. Leave the beam in a raised and locked position, and arrest the pans.

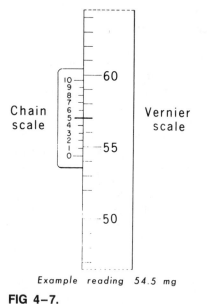

Chain scale

Vernier scale

Example reading 54.5 mg

FIG 4–7.
Reading obtained with a vernier scale.

or by dropping, can result in an alteration of the actual and true mass of the weight. Weights come in units ranging from a 50-g to a 100-mg weight. The values of the weights are stamped directly on top of them. In the electronic analytical balance, the weights are inside the instrument and are not seen by the operator unless there is need to remove the casing for repair or adjustment. The weights are added by manipulating specific dials calibrated for the weighing process. The built-in weights are on the same end of the beam as the sample pan and are counterbalanced by a fixed weight at the opposite end; they are removed from above the pan when an object is weighed. There is always a constant load on the beam, and the projected scale has the same weight regardless of the load. The total weight of an object is registered automatically by a digital counter or in conjunction with an optical scale.

7. *Pan arrest*. This is a means of arresting the pan so that sudden movement or addition of weights or chemical will not injure the delicate knife-edges. The pan arrests (usually found under the pans) can absorb any shock due to weight inequalities, so that the knife-edges are not subjected to this shock. The pan must be released to swing freely during actual weighing. In the electronic analytical balance the arresting mechanism for both the pan and the beam is operated by a single lever. Partial

---

Procedure 4–4. Weighing With an Electronic Analytical Balance

1. Before doing any weighing, make certain that the balance is properly leveled. Observe the spirit level (leveling bubble), and adjust the leveling screws on the legs of the balance if necessary.

2. To check the zero point adjustment, fully release the balance and turn the adjustment knob clockwise as far as it will go. The optical scale zero should indicate three divisions below zero on the vernier scale. Using the same adjustment knob, adjust the optical scale zero so that it aligns exactly with the zero line on the vernier scale. Arrest the balance.

3. With the balance arrested, place the weighing vessel on the pan, using tongs if possible, so that no humidity or heat is brought into the weighing chamber by the hands. Close the balance window.

4. Weigh the vessel in the following manner: Partially release the balance and turn the 100-g weight control knob clockwise. When the scale moves up, turn the knob back one step. Repeat this operation with the 10-g, 1.0-g, and 0.1-g knobs, in that order. Arrest the balance. After a short pause, release the balance, and allow the scale to come to rest. Read the result and arrest the balance. With the balance arrested, unload the pan and bring all knobs back to zero.

5. Add the weight of the sample desired to the weight of the vessel just weighed to get the total to be weighed. Set the knobs (100, 10, 1.0, and 0.1 g) to the correct total weight needed. When the 0.1-g knob has been set at its proper reading, the balance should be placed in partial release. Slowly add the chemical to the vessel until the optical scale begins to move downward. When the optical scale starts downward, fully release the beam, and continue to add the chemical until the optical scale registers the exact position desired. To obtain the reading to the nearest 0.1 mg (the sensitivity of most analytical balances), the vernier scale must be used in much the same manner as in the manual analytical balance readings.

6. With the balance arrested, unload the pan, and bring all the knobs back to zero. Clean up any spilled chemical in the balance area.

release or full release can be obtained, depending on how the lever is moved.

8. *Damping device*. This is necessary to arrest the swing of the beam in the shortest practical time, thus cutting down the time consumed in the weighing process.

9. *Vernier scale*. This is the small scale used to obtain precise readings to the nearest 0.1 mg. It is used in conjunction with the large reading scale to obtain the necessary readings.

10. *Reading scale*. In the manual analytical balance, this scale is actually the reading scale for the chain that is used for weighing 100 mg or less. It is used in conjunction with the vernier scale to obtain readings to the nearest 0.1 mg. In the electronic analytical balance, this is usually a lighted optical scale, giving a high magnification and sharp definition for easier reading. The total weight of the object in question is registered automatically on this viewing scale.

Torsion Balance

Torsion balances are mechanical and are used mainly for weighing chemicals in the laboratory. They are sensitive, responsive instruments with an exceptionally long service life, during which there is no significant deterioration in performance. In normal use, they require very little maintenance. The unique attribute of the torsion balance movement, which is assembled as a single flexible structure by means of highly tensed torsion bands of watch-spring alloy, is that the use of knife-edges, bearings, and other loose parts that would become dull, misaligned, and soiled is eliminated. Having no knife-edges to dull or other loose parts to be adjusted accounts for the popularity of the torsion balance. Little or no adjustment is required, and this is important in a laboratory, where time is important. (Procedure 4–5).

Use and Basic Parts

The torsion balance has high sensitivity under a heavy load, permits fast weighing, and is relatively inexpensive. Care must be taken to avoid overloading these balances. Some models have a dial-controlled torque spring to eliminate the use of smaller loose weights. Other models are offered with dial-controlled built-in weights, which may further reduce the number of loose weights required. Many weighing determinations can be completed in about one-fifth the time formerly required. A sliding tare weight is provided to counterbalance the weighing vessel used. The beam is operated by a lever on the balance case. Some torsion balances are enclosed completely in glass or metal cases. Several of these balances have a damping feature, which brings the balance to equilibrium quickly. One such damping device is an oil dashpot, which is filled at the factory with silicon oil. Weighing can be done more rapidly on torsion balances with damping devices than on those lacking them.

There is usually a means by which the torsion balance can be arrested. This need only be done when the balance is to be moved to a new location or otherwise transported.

The sensitivity of the torsion balance varies with the model chosen. For most clinical laboratories, however, balances with a sensitivity of readings to the nearest 0.01 g are satisfactory. The manufacturer supplies a complete manual with directions for setting up, proper use, and care of the particular torsion balance. These directions should be followed closely.

Procedure 4–5. Weighing With a Torsion Balance

1. Check to be sure that the balance is level, and adjust the leveling screws if necessary.
2. Check the zero adjustment. The optical reading scale should read zero with the pan empty and clean; adjust the optical zero with the small control knob if necessary.
3. Place the weighing vessel on the pan. Turn the weight control knob until the optical reading scale reads zero.
4. Add the chemical to the vessel until the desired weight registers on the optical scale. A vernier scale is present on most models so that the weight may be read to the accuracy needed. Torsion balances used in clinical laboratories have an accuracy of either 0.1 or 0.01 g.
5. Remove the vessel with the weighed chemical from the pan. Turn the control knob to zero, and wipe up any spilled chemical immediately.

Top-Loading Balance

A single-pan top-loading balance is one of the most commonly used balances in the laboratory. It is usually electronic and is self-balancing. It is much faster and easier to use than some of the balances described above. A substance can be weighed in just a few seconds. These balances are usually modified torsion or substitution balances. Top-loading balances are used when the substance being weighed does not require as much analytic precision, as when reagents of a large volume are being prepared.

Triple-Beam Balance

Another common piece of laboratory apparatus used for weighing is the triple-beam or "trip" balance (Fig 4–8). This mechanical balance is less sensitive, with an accuracy to the nearest 0.1 g. Whenever reagents are to be prepared with an accuracy of 0.1 g or less, the triple-beam balance can be used. As the words *triple-beam* and *trip* suggest, three beams are present on the balance. Each beam provides a different weighing scale. Scales reading from 0 to 100 g, 0 to 500 g, and 0 to 10 g are usually provided on the triple-beam balance. These scales are provided with movable weights. The two larger scales have weights that lock into accurately milled notches at each calibration to ensure absolute accuracy at each position.

Some models of the triple-beam balance (called the *Harvard triple-beam* balance) have two pans, and some have a single pan. The principle of the weighing process is the same whether there are two pans or only one. Two-pan balances are used when two objects must be balanced against each other, as in balancing tubes for use in the centrifuge. One-pan balances are used a great deal in the laboratory for preparing reagents and chemical solutions.

A special type of triple-beam balance is known as the *Cent-O-Gram* balance. This balance also has three beams, but they are tiered on three levels, so that the readings can be obtained from a single eye level. The three beams on the Cent-O-Gram provide different weighing scales. The center beam is graduated to 10 g in 1-g notches. As the name implies, the sensitivity of this balance is to the nearest 0.01 g. The Cent-O-Gram balance has a lever for arresting the balance when placing objects on the pan.

On any type of triple-beam balance, the balance position of an object on the pan can be determined by observing the swing of the pointer. A swing of an equal number of divisions on either side of the zero mark on the dial indicates that the scale is balanced. It is not necessary to wait for the oscillation to stop to determine the correct weight. This observation enables the weighing process to be simple and rapid. (Procedure 4–6).

Use and Basic Parts

Some type of less sensitive balance such as the triple-beam or torsion balance is an essential piece of equipment for every clinical laboratory, as many reagents are prepared that do not need the accuracy of the analytical balance. When an accuracy of more than 0.1 g is not needed, the triple-beam balance can be used. It can

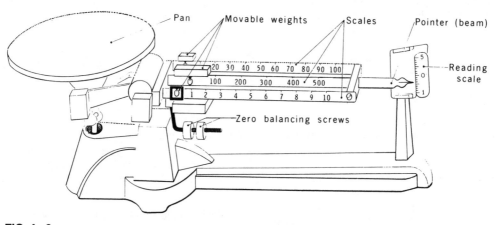

FIG 4–8.
Triple-beam balance.

be operated simply and rapidly and gives accurate weighings when used properly. Even a balance with less sensitivity must be used carefully and according to the directions provided with the particular model.

The triple-beam balance should be placed on a reasonably flat and level surface. The beam should be near zero balance, with all the movable weights at their zero points. A final zero balance is attained by adjusting the balancing screws. It is advisable to check the zero balance periodically, especially if the balance has been moved. If an object is to be weighed, the balance must be set at zero before the weighing is begun. If a vessel is weighed in preparation for the addition of a chemical, it is not necessary to set the balance at the exact zero reading.

Parts basic to triple-beam balances are:

1. *Pan*. This is where the object or weighing vessel holding the substance to be weighed is placed.

2. *Beam*. The beam is a lever supported by a knife plane bearing at the center post. The length of beam to the right of the knife plane is graduated for placement of a sliding weight and ends in a pointer. The other end of the beam is attached to the pan guide with a knife-edge contact.

3. *Movable weights or poises*. These are sliding weights attached to the beam that are moved to bring the balance into equilibrium. The trip balance has three beams, and various weight increments are added as the poises are advanced toward the pointer ends of the beams.

4. *Reading scale*. This is a scale located at the end of the beam pointer that shows when the balance is in equilibrium.

5. *Balancing screws or spindle*. This is a pair of threaded weights that are used to bring the empty balance into equilibrium.

Measurement of Volume: Pipetting and Titration

PIPETTING

Pipettes—An Overview and Uses

Pipettes are a type of volumetric glassware used extensively in the laboratory. Many kinds are available. Care and discretion should be used in selecting pipettes for clinical laboratory use, since their accuracy is one of the determining factors in the accuracy of the procedures carried out. A pipette is a cylindrical glass tube used in measuring fluids. It is calibrated to deliver, or transfer, a specified volume from one vessel to another.

Pipettes used in volumetric measurement in the laboratory must be free from all grease and dirt. For that reason, a special analytic cleaning solution is used. For a description of cleaning solutions, see Cleaning Laboratory Glassware and Plasticware.

Since the accuracy of laboratory determinations depends to such a large extent on the equipment used and since pipetting is a principal means of volume measurement, it is imperative that any pipettes used in the clinical laboratory be of the finest quality and be manufactured and calibrated by a reputable company. Care and discretion should be used in the selection of laboratory pipettes whether manual or automatic.

Several types of pipettes are used commonly in the

Procedure 4–6. Weighing With a Triple-Beam Balance

1. Place the weighing vessel on the balance pan without previously bringing the balance to zero.
2. With the weighing vessel on the pan, bring the balance to zero by adjusting the movable weights on the three scales. Record the sum of the weights required for balance.
3. To the recorded weight add the amount of chemical to be weighed. For example, if the reagent to be prepared requires 10.5 g of NaCl and the weighing vessel weighs 35.5 g, the total weight is 46.0 g. Move the movable weights on the scales to give this total weight.
4. Gradually add the chemical until the pointer of the balance rests exactly at the zero mark on the vertical reading scale. Remove the weighing vessel and return the movable weights to their zero positions. Transfer the chemical quantitatively to the flask for dilution.
5. Wipe up any spilled chemical immediately from the balance area.

laboratory. It is necessary that their uses be understood and experience in how to handle them in clinical determinations be gained (see Pipettes under Laboratory Glassware and Plasticware). Practice, again, is the key to success in the use of laboratory pipettes; only through practice will anyone become proficient in pipetting.

There are two categories of manual pipettes: to-contain (TC) and to-deliver (TD). TC pipettes are calibrated to contain a specified amount of liquid but are not necessarily calibrated to deliver that exact amount. A small amount of fluid will cling to the inside wall of the TC pipette, and when these pipettes are used, they should be rinsed out with a diluting fluid to ensure that the entire contents have been emptied. TD pipettes are calibrated to deliver the amount of fluid designated on the pipette; this volume will flow out of the pipette by gravity when the pipette is held in a vertical position with its tip against the inside wall of the receiving vessel. A small amount of fluid will remain in the tip of the pipette; this amount is to be left in the tip as the calibrated portion has been delivered into the receiving vessel. There is another category of pipette, called *blowout*. The calibration of these pipettes is similar to that of TD pipettes, except that the drop remaining in the tip of the pipette must be blown out into the receiving vessel. If a pipette is to be blown out, an etched ring will be seen near the suction opening (see discussion of serologic and Ostwald pipettes above). A mechanical device must be used to blow out the entire contents of the pipette.

Pipetting Technique Using Manual Pipettes

It is important to develop a good technique for handling pipettes (Fig 4–9). It is only through practice that this is accomplished, however (Procedure 4–7). With few exceptions, the same general steps apply to pipetting with any of the manual pipettes described under Laboratory Glassware and Plasticware.

General Considerations in Pipetting With Manual Pipettes

Laboratory accidents frequently result from improper pipetting techniques. The greatest potential hazard is when mouth pipetting is done instead of mechanical suction. Caustic reagents, contaminated specimens, or poisonous solutions are all pipetted at one time or another in the laboratory, and every precaution must be

---

Procedure 4–7. Pipetting With Manual Pipettes

1. Check the pipette to ascertain its correct size, being careful also to check for broken delivery or suction tips.
2. Wearing protective gloves, hold the pipette lightly between the thumb and the last three fingers, leaving the index finger free.
3. Place the tip of the pipette well below the surface of the liquid to be pipetted.
4. Using mechanical suction or an aspirator bulb, carefully draw the liquid up into the pipette until the level of liquid is well above the calibration mark.
5. Quickly cover the suction opening at the top of the pipette with the index finger.
6. Wipe the outside of the pipette dry with a piece of gauze or tissue to remove excess fluid.
7. Hold the pipette in a vertical position with the delivery tip against the inside of the original vessel. Carefully allow the liquid in the pipette to drain by gravity until the *bottom of the meniscus* is exactly at the calibration mark. (The meniscus is the concave or convex surface of a column of liquid as seen in a laboratory pipette, buret, or other measuring device.) To do this, do not entirely remove the index finger from the suction-hole end of the pipette, but, by rolling the finger slightly over the opening, allow a slow drainage to take place.
8. While still holding the pipette in a vertical position, touch the tip of the pipette to the inside wall of the receiving vessel. Remove the index finger from the top of the pipette to permit free drainage. Remember to keep the pipette in a vertical position for correct drainage. In TD pipettes, a small amount of fluid will remain in the delivery tip.
9. To be certain that the drainage is as complete as possible, touch the delivery tip of the pipette to another area on the inside wall of the receiving vessel.
10. Remove the pipette from the receiving vessel and place it in the appropriate place for washing (see under Cleaning Laboratory Glassware and Plasticware).

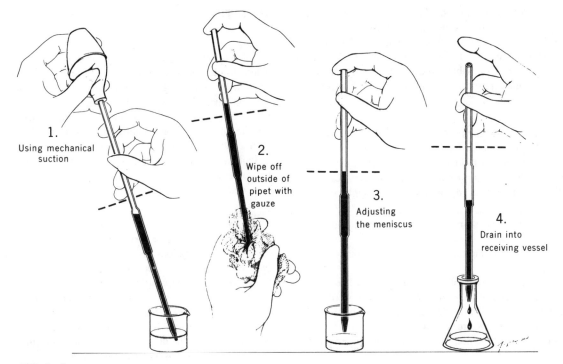

FIG 4–9.
Pipetting technique.

taken to ensure the safety of the person doing the work (see Chapter 1).

After the pipette has been filled above the top graduation mark, removed from the vessel, and held in a vertical position, the meniscus must be adjusted. The pipette should be held in such a way that the calibration mark is at eye level. The delivery tip is touched to the *inside wall* of the original vessel, not the liquid, and the meniscus of the liquid in the pipette is eased, or adjusted, down to the calibration mark.

When clear solutions are used, the bottom of the meniscus is read. For colored or viscous solutions, the top of the meniscus is read. All readings must be made with the eye at the level of the meniscus (Fig 4–10).

Before the measured liquid in the pipette is allowed to drain into the receiving vessel, any liquid adhering to the outside of the pipette must be wiped off with a clean piece of gauze or tissue. If this is not done, any drops present on the outside of the pipette might drain into the receiving vessel along with the measured volume. This would make the volume greater than that specified, and an error would result.

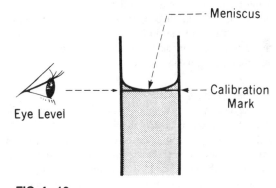

FIG 4–10.
Reading the meniscus.

Pipetting Technique Using Automatic Pipettes

Automatic pipettes allow fast, repetitive measurement and delivery of solutions of equal volumes. There are several commercially available types of automatic pipettes, either of the sampling type or of the sampling-diluting type (see Automatic Measuring Devices under

Laboratory Glassware and Plasticware). The sampling types are mechanically operated and use a piston-operated plunger. These are adjustable so that varying amounts of reagent or sample can be delivered with the same device. Disposable and exchangeable tips are available for these pipettes. Automatic pipettes must be calibrated before use.

Micropipettors

Micropipettors contain or deliver from 1 to 500 μL. It is important to follow the manufacturer's instructions for the device being used as each one may be slightly different. In general, the following steps apply:

1. Attach the proper tip to the pipettor and set the delivery volume.
2. Depress the piston to a stop position on the pipettor.
3. Place the tip into the solution and allow the piston to slowly rise back to its original position (this fills the pipettor tip with the desired volume of solution).
4. Some tips are wiped with a dry gauze at this step, and some are not. Follow the manufacturer's directions.
5. Place the tip on the wall of the receiving vessel and depress the piston, first to a stop position where the liquid is allowed to drain, and then to a second stop position where the full dispensing of the liquid takes place.
6. Dispose of the tip in the waste disposal receptacle. Some pipettors automatically eject the used tips, thus minimizing biohazard exposure.

Repipettors

Several types of repipettors or dispensers are available which allow repeated volumes of a specific reagent to be delivered to a solution or receiving vessel. These devices are useful for serial dispensing of relatively small volumes of the same liquid. The volume to be dispensed is set on the pipettor dispenser device which generally is attached by tubing to a reagent bottle containing the reagent to be dispensed. The dispenser consists of a plunger, a valve system, and the dispensing tip. Once the dispensing device is primed with liquid, pressing on the plunger allows the selected volume of liquid to be dispensed into the receiving vessel. When the plunger returns to the original position, usually by means of a spring-activated device, the dispenser chamber is refilled with the liquid being measured.

TITRATION

Titration is a method of quantitative analysis, a volumetric technique measuring the concentration of one solution by comparing it with a measured volume of a solution whose concentration is known. If the concentration of a solution is unknown, it can be found by measuring the volume of the unknown solution that will react with a measured amount of the solution of known concentration (called a standard solution). This process is known as titration.

Use

In the clinical laboratory, titration is used to determine the concentrations of acids and bases, as the analytic tool for certain laboratory procedures with body fluids, and in the preparation of some reagents.

This technique is often used to determine the concentration of an unknown acid or an unknown base by means of comparison with a known base or a known acid. In this case the quantity of hydronium ions that react with hydroxyl ions to form water is measured. However, numerous reactions, other than the neutralization reaction between an acid and a base, are used in titrations to determine the concentration of a solution.

The titration technique has numerous other uses in the clinical laboratory. It is the means of checking the concentrations of new reagents before they are used in the clinical laboratory. When weaker acids or bases are prepared from more concentrated solutions, the actual normality of the new solution must be determined by titration. (Procedure 4–8).

Expression of Normality or Equivalents

When titration is used to determine concentration, the concentration is traditionally expressed in terms of normality or equivalents. Normality is employed because it is a unit that provides a basis for direct comparison of strength for all solutions. Normality is the number of gram-equivalents per liter of solution. A gram-equivalent is the amount of a compound that will liberate, combine with, or replace one gram-atom of hydrogen. Therefore, 1 equivalent of any compound will react with exactly 1 equivalent of any other compound. For example, 1 equivalent of any acid will exactly neutralize 1 equivalent of any base. It is very convenient to have laboratory solutions of such concentrations that any chosen volume of one reagent reacts with an equal volume of another reagent. The system of equivalents or equivalent weights provides this useful tool. The equivalent weight of a substance is calculated by dividing the gram-molecular weight of the substance by the sum of the positive valences. A solution that contains 1 gram-equivalent weight of substance in 1 L of solution is called a normal (1N) solution (see Chapter 6).

Essential Components for Titration

In any titration procedure there are certain components that must always be present: (1) a standard solution of known concentration, (2) an accurately measured volume of the standard solution or unknown, (3) an indicator to show when the reaction has reached completion, and (4) a buret (or similar device) to measure the volume of solution required to reach the end point.

Standard Solutions

Standard solutions of a desired normality may be prepared by weighing on the analytical balance the exact amount of substance calculated to give that normality, dissolving this in a small amount of deionized water, and then diluting the solution to the number of liters required in the original calculation. Standard solutions prepared in this way (by direct weighing on the analytical balance) are known as primary standards. The chemical substances used in the preparation of standard solutions must be pure, must have a high molecular weight, and must not take up or give off moisture. Oxalic acid meets these requirements and is often used as a primary standard. A solution of hydrochloric acid prepared from constant-boiling HCl is also often used as a primary standard. Bases are not often used as primary standards because they take up moisture when exposed to the air, which makes the measurement inaccurate.

Indicator for Reaction

The point at which equal concentrations of the standard and the unknown are present is called the *end point* of the titration. In the case of acid-base titrations, the end point is where neutralization occurs. Various means of detecting the end point are used, depending on the procedure. Sometimes the formation of a precipitate indicates that the end point has been reached. A change in color of one of the reacting solutions can also indicate the end point. The most common method of detecting the end point is through the use of an indicator solution. An indicator solution is a third solution added in the titration procedure (in addition to the standard solution and the unknown solution). The indicator solution is added in measured amounts to the titration flask. Most indicators are solids dissolved in water or alcohol. Phenolphthalein (0.1%) is commonly used as the indicator in acid-base titrations. Phenolphthalein is made up in a solution of alcohol. It is generally best to arrange the titration procedure so that one titrates from a colorless solution to the first sign of a permanent color rather than from a colored to a colorless solution. Phenolphthalein is colorless in an acid solution and red in an alkaline solution. When one is near the end point, the addition of a single drop from the buret may overrun the true end point considerably. This can cause significant error in the titration of small amounts of solutions. To avoid this *drop error,* the titrating solution should be added in split drops as the end point approaches. It is possible to control the flow from the buret with careful manipulation of the stopcock so that only part of a drop goes into the titration flask.

Burets

The device that is most often employed to measure the volume required to reach completion of the reaction in a particular titration procedure is the buret. The buret is basically a graduated pipette with a stopcock near the delivery tip to facilitate better control and delivery of the solution (Fig 4–11). Burets may be obtained in many different capacities and tolerances. The particular buret capacity and tolerance used in a particular procedure will be determined by the degree of accuracy that is desired. To ensure that the buret used is employed with maximum accuracy, a very specific technique or procedure must be followed. Mastery of this technique will come only with practice. It is essential that chemically clean, well-calibrated volumetric equipment be used throughout the procedure to ensure reliable results (see Burets under Laboratory Glassware and Plasticware).

Calculations

To find the concentration of a solution, the following information must be available: a standard solution of known concentration, the volume of the standard solution, and the volume of the undetermined solution re-

---

Procedure 4–8. Titration

---

1. Use the buret clamp to fasten the buret, which must be clean and free from chips or cracks, to the buret stand, which will support it during the titration procedure. Fasten the clamp to the stand about halfway up the rod.

2. Grease the buret stopcock lightly. The stopcock should turn easily and smoothly, but an excess of lubricant will plug the stopcock capillary bore and prevent emptying of the buret. To grease a clean stopcock properly, apply a bit of grease with the fingertip down the two sides of the stopcock away from the capillary bore. Then insert the stopcock in the buret and rotate it until a smooth covering of the whole stopcock is obtained. If the buret is equipped with a Teflon plug, the stopcock need not be lubricated.

3. Rinse the buret with the titrant. In the case of an acid-base titration with phenolphthalein as the indicator, the titrant (or solution to be added and measured by means of the buret) will always be the base. In rinsing the buret, fill it completely with the titrant, and then let it drain. Discard the rinse solution. Fill the buret slowly and carefully to prevent air bubbles from forming in the narrow buret tube. It is essential that the buret be absolutely clean if the results are to be accurate. A clean buret will drain without any solution clinging to its sides; if the buret is dirty, there will be droplets of liquid clinging to the sides. After rinsing the buret several times with the titrant solution, fill it past the zero mark, and then bring the meniscus exactly to the zero mark by draining, using the stopcock to control the flow (see Fig 4–11).

4. Into an Erlenmeyer flask, pipette the stated amount of the second solution to be employed in the titration. Pipette this solution with a volumetric pipette, using great care to ensure maximal accuracy.

5. Add the required amount of the indicator solution employed to show when the titration reaction has reached completion. (At this point, approximately 5 to 10 mL of water is often added to the Erlenmeyer flask to dilute the indicator and make the end point more visible. The volume of this diluent is not critical, since it does not enter into the reaction or affect the volumes of the solutions that are being titrated.)

6. Titrate each flask in the following manner:

   a. Inspect the buret to be sure that there are no air bubbles trapped in the capillary tube or tip. Air bubbles will add to the apparent volume required to reach the end point, leading to erroneous results. If bubbles are present, drain the buret and refill it with the titrant until there are no bubbles.

   b. Inspect to see that the meniscus is exactly at zero, or record the actual buret reading immediately before beginning the titration.

   c. Add the solution in the buret to the flask by rotating the stopcock carefully. A right-handed person encircles the buret stopcock with the left hand, using the right hand to swirl the flask during the titration (see Fig 4–11). This will be awkward at first, but when mastered it will become natural.

   d. With the buret tip well within the titration flask, the titrant may be added fairly rapidly at first, but as the reaction nears completion, the titrant is added drop by drop and finally by only portions of drops (split drops). Clues that the reaction is nearing completion depend on the particular reaction and indicator being employed. In the case of an acid-base titration with phenolphthalein as the indicator, there is a change from a colorless to a red solution. The phenolphthalein is colorless in acid solutions and red in alkaline solutions. In the neutralization reaction itself hydronium ions react with hydroxyl ions to form water. The reaction begins with an excess of hydronium ions in the Erlenmeyer flask, and the titration is performed until all the hydronium ions have been neutralized by the hydroxyl ions added from the buret. The titration should be stopped at the actual point of neutralization, or as close to it as possible.

   In practice, a pink color will appear when the alkali is added to the acid. This color will disappear on shaking. As the titration nears

Continued.

completion, the pink color will remain for a longer time. The base is then added slowly, by split drops, until a faint pink color remains. When the pink color no longer disappears but remains for more than 30 seconds, the end point (or neutralization) has been achieved. It is essential that any titration, using any indicator, be stopped at the actual end point, which is the first faint but permanent color change, or the results will be inaccurate.

e. Immediately on reaching the end point, record the buret reading. Be sure to record a figure that is significant considering the tolerance of the particular buret being used.

7. Clean the buret by rinsing thoroughly with tap water and then with deionized water. Remove any grease from the stopcock with ether. The titrant should not be left standing in the buret. Alkali will "freeze" the stopcock to the buret, and the concentration of the titrant will increase because of evaporation. When the buret is clean, it can be stored either in an inverted position on the buret clamp or in an upright position filled with deionized water.

8. Use the buret readings obtained in the titration procedure to determine the concentration of the unknown solution.

quired to reach completion in the particular reaction. As mentioned previously, the concentration is usually expressed in terms of normality, which permits direct comparison of solutions. Normality is the number of gram-equivalents per liter of solution, or milliequivalents per milliliter of solution. However, in practice, 1 L of a solution is rarely used; instead, parts of 1 L are used. Therefore, the number of equivalents is actually the normality of the solution times the volume that is used in the titration. All the ingredients required for the equation to determine the concentration of a solution in any titration are now present. If the equivalents of solution 1 are equal to the equivalents of solution 2, and if the number of equivalents of a particular solution is actually the normality of the solution times the volume, it follows that the normality of solution 1 times the volume of solution 1 is equal to the normality of solution 2 times the volume of solution 2. Or in equation form:

Equivalents of solution 1

$$= \text{equivalents of solution 2}$$

or

$$N_1 \times V_1 = N_2 \times V_2$$

In the case of a typical acid-base titration, assume that 2 mL of a standard 0.1000N HCl solution required 1.50 mL of NaOH, added from a buret, to reach the first permanent pink color. What is the normality of NaOH?

$$N_{acid} \times V_{acid} = N_{base} \times V_{base}$$

$$0.1000N \times 2 \text{ mL} = N_{base} \times 1.50 \text{ mL}$$

$$N_{base} = \frac{0.1000N \times 2 \text{ mL}}{1.50 \text{ mL}} = 0.1333$$

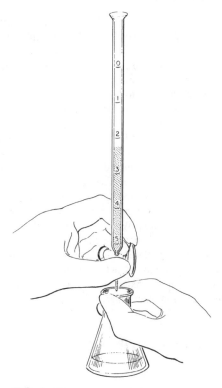

FIG 4–11.
Method of manual titration.

That is, the normality of the sodium hydroxide is 0.1333.

General Considerations for Titration

Chemically clean, well-calibrated volumetric equipment, including flasks, pipettes, and burets, must be used in every titration procedure. Accurately prepared standard solutions are essential for accurate results. These are weighed analytically and diluted volumetrically. Indicators must be employed to show when the particular reaction has reached completion. These are often color indicators, which change from colorless to a faint permanent color when the reaction has reached completion. However, such instruments as pH meters may also be employed, where the end point is a particular hydronium ion concentration as recorded on the pH meter (see under pH in Chapter 13).

Acid-Base Titration

In acid-base titrations in the clinical laboratory, the most commonly used alkali is 0.1N sodium hydroxide (NaOH). This is relatively stable and can be used to determine the concentration of an acid. However, NaOH is not absolutely stable and it should be checked daily against a standard acid to be considered reliable.

The acids most commonly used in titration are oxalic acid, hydrochloric acid (HCl), sulfuric acid (H_2SO_4), and nitric acid (HNO_3). A 0.1N solution of HCl made from constant-boiling HCl may be used as the reference, or primary standard, in the clinical laboratory. Constant-boiling HCl is obtained by distillation and collection of the constant-boiling mixture. The constant-boiling acid is then weighed on an analytical balance and diluted volumetrically. When prepared in this manner, using constant-boiling acid weighed analytically, the primary standard 0.1000N HCl is accurate within ±0.0004. Further standardization is not necessary. The acid standard prepared in this manner is used for the standardization of alkalis and other reagents.

Laboratory Centrifuges

Centrifugation is used in the separation of a solid material from a liquid by application of increased gravitational force by rapid rotating or spinning. It is also used in recovering solid materials from suspensions, as in the microscopic examination of urine. The solid material or sediment packed at the bottom of the centrifuge tube is sometimes called the precipitate, and the liquid or top portion is called the supernatant. Another important use for the centrifuge is in the separation of serum or plasma from cells in blood specimens. The suspended particles, solid material, or blood cells usually collect at the bottom of the centrifuge tube because the particles are heavier than the liquid. Occasionally the particles are lighter than the liquid and will collect on the surface of the liquid when centrifuged. Centrifugation is employed in many areas of the clinical laboratory, in chemistry, urinalysis, hematology, and blood banking, among others. Proper use of the centrifuge is important for anyone engaged in laboratory work.

TYPES OF CENTRIFUGES

Centrifuges facilitate the separation of particles in suspension by the application of centrifugal force. Several types of centrifuges will usually be found in the same laboratory, each designed for special uses. There are table-model and floor-model centrifuges, some small and others very large; there are refrigerated centrifuges, ultracentrifuges, cytocentrifuges, and other centrifuges adapted for special procedures.

Two traditional types of centrifuges are used in doing routine laboratory determinations. One is a conventional horizontal centrifuge and the other is a fixed angle-head centrifuge. For the horizontal-type centrifuge, the cups holding the tubes of material to be centrifuged occupy a vertical position when the centrifuge is at rest, but assume a horizontal position when the centrifuge revolves. For the angle-head centrifuge, the cups are held in a rigid position at a fixed angle. This position makes the process of centrifuging more rapid than it is with the horizontal centrifuge. There is also less chance that the sediment will be disturbed when the centrifuge stops. Both types of centrifuge may be purchased as table or floor models.

A cytocentrifuge utilizes a very high torque and a low inertia motor to rapidly spread monolayers of cells across a special slide for critical morphologic studies. This type of preparation can be used for blood, urine, body fluid, or any other liquid specimen that can be spread on a slide. An advantage of this technology is that only a small amount of sample is used producing evenly distributed cells which can then be stained for microscopic study. The slide produced can be saved and examined at a later time, in comparison with "wet" preparations which must be examined immediately.

Refrigerated centrifuges are available with internal refrigeration temperatures ranging from -15 to $-25°$ C during centrifugation. This permits centrifugation at higher speeds while protecting the specimens from the heat that is generated by the rotors of the centrifuge. The temperature of any refrigerated centrifuge should be checked regularly and the thermometers checked periodically for accuracy.

CENTRIFUGE SPEED

Directions for use of a centrifuge are most frequently given in terms of speed, or revolutions per minute. The number of revolutions per minute (rpm) and the centrifugal force generated is expressed as **relative centrifugal force (RCF)**. The number of revolutions per minute is related to the relative centrifugal force by the following formula:

$$RCF = 1.12 \times 10^{-5} \times r \times (rpm)^2$$

where r is the radius of the centrifuge expressed in centimeters. This is equal to the distance from the center of the centrifuge head to the bottom of the tube holder in the centrifuge bucket.

General laboratory centrifuges operate at speeds of up to 6,000 rpm, generating RCF up to 7,300 times the force of gravity (g). The top speed of most conventional centrifuges is about 3,000 rpm. Conventional laboratory centrifuges of the horizontal type attain speeds of up to 3,000 rpm—about 1,700 g—without excessive heat production caused by friction between the head of the centrifuge and the air. Angle-head centrifuges produce less heat and may attain speeds of 7,000 rpm (about 9,000 g).

The microhematocrit centrifuge used in many hematology laboratories for packing red blood cells attains a speed of about 10,000 to 15,000 rpm with an RCF of up to 14,000 g. Ultracentrifuges are generally used for research projects, but for certain clinical uses, a small air-driven ultracentrifuge is available which operates at

90,000 to 100,000 rpm and generates a maximum RCF of 178,000 g.

A rheostat is used to set the desired speed; the setting on the rheostat dial does not necessarily correspond directly to revolutions per minute. The setting speeds on the rheostat can also change with variations in weight load and general aging of the centrifuge.

The College of American Pathologists recommends that the number of revolutions per minute for a centrifuge used in chemistry laboratories be checked every 3 months. This periodic check can most easily be done by using a photoelectric tachometer or strobe tachometer. Timers and speed controls must also be checked on a periodic basis with any corrections posted near the controls for the centrifuge.

USE OF CENTRIFUGES

A primary use for centrifuges in clinical laboratories is to process blood specimens. Separation of cells or clotted blood from plasma or serum is done on an ongoing basis in the handling and processing of the many specimens needed for the various divisions of the clinical laboratory. The relative centrifugal force is not critical for the separation of serum from clot for most laboratory determinations and a force of at least 1,000 g for 10 minutes will usually give a good separation. When serum separator collection tubes are used that contain a silicon gel needing displacement up the side of the tube, a greater centrifugal force is needed to displace this gel— 1,000 to 1,300 g for 10 minutes. An RCF less than 1,000 g may result in an incomplete displacement of the gel. It is always important to follow the manufacturer's directions when using special collection tubes or serum separator devices. These may require different conditions for centrifugation (see Processing Blood for Serum and Serum Separator Devices in Chapter 2).

In the hematology laboratory, a table-top version of the centrifuge has been specially adapted for determination of microhematocrit values. This centrifuge accelerates rapidly to a force of about 12,000 g and can be stopped in seconds. Centrifugation is needed to prepare urinary sediment for microscopic examination. The urine specimen is centrifuged, the supernatant decanted, and the remaining sediment examined. Refrigerated centrifuges are utilized in the blood bank and for other temperature-sensitive laboratory procedures. Ultracentrifuges, which can generate G forces in the hundreds of thousands, are used in laboratories where tissue receptor assays and other assays requiring high-speed centrifugation are needed.

Technical Factors in Using Centrifuges

The most important rule to remember in using any centrifuge is: *Always balance the tubes placed in the centrifuge.* That is, in the centrifuge cup opposite the material to be centrifuged, place a container of equivalent size and shape with an equal volume of liquid of the same specific gravity as the load. For most laboratory determinations, water may be placed in the balance load.

Tubes being centrifuged must be capped. Open tubes of blood should never be centrifuged because of the risk of aerosol spread of infection (see under Protection from Aerosols in Chapter 1). Aerosols produced from the heat and vibration generated during the centrifugation process can increase the risk of infection to the laboratory personnel. Some evaporation of the sample can occur during centrifugation in uncapped specimen tubes.

Special centrifuge tubes can be used. These are tubes constructed to withstand the force exerted by the centrifuge. They have thicker glass walls or are made of a stronger, more resistant glass. Some of these tubes are conical, and some have round bottoms. Some are disposable and others must be washed.

Before placing the centrifuge tubes in the cups or holders, check the cups to make certain that the rubber cushions are in place. If some cushions are missing, the centrifuge will not be properly balanced. Without the cushions, the tubes are more likely to break.

Whenever a tube breaks in the centrifuge cup, it is most important that both the cup and the rubber cushion in the cup be cleaned well to prevent further breakage by glass particles left behind.

Covers specially made for the centrifuge should be used except in certain specified instances. Using the cover prevents possible danger from aerosol spread and from flying glass should tubes break in the centrifuge. Keep the centrifuge cover closed at all times, even when not using the machine. In addition to the danger from broken glass, using the centrifuge without the cover in

place may cause the revolving parts of the centrifuge to vibrate, which causes excessive wear of the machine.

Do not try to stop the centrifuge with your hands. It is generally best to let the machine stop by itself. A brake may be applied if the centrifuge is equipped with one. The brake should be used with caution, as braking may cause some resuspension of the sediment. Many laboratories discourage use of the brake except where it is evident that a tube or tubes have broken in the centrifuge.

Centrifuges should be checked, cleaned, and lubricated regularly to ensure proper operation.

BIBLIOGRAPHY

Commission on Laboratory Inspection and Accreditation: *Reagent Water Specifications.* Chicago, College of American Pathologists, 1985.

Henry JB (ed): *Clinical Diagnosis and Management by Laboratory Methods,* ed 18. Philadelphia, WB Saunders Co, 1991.

International System of Units. Washington, DC, National Bureau of Standards, 1972, special publication No. 330.

Kaplan LA, Pesce AJ: *Clinical Chemistry Theory, Analysis, and Correlation,* ed. 2. St Louis, Mosby–Year Book, Inc, 1989.

National Bureau of Standards: *Standard Reference Materials, Summary of the Clinical Laboratory Standards.* Washington, DC, US Department of Commerce, 1981, NBS special publication.

National Bureau of Standards: *Testing of Glass Volumetric Apparatus.* Washington, DC, US Department of Commerce, 1959, NBS Circ 602.

Preparation and Testing of Reagent Water in the Clinical Laboratory, Tentative Guidelines, ed 2. Villanova, Pa, National Committee for Clinical Laboratory Standards. 1988; 8(December) C3-T2.

Quantities and Units: SI, Committee Report, Villanova, Pa, National Committee for Clinical Laboratory Standards. 1983; 3(March):C11-CR.

Tietz NW (ed.): *Fundamentals of Clinical Chemistry,* ed 3. Philadelphia, WB Saunders Co, 1987.

Tietz NW (ed): *Textbook of Clinical Chemistry,* Philadelphia, WB Saunders Co, 1986.

5 Photometry (Including Absorbance Spectrophotometry and Flame Emission Photometry)

Key Terms	
Absorbance spectrophotometry	Percent transmittance units
Absorbed light	Photoelectric cell
Beer's law	Photometry
Cuvettes	Spectrophotometers or colorimeters
Flame emission photometry	Standard solutions
Galvonometer	Transmitted light
Internal standard	Visual colorimeter
Optical density (OD)	Wavelength of light

ABSORBANCE SPECTROPHOTOMETRY

Use of Spectrophotometry

In the clinical laboratory there is a continual need for the use of quantitative techniques. By using a quantitative method, the exact amount of an unknown substance can be determined accurately, and this is the basis for many laboratory determinations, especially in the chemistry department. Various methods for measuring substances quantitatively have been discussed in Chapter 4. One of the techniques used most frequently in the clinical laboratory is **photometry** or specifically, **absorbance spectrophotometry.** Photometry, or colorimetry, employs color and color variation to determine the concentrations of substances.

Spectrophotometry is perhaps the most frequently used quantitative method in the laboratory (although not as accurate as titration), and it is imperative that any person doing clinical laboratory techniques know and understand thoroughly the principles of photometry in general. Probably no measurement technique is used as much but understood as little as photometry. Although spectrophotometry is often less precise than other procedures, it has the advantage of being very simple to use. In most laboratories today there is a need for greater efficiency, and through the use of spectrophotometry the results of certain tests can be obtained simply and quickly.

Principle of Spectrophotometry

The use of absorbance spectrophotometry, or colorimetry, as a means of quantitative measurement depends primarily on two factors, the color itself and the intensity of the color. Any substance to be measured by spectrophotometry must be colored to begin with or must be capable of being colored. An example of a substance that is colored to begin with is hemoglobin (determined by use of spectrophotometry in the hematology laboratory). Sugar, specifically glucose, is an example of a substance that is not colored to begin with but is capable of being colored by the use of certain reagents and reactions. Sugar content can therefore be measured by spectrophotometry.

When using spectrophotometry as a method for quantitative measurement, the unknown colored substance is compared with a similar substance of known strength (a standard solution), based on the principle that the intensity of the color is directly proportional to the concentration of the substance present.

The absorbance units or values for several different concentrations of a standard solution are determined by spectrophotometry and are plotted on graph paper. The resulting graph is known as a standard calibration curve or a **Beer's law** plot. Unknown specimens can then be read in the spectrophotometer and, using their absorbance values, their concentrations determined from the calibration curve. **Standard solutions** are discussed further in Chapter 10.

The Nature of Light

To understand the use of absorbance spectrophotometry (and photometry in general), one must first understand the fundamentals of color. To understand color, one must also understand the nature of light and its effect on color as we see it. Light is a type of radiant energy and it travels in the form of waves. The distance between waves is the **wavelength of light.** The term *light* is used to describe radiant energy with wavelengths visible to the human eye and with wavelengths bordering on those visible to the human eye. The human eye responds to radiant energy, or light, with wavelengths between about 400 and 750 nm. A nanometer is 1×10^{-9} m. With modern photometric apparatus, shorter (ultraviolet) or longer (infrared) wavelengths can be measured.

The wavelength of light determines the color of the light seen by the human eye. Every color that is seen is light of a particular wavelength. A combination, or mixture, of light energy of different wavelengths is known as daylight, or *white light*. When light is passed through a filter, prism, or diffraction grating, it can be broken into a spectrum of visible colors ranging from violet to red. The visible spectrum consists of the following range of colors: violet, blue, green, yellow, orange, and red. If white light is diffracted or partially absorbed by a filter or prism, it becomes visible as certain colors. The different portions of the spectrum may be identified by wavelengths ranging from 400 to 750 nm for the visible colors. Wavelengths below 400 nm are ultraviolet and those above 750 nm are infrared; these light waves are not visible to the human eye.

The color of light seen in the visible spectrum depends on the wavelength that is not absorbed. When light is not absorbed, it is transmitted. A colored solution has color because of its physical properties, which result in its absorbing certain wavelengths and transmitting others. When white light is passed through a solution, part of the light is absorbed and that remaining is **transmitted light.** A rainbow is seen when there are droplets of moisture in the air that refract or filter certain rays of the sun and allow others to pass through. The colors of the rainbow range from red to violet—the visible spectrum.

Absorbance and Transmittance of Light—Beer's Law

Many solutions contain particles that absorb certain wavelengths and transmit others. Solutions appear to the human eye to have characteristic colors. The wavelength of light transmitted by the solution is recognized as color by the eye. The following are the visible colors of the spectrum and their respective wavelength ranges: violet (400–440 nm), blue (440–500 nm), green (500–580 nm), yellow (580–600 nm), orange (600–620 nm), and red (620–750 nm). A blue solution appears blue because particles in the solution absorb all the wavelengths except blue; the blue is the color transmitted and seen. A red solution appears red because all other wavelengths except red have been absorbed by the solution, while the red wavelength passes through.

Measurement by spectrophotometry is based on the reaction between the substance to be measured and a reagent, or chemical, used to produce color. The amount of color produced in a reaction between the substance to be measured and the reagent depends on the concentration of the substance. Therefore, the intensity of the color is proportional to the concentration of the substance. Beer's law states this relationship: color intensity at a constant depth is directly proportional to concentration. Beer's law is the basis for the use of photometry in quantitative measurement. Using this law, if one saw a solution with a very intense red color, one would be correct in assuming that the solution had a high concentration of the substance that made it red. Another way of describing Beer's law is that any increase in the concentration of a color-producing substance will increase the amount of color seen.

As the law states, the depth at which the color is determined must be constant. The depth of the solution is regulated by the cuvette or tube used to hold it. Increasing the depth of the solution through which the light must pass (by using a cuvette with a larger diameter) is the same as placing more particles between the light and the eye, thereby creating an apparent increase in the concentration, or intensity, of color. To avoid this alteration of the actual concentration, only cuvettes with a constant diameter can be used or a flow-through apparatus used which eliminates the use of cuvettes.

Expressions of Light Transmitted or Absorbed

There are two common methods of expressing the amount of light transmitted (or absorbed) by a solution. The units used to express the readings obtained by the electronic measuring device (see under Parts Essential to All Spectrophotometers) are either absorbance units or **percent transmittance units.** Another term for **absorbed light** is **optical density (OD).** The term *optical density* is generally outdated. Most spectrophotometers give the readings in both units. Absorbance units are difficult to read directly from the reading scale because it is divided logarithmically rather than in equal divisions. Absorbance values are directly proportional to the concentration and therefore they may be plotted on linear graph paper to give a straight line (see under Standardization of a Procedure and Use of a Standard Curve in Chapter 10). Most spectrophotometers also give the percent transmittance readings on the viewing scale. Percent transmittance is the amount of light that passes through a colored solution compared with the amount of light that passes through a blank solution (see under Means of Ensuring Reliable Laboratory Results—Quality Control Program, in Chapter 7). Percent transmittance varies from 0 to 100 (it is usually abbreviated %T), with equal divisions on the viewing scale. As the concentration of the colored solution increases, the amount of light absorbed increases and the percentage of the light transmitted decreases. The transmitted light does not decrease in direct proportion to the concentration or color intensity of the solution being measured. There is a logarithmic relationship between percent transmittance and concentration (see under Standardization of a Procedure and Use of a Standard Curve in Chapter 10). Absorbance and percent transmittance are related in the following way: absorbance = 2 minus the logarithm of the percent transmittance, or $A = 2 - \log \%T$. Therefore, 2 is the logarithm of 100%T. It is possible to obtain a convenient conversion table for transmittance and absorbance from a standard chemistry reference textbook.

Instruments Used in Spectrophotometry

The instrument used to show the quantitative relationship between the colors of the undetermined solution and the standard solution is called a spectrophotometer, or colorimeter.

Most of the instruments used in photometry have some means of isolating a narrow wavelength, or range, of the color spectrum for measurements. Instruments using filters for this purpose are referred to as *filter photometers,* while those using prisms or gratings are called **spectrophotometers or photoelectric colorimeters.** Both types are used frequently in the clinical laboratory. In older colorimetric procedures, visual comparison of the color of an unknown with that of a standard was used. In general, visual colorimetry has been replaced by the more specific and accurate photoelectric methods.

One current application of visual colorimetry is employed in the various dry reagent strip tests which are so prevalent in many clinical chemistry tests—dry reagent strip tests used in urinalysis, for example. These strips can be read visually, although instruments are also available to electronically read the color developed.

There are many types of spectrophotometers in common use in the clinical laboratory. The principle of most of these instruments is the same, in that the amount of light transmitted by the standard solution is compared with the amount of light transmitted by the solution of unknown concentration.

Precise, accurate methods are needed to accomplish the numerous determinations required in today's clinical laboratory. The spectrophotometer is one piece of equipment that is essential and can be considered to be of prime importance. Spectrophotometers are also known as *photoelectric colorimeters* or *photometers.* The many available spectrophotometers have their own technical variations, but all operate according to the same general principles.

Several types of spectrophotometers are available. For teaching purposes, the Coleman Junior Spectrophotometer has proved to be very satisfactory (Fig 5–1). In general, photometers employing filters are called *filter photometers,* and those with diffraction gratings are called *spectrophotometers.* Photometers utilize an electronic device to compare the actual color intensities of the solutions measured. As the name implies, a spectrophotometer is really two instruments in a single case: a spectrometer, a device for producing light of a specific wavelength, the monochromator; and a photometer, a device for measuring light intensity. Because of its widespread use, the operation of the Coleman Junior Spectrophotometer is described in Procedure 5–1. Any spectrophotometric instrument should be used only by following the manufacturer's instructions.

In the automated analyzing instruments used in many laboratories, a photometer is still a necessary com-

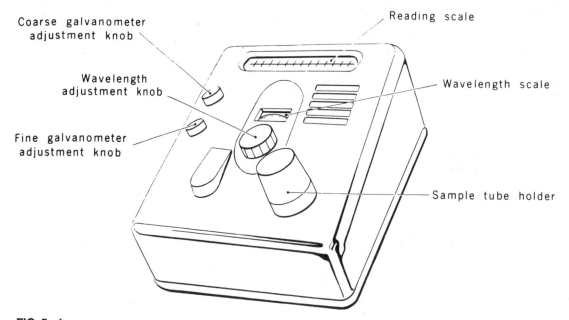

FIG 5–1.
Coleman Junior spectrophotometer.

ponent, so absorbance values for unknown and standard solutions can be determined. Some instruments contain a filter wheel which allows for the measurement of absorbance at any wavelength for which there is a filter on the wheel. Microprocessors control the location of the correct filter for the particular analyte being measured. From the absorbance information, the computer microprocessor calculates the unknown concentration.

Parts Essential to All Spectrophotometers

There are parts necessary to all spectrophotometers (Fig 5–2). These are:

1. *Light source.* Each spectrophotometer must have a light source. This can be a light bulb constructed to give the optimum amount of light. The light source must be steady and constant; therefore, use of a voltage regulator or electronic power supply is recommended. The light source may be movable or stationary.

2. *Wavelength isolator.* Before the light from the light source reaches the sample of solution to be measured, the interfering wavelengths must be removed. A system of isolating a desired wavelength and excluding others is called a *monochromator*. In doing this the light is actually being reduced to a particular wavelength. Filters can be used to accomplish this. Some are very simple, composed of one or two pieces of colored glass. Some are more complicated. The more complicated filters are found in the better spectrophotometers. The filter must transmit a color that the solution *can* absorb. A red filter transmits red, and a green filter transmits green. Filters are available to cover almost any point in the visible spectrum, and each filter has inscribed on it a number that indicates the wavelength of light that it trans-

mits. For example, a filter inscribed with 540 nm absorbs all light except that of wavelengths around 540 nm. Since the filter must transmit a color that the solution can absorb, for a red solution the filter chosen should not be red (all colors *except* red are absorbed). The wavelength of light transmitted is, then, the important thing to consider in choosing the correct filter for a procedure.

Light of a desired wavelength can also be provided by other means. One of the more commonly used instruments employs a diffraction grating with a special plate and slit to reduce the spectrum to the desired wavelength. The grating consists of a highly polished surface with numerous lines on it that break up white light into the spectrum. By moving the spectrum behind a slit (the light source must be movable), only one particular portion of the spectrum is allowed to pass through the narrow slit. The particular band of light, or wavelength, that is transmitted through the slit is indicated on a viewing scale on the machine. Certain wavelengths are more desirable than others for a particular color and procedure. The wavelength chosen is determined by running an absorption curve and selecting the correct wavelength after inspecting the curve obtained. Only when new methods are being developed is it necessary to run an absorption curve.

3. *Cuvettes, absorption cells, or photometer tubes.* Any light (of the wavelength selected) coming from the filter or diffraction grating will next pass on to the solution in the **cuvette.** Glass cuvettes are relatively inexpensive and are satisfactory, provided they are matched or calibrated. Calibrated cuvettes are tubes that have been optically matched so that the same solution in each will give the same reading on the photometer. In using calibrated cuvettes, the depth factor of Beer's law is kept constant. The means by which these tubes can be ob-

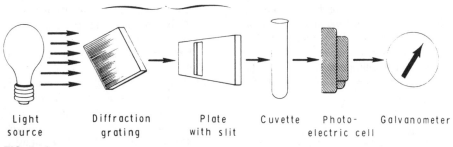

or filter

| Light source | Diffraction grating | Plate with slit | Cuvette | Photo- electric cell | Galvanometer |

FIG 5–2.
Parts essential to all spectrophotometers.

Procedure 5–1. Operation of the Coleman Junior Spectrophotometer*

1. Mount the selected scale panel in the galvanometer viewing window. A general purpose scale panel is usually used. There are several types of scale panels available, depending on the use to which the spectrophotometer is to be put. The scale panel is calibrated both in percent transmittance and absorbance (optical density).

2. Insert in the cuvette well the cuvette adapter of the proper size to accommodate the type of cuvette specified in the analytic procedure.

3. Turn on the switch located on the back of the instrument. Allow the instrument to warm up for 5 minutes.

4. Verify the galvanometer zero setting, and readjust if necessary. The indicator line on the galvanometer spot should register at zero on the percent transmittance scale. The zero adjustment level for this instrument is located under the raised housing just to the left of the cuvette well. If the spectrophotometer is not disturbed and its position is not altered, this galvanometer adjustment remains very stable.

   a. To check the zero position, darken the photoelectric cell by inserting a cuvette adapter in the cuvette well turned 90 degrees from the calibration marker. In this position, the body of the adapter completely blocks the pathway of light. A piece of opaque paper may also be slipped in the adapter well; in this way the light pathway is also completely stopped.

   b. Cover the well with the light shield or other suitable cover.

   c. With a pencil point move the galvanometer adjusting lever so that the indicator line on the galvanometer spot reads zero on the left zero index of the selected scale panel.

   d. Complete the adjustment by sliding the scale panel until the index is *exactly* at zero on the scale.

   *From *Operating Directions for the Coleman Model 6A and 6C Junior Spectrophotometer*. Maywood, Ill., Coleman Instruments Corp, September 1966.

5. Adjust the wavelength knob so that the specific wavelength is set. Different procedures will call for different wavelengths. The wavelength to be used will be specified in the procedure.

6. Cuvettes used for reading in the spectrophotometer must be free from scratches. Before placing the cuvette in the adapter for reading, it must be free of finger marks and bubbles; the spectrophotometer does not recognize the cause of light impediment and will respond similarly to a scratched tube, lint, bubbles, finger marks, and the absorbance of the solution being examined. Therefore, wipe the cuvettes with a clean, dry, soft cloth or gauze before reading.

   All cuvettes must contain a certain volume of solution, called the *minimum volume*. Various sized cuvettes need various minimum volumes to ensure that the light passes through the solution rather than through the empty space in the tube.

7. Place the cuvette containing the reagent blank in the adapter first. For more information on the use of blank solutions, see Chapter 7. The calibration mark (or trademark, if precalibrated Coleman cuvettes are used) must face the light source to ensure constancy of the light path. Adjust the galvanometer control knobs (labeled *GALV Coarse* and *GALV Fine*) until the galvanometer index on the viewing scale reads 100%T for the "blank" tube.

8. Remove the blank tube.

9. Place the next polished cuvette containing the solution to be read in the adapter well, again taking note of the calibration mark. Place this mark in a position facing the light source.

10. Record the galvanometer reading to the nearest $\frac{1}{4}$%T reading.

11. Remove the cuvette, and reinsert the blank tube.

12. Observe the reading for the blank tube on the galvanometer scale. It should still read 100%T. If it does, remove the blank tube and proceed with the next tube to be read. If the blank tube does not read exactly 100%T, adjust it to read 100%T with the *GALV Coarse* and *GALV Fine*

Continued.

knobs. Then read the next tube. The blank tube should be reinserted between all readings, and it should always read 100%T.

13. Read all tubes, and record results to the nearest $\frac{1}{4}$%T reading. Fractional parts (in fourths) of percent transmittance readings are recorded with the numerator figure only. For example, if a reading is $75\frac{1}{2}$ ($=75\frac{2}{4}$), the result is recorded as 75^2%T. For a reading of $75\frac{3}{4}$ the result is recorded as 75^3, and for a reading of $75\frac{1}{4}$ the result is recorded as 75^1.

14. When finished, return the galvanometer index to the original position by turning both the *GALV Coarse* and *GALV Fine* knobs completely counterclockwise, and turn off the machine switch.

15. Clean up the area around the instrument, wipe up anything spilled on the machine, and cover the spectrophotometer with the protective cover provided. For cleaning cuvettes see under Cleaning Laboratory Glassware and Plasticware, in Chapter 4.

tained is discussed under Calibration of Cuvettes for the Spectrophotometer. Depending on the concentration and thus the color of the solution, a certain amount of light will be absorbed by the solution, and the remainder will be transmitted. The light not absorbed by the solution is transmitted. This light next passes on to an electronic measuring device of some type. Alternatively, to eliminate the cuvette entirely, a flow-through apparatus can be used. (See Procedure 5–1.)

4. *Electronic measuring device.* In the more common spectrophotometers, the electronic measuring device consists of a **photoelectric cell** and a **galvanometer.** The amount of light transmitted by the solution in the cuvette is measured by a photoelectric cell. This cell is a most sensitive instrument, producing electrons in proportion to the amount of light hitting it. The electrons are passed on to a galvanometer, where they are measured. The galvanometer records the amount of current (in the form of electrons) that it receives from the photoelectric cell on a special viewing scale on the spectrophotometer. The results are reported in terms of percent transmittance. In some cases, the readings are made in terms of absorbance. The percent transmittance is dependent on the

concentration of the solution and its depth. If the solution is very concentrated (the color appearing intense), less light will be transmitted than if it is dilute (pale). Therefore, the reading on the galvanometer viewing scale will be lower for a more concentrated solution than for a dilute solution. This is the basis for the comparison of color intensity with the spectrophotometer.

Flow-Through Adaptation

A special adaptation available for Coleman Junior Spectrophotometers is called a Coleman Vacuvette Cell Assembly. This is designed to increase the speed with which samples can be introduced into and discharged from the photometer. Another name for an assembly of this kind is a *flow-through apparatus.* Instead of using separate cuvettes for each sample read in the photometer, the sample is poured directly into a specially designed cuvette incorporating a funnel for easy pouring. The sample is read in the same way as in the regular cuvette method and is then evacuated from the photometer by means of a capillary tubing attached to a discard bottle. When a suitable vacuum system is attached to the cuvette-capillary tubing assembly, rapid and automatic discarding of the sample is possible. This assembly apparatus must be periodically cleaned to maintain its proper operation. A flow-through apparatus can be used for reading samples when the sample can be discarded. It cannot be used to read multiple values on the same sample because the sample is lost once it is poured into the special cuvette. The Coleman Instruments manufactures this specially designed cuvette in various sizes so that varying amounts of sample may be read in the photometer. This device is another example of how many laboratory functions have been made more efficient so that time can be saved and results can be sent out more quickly.

Care and Handling of Spectrophotometers

When using a spectrophotometer, error caused by color in the reagents used must be eliminated. Since color is so important and since the color produced by the undetermined substance is the desired one, any color resulting from the reagents themselves or from interactions between the reagents could cause confusion and error. By using a blank solution, a correction can be made for any color because of the reagents used. The blank solution contains the same reagents as the unknown and standard tubes with the exception of the substance being measured. The use of blank solutions is discussed further in Chapter 7.

A spectrophotometer, as is the case with any expensive, delicate instrument, must be handled with care. The manufacturer supplies a manual of complete instructions on the care and use of a particular machine. Care should be taken not to spill reagents on the spectrophotometer. Spillage could damage the delicate instrument, especially the photoelectric cell. Any reagents spilled must be wiped up immediately. Spectrophotometers with filters should not be operated without the filter in place, since the unfiltered light from the light source may damage the photoelectric cell and the galvanometer. A spectrophotometer should be placed on a table with good support, where it will not be bumped or jarred.

Tests of Quality Control for Spectrophotometers

The spectrophotometer must be tested periodically to ensure that it is functioning properly. Wavelength calibration can be checked by use of a rare-earth glass filter such as didymium. The wavelength calibration can also be checked by use of a stable chromogen solution. Calibration at two wavelengths is necessary for instruments with diffraction gratings and at three wavelengths for instruments with prisms.

Photoelectric accuracy can be checked by reading standard solutions of potassium dichromate or potassium nitrate. As an alternative, the National Bureau of Standards (NBS) has sets of three neutral-density glass filters that have known absorbance at four wavelengths for each filter. These filters are not completely stable, however, and require periodic recalibration.

Calibration of Cuvettes for the Spectrophotometer

If cuvettes are used, it is essential that their diameters be uniform, that is, it is necessary that the depth of the cuvettes or tubes used in the spectrophotometer be constant for Beer's law to apply. The quality of disposable glass test tubes is so good that in many cases, these can be used in place of the calibrated cuvettes.

Cuvettes for the spectrophotometer can be purchased precalibrated, but these are expensive. Precalibrated cuvettes must also be checked before being put into actual use in the laboratory. Most laboratories, especially those involved with teaching, calibrate cuvettes for the spectrophotometer. As noted previously, these cuvettes have been optically matched so that the same solution in each will give the same percent transmittance reading on the galvanometer viewing scale.

In calibrating cuvettes for use in spectrophotometry (Procedure 5–2), the cuvette is carefully checked to see that the solution gives the same reading in that cuvette as it did in a previously calibrated cuvette. To check cuvettes for uniformity, the same solution, such as a stable solution of copper sulfate or cyanmethemoglobin, is read in many cuvettes. Readings are taken and cuvettes that match within an established tolerance are reserved for use. Since cuvettes may not be perfectly round, they are rotated in the cuvette well to observe any changes in reading with the position in the well. The cuvette is etched at the point where the reading corresponds with the established tolerance for the absorption reading. Those that do not agree or do not correspond are not used for spectrophotometry. Different-sized cuvettes can be used, depending on the spectrophotometer. One of the more common sizes of cuvettes, especially for the Coleman Junior Spectrophotometer, is 19 × 105 mm. The Coleman Junior Spectrophotometer can be adapted to use several different-sized cuvettes in the same machine. For each size, a special cuvette adapter is used, enabling the cuvette to fit securely in the cuvette holder. Only when the cuvette fits securely will the readings obtained be precise and accurate.

VISUAL COLORIMETRY

Before photometers and spectrophotometers became readily available for quantitative measurements, another type of color-comparing device was in common use. This device utilized the human eye to compare color intensity differences and was called a **visual colorimeter.** This type of visual colorimetry is now used only rarely and has been replaced by photometry and spectrophotometry. In visual colorimetry, the human eye acts as the instrument for color comparison (in the spectrophotometer, the photoelectric cell and galvanometer accomplish this). As previously discussed, some forms of visual colorimetry are currently employed in the various tests utilizing dry reagent strip chemistry.

The human eye is a poor instrument for measuring

Procedure 5–2. Calibrating Cuvettes

---

1. Use only clean, dry cuvettes for calibration.
2. Filter a portion of the chosen colored solution to be placed in the cuvettes. One solution used frequently for calibration is 5% copper sulfate. Filter enough solution to fill the cuvettes to be calibrated. The cuvettes should be filled to approximately the same level.
3. Fill the uncalibrated cuvettes to approximately the same level with the filtered solution.
4. Polish the cuvettes with a gauze or tissue.
5. Calibrate the new cuvettes against previously calibrated tubes.
   a. Fill four or five calibrated cuvettes with the same filtered solution to approximately the same level. Polish the cuvettes thoroughly and read in the spectrophotometer, noting the readings in percent transmittance for each (see steps 6–9).
   b. Read the uncalibrated cuvettes in the same manner, following the directions given in the next steps.
6. Set the wavelength at 550 nm (or other suitable wavelength chosen for this procedure).
7. Prepare the spectrophotometer for reading cuvettes by following the directions for the particular instrument being used.
8. Pick an arbitrary setting on the galvanometer reading scale against which to read the cuvettes. Usually a setting near the center of the viewing scale is chosen (50%, 60%, or 70%T, for example).
9. Read the previously calibrated cuvettes first,

checking the arbitrary setting between each reading. Adjust and reread, if necessary. Record these readings. All the readings for the previously calibrated cuvettes should be within $\frac{1}{2}\%T$ of one another on the galvanometer scale.

10. To calibrate the new cuvettes:
    a. Check the arbitrary center setting; adjust if necessary.
    b. Place the polished uncalibrated cuvette in the tube holder; note the reading on the galvanometer viewing scale.
    c. If the reading is the same as for the standard cuvettes read previously, mark the cuvette with a wax pencil at the place corresponding to the mark on the calibrated cuvettes (that is, the side of the cuvette facing the light source); this mark will later be permanently etched on the cuvette.
    d. If the reading is not the same as for the precalibrated cuvettes, slowly rotate the cuvette in the holder until the same reading is obtained. Mark the cuvette with a wax pencil as in step 10c. If the reading is not obtained after a complete rotation in the cuvette holder, the new cuvette cannot be used with this particular set of calibrated cuvettes. Set it aside to be calibrated with a different set.
    e. Etch the cuvettes with a glass etcher, making a well-defined mark where the wax pencil mark was made. The cuvettes are now ready to be washed and used.

---

light intensity. It is difficult for the human eye to measure accurately shades of color or intensity. There is an error of 5% or more even with experience and proper technique, which is one of the reasons why the early visual colorimetry techniques are inadequate for today's laboratory procedures. Interfering spectra will often cause an even greater error. Such interference often can be reduced or eliminated by the use of a filter.

The visual colorimeter has several other disadvantages. One of these is that more time is required to carry out the desired procedure. In the modern laboratory,

many tests are run and speed is important. The temperature of the surrounding area and the order of adding the reagents can also affect the visual colorimeter. In using visual colorimetry, there is a need for deep colors, which requires a larger quantity of the specimen and more reagents. It is not always possible to obtain enough specimen (blood, for example) to run the test satisfactorily with a visual colorimeter.

The names of some of the visual colorimeters used in years past are the Klett, Duboscq, and Dennison colorimeters.

FLAME EMISSION PHOTOMETRY

Use and Principle of Flame Emission Photometry

Flame emission photometry is used most commonly for the quantitative measurement of lithium, sodium, and potassium in body fluids. In flame emission analysis by emission photometry, a solution containing metal ions is sprayed into a flame. The metal ions are energized to emit light of a characteristic color. Atoms of many metallic elements, when given sufficient energy (such as that supplied by a hot flame), will emit this energy at wavelengths characteristic of the elements. Lithium produces a red, sodium a yellow, potassium a violet, and magnesium a blue color in a flame. Sodium and potassium are the metal ions most commonly measured in biological specimens, but lithium, which is not normally present in serum, may also be measured in connection with the use of lithium salts in the treatment of some psychiatric disorders. The intensity of the color is proportional to the amount of the element burned in the flame. Flame photometers are laboratory instruments that make use of this principle. Details of the operation of a specific flame photometer should be obtained from the manufacturer, but there are a few general principles and components that are common to most instruments.

Essential Parts of Flame Photometer

An atomizer is needed to spray the sample as fine droplets into the flame. Another name for atomizer is nebulizer (Fig 5–3). The atomizer creates a fine spray of the sample and feeds this spray into a burner. The fine spray is produced by combining a stream of sample with a stream of air. A total-consumption burner feeds the entire sample directly into the flame. A premix atomizer mixes the fuel gases and the sample in a mixing chamber before sending this mixture to the flame. Both types of atomizers are available in modern machines.

In most flame photometers the fuel usually consists of various combinations of acetylene, propane, oxygen, natural gas, and compressed air. The combinations and types of fuel used determine the temperature of the flame. For sodium and potassium determinations, a propane-compressed air flame appears entirely adequate. The atomizer and the flame are critical components of a flame photometer. The most important variable in the flame itself is the temperature, since the energy emitted by the metal ions is measured and the number of energized metal ions is dependent on the temperature of the flame. Frequent standardization of flame photometers is essential because thermal changes occur and affect the operation of the instrument and subsequent measurements with it.

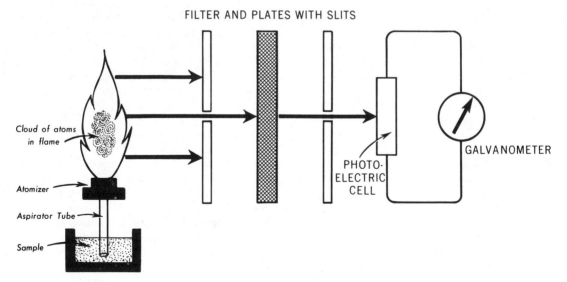

FIG 5–3.
Essential parts of a flame emission photometer.

Flame photometers must also have a filter, prism, grating, or other device for selecting light of the appropriate wavelength for the element to be measured. These devices spread or disperse the light into its spectral components. The desired wavelength is selected by means of a narrow slit. In this respect the flame photometer is similar to the spectrophotometer. In fact, the light source described for the spectrophotometer has been replaced with an atomizer-flame combination in the flame photometer. The flame photometer must also have an electronic measuring device to detect the intensity of the emitted light. Photocells or phototubes are used to detect the light intensity by converting the light into an electrical current. The amount of current generated is proportional to the quantity of light that reaches the detector. The amount of current is measured by a galvanometer or other recording device (see under Absorbance Spectrophotometry).

Types of Flame Photometers

An example of a flame photometer that operates on an absolute or direct principle is one where the intensity of color is proportional to the amount of the element burned in the flame. When measuring an unknown sample, its intensity of color is compared with that of a standard solution of the element being measured. For example, a standard solution of potassium is used for measuring potassium.

In another commonly used method of flame photometry, the principle of the **internal standard** is applied. Most modern flame photometers employ an internal standard. In this method, another element, usually lithium, is added to all solutions analyzed—blanks, standards, and unknowns. Lithium is usually absent from biological fluids and it has a high emission intensity. It also emits at a wavelength sufficiently distant from that of potassium or sodium to permit spectral isolation. In flame photometry using the internal standard principle, the emission of the unknown element (sodium or potassium) is compared with that of the reference element lithium. By measuring the ratios of the emissions, any change in gas or air pressure, line voltage, flame temperature, rate of atomization, or other small variable will be minimized because both the unknown element and the reference element are affected simultaneously. A specially designed adaptation of the machine is used for this purpose, and the ratio of the reference lithium and unknown metal emissions is measured by two detectors. Two filter systems are set up, one for the unknown and one for the lithium reference. Lithium does not function as a "true" standard in its use as a reference solution. Therefore, various known concentrations of potassium or sodium are prepared and used to establish calibration curves. The use of lithium as the reference solution can cause problems, however, because lithium salts are given to patients treated for manic-depressive states. In these patients, the lithium level must be measured.

BIBLIOGRAPHY

Henry JB (ed): *Clinical Diagnosis and Management by Laboratory Methods,* ed. 18. Philadelphia, WB Saunders Co, 1991.

Kaplan LA, Pesce AJ: *Clinical Chemistry Theory, Analysis, and Correlation,* ed 2. St Louis, Mosby–Year Book, Inc, 1989.

Tietz NW (ed): *Textbook of Clinical Chemistry.* Philadelphia, WB Saunders Co, 1986.

Tietz NW (ed): *Fundamentals of Clinical Chemistry,* ed 3. Philadelphia, WB Saunders Co, 1987.

6 Laboratory Mathematics

Key Terms

Density	Proportions
Dilutions	Ratio
Dilution factor	Rounding off
Equivalent	Serial dilutions
Exponents	Significant figures
Molarity	Weight per unit volume
Normality	Weight per unit weight
Osmolarity	Volume per unit volume
Percent solution	

It is important for any person involved in doing clinical laboratory analyses to understand not only how the necessary calculations are done but why the mathematical concepts work as they do. The principles on which a particular formula is based must be understood and not only the formula itself. When principles are understood thoroughly, modifications can be made, if necessary.

A sound background in basic mathematics (including algebra), an understanding of the units in which quantities are expressed, and a knowledge of the methods of analysis are all necessary in performing laboratory calculations. There are no simple formulas for solving all such problems, but certain fundamentals are a part of many of the problems encountered in a clinical laboratory.

PROPORTIONS AND RATIOS

The use of **proportions** involves a commonsense approach to problem solving. Proportions are devices used to determine a quantity from a given **ratio.** A ratio is an amount of something compared to an amount of something else.

Ratios always describe a relative amount and at least two values are always involved. For example, 5 g of something dissolved in 100 mL of something else can be expressed by the ratio 5/100, 5:100, or 5 ÷ 100, or by the decimal 0.05. Proportion is a means of saying that two ratios are equal. Thus, the ratio 5:100 is equal or proportional to the ratio 1/20. This proportion can be expressed as 5:100 = 1:20. In the laboratory, proportions and ratios are useful when it is necessary to make more (or less) of the same thing. However, ratios and proportions can be used only when the concentration (or any other kind of relationship) does not change.

An *example* of a proportion or ratio problem is: A formula calls for 5 g of sodium chloride (NaCl) in 1000 mL of solution. If only 500 mL of solution is needed, how much NaCl is required?

$$\frac{5\ g}{1,000\ mL} = \frac{x\ g}{500\ mL}$$

$$x = \frac{5\ g \times 500\ mL}{1,000\ mL}$$

$$x = 2.5\ g\ NaCl$$

In setting up ratio and proportion problems, the two ratios being compared must be written in the same order and they must be in the same units.

When specimens are diluted in the various laboratory analyses, the ratio principle is applied. This use of **dilutions** is described later in this section.

Relating Concentrations of Solutions

To relate different concentrations of solutions that contain the same amount of substance (or solute) a basic relationship, or ratio, is used. The volume of one solution (V_1) times the concentration of that solution (C_1) equals the volume of the second solution (V_2) times the concentration of the second solution (C_2), or $V_1 \times C_1 = V_2 \times C_2$. If any three of the values are known, the fourth may be determined. This relationship shows that when a solution is diluted, the volume is increased as the concentration is decreased. However, the total amount of substance (or solute) remains unchanged. Several applications of this relationship are used in the clinical laboratory, some of them being in titrations (see under Titration in Chapter 4); in dilution of specimens, and in the preparation of weaker solutions from stronger solutions.

An *example* of making a less concentrated solution from one more concentrated is: A sodium hydroxide (NaOH) solution is available that has a concentration of 10 g of NaOH per deciliter (dL) of solution (1 dL = 100 mL). To calculate the volume of the 10 g/dL NaOH solution required to prepare 1,000 mL of 2 g/dL NaOH:

$$V_1 \times C_1 = V_2 \times C_2$$

$$x\ mL \times 10\ g/dL = 1,000\ mL \times 2\ g/dL$$

$$x = \frac{2\ g/dL \times 1,000\ mL}{10\ g/dL} = 200\ mL$$

Note that this relationship is not a direct proportion; instead, it is an inverse proportion. As this is a proportion problem, it is important to remember that the concentrations and volumes on both sides of the equation must be expressed in the same units.

DILUTIONS

It is often necessary to dilute specimens being analyzed or to make weaker solutions from stronger solutions in various laboratory procedures. It is therefore necessary to be capable of working with various dilution problems and dilution factors. In these problems one must often be able to determine the concentration of material in each solution, the actual amount of material in each solution, and the total volume of each solution. All dilutions are a kind of ratio. Dilution is an indication of *relative* concentration.

Diluting Specimens

In most laboratory determinations, a small sample is taken for analysis, and the final result is expressed as concentration per some convenient standard volume. In a certain procedure, 0.5 mL of blood is diluted to a total of 10 mL with various reagents, and 1 mL of this dilution is then analyzed for a particular chemical constituent. The final result is to be expressed in terms of the concentration of that substance per 100 mL of blood.

Dilution Factor

A **dilution factor** is used to correct for having used a diluted sample in a determination rather than the undiluted sample. The result (answer) using the dilution must be multiplied by the reciprocal of the dilution made.

For example, a dilution factor by which all determination answers are multiplied to give the concentration per 100 mL of sample (blood) may be calculated as follows:

First determine the volume of blood that is actually analyzed in the procedure. By use of a simple proportion, it is evident that 0.5 mL of blood diluted to 10 mL is equivalent to 1 mL of blood diluted to 20 mL.

$$\frac{0.5 \text{ mL blood}}{10 \text{ mL solution}} = \frac{1 \text{ mL blood}}{x \text{ mL solution}}$$

$$x = \frac{1 \text{ mL} \times 10 \text{ mL}}{0.5 \text{ mL}} = 20 \text{ mL}$$

In other words, there is a 1:20 dilution of blood in this procedure—that is, 1 mL of blood diluted to a total volume of 20 mL with the desired diluent (usually saline or deionized water) or reagents. This is the same as 1 mL of blood plus 19 mL of diluent.

The concentration of specimen (blood) in each milliliter of solution may be determined, by the use of an-

other simple proportion, to be 0.05 mL of blood per milliliter of solution:

$$\frac{1 \text{ mL blood}}{20 \text{ mL solution}} = \frac{x \text{ mL blood}}{1 \text{ mL solution}}$$

$$x = \frac{1 \text{ mL} \times 1 \text{ mL}}{20 \text{ mL}} = 0.05 \text{ mL}$$

Since 1 mL of the 1:20 dilution of blood is analyzed in the remaining steps of the procedure, 0.05 mL of blood is actually analyzed (1 mL of the dilution used × 0.05 mL/mL = 0.05 mL of blood analyzed).

To relate the concentration of the substance measured in the procedure to the concentration in 100 mL of blood (the units in which the result is to be expressed) another proportion may be used.

$$\frac{100 \text{ mL (volume of blood desired)}}{0.05 \text{ mL (volume of blood used)}}$$
$$= \frac{\text{concentration desired}}{\text{concentration used or determined}}$$

$$\text{Concentration desired}$$
$$= \frac{100 \text{ mL} \times \text{concentration determined}}{0.05 \text{ mL}}$$

$$\text{Concentration desired} = 2,000 \times \text{value determined}$$

In other words, the concentration of the substance being measured in the volume of blood actually tested (0.05 mL) must be multiplied by 2,000 in order to report the concentration per 100 mL of blood.

The preceding material may be summarized by the following statement and equations. In reporting results obtained from laboratory determinations, one must first determine the amount of specimen actually analyzed in the procedure and then calculate the factor that will express the concentration in the desired terms of measurement. Thus, in the previous example the following equations may be used:

$$\frac{0.5 \text{ mL (volume of blood used)}}{10 \text{ mL (volume of total dilution)}}$$
$$= \frac{x \text{ mL (volume of blood analyzed)}}{1 \text{ mL (volume of dilution used)}}$$

$$x = 0.05 \text{ mL (volume of blood actually analyzed)}$$

$$\frac{\text{100 mL (volume of blood required for expression of result)}}{\text{0.05 mL (volume of blood actually analyzed)}}$$
$$= 2,000 \text{ (dilution factor)}$$

Single Dilutions

When the concentration of a particular substance in a specimen is too great to be accurately determined, or when there is less specimen available for analysis than the procedure requires, it may be necessary to dilute the original specimen, or to further dilute the initial dilution (or filtrate). Such dilutions are usually expressed as a ratio, such as 1:2, 1:5, or 1:10, or as a fraction, $\frac{1}{2}$, $\frac{1}{5}$, or $\frac{1}{10}$. These ratios or fractions refer to 1 unit of the original specimen diluted to a final volume of 2, 5, or 10 units, respectively. A dilution therefore refers to the volume of concentrate in the total volume of final solution. A dilution is an expression of concentration; it indicates the relative amount of substance in solution. Dilutions can be made singly or in series.

To calculate the concentration of a single dilution, multiply the original concentration by the dilution expressed as a fraction.

Calculation of the Concentration of a Single Dilution

A specimen contains 500 mg of substance per deciliter of blood. A 1:5 dilution of this specimen is prepared by volumetrically measuring 1 mL of the specimen and adding 4 mL of diluent (usually distilled water or saline). The concentration of substance in the dilution is

$$500 \text{ mg/dL} \times \frac{1}{5} = 100 \text{ mg/dL}$$

Note that the concentration of the final solution (or dilution) is expressed in the same units as that of the original solution.

To obtain a dilution factor that can be applied to the determination answer in order to express it as a concentration per standard volume, proceed as follows. Rather than multiply by the dilution expressed as a fraction, multiply the determination value by the reciprocal of the dilution fraction. In the case of a 1:5 dilution, the dilution factor that would be applied to values obtained in the procedure would be 5, since the original specimen was five times more concentrated than the diluted specimen tested in the procedure.

Use of Dilution Factors

A 1:5 dilution.of a specimen is prepared and an aliquot (one of a number of equal parts) of the dilution is analyzed for a particular substance. The concentration of the substance in the aliquot is multiplied by 5 to determine its concentration in the original specimen. If the concentration of the dilution is 100 mg/dL, the concentration of the original specimen is

100 mg/dL × 5 (the dilution factor)
$$= 500 \text{ mg/dL in blood}$$

Serial Dilutions

As mentioned previously, dilutions can be made singly or in series, where the original solution is further diluted. A general rule for calculating the concentrations of solutions obtained by dilution in series is to multiply the original concentration by the first dilution (expressed as a fraction), this by the second dilution, and so on until the desired concentration is known.

Several laboratory procedures, especially serologic ones, make use of a dilution series where all dilutions, including or following the first one, are the same. Such dilutions are referred to as **serial dilutions**. A complete dilution series usually contains five or ten tubes, although any single dilution may be made directly from an undiluted specimen or substance. In calculating the dilution or concentration of substance or serum in each tube of the dilution series, the rules previously discussed apply.

A five-tube twofold dilution may be prepared as follows (see Fig 6–1): A serum specimen is diluted 1:2 with buffer. A series of five tubes are prepared where each succeeding tube is rediluted 1:2. This is accomplished by placing 1 mL of diluent into each of four tubes (tubes 2–5). Tube 1 contains 1 mL of undiluted serum. Tube 2 contains 1 mL of undiluted serum plus 1 mL of diluent, resulting in a 1:2 dilution of serum. A 1-mL portion of the 1:2 dilution of serum is placed in tube 3, resulting in a 1:4 dilution of serum ($\frac{1}{2} \times \frac{1}{2} = \frac{1}{4}$). A 1-mL portion of the 1:4 dilution from tube 3 is placed in tube 4, resulting in a 1:8 dilution ($\frac{1}{4} \times \frac{1}{2} = \frac{1}{8}$). Finally, 1 mL of the 1:8 dilution from tube 4 is added to tube 5, resulting in a 1:16 dilution ($\frac{1}{8} \times \frac{1}{2} = \frac{1}{16}$). One milliliter of the final dilution is discarded so that the volumes in all the tubes are equal. Note that each tube is diluted twice as much as the previous tube and that the final volume in

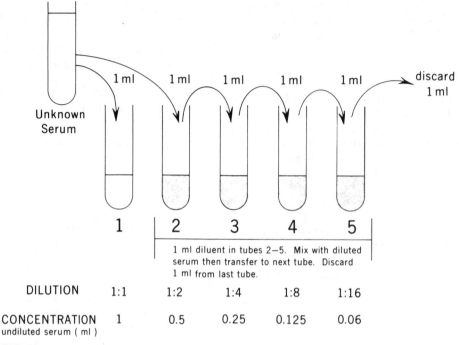

FIG 6–1.
Five-tube twofold dilution.

each tube is the same. The undiluted serum may also be given a dilution value, namely 1:1.

The concentration of serum in terms of milliliters in each tube is calculated by multiplying the previous concentration (mL) by the succeeding dilution. In this example tube 1 contains 1 mL of serum, tube 2 contains 1 mL × $\frac{1}{2}$ = 0.5 mL of serum, and tubes 3 to 5 contain 0.25, 0.125, and 0.06 mL of serum, respectively.

Other serial dilutions might be fivefold or tenfold, where each succeeding tube is diluted five or ten times. A fivefold series would begin with 1 mL of serum in 4 mL of diluent and a total volume of 5 mL in each tube, while a tenfold series would begin with 1 mL of serum in 9 mL of diluent and a total volume of 10 mL in each tube. Other systems might begin with a 1:2 dilution and then dilute five succeeding tubes 1:10. The dilutions in such a series would be 1:2, 1:20 ($\frac{1}{2} \times \frac{1}{10} = \frac{1}{20}$), 1:200 ($\frac{1}{20} \times \frac{1}{10} = \frac{1}{200}$), 1:2,000, 1:20,000, and 1:200,000.

Calculation of the Concentration After a Series of Dilutions

A working solution is prepared from a stock solution. In so doing, a stock solution with a concentration of 100 mg/dL is diluted 1:10 by volumetrically adding 1 mL of it to 9 mL of diluent. The diluted solution (intermediate solution) is further diluted 1:100 by volumetrically measuring 1 mL of intermediate solution and diluting to the mark in a 100-mL volumetric flask. The concentration of the final or working solution is

$$100 \text{ mg/dL} \times \frac{1}{10} \times \frac{1}{100} = 0.1 \text{ mg/dL}$$

SIGNIFICANT FIGURES

Using more digits than are necessary to calculate and report the results of a laboratory determination has several disadvantages. It is important that the number used contain only the digits necessary for the precision of the determination. Using more digits than necessary is misleading in that it ascribes more accuracy to the determination than is actually the case. There is also the danger of overlooking a decimal point and making an error in judging the magnitude of the answer. Digits in a number that are needed to express the precision of the measurement from which the number is derived are known as **significant figures.** A significant figure is one that is known to be reasonably reliable. Judgment must be exercised in determining how many figures should be used. Some rules to assist in making such decisions are:

1. Use the known accuracy of the method to determine the number of digits that are significant in the answer, and, as a general rule, retain one more figure than this. An *example* is: A urea nitrogen result was reported as 11.2 mg/dL. This would indicate that the result is accurate to the nearest tenth and that the exact value lies between 11.15 and 11.25. In reality, the accuracy of most urea nitrogen methods is ±10%, so that the result reported as 11.2 mg/dL could actually vary from 10 to 12 mg/dL and should be reported as 11 mg/dL. In addition, if the decimal point were omitted or overlooked, the result could be taken as 112 mg/dL.

2. Take the accuracy of the least accurate measurement, or the measurement with the least number of significant figures, as the accuracy of the final result. In doing so, certain things must be done in the addition and subtraction or multiplication and division of numerals. An *example* of addition or subtraction is:
In order to add

$$\begin{array}{r} 206.1 \\ 7.56 \\ \underline{0.8764} \end{array}$$

rewrite it as

$$\begin{array}{r} 206.1 \\ 7.6 \\ \underline{0.9} \end{array}$$

In this example, the least accurate figure is accurate to one decimal place; this is therefore the determining factor. In determining the least accurate figure, the following rule is utilized: In a column of addition or subtraction, in which the decimal points are placed one above the other, the number of significant figures in the final answer is determined by the first digit encountered going from left to right that terminates any one numeral.

An *example* of multiplication or division is:
In the multiplication of

$$32,500 \times 0.00125$$

the result should be reported as 40.6. In this example, the final product should be reported to three significant figures since each factor in the problem has three significant figures. This is determined by utilizing the following general rule: The number of significant figures in the final product or quotient should not exceed the least number of significant figures in any one factor.

Rounding Off Numbers

Test results sometimes produce insignificant digits. It is then necessary to *round off* the numbers to a chosen number of significant value in order not to imply an accuracy of precision greater than the test is capable of delivering.

The following general rule may be used in rounding off decimal values to the proper place: When the digit next to the last one to be retained is less than 5, the last digit should be left unchanged. When the digit next to the last one to be retained is greater than 5, the last digit is increased by 1. If the additional digit is 5, the last digit reported is changed to the nearest even number. *Examples* are:

2.31463 g is rounded off to 2.3146 g.
5.34659 g is rounded off to 5.3466 g.
23.5 mg is rounded off to 24 mg.
24.5 mg is rounded off to 24 mg.

EXPONENTS

Exponents are used to indicate that a number must be multiplied by itself as many times as is indicated by the exponent. The number which is to be multiplied by itself is called the *base*. Usually the exponent is written as a small superscript figure to the immediate right of the base figure and is sometimes referred to as the *power* of the base. The exponent figure can either have a plus or a minus sign before it. The plus sign is usually implied and does not actually appear. An exponent indicates the number of times the base is to be multiplied by itself.

Examples of exponents with no sign or a plus sign (positive exponents) are:

$$10^2 = 10 \times 10 = 100$$

$$10^5 = 10 \times 10 \times 10 \times 10 \times 10$$
$$= 100,000$$

Examples of exponents with a minus sign (negative exponents) are:

$$10^{-1} = \frac{1}{10} = 0.1$$

$$10^{-4} = \frac{1}{10} \times \frac{1}{10} \times \frac{1}{10} \times \frac{1}{10} = \frac{1}{10,000} = 0.0001$$

EXPRESSIONS OF SOLUTION CONCENTRATION

Solution concentration is expressed in several different ways. The most common methods used in clinical laboratories involve either **weight per unit weight** (w/w), also known as mass per unit mass (m/m); **weight per unit volume** (w/v), also known as mass per unit volume (m/v); or **volume per unit volume** (v/v). *Weight* is the term commonly used, although *mass* is really what is being measured. Mass is the amount of matter in something and weight is the force of gravity on something. The most accurate measurement is weight per unit weight since weight (or mass) does not vary with temperature as does volume. Probably the most common measurement is weight per unit volume. The least accurate measurement is volume per unit volume because of the changes in volume due to temperature changes. Volume per unit volume is used in the preparation of a liquid solution from another liquid substance. A few concentrations are expressed as a proper name, such as Wright's stain (used in hematology) or the Sudan III stain (used to demonstrate fat).

Proper Name

There are very few instances where a solution is described by a proper name as far as its concentration is concerned. In Chapter 11 (Hematology), the use of Wright's stain is discussed. This solution is prepared with specific amounts of ingredients according to a series of instructions or directions. When Wright's stain is needed, one knows exactly what is meant and what chemicals in which amounts are used in its preparation.

Weight (Mass) per Unit Volume (w/v)

The most common way of expressing concentration is by *weight (mass) per unit volume (w/v)*. When weight (mass) per unit volume is used, the amount of solute (the substance that goes into solution) per volume of solution is expressed. Weight per unit volume is used most often when a solid chemical is diluted in a liquid. The usual way to express weight per unit volume is as grams per liter (g/L) or milligrams per milliliter (mg/mL). If a concentration for a certain solution is given as 10 g/L, it means that there are 10 g of solute for every liter of solution. If a solution with a concentration of 10 mg/mL is desired and 100 mL of this solution is to be prepared, the use of a proportion formula can be applied. An *example* follows:

$$\frac{10 \text{ mg}}{1 \text{ mL}} = \frac{x \text{ mg}}{100 \text{ mL}}$$

$$x = 1,000 \text{ mg, or } 1 \text{ g}$$

One gram of the desired solute is weighed and diluted to 100 mL (see under Reagents Used in Laboratory Assays, in Chapter 4).

In working with *standard solutions* it will be seen that their concentrations, almost without exception, are expressed as milligrams per milliliter (mg/mL).

Volume per Unit Volume (v/v)

Another way of expressing concentration is by *volume per unit volume (v/v)*. Volume per unit volume is used to express concentration when a liquid chemical is diluted with another liquid; the concentration is expressed as the number of milliliters of liquid chemical per unit volume of solution. The usual way to express volume per unit volume is as milliliters per milliliter (mL/mL) or milliliters per liter (mL/L). The number of milliliters of liquid chemical in 1 mL or 1 L of solution utilizes the volume per unit volume expression of concentration. If 10 mL of alcohol is diluted to 100 mL with water, the concentration is expressed as 10 mL/100 mL, or 10 mL/dl, or 0.1 mL/mL, or 100 mL/L. If a solution with a concentration of 0.5 mL/mL is desired and 1 L is to be prepared, a proportion can again be used to solve the problem. An *example* follows:

$$\frac{0.5 \text{ mL}}{1 \text{ mL}} = \frac{x \text{ mL}}{1,000 \text{ mL}}$$

$$x = 500 \text{ mL}$$

Thus 500 mL of the liquid chemical is measured accurately and diluted to 1,000 mL (1 L).

To express concentration in milliliters per liter, one needs to know how many milliliters of liquid chemical there are in 1 L of the solution.

Any chemical (liquid or solid) can be made into a solution by diluting it with a solvent. The usual solvent is deionized or distilled water (see under Laboratory Reagent Water, in Chapter 4). If the desired chemical is a liquid, the amount needed is measured in milliliters or liters (on occasion liquids are weighed, but the usual method is to measure their volume); if the desired chemical is a solid, the amount needed is weighed in grams or milligrams.

Weight per Unit Weight (w/w)

Another way of expressing concentration is by *weight per unit weight* (or *mass per unit mass (m/m)*. This expression is not commonly used. Not many reagents are prepared by using only solid chemicals and no liquid solvent. When the desired chemical is a solid and it is mixed with, or diluted with, another solid, the expression of concentration is mass per unit mass. The usual ways to express mass per unit mass is as milligrams per milligram (mg/mg), grams per gram (g/g), or grams per kilogram (g/kg). The number of milligrams or grams of one solid in the total number of milligrams or grams of the dry mixture is the mass per unit mass.

Percent

Another expression of concentration is the **percent solution** *(%)*, although in the SI system the preferred units are kilograms (or fractions thereof) per liter (w/v) or milliliters per liter (v/v). A description of the percent solution follows, as this expression of concentration is still used in some instances. Percent is defined as *parts per hundred parts* (the part can be any particular unit). Unless otherwise stated, a percent solution usually means grams or milliliters of solute per 100 mL of solution (g/100 mL or mL/100 mL). Recall that 100 mL is equal to 1 deciliter (dL). Percent solutions can be prepared by using either liquid or solid chemicals. Percent solutions can be expressed either as weight per unit volume percent (w/v%) or volume per unit volume percent (v/v%), depending on the state of the solute (chemical) used—that is, whether it is a solid or a liquid. When a solid chemical is dissolved in a liquid, percent means *grams of solid in 100 mL of solution*. If 10 g of NaCl is diluted to 100 mL with deionized water, the concentration is expressed as 10% (10 g/dL). If 2.5 g is diluted to 100 mL, the concentration is 2.5% (2.5 g/dL). The following is an *example* of concentration expressed in percent:

Ten grams of NaOH is diluted to 200 mL with water. What is the concentration in percent? A proportion can be set up to solve this problem.

$$\frac{10 \text{ g}}{200 \text{ mL}} = \frac{x \text{ g}}{100 \text{ mL}}$$

$$x = 5\% \text{ solution (preferably expressed as 5 g/dL)}$$

Remember that the percent expression is based on how much solute is present in *100 mL (or 1 dL)* of the solution.

When specifically stated, some concentrations of solutions are expressed as the milligrams of solute in 100 mL of solution (mg%). When this is used, *mg%* is always stated. If 25 mg of a chemical is diluted to 100 mL, the concentration in milligrams percent would be expressed as 25 mg% (preferably expressed as 25 mg/dL).

If a liquid chemical is used to prepare a percent solution, the concentration is expressed as volume per unit volume percent, or milliliters of solute per 100 mL of solution. If 10 mL of hydrochloric acid (HCl) is diluted to 100 mL with water, the concentration is 10% (preferably expressed as 10 ml/dL). If 10 mL of the same acid is diluted to 1 L (1,000 mL), the concentration is 1% (preferably expressed as 1 mL/dL).

Molarity

The **molarity** of a solution is defined as the gram-molecular mass (or weight) of a compound per liter of solution. This is a weight per unit volume method of expressing concentration. Another way to define molarity is as the number of moles per liter (mol/L) of solution. A *mole* is the molecular weight of a compound in grams (1 mole equals 1 gram-molecular weight). The number of moles of a compound equals the number of grams divided by the gram-molecular weight of that compound. One gram-molecular weight equals the sum of all atomic weights in a molecule of the compound, expressed in grams.

To determine the gram-molecular weight of a compound, the correct formula must be known. When this formula is known, the sum of all the atomic weights in the compound can be found by consulting a periodic table of the elements or a chart with the atomic masses of the elements.

Examples of Molarity Calculations

1. Sodium chloride has one sodium ion and one chloride ion; the formula is written NaCl. The gram-molecular weight is derived by finding the sum of the atomic weights:

$$Na = 23$$

$$Cl = 35.5$$

$$\text{Gram-molecular weight} = 58.5$$

If the gram-molecular weight of NaCl is 58.5 g, a 1 molar (1M) solution of NaCl would contain 58.5 g of NaCl per liter of solution, because molarity equals moles per liter, and 1 mol of NaCl equals 58.5 g.

2. For barium sulfate ($BaSO_4$), the gram-molecular weight equals 233 (the formula indicates that there are one barium, one sulfate, and four oxygen ions).

$$1\ Ba = 137 \times 1 = 137$$

$$1\ S = 32 \times 1 = 32$$

$$4\ O = 16 \times 4 = \underline{\ \ 64\ }$$

$$233$$

Since the gram-molecular weight is 233, a 1M solution of $BaSO_4$ would contain 233 g of $BaSO_4$ per liter of solution.

The quantities of solutions needed will not always be in units of whole liters, and often concentrations using fractions or multiples of a 1M concentration will be desired. Parts of a molar solution are expressed as decimals. If a 1M solution of NaCl contains 58.5 g of NaCl per liter of solution, a 0.5M solution would contain one-half of 58.5 g, or 29 g/L, and a 3M solution would contain 3×58.5 g, or 175.5 g/L.

What is the molarity of a solution containing 10 g of NaCl per liter? Molarity equals the number of moles per liter, and the number of moles equals the grams divided by the gram-molecular weight.

Step 1: Find the gram-molecular weight of NaCl. It is 58.5 g (Na = 23 and Cl = 35.5).

Step 2: Find the moles per liter.

$$\frac{10\ \text{g/L}}{x} = \frac{58.5\ \text{g/L}}{1\ \text{mol}}$$

$$x = \frac{10\ \text{g/L} \times 1\ \text{mol}}{58.5\ \text{g/L}} = 0.171\ \text{mol NaCl}$$

Step 3: Knowing that the number of moles per liter of solution equals the molarity, the solution in the example is therefore 0.171M

Equations might prove useful to some in working with molarity solutions. However, all of these equations can be derived by applying a common sense proportion approach to molarity problems, as described above under Proportions and Ratios. Some of these equations are listed below.

1. Molarity $= \dfrac{\text{moles of solute}}{\text{liters of solution}}$

2. Molarity
$= \dfrac{\text{grams of solute}}{\text{gram-molecular weight}} \times \dfrac{1}{\text{liters of solution}}$

3. Moles of solute = molarity × liters of solution

4. Grams of solute = molarity × gram-molecular weight × liters of solution

Note: These equations are all on the basis of 1 L of solution; if something other than 1 L is used, refer back to the 1-L basis (500 mL = 0.5 L, or 2,000 mL = 2 L, for example).

Molarity does not provide a basis for direct comparison of strength for all solutions. An example of this is that 1 L of 1M NaOH will exactly neutralize 1 L of 1M HCl, but it will neutralize only 0.5 L of 1M sulfuric acid (H_2SO_4). It is therefore more convenient to choose a unit of concentration that *will* provide a basis for direct comparison of strengths of solutions. Such a unit is referred to as an **equivalent** (or equivalent weight or mass), and this term is used in describing the next unit of concentration to be discussed—**normality.**

Normality

Normality is defined as the number of equivalent weights per liter of solution. The *equivalent* (equiv) weight is the mass in grams that will liberate, combine with, or replace one gram-atom (g atom) of hydrogen ion (H^+). By using equivalents, the numbers of units of all substances involved in a reaction are made numerically equal. It is expressed as a weight per unit volume concentration.

Examples of Normality Calculation

Reaction 1:

1 equiv NaOH + 1 equiv HCl →
$$1 \text{ equiv } H_2O + 1 \text{ equiv NaCl}$$

Reaction 2:

1 equiv NaOH + 1 equiv H_2SO_4 →
$$1 \text{ equiv } H_2O + 1 \text{ equiv } Na_2SO_4$$

The balanced equation for this reaction is

$$2NaOH + 1H_2SO_4 \rightarrow 2H_2O + 1Na_2SO_4$$

This same reaction expressed using moles is

1 mol NaOH + 0.5 mol H_2SO_4 →
$$1 \text{ mol } H_2O + 0.5 \text{ mol } NaSO_4$$

One equivalent of any acid will neutralize one equivalent of any base.

In discussing molarity, the term *moles per liter* (mol/L) is used; in units of normality, the terms *equivalents per liter* (equiv/L), *milliequivalents per milliliter* (mEq/mL), and *milliequivalents per liter* (mEq/L) are used. The normality of a solution is defined as the number of gram-equivalents (or equivalent weights) per liter of solution, or the number of milliequivalents per milliliter of solution.

Equivalent Weight

The *equivalent weight* (or mass) is the weight in grams that will liberate, combine with, or replace one gram-atom of hydrogen. The equivalent weight may be found by dividing the gram-molecular weight by the total combining power, or valence, of the positive ion (ions) of the substance. As a general rule, the equivalent weight of a compound or substance (element) is equal to the molecular weight divided by the valence. The SI system prefers the use of molarity (mol/L) to express the amount of substance in chemical units. A disadvantage of the concept of normality is that a particular solution may have more than one normality depending on the reaction in which it is used, while it will always have the same molarity since there is only one molecular weight for any substance.

Examples of Equivalent Weights.—Hydrochloric acid has one atom of H^+ and one atom of Cl^-; therefore, the gram-equivalent weight equals the molecular weight.

Hydrogen sulfide (H_2S) has two atoms of H^+ and only one atom of S^{2-}, *or* one atom of H^+ and $\frac{1}{2}$ atom of S^{2-}; therefore, the equivalent weight equals one-half the molecular weight or

$$\frac{\text{Molecular weight}}{\text{Total positive valence}} = \frac{34}{2} = 17$$

NaCl has one atom of Cl^- and one atom of Na^+ (Na^+ replaces H^+); therefore, the gram-equivalent weight equals the gram-molecular weight.

A liter of a 1N solution of H_2SO_4 contains the same number of equivalents as 1 L of 1N HCl, or 1N NaOH, or 1N barium hydroxide [$Ba(OH)_2$]. Again, equations might prove useful in working with normality solutions. Some of these are

$$\text{Normality} = \frac{\text{equivalents of solute}}{\text{liters of solution}}$$

$$\text{Normality} = \frac{\text{grams of solute}}{\text{GMW/combining power (valence)}} \times \frac{1}{\text{liters of solution}}$$

where GMW is gram-molecular weight

$$\text{Normality} = \frac{\text{moles}}{\text{combining power}} \times \frac{1}{\text{liters of solution}}$$

$$\text{Normality} = \frac{\text{grams of solute}}{\text{equivalent weight}} \times \frac{1}{\text{liters of solution}}$$

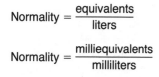

$$\text{Normality} = \frac{\text{equivalents}}{\text{liters}}$$

$$\text{Normality} = \frac{\text{milliequivalents}}{\text{milliliters}}$$

Interconversion of Molarity and Normality

On occasion, it is necessary to convert an expression of concentration in molarity to one in normality and vice versa. Two simple formulas are available for this purpose:

$$\text{Molarity} = \frac{\text{normality}}{\text{total positive combining power (valence)}}$$

$$\text{Normality} = \text{molarity} \\ \times \text{total positive combining power}$$

To prepare 1 L of a 2N NaCl solution, first calculate the gram-molecular weight, using the known formula for the compound: Na = 23, Cl = 35.5, the gram-molecular weight thus being 58.5 g. In working with normality problems, the gram-equivalent weight is used; therefore, the next step is to calculate this. The gram-equivalent weight equals the gram-molecular weight divided by the valence, or 58.5 g divided by 1; the gram-equivalent weight is therefore 58.5 g. For 1 L of a 1N solution of this compound, 58.5 g would be weighed; for 1 L of a 2N solution, 58.5 g × 2, or 117 g, of NaCl is needed per liter. An *example* of another such problem follows.

Prepare 200 mL of a 0.5N calcium chloride (CaCl$_2$) solution.

Step 1: Calculate the gram-molecular weight.

Ca = 40 × 1 = 40

Cl = 35.5 × 2 = 71

111 g = gram-molecular weight

Step 2: Calculate the gram-equivalent weight.

$$\text{Equivalent weight} = \frac{\text{GMW}}{\text{valence}} = \frac{111}{2} = 55.5 \text{ g}$$

Step 3: Solve for normality. A 1N solution would contain 55.5 g/L. A 0.5N solution would contain only half

as much chemical per liter of solution, or 27.8 g. A proportion could be set up to solve this:

$$\frac{55.5 \text{ g/L}}{1\text{N solution}} = \frac{x \text{ g/L}}{0.5\text{N solution}}$$

$$x = 27.8 \text{ g}$$

However, only 200 mL of this solution is needed. Therefore another proportion could be set up for this:

$$\frac{27.8 \text{ g}}{1,000 \text{ mL}} = \frac{x \text{ g}}{200 \text{ mL}}$$

$$x = 5.6 \text{ g}$$

Step 4: In the actual preparation of solution, 5.6 g of CaCl$_2$ is weighed and diluted to 200 mL volumetrically (see under in Reagents Used in Laboratory Assays, in Chapter 4).

OSMOLARITY

Osmolarity is defined as the number of osmoles of solute per liter of solution. An *osmole* (osm) is the amount of a substance that will produce 1 mol of particles having osmotic activity. An osmole of any substance is equal to 1 gram-molecular weight (1 mol) of the substance divided by the number of particles formed by the dissociation of the molecules of the substance. For those materials which do not ionize, 1 osm is equal to 1 mol. This gives an estimate of the osmotic activity of the solution—the relative number of particles dissolved in the solution. Osmolarity is an expression of weight per unit volume concentration.

For a solution of glucose, a substance which does not ionize or dissociate in aqueous solution, 1 osm of glucose is equal to 1 mol of glucose. For solutions which do ionize, as for a solution of sodium chloride, 1 osm of sodium chloride is equal to 1 gram-molecular weight divided by the number of particles formed upon ionization. Sodium chloride completely ionizes in water to form one sodium ion and one chloride ion, or a total of two particles. The molecular weight of NaCl is 58.5. To calculate the osmolarity of NaCl, the following formula is used:

$$1 \text{ osm NaCl} = \frac{58.5}{2} = 29.25 \text{ g}$$

DENSITY

Density is defined as the amount of matter per unit volume of a substance. All substances have this property, not only solutions. An example of the expression of density is the specific gravity of a substance. *Specific gravity* is defined as the ratio between the mass of a substance relative to the mass of an equal volume of water, or:

$$\text{Specific gravity} = \frac{\text{mass of substance}}{\text{mass of equal volume of water}}$$

See under Specific Gravity, in Chapter 13.

BIBLIOGRAPHY

Campbell JM, Campbell JB: *Laboratory Mathematics: Medical and Biological Applications,* ed 4. St Louis, Mosby–Year Book, Inc, 1990.

7 Quality Assurance in the Clinical Laboratory

Key Terms

Accuracy	Precision
Blank solution	Problem solving mechanisms
CLIA 88	Quality assurance programs
Control specimen	Quality control
Department of Health and Human Services (HHS)	Quality control charts
Gaussian curve	Proficiency testing
Health Care Financing Administration (HCFA)	Reference range
Joint Commission of Accreditation of Healthcare Organizations (JCAHO)	Reference values
	Reliability
Laboratory procedure manual	Standard deviation (SD)
95% confidence interval	Standard solution

Analytic results obtained through laboratory determinations are used by the physician both to discover the existence of disease in a patient and to follow the progress of treatment. In turn, it is the responsibility of the clinical laboratory to both patient and physician to ensure that the results reported are reliable and to give the physician an estimate of what constitutes "normal".

STANDARDS SET BY THE JOINT COMMISSION OF ACCREDITATION OF HEALTHCARE ORGANIZATIONS

The public's focus on health care delivery is relevant to most areas of work done in clinical laboratories. Agencies from public and medical communities, as well as from the government are continually reexamining health care facilities. Standards have been set by the Joint Commission of Accreditation of Healthcare Organizations (JCAHO) reflecting the commission's focus on quality assurance programs. These standards require the monitoring and evaluation of quality and appropriateness of services to patients and the resolution of any identified problems. JCAHO has published a ten-step monitoring process for quality assurance programs. These steps are:

1. Assign responsibility for a quality assurance plan.

2. Define the scope of patient care.
3. Identify the important aspects of care.
4. Construct indicators.
5. Define the thresholds for evaluation.
6. Collect and organize the data.
7. Evaluate the data.
8. Develop a corrective action plan.
9. Assess actions; document improvement.
10. Communicate relevant information.

No concern is of greater importance than that of quality assurance. As defined by the JCAHO ten-step plan, quality assurance is an overall and continuing process for the hospital or health care facility to monitor all areas that contribute to providing only the highest quality and most appropriate care for the patient. Quality assurance requires a planned, systematic process of monitoring all aspects of patient care. As part of the health care team, the clinical laboratory must also have an ongoing quality assurance process for monitoring its analytic results. The analytic result of the test or tests done on a clinical specimen must be as accurate as possible so the physician can rely on the data and use them in the diagnostic and treatment plan for the patient. This is the service provided by the clinical laboratory to the total health care plan for the patient. An ongoing, active, comprehensive **quality assurance program** is an essential component for hospital accreditation. Because quality assurance has become so important, other regulatory groups, such as the College of American Pathologists (CAP), have included quality assurance activities as necessary components of accreditation standards.

GOVERNMENTAL REGULATION OF LABORATORIES

Quality assurance programs are now also a requirement in the federal government's implementation of the Clinical Laboratory Improvement Amendments of 1988 **(CLIA 88).** Standards are for all laboratories with the intent that the medical community's ability to provide good-quality patient care will be greatly enhanced. Included in the CLIA 88 provisions are requirements for **quality control** and assurance, for the use of **proficiency testing,** and for certain levels of personnel to perform and supervise the work in the laboratory.

The **Health Care Financing Administration (HCFA)** under the US **Department of Health and Human Services (HHS)** has established regulations to implement CLIA 88. Any facility performing quantitative, qualitative, or screening test procedures or examinations on materials derived from the human body are regulated by CLIA 88. This includes hospital laboratories of all sizes; physician office laboratories; nursing home facilities; clinics; industrial laboratories; city, state, and county laboratories; pharmacies and health fairs; and independent laboratories, to list but some.

Based on the complexity of tests performed by a laboratory, a three-tiered grouping has been devised, with varying degrees of regulation for each level. The law contains a provision to exempt certain laboratories from meeting standards for personnel and from using quality control programs, proficiency testing, or quality assurance programs. These laboratories are defined as those that perform only simple routine tests which, as determined by HHS, have an insignificant risk of an erroneous result. These laboratories receive a "certificate of waiver." The remaining two levels, levels I and II, are more regulated, with some minimal personnel standards required, as well as proficiency testing and quality control and assurance programs. The level to which the laboratory is assigned depends on the complexity of the tests performed. The criteria for classification of the three tiers include risk of harm to the patient, the likelihood of erroneous results, type of testing method used, degree of independent judgment needed, and interpretation and availability of home use for the particular test in question. A panel of experts will periodically review the test complexity criteria for the three categories and make suggestions for any changes needed.

A laboratory that wishes to receive payment for its services from Medicare or Medicaid must be licensed under the Public Health Service Act. To be licensed, the laboratory must meet the conditions for participation in those programs. HCFA has the administrative responsibility for both the Medicare and CLIA 88 programs. Facilities accredited by approved private accreditation agencies, such as CAP, must also follow the regulations for licensure under CLIA 88. States with equivalent CLIA 88 regulations will be reviewed individually as to possible waiver for CLIA 88 licensure.

COMPONENTS OF QUALITY ASSURANCE PROGRAMS

Commitment

It is essential that all persons working in the clinical laboratory be totally committed to the concepts of the quality assurance process as it is defined by the specific health care facility. The importance of sufficient planning time dedicated to the topic of quality assurance and the priority given to the attention to the program implemented in the total laboratory operation is critical. All persons working in the clinical laboratory must be willing to work together to make the quality of service to the patient their top priority. Because the total laboratory staff must be involved in carrying out any quality assurance process, it is important to develop a comprehensive program to include all levels of laboratorians.

Facilities and Resources

The physical location and layout of the laboratory is an important aspect of quality assurance. Since the product of the laboratory is the analytic result for the patient's specimen, it is vital that the physical laboratory site be conducive to good performance by the laboratorians working there. A safe working site with adequate, properly maintained equipment and supplies is essential to ensure that high-quality of analytic results is a reasonable expectation.

Technical Competence

The competence of personnel is an important determinant of the quality of the laboratory result. Crucial to any quality assurance process is the maintenance of a high level of performance by the laboratorian doing the analyses. Only well-trained, competent personnel should be carrying out the testing processes. In addition to the actual performance of analytic procedures, competent laboratory personnel must be able to perform quality control activities, maintain instruments, and keep accurate and systematic records of reagents and control specimens, equipment maintenance, and patient and analytic data. For new laboratory personnel, a thorough orientation to the laboratory procedures and policies is vital.

Periodic opportunities for personal upgrading of technical skills and for obtaining new relevant information should be made available to all persons working in the laboratory. This can be accomplished through in-service training classes, opportunities to attend continuing education courses, and by encouraging independent study habits by means of scientific journals and audiovisual materials.

Personnel performance should be monitored with periodic evaluations and reports. Quality assurance demands that the results of daily work be monitored by a supervisor and that all analytic reports produced during a particular shift be evaluated for errors and omissions. Quality control measures are used to monitor possible human error in performing laboratory analyses. Quality control is one aspect of the quality assurance process and is discussed in more detail below.

Quality Assurance Procedures

Quality assurance programs monitor test requesting procedures; patient identification, specimen procurement, and labeling; specimen transportation and processing procedures; laboratory personnel performance; laboratory instrumentation, reagents, and analytic test procedures; turnaround times; and the accuracy of the final result. Complete documentation of all procedures which are involved in obtaining the final analytic result for the patient sample must be maintained and monitored in a system-

atic manner. Some of these procedures are described in the following paragraphs.

Test Requesting

The request form for each patient's laboratory work must be completed by the physician directing the patient's care. The form must include the patient identification data, the time and date for the specimen collection, the source of the specimen, and the requested analyses to be done. The complete request form must accompany the specimen. It is of interest to the laboratory to note the time of receipt of the specimen. This information is necessary for the monitoring of turnaround times—the interval between receipt of the specimen in the laboratory and release of the analytic result when the test has been completed and the result verified. The request form must be clean and legible. The information on the accompanying specimen container must match exactly the patient identification on the request slip. The information needed by the physician to assist in ordering tests is included in the handbook described in the following section.

Patient Identification, Specimen Procurement, and Labeling

A process of educating physicians, nurses, laboratorians, and other health care personnel who are involved in collecting clinical specimens is extremely important. A handbook of specimen requirement information, in an easily accessible format and location, is one of the first steps in establishing a quality assurance program for the clinical laboratory. This information must be made available on the patient care units or any other place where patient specimens are collected and it must be kept current. Information about obtaining appropriate specimens, special collection requirements for special kinds of tests, ordering tests correctly, and transporting and processing specimens appropriately is included in this handbook. Any changes in content must be communicated to those persons needing this information.

Patients must be carefully identified. For hospitalized patients, the most convenient way to do this is to have the patient wear a wristband with the necessary information printed on it.

Using established specimen requirement information, the clinical specimens must be properly labeled or identified once they have been obtained from the patient. The practice of using universal precautions in collecting specimens cannot be overemphasized. All specimens should be handled as though they contain a hazardous agent or pathogen. (See Universal Precautions, in Chapter 1.)

The laboratory can accept only properly labeled specimens. Computer-generated labels assist in making certain that proper patient identification is noted on each specimen container sent to the laboratory. Improperly labeled or nonlabeled specimens cannot be accepted by the laboratory. All containers must be labeled by the person doing the collection to make certain that the specimen has been collected from the patient whose identification is noted on the label. An important rule to remember is: The analytic result can only be as good as the specimen received (see Chapter 2).

Specimen Transportation and Processing

Specimens must be transported to the laboratory in a safe, timely, and efficient manner. It is important that a central receiving and processing area be set aside in the laboratory to monitor and record all incoming specimens and the requests accompanying them. The documentation of specimen arrival times in the laboratory as well as other specific test request data is an important aspect of laboratory organization and an essential part of the quality assurance process. It is important that the specimen status can be determined at any time—that is, where in the laboratory processing system a given specimen can be found. Turnaround time is an important factor and specimen processing, analyses, and reporting of results within an acceptable time frame is a part of the quality assurance process as a whole (see Chapter 2).

Quality Control

Quality control activities include monitoring the performance of laboratory instruments, reagents, products, and equipment. In the process of quality assurance, it is important to document the performance of quality control measures. The written record of quality control activities for each procedure or function should also include details of deviation from the usual results, problems, or failures in functioning or in the analytic procedure, as well as any corrective action taken in response to these problems.

Instruments for quality control can include preventive maintenance records, temperature charts, and other records of performance such as **quality control charts** for specific analytic procedures. All products and reagents used in the analytic procedures must be carefully

checked before actual use in testing patient samples. Use of quality control specimens, proficiency testing, and standards depends upon the specific requirements of the accrediting agency of the health care facility. General use of control specimens, proficiency testing programs, and reference values are described later in this chapter.

Sometimes laboratories are asked to assist other departments in the health care facility in their quality control measures. This could include checking the effectiveness of autoclaves in surgery or in the laundry, or providing aseptic checks for the pharmacy, blood bank, or dialysis service.

External quality control activities include periodic inspections by the various accrediting agencies involved in the regulation of clinical laboratories. It is for these inspections that the well-monitored, well-documented quality assurance records are maintained.

Laboratory Procedure Manuals

A complete **laboratory procedure manual** for all analytic procedures performed within the laboratory must be provided. The manual should contain information about patient preparation (if needed); specimen requirements and special collection or processing details; test request information; other criteria for performing the test; procedural information (how to perform the test), including the reagents and control specimens used, and the calibration of instruments and maintenance checks performed; quality control data; details about reference values; and reporting of results for each clinical analysis done. These manuals must be reviewed regularly by the supervisory staff and updated, as needed. In the process of quality assurance, the documentation of laboratory procedural information is as important as documentation of quality control activities, specimen receiving data, or the reporting of the laboratory result itself. The National Committee for Clinical Laboratory Standards (NCCLS) has set guidelines for writing laboratory procedure manuals.

Problem Solving Mechanisms

Since an important aspect of quality assurance is documentation, any problem or situation that might affect the outcome of a test result must be recorded and reported. All such incidents must be documented in writing, including the changes proposed and their implementation, and follow-up monitored. These incidents can involve specimens that are improperly collected, labeled, or transported to the laboratory, or problems concerning prolonged turnaround times for test results. Errors in procedure are the responsibility of the laboratory personnel. Quality control measures are used to ascertain the confidence level for the specific analytic result obtained. There must be a reasonable attempt to correct the problem or the laboratory impropriety and all steps in this process must be documented.

Test Result and Information Processing Systems

With the use of laboratory computer systems and information processing, record-keeping can be done in a fast, efficient manner. Quality assurance programs require documentation and computer record-keeping capability assists in doing this. Patient test results, by dates performed, as well as quality control data for the same dates, must be recorded. When control results are within the acceptable limits established by the laboratory, these data provide the necessary link between the control and patient data, thus giving reassurance that the patient results are reliable, valid, and reportable. This information is necessary to document that uniform protocols have been established and that they are being followed. The data can also support the proper functioning capabilities of the test systems being used at the time patient results are produced.

RELIABILITY DESCRIPTORS

When describing the **reliability** of a particular procedure, two terms are commonly used: **accuracy** and **precision.** The reliability of a procedure depends on a combination of these two factors, although they are different and are not dependent on each other. Variance is another general term that describes the factors or fluctuations that affect the measurement of the substance in question.

Accuracy vs. Precision

The *accuracy* of a procedure refers to the closeness of the result obtained to the true or actual value, while *precision* refers to repeatability or reproducibility—that is, the ability to get the same value in subsequent tests on the same sample. It is possible to have great precision, where all laboratory personnel performing the same pro-

cedure arrive at the same answer, but without accuracy if the answer does not represent the actual value being tested for. On the other hand, a procedure may be extremely accurate, yet so difficult to perform that individual laboratory personnel are unable to arrive at values that are close enough to be clinically meaningful.

In very general terms, accuracy can be aided by the use of properly standardized procedures, statistically valid comparisons of new methods with established reference methods, the use of samples of known values (controls), and participation in proficiency testing programs.

Precision can be measured by the proper inclusion of standards, reference samples, or control solutions; statistically valid replicate determinations of a single sample; or duplicate determinations of sufficient numbers of unknown samples. Day-to-day and between-run precision is measured by inclusion of blind samples and control specimens.

Sources of Variance or Error

In general, it is impossible to obtain exactly the same result each time a determination is performed on a particular specimen. This may be described as the variance (or error) of a procedure. These factors include limitations of the procedure itself and limitations related to the sampling mechanism used.

Sampling Factors

One of the major difficulties in guaranteeing reliable results involves the sampling procedure. Only a very small amount of sample is taken, for example, 5 to 10 mL of a total blood volume of 5 to 6 L, approximately one-thousandth of the total blood volume. Other sources of variance that involve the sample include the time of day at which the sample is obtained, the patient's position (lying down or seated), the patient's state of physical activity (in bed, ambulatory, or physically active), the interval since last eating (fasting or not), and the time interval and storage conditions between obtaining the specimen and processing by the laboratory. The aging of the sample is another source of error.

Procedural Factors

Still other sources of variance involve aging of chemicals or reagents; personal bias or limited experience of the person performing the determination; and laboratory bias because of variations in standards, reagents, environment, methods, or apparatus. There may also be experimental error resulting from changes in the method used for a particular determination, changes in instruments, or changes in personnel.

Reference Values

Definition of "Normal"

Before physicians can determine whether a patient is diseased, they must have an idea of what is normal. This is not an easy task, yet it is the responsibility of the clinical laboratory to supply the physician with this information. Much attention is being paid to the description of what constitutes normal, yet our knowledge remains quite limited. Many factors enter into this determination. There are variations because of such factors as age, sex, race, geographic location, and ethnic, cultural, and economic characteristics, plus internal factors related to the actual analytic methods and practices used by a particular laboratory. To complicate matters, an individual may show daily physiologic variations within his or her normal range, to say nothing of normal changes with age. Biometrics (the science of statistics applied to biological observations) is a rapidly expanding field that attempts to describe these variations. The selection of a group on which to base "normals" is another problem confronting the individual laboratory. Traditionally, normals have been defined by testing such groups as blood donors, persons who are working and "feeling healthy," medical students, student nurses, and medical technologists. Many of the old established normals reported in the medical literature have questionable validity because of such factors as poor sampling techniques, questionable selection of the normal group, and questionable use of clinical methods. In developing normal values or **reference values,** the proper statistical tools of sampling, selection of the normal comparison group, and analysis of data must be used. Such statistical tools are relatively well defined, but a discussion of them here is beyond the scope of this text.

Reference Range Statistics

Statistically, the **reference range** for a particular measurement is in most cases related to a normal bell-shaped curve (Fig 7–1). This **gaussian curve** or distribution has been shown to be correct for virtually all types of biological, chemical, and physical measurements. A statistically valid series of individuals who are

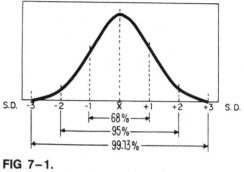

FIG 7–1.
Normal bell-shaped gaussian curve.

thought to represent a normal healthy group are measured and the average value is calculated. This mathematical average is defined as the mean ($\overline{X}$). The distribution of all values around the average for the particular group measured is described statistically by the **standard deviation (SD).**

Standard Deviation.—In any normal population, 68% of the values will be clustered above and below the average and defined statistically as falling within the first standard deviation (± 1 SD). The second standard deviation represents 95% of the values falling equally above and below the average; while 99.7% will be included within the third standard deviation (± 3 SD). (Again, variations occur equally above and below the average value [or mean] for any measurement.) Thus, in determining reference values for a particular measurement, a statistically valid series of people are chosen and assumed to represent a healthy population. These people are then tested and the results are averaged. The term *reference range* therefore means the range of values that includes 95% of the test results for a healthy reference population. The term replaces "normal values" or "normal range." The limits (or range) of normal are defined in terms of the standard deviation from the average value.

In evaluating an individual's state of health, values outside the third standard deviation value are considered clearly abnormal. When the distribution is gaussian, the reference range closely approximates the mean ± 2 SD. Values within the first (68%) and second (95%) standard deviation limits are considered normal, while those between the second (95%) and third (99.7%) standard deviation limits are questionable. Thus, normal or reference values are stated as a range of values. This stated range is in terms of standard deviation units.

Confidence Intervals.—When the reference range is expressed using 2 SD on either side of the mean, with 95% of the values falling above and below the mean (see Fig 7–1), the term **confidence interval** or confidence limits is used. This interval should be kept in mind when there are day-to-day shifts in values for a particular analytic procedure. The 95% confidence interval is used, in part, to account for certain unavoidable error due to sampling variability and imprecision of the methods themselves.

As an example, for a population study, the 95% confidence interval can be interpreted in the following way: If the procedure or experiment is repeated many times and a 95% confidence interval is constructed each time for the parameter being studied, then 95% of these intervals will actually include the true population parameter and 5% will not.

Reference Values for a Specific Laboratory

It is important to realize that reference values will vary with innumerable factors, but especially between laboratories and between geographic locations. Thus, it is necessary for each laboratory to give the physician information concerning the range of reference values for that particular laboratory. The values will be related to an overall normal, yet they may be more refined or narrow and they may be skewed in the particular situation in question. Although several textbooks are available that describe reference values for virtually all laboratory measurements, and generally accepted reference values are given in such books, the most important indicator of disease is the situation in the clinician's particular institution and locale.

It is hoped that increasing standards and improving the quality of all clinical laboratories will bring all of these reference values closer to an overall value, while parameters describing what constitutes a physiologically normal situation will become established as biometry is further advanced.

ENSURING RELIABLE RESULTS: THE QUALITY CONTROL PROGRAM

Some type of control system to ensure reliable results in the clinical laboratory is essential, a fact that has been proved by numerous laboratory accuracy surveys. A means of ensuring that a particular procedure is performed in such a way that the day-to-day results are within the established precision for the procedure and that the values reported to the physician represent the true clinical condition of the patient is essential for quality assurance. Control of laboratory error is influenced and maintained by several factors. The physician depends on the laboratory values and might be misled if these values are not those expected from the clinical diagnosis. Thus, the laboratory must be sure that the results it gives for any analysis are clinically correct. This is done primarily through the use of a *quality control program,* which makes use of standards and control samples. Other factors influencing the control of laboratory variance are expanding state and federal regulations and participation in various proficiency testing programs, either voluntarily or because of legal mandate.

The control system that is used in most laboratories is the quality control program. The quality control program for the laboratory makes use of a **control specimen,** which is similar in composition to the unknown specimen and is included in every batch or run. It must be carried through the entire test procedure, treated in exactly the same way as any unknown specimen, and is affected by any or all of the variables that affect the unknown specimen. Control specimens have long been routinely included in the clinical chemistry laboratory as well as in routine hemoglobin determinations. All clinical laboratory departments, such as the urinalysis laboratory, now recognize the need for quality control programs and specimens as a part of the quality assurance process.

The quality control program established by a laboratory involves more than only the use of control samples. The use of standards, blanks, duplicates, and recoveries are a part of the quality control program and are discussed separately. The use of automated procedures in place of manual methods often requires the inclusion of additional standards and controls, both between specimens and at the end of the run.

In controlling the reliability of laboratory determinations, the objective is to reject results when there is evidence that more than the permitted amount of error has occurred. The clinical laboratory has several ways of controlling the reliability of the results it turns out. When chemical determinations are performed, the term *batch* or *run* is often used. A batch or run is a collection of any number of specimens to be analyzed plus any or all of the following aids for ensuring reliable results—that is, controlling the variance of the procedure: standard solutions, blanks (these are used only for photometric procedures), control specimens, duplicates, and recoveries (these are used only occasionally).

Proficiency testing programs are still another means for verification of laboratory accuracy. Periodically a specimen is tested which has been provided by a government agency, professional society, or commercial company. The identical sample is sent to a group of laboratories participating in the proficiency testing program, the laboratory analyzes the specimen, reports the results to the agency, and is evaluated and graded on those results in comparison to those from other laboratories. In this way, quality control between laboratories is monitored.

Standard Solutions

To determine the concentration of a substance in a specimen, there must be a basis of comparison. For analyses that result in a colored solution, a spectrophotometer is used to make this comparison (see Chapter 5). The buret is also used in the clinical laboratory for comparison, in titration for volumetric analysis (see Measurement of Volume: Pipetting and Titration, in Chapter 4).

A **standard solution** is one that contains a known, exact amount of the substance being measured in the sample. The standard solution is measured accurately and then treated as if it were a specimen with contents to be determined. Standard solutions are prepared from high-quality chemicals that have been dried and placed in a desiccator. The standard chemical is weighed on the analytical balance and diluted volumetrically. This standard solution is usually most stable in a concentrated form, in which case it is usually referred to as a *stock* standard. Working standards (a more dilute form of the stock standard) are prepared from the stock, and sometimes an intermediate form is prepared. The working standard is the one employed in the actual determination. Stock and working standards are usually stored in the refrigerator. The accuracy of the procedure is absolutely dependent on the standard solution used; therefore extreme care must be taken whenever these solutions are prepared or used in a clinical laboratory.

Standards Used in Spectrophotometry

To use the standard solution as a basis of comparison in quantitative analysis with the spectrophotometer, a series of calibrated cuvettes (or tubes) are prepared. Each cuvette has a different amount of the standard solution.

In this way, a series of cuvettes is available containing various known amounts of the standard. Standard cuvettes are carried through the same developmental steps (usually from the filtrate stage) as cuvettes containing specimens to be measured. This set of standard cuvettes is read in the spectrophotometer and the galvanometer readings are recorded. These readings can be recorded in percent transmittance or in absorbance units (see Chapter 5). Standard solutions are also included in automated analytic methods.

Blanks

For every procedure using the spectrophotometer, a **blank solution** must be included in the batch. The blank contains reagents used in the procedure, but it does not contain the substance to be measured. It is treated with the same reagents and processed along with the undetermined specimens and the standards. The blank solution is set to read 100% *T* on the galvanometer viewing scale. In other words, the blank tube is set to transmit 100% of the light. The other cuvettes in the same batch (undetermined specimens and standards, for example) transmit only a fraction of this light, because they contain particles that absorb light (particles of the unknown substance), and thus only part of the 100% is transmitted. Using a blank solution corrects for any color that may be present because of the reagents used or an interaction between those reagents.

Control Specimens

The use of control specimens is based on the fact that repeated determinations on the same or different portions (or aliquots) of the same sample will not, as a rule, give identical values for any particular constituent. There are many factors that can produce variations in laboratory analyses. However, with a properly designed control system, it is possible to be aware of the variables and to keep them under control.

For the control specimen to have meaning in terms of the reliability of all results reported by the laboratory, it must be treated exactly like any unknown specimen. It does the patient and physician no good to have the control specimen within the allowable range if the value reported for the unknown is not accurate and precise. The use of quality control specimens is an indication of the overall reliability (both accuracy and precision) of the results reported by the laboratory, a part of the quality assurance process.

If the value of the control specimen for a particular method is not within the predetermined acceptable range, it must be assumed that the values obtained for the unknown specimens are also incorrect. After the procedure has been reviewed for any indication of error, and the error has been found and corrected, the batch must be repeated until the control value falls in the acceptable range.

If the control value in a determination is out of the acceptable range (out of control), one or more of the following factors may be responsible: (1) deterioration of reagents or standards, (2) faulty instrument or equipment, (3) dirty glassware, (4) lack of attention to timing or incubation temperature, (5) use of a method not suited to the needs and facilities of the laboratory, (6) use of poor technique by the person doing the test owing to carelessness or lack of proper training, and (7) statistics: a certain percentage of all determinations will be statistically out of control.

The control sample may be obtained commercially or prepared by the individual laboratory. The most important consideration is that it be routinely included with each group of laboratory determinations, or in certain instances at least each day, by each person performing the determinations.

Commercial Control Specimens

Commercially prepared controls can be purchased from a manufacturer. These control solutions are obtained in small samples, called *aliquots,* prepared originally from a large pooled supply of serum or plasma. Commercial controls are usually obtained in a lyophilized (or dried) form. Care must be taken in reconstituting the material to add exactly the correct amount of diluent (usually deionized or distilled water) and to make certain that the material is completely dissolved and well mixed. Commercial control solutions generally have an expiration date, the date by which they must be used in order to give reliable results. Controls should not be used after the expiration date. Reconstituted control solutions must be used within a relatively short period of time, which is generally specified by the manufacturer. Commercial control material may be purchased either assayed or unassayed. Assayed control preparations have been tested by the manufacturer and stated values are given for each of the constituents. The manufacturer should provide information concerning the analytic method and

statistical procedures used in arriving at the stated values, so that the laboratory can determine the appropriateness of the material for its particular methods and practices. If unassayed control preparations are used, the laboratory will have to establish its own range of acceptable results for each constituent being measured. The method of arriving at this acceptable range is the same as that used in establishing limits for "laboratory-made" control solutions, to be described next. Tentative standards for manufacturers of control preparations were established in 1972 by the NCCLS.

Control Solutions Prepared by the Laboratory

Control solutions can also be prepared by the individual laboratory. In the case of control specimens for certain chemistry determinations, serum or plasma is pooled using blood obtained from known donors. The blood is tested for hepatitis B and human immunodeficiency virus (HIV) pathogens. Only disease-free blood is used. Blood is processed and serum frozen. In most laboratories, the commercially prepared product is preferable. After a sufficient pool of the serum or plasma has accumulated, the control specimens for daily use can be made. Only normal serum or plasma is used (i.e., not lipemic or hemolyzed). When enough serum has been saved, it is thawed and mixed thoroughly. After thorough mixing, the pool is divided into aliquots of a convenient size. Aliquots of 2 to 3 mL in a small tube or vial are satisfactory. These samples are then stored in a freezer. Every effort must be made to exclude serum from the pool from patients with blood-born diseases.

Determination of Control Range

Once a control solution has been prepared or purchased, it is necessary for the laboratory to determine the acceptable control range for a particular analysis. There are various ways of establishing such a range, and one commonly employed method will be described; however, any method must adhere to statistically acceptable methods. In establishing the control range, an aliquot of the pooled serum or a commercial control specimen is processed along with the regular batch of tests for 15 to 25 days. It is imperative to thoroughly mix the thawed aliquot since the sample layers as it freezes. In testing the control sample it is important that it be treated exactly like an unknown specimen; it must not be treated any more or less carefully than the unknown specimen.

As mentioned previously, repeated determinations on different aliquots of the same sample will not give identical values for any particular constituent. However, it has been shown that if a sufficient number of repeated determinations are made, the values obtained will fall into a normal bell-shaped curve, as described above (see Fig 7–1). When a statistically sufficient number of determinations have been run (the number is different for averaged duplicate determinations and single tests) the mathematical mean ($\bar{x}$) or average value can be calculated. The acceptable limits or variation from the mean for the control solution are then calculated on the basis of the standard deviation from the mean, using certain statistical formulas. Most laboratories use 2 SD above and below the mean as the allowable range of the control specimen, while others use this range as a warning limit. Referring back to the normal bell-shaped curve (see Fig 7–1), setting 2 SD as the allowable range for the control sample means that 95% of all determinations on that sample will fall within the allowable range, while 5% will be out of control. It may not be desirable to disallow this many batches, so the third standard deviation may be chosen as the limit of control, or the action limit. Once the range of acceptable results has been established, one of the control specimens is included in each batch of determinations. If the control value is not within the limits established, the procedure must be repeated, and no patient results may be given to the physician until the control value is within the allowable range.

Quality Control Chart

It is conventional in most laboratories to plot the daily control specimen values on a quality control chart, as shown in Figure 7–2. The control chart is made on a rectangular sheet of linear graph paper. Monthly control charts are prepared, with the days of the month marked on the horizontal axis and units of concentration for the determination in question marked on the vertical axis. The mean value for the determination in question is then indicated on the chart in addition to the limits of acceptable error. The 2- and 3-SD values might be indicated with the 2-SD value as a warning limit and the 3-SD value as an action limit. Each day the control value is plotted on the chart, and any value falling out of control can easily be seen.

Glucose — Alkaline Ferricyanide — Autoanalyzer

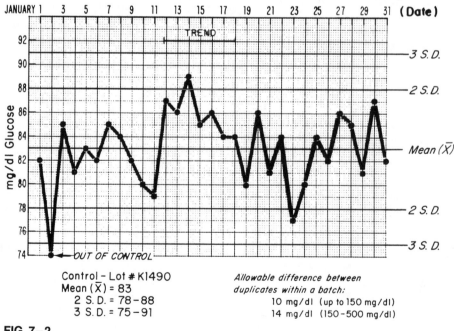

Control – Lot # K1490
Mean ($\bar{X}$) = 83
2 S.D. = 78 – 88
3 S.D. = 75 – 91

Allowable difference between
duplicates within a batch:
   10 mg/dl (up to 150 mg/dl)
   14 mg/dl (150 – 500 mg/dl)

FIG 7–2.
Monthly quality control chart.

The control chart serves as visual documentation of the information derived from using control specimens. A different control chart is plotted for each substance being determined. It is possible to observe trends leading toward trouble by plotting the control values daily. When procedural changes such as the addition of new reagents, standards, or instruments are made, they are also noted on the control chart. Such a chart can assist in preventing difficulties and can aid in trouble-shooting. If all is going well, the plotted control values should be distributed equally above and below the established mean value. A regular weekly visual inspection of the control chart is particularly useful for observing trends before control specimen values are actually out of the established acceptable limits. Generally, an excess of more than five control value results on one side of the mean indicates a trend, although not all such trends need action. The use of quality control programs, including the control chart, is a part of the laboratory quality assurance process.

Duplicate Determinations

In each batch of determinations, one of the specimens is measured in duplicate. This specimen is chosen at random from those to be tested. Often control specimens are measured in duplicate. If this is done, the allowable range for duplicates is less than that for single determinations. The use of duplicates checks the technique used—that is, the precision, or repeatability, of the method. Duplicates do not measure accuracy. It is possible to have grossly inaccurate duplicate results that agree perfectly. The allowable difference between duplicate determinations varies and must be established for each determination performed by the laboratory. This is done using certain statistical formulas; the standard deviation is calculated from the differences between a certain number of duplicate determinations. Duplicate determinations are also part of a quality control and assurance program.

Recovery Solutions

Recovery solutions are used as an indicator of the accuracy of a particular determination. To any specimen in the batch (or to a control solution), in addition to the regular specimens, a measured amount of the pure substance being analyzed is added. Theoretically, the amount of substance added should be recovered at the end of the determination if the method is an accurate

one. Recoveries are not used routinely with most procedures, but are often used to evaluate a new procedure. One method to be discussed in this text, the blood urea nitrogen determination, uses a recovery solution as part of the regular batch. Recovery solutions are another part of a quality control program.

Other Components of Quality Control

Specimen Appearance

First, consider the specimen itself—how it is collected, transported to the laboratory, received, identified, processed, and stored. The specimen should be visually inspected for hemolysis or lipemia, as these might affect or invalidate certain determinations. Certainly their presence should be recorded with the final result. In photometric procedures, the laboratorian should observe the final solution in the cuvette for turbidity or inappropriate color development.

Validating New Procedures

Another part of the quality control program concerns the way new procedures are validated before they are included among the methods routinely used by the laboratory. Each laboratory must determine the reproducibility (or confidence limits) for each procedure used and establish acceptable limits of variation for control specimens. The quality control program includes calculation of the mean (or average value) and standard deviation and the preparation of control charts for each procedure.

Control of Human Error

The program should include a means of independent monitoring to minimize bias on the part of the person doing the tests. This may be done by using blind controls, such as commercial control solutions labeled as patient unknowns, or dividing patient specimens into different aliquots to be processed blindly and independently on the same day, or carried over to another day if the constituent is stable.

Correlation of Test Results

Another valuable quality control technique is to look at the data generated for each patient and inspect them for relationships between the results obtained by the laboratory. There are many relationships, such as the mathematical relationship between anions and cations in the electrolyte report, the correlation between protein and casts in urine, and the relationship between hemoglobin and the hematocrit and the appearance of the blood smear in hematologic studies.

Evaluation of Procedures

Each laboratory must have an assessment routine for all procedures to be done on a daily, weekly, and monthly basis to detect problems such as trends and shifts of the established mean value. When such problems are indicated, it is most important that they be corrected as soon as possible. Many of the components of the quality control program are the responsibility of the laboratory supervisor or director. However, every person working in the laboratory has an important role in ensuring reliable laboratory results, either by running the control specimen or by calling potential problems to the attention of the supervisor.

Proficiency Testing

In addition to the use of internal quality control programs, each laboratory should participate in at least one external control program. These are known as proficiency testing programs and are a required provision of the CLIA 88 regulations.

Proficiency surveys are a means of establishing quality control between laboratories. Both state and national agencies have established programs to help laboratories maintain their quality control programs. Proficiency testing programs are available through CAP, the Centers for Disease Control (CDC), and various state health departments. These proficiency testing programs periodically send specimens to laboratories that participate in the program. The laboratory analyzes the sample, using its routine procedures, and sends the results to the program administrator. Each participating laboratory is furnished with an evaluation of its results compared with those of all other laboratories participating in the survey. Participation in at least one proficiency survey is an important part of a laboratory's quality control program.

BIBLIOGRAPHY

Accreditation Manual for Hospitals. Chicago, Joint Commission on Accreditation of Healthcare Organizations, 1987.

Approved Guidelines for Clinical Laboratory Procedure Manuals. Villanova, Pa, National Committee for Clinical Laboratory Standards, 1984;4(February):GP2-A.

Henry JB (ed): *Clinical Diagnosis and Management by Laboratory Methods,* ed 18. Philadelphia, WB Saunders Co, 1991.

Meisenheimer CG: *Quality Assurance, a Complete Guide to Effective Programs*. Rockville, Md, Aspen Publications, 1985.

Monitoring and Evaluation, Pathology and Laboratory Services. Chicago, Joint Commission on Accreditation of Healthcare Organizations, 1987.

Revision of the laboratory regulations for Medicare, Medicaid and Clinical Laboratories Improvement Act of 1967 programs, final rule. *Federal Register* 1990;55:50(March 14).

Standards for Accreditation. Northfield, Ill, College of American Pathologists, 1987.

Tietz NW (ed): *Textbook of Clinical Chemistry,* Philadelphia, Pa, WB Saunders Co, 1986.

8 Automation in the Clinical Laboratory

Key Terms

Analog computation	Discrete-sample analyzer
Automatic cell counters	Dry film reagent technology
Automated differential counters	Flow cytometers
Batch analyzer	Interfacing data
Continuous-flow analyzer	Light-emitting diodes
Cathode-ray tube	Random access analyzer
Digital computation	Wet reagent chemistry

One of the major technologic changes in the clinical laboratory has been the introduction of automated analysis. An automated analytic instrument provides a means of transfer of a specimen within its complex assembly to a series of self-acting components each of which carries out a specific process or stage of the process, ending in the analytic result being produced. In general, laboratory automation has centered on handling the sample after it has been received in the laboratory, culminating in the transfer of the analytic data back to the requesting physician.

USE OF AUTOMATION

The demand for laboratory data has grown to such an extent, through the use of the data by physicians in the diagnosis and treatment of disease, that automation has become essential to process the increasing number of requests for laboratory determinations. Physicians have become more and more dependent on the clinical laboratory for accurate, fast results. Automation provides a means by which an increased workload can be processed rapidly and reproducibly. It does not necessarily improve the accuracy of the results.

The first practical automated system was introduced into the clinical laboratory in 1957. Numerous other instruments for automation have been devised since that first system, employing the *continuous-flow* principle, was conceived by L.T. Skeggs. This system was introduced commercially as the AutoAnalyzer (Technicon Instruments Corp., Tarrytown, N.Y.) and has since been used extensively by many laboratories. It has undergone several refinements and modifications, so that the latest units have much more versatility than the original instrument. In the **continuous-flow analyzer,** samples flow in sequence through a channel. Another group of instruments employs the principle of *discrete-sample processing*. The **discrete-sample analyzer** processes each specimen separately, generally in steps, somewhat as in the conventional manual method. A third group makes use of *centrifugal force* to transfer and mix samples and reagents.

Originally, automation was used for the tests done most frequently in the clinical laboratory. Automation is used in many areas of the laboratory, and in many larger laboratories today, very few procedures are done manually. Perhaps the chemistry department is the area in which the advent of automation has made the greatest difference. In hematology, automation has also made a great change in the work done. Electronic cell counters have replaced manual counting of blood cells in many laboratories. There is an automated system for Wright's staining of blood smears. For coagulation studies several automated and semiautomated units are available. Prothrombin time and activated partial thromboplastin time determinations can be done automatically on various instruments. Semiautomatic instruments are also used, especially for dilution. Several instruments are available for precise and convenient diluting, which both aspirate the sample and wash it out with the diluent. Some automatic diluters dispense and dilute in separate processes. There also are automated instruments for performing routine urinalysis determinations.

If an automated system is basically sound and in good working order, there are many advantages to its use: large numbers of samples may be processed with minimal technician time, two or more methods may be performed simultaneously, precision is superior to that of a manual method, and calculations may not be required. Sometimes the automatic systems are so impressive in their appearance that laboratory personnel put too much faith in them and are misled about their shortcomings. These machines must be understood and their potential problems noted and remembered.

The fact that automation has found its way into the clinical laboratory does not mean that the person responsible for the work is not important. There still are many laboratories where manual procedures are used, especially in smaller hospitals, where the number of laboratory determinations does not always justify the purchase of an automated system. Many smaller hospital laboratories do lease these units, however, and so the size of the hospital does not always limit the use of automated equipment. Back-up manual procedures are always necessary in case of equipment failure, and these procedures must be set up and ready to use when needed. The emphasis in the laboratory has turned to faster turnaround times for results, with accuracy and precision maintained. Automation has enabled the laboratory to accommodate the increased demand for increased numbers of tests.

Disadvantages of Automation

Some problems that may arise with many automated units are: (1) there may be limitations in the methodology that can be used (sometimes a compromise must be made that results in less accurate, although often more precise, values than are obtained with manual methods); (2) with automation, laboratorians are often discouraged from making observations and using their own judgment about potential problems; (3) many systems are impractical for small numbers of samples, and therefore manual methods are still necessary as back-up procedures for emergency individual analyses; (4) back-up procedures must be available in case of instrument failures; (5) automated systems are expensive to purchase and maintain—regular maintenance requires technician time as well as the time of trained service personnel; and (6) there is often an accumulation of irrelevant data because it is so easy to produce the results—tests are run that are not always necessary.

COMPONENTS OF AN AUTOMATED LABORATORY ANALYZER

Automation can be applied to any or all of the steps used to perform any manual assay. Automated systems include some kind of device for sampling the patient's specimen or other samples to be tested (such as blanks, controls, and standard solutions), a mechanism to add the necessary amounts of reagents in the proper sequence, incubation modules when needed for the specific reaction, monitoring or measuring devices such as photometric technology to quantitate the extent of the reaction, and a recording mechanism to provide the final reading or permanent record of the analytic result. Most analyzers are capable of processing serum, plasma, urine, and cerebrospinal fluid, but not whole blood. A few instruments are designed to process whole blood.

The steps included in the analytic process can be performed manually or with automated instruments. Generally the automated analyzers employ the same steps as do the manual methods, using the same reagents and principles. The precision is greater in automated systems, however, because the operation of the instrument is under better control and manual intervention has been replaced by mechanical intervention. Automated systems perform essentially the same types of analyses, most of them being chemistry tests, as do the manual methods. Almost any manual method can be adapted to one that is automated. As with any piece of laboratory apparatus, the manufacturer's directions must always be followed

carefully. Automation of analyses generates test results rapidly and accurately and provides data which can be sent to the requesting physician in time to affect medical decisions concerning the patient.

General Functions Provided by Automated Analyzers

Whether a laboratory determination is done manually or automatically, certain individual steps are necessary. It is generally advisable to perform as many steps as possible without manual intervention to increase efficiency. Several of these steps can be automated for faster and more accurate results. Some methods and procedures have been partially automated, or semiautomated, by use of mechanical pipetting and diluting devices. Full automation reduces the possibility of human errors that arise from repetitive and boring manipulations done by laboratorians such as pipetting errors in routine procedures.

Collection and Preparation of the Sample

The specimen must be collected properly, labeled, and transported to the laboratory for analysis. Specimen handling and processing is a vital step in the total analytic process (see Chapter 2). Automation of specimen preparation steps can include the use of bar-coded labels on samples which allow electronic identification of the sample and the tests requested. This can prevent clerical errors from improperly entering patient data for analysis.

Sample and Reagent Measurements and Mixing

Automated instruments measure, aspirate, and introduce samples into the analyzer reagents. Automation combines reagents and sample in a prescribed manner to yield a specific final concentration. It is important that the proper amounts of reagents be introduced to the sample in specific sequences for the analysis to be carried through correctly. Mixing of reagents and sample can be done by stirring, agitation, or by some other device.

Incubation

In automated analyzers, incubation is simply a waiting period in which the test mixture is allowed time to react. This is done at a specified, constant temperature controlled by the analyzer.

Monitoring or Sensing the Reaction Result

This can be done by optical, thermal, or electrical means. Chemical reactions can be monitored either at one time point or at many. Some measurements can be done in the vessel, cell, or cuvette where the reaction has taken place; this is known as *in situ monitoring*. If the sample has been transferred from the reaction vessel to the sensing device, the monitoring is external. Different instruments employ different monitoring mechanisms.

Quantitating the Reaction Result

Quantitating by automated computation can be done by either the digital or analog format.

Analog Computation.—The analog microprocessor uses an electrical signal from the sensor, as from the photoelectric cell, and compares it with a reference signal, as for the blank solution. It then compares the two signals and takes the logarithm of the result as the final result for the unknown sample.

Digital Computation.—**Digital computation** is usually restricted to certain mathematical functions (such as addition or subtraction). A digital computer needs an analog-to-digital converter in order to process the signals received from the many types of sensing or monitoring devices used in the automated instruments. This converter changes the voltage or current signal into a digital form which can then be processed by the computer.

Visualizing the Result

A common and easy way to visualize an instrument readout is with the use of a television monitor (**cathode-ray tube**) or **light-emitting diodes.** Data can be visualized before results are accepted. This visualized readout can be converted to hard copy by means of a paper or tape printout. This data printout information must then be transferred or transcribed to laboratory report slips or other permanent records. If the data (results) are interfaced with a laboratory computer, this transcription process is done quickly and without errors, which may occur when transcription is done manually.

Standardization

To ensure the accuracy of results obtained with automated systems, there must be frequent standardization of methods. Once the standardization has been done, a well-designed automated system maintains or reproduces the prescribed conditions with great precision. Frequent standardization and running of control specimens is essential to ensure this accuracy and precision.

KINDS OF AUTOMATED ANALYZERS

Many analyzers are being manufactured for use in the clinical laboratory. The choice of which type of instrument to use is dependent on several factors: the volume of determinations done in the laboratory, the type of data profile to be generated, the level of staffing, the initial cost of the instrument and of its upkeep and operation, and the amount of time it takes for each analysis. Versatility and flexibility are often just as important as high volume and speed of testing. Some of the most common instruments or categories of instruments are described in the following paragraphs.

Automation in the Chemistry Laboratory

Automated Batch Analyzers

These instruments can analyze a batch of samples simultaneously for one particular analyte at a time. **Batch analyzers** can also be designed to analyze a number of different analytes. They are controlled by a microprocessor which can change the program for each different analyte to be measured. It is possible to have a batch analyzer capable of measuring 30 or more analytes, one analyte at a time. For these systems, generally there is a reagent delivery apparatus for each reagent needed. This type of analyzer does not require that every sample be tested for every analyte.

Random Access Analyzer

The **random access analyzer** does all the selected determinations on a patient sample before it goes on to the next sample. The microprocessor enables the analyzer to perform up to 30 determinations. Ordering of selected tests from the menu is done and the testing begun, leaving the unordered tests undone. A sampling device begins the process by measuring the exact amount of sample into the required cells. The microprocessor controls the addition of the proper diluents and reagents to each cell. After the proper reacting period, the microprocessor begins the spectrophotometric measurements of the various cells, the results are calculated, and control values checked. The results are then reported. Some analyzers of this type have a circular configuration utilizing an analytic turntable device for the various cells. Other random access analyzers have a parallel configuration.

DuPont ACA

The *automated clinical analyzers (ACA)* introduced by DuPont are designed to perform analyses in prepackaged plastic bags. They are discrete, selective analyzers. The sample is automatically discharged into the pack, the reagents which are compartmentalized in the pack are released and mixed with the sample, and the functions which are necessary to carry out a particular analysis are carried out. For some methods, measurement is made photoelectrically and for end-point methods, the measurement is done bichromatically. This instrument requires a separate reagent pack for each test. At present, these packs are available only from DuPont. They must be refrigerated and the cost per test is relatively expensive. The reagent packs allow introduction of the sample to various reagent compartments where different stages of reagent mixing and reactions occur, depending on the analysis to be done. The pack moves to the photometer where the amount of absorbance for the particular constituent being measured is noted electronically. The instrument's computer calculates the concentration for the unknown along with that for the necessary controls and standards.

The DuPont ACA can serve as a general chemistry analyzer in small-sized hospital laboratories. It can also be used in medium-sized laboratories as a specialty analyzer. Any combination of tests can be run on any sample at any time.

Eastman Kodak Ektachem Analyzer

There are various models of these discrete, selective analyzers, using a random access design. They utilize dry film technology where the dry reagents are impregnated into a slide. A thin layer of gelatin is mounted on plastic slides to which the dry reagent is added. The addition of the sample provides the necessary solvent (water) to rehydrate the dry reagents. The slides are composed of multiple layers of film, some of which serve as ultrafilters for the sample. Others provide reactive reagents for the particular analysis being performed. The reagent slides must be stored at refrigerated temperature and are relatively expensive.

Samples are placed in cups on a turntable. The sample cups are covered with a top which can be penetrated by the automatic robotic device attached to a disposable pipette. This robotic device applies the measured sample to the selected dry reagent slide. Depending on the method to be performed, slides are automatically dispensed from method-specific cartridges. Slides are incubated while color development takes place. For methods utilizing reflectance photometry, after the reaction has taken place on the slide and incubation has occurred, reflected radiant energy is read with the measured energy being relayed to a microprocessor. The reflected energy is converted into concentration units. Printouts are available with results for unknown samples and controls.

Beckman ASTRA

This discrete, selective analyzer is used to process high-volume tests such as glucose, creatinine, blood urea nitrogen (BUN), potassium, chloride, and sodium determinations in a very short period of time. One model can process up to 72 samples per hour and up to 648 tests per hour.

Automated Analyzers for the Physician's Office

Since physician office laboratories are performing many tests, and since the number of these laboratories is expected to increase over the next few years, there have been many automated or semiautomated analyzers introduced for use outside the traditional hospital laboratory setting. The criteria used by the physician to select the appropriate instrument(s) for a particular laboratory include the type of practice or specialty, the volume of tests to be done, whether single tests or chemistry profiles are needed, the turnaround time available, and the cost of the analyzer and its reagents.

In a physician's office laboratory, ideally the specimen to be tested would be whole blood and the automatic pipetting of the specimen and necessary reagents would be done by the analyzer, eliminating as much interaction by laboratory personnel as possible. The use of instruments with stable calibration curves is important and a quality control program should be available from the manufacturer. The analyzing instruments should be interfaced with a computer, if possible, to provide the necessary documentation of laboratory results. Quality control information can also be stored in the computer. The instrument should be easy to use and, because in many physician office laboratories there will be persons working there who have little or no laboratory training, the instrument should require only a limited user training period. The reagents, whether wet or dry, should be bar-coded, prepackaged, and stable for at least 6 months.

Dry Reagent Systems

There are several systems available which utilize dry reagent technology. They include the Seralyzer system (Ames Division, Miles Laboratories), the Kodak DT system (Kodak Ektachem), the ChemPro system (Sentech), the ANALYST system (DuPont DeNemours), and the Reflotron system (Boehringer Mannheim Diagnostics). Each has slightly different testing reagents, but the principle of use is similar. The Reflotron system is described here.

Reflotron System.—The solid phase reagent test tabs used in this system are bar-coded to identify the tests, the reaction parameters, and the calibration curves for each assay. The manufacturer establishes the calibration curve for each lot of reagent strips, eliminating the need for calibration by the laboratory. The reagent strips have a shelf life of from 1 to 2 years. In using this system, whole blood from a finger or heel stick can be used for analysis. The blood is placed on the reagent strip, made up of a glass fiber pad which separates the plasma from the red cells. The separation of cells from plasma is accomplished by capillary action, leaving the required plasma to react with the reagent in the strip at a temperature of 37° C. Excess plasma is removed from the reaction site. The analyte concentration is determined by reflectance photometry and recorded visually or interfaced with a laboratory computer.

Wet Chemistry Reagent Systems

One system utilizing **wet reagent chemistry** is the Vision system (Abbott Diagnostics Co.). Another is the GEMSTAR (Electronucleonics Co.). The Vision system is described.

Vision System.—This automated system uses specially designed reagent packs which are disposable. The reagent pack is a self-contained unit with a cuvette, liquid reagents, and bar codes to identify the assay to be done. Blood can be obtained by finger or heel stick and placed in a special tube provided by the manufacturer. This special tube can then be inserted into the reagent pack, eliminating the step of pipetting the sample from the capillary tube into the analyzer. Two drops of blood,

serum, or plasma are placed in the multichambered reagent pack and the packs are placed in the ten-position rotor in the analyzer. The red cells, if whole blood is used, are separated from plasma using centrifugal force. Next the packs are rotated at a 90-degree angle allowing the premeasured amount of sample and the reagents to be transferred into the cuvette. The reaction occurs at 37° C, is monitored, and the absorbances are measured bichromatically. The reagents for this system are stable for several months and one to ten analytes can be measured. The Vision system is suitable for doing batches of tests, profiles, or stat procedures.

Automation in the Hematology Laboratory

The best sources for information about the various instruments available are found in the manufacturers' product information literature. The continual advances in commercial instruments for hematologic use and their variety preclude an adequate description of them in this chapter.

Automatic Cell Counters

Automatic cell counters are used extensively in hematology to identify and enumerate the blood cells in a given patient sample. Even the simplest instruments can identify and count red blood cells, white blood cells, and platelets. In more sophisticated instruments, the types of white blood cells can be identified and counted. These instruments are known as **flow cytometers.**

Automated cell counters are of two types, those using electrical resistance and those using optical methods with focused laser beams. Both types of instrument count thousands of cells in a few seconds, decrease the coefficient of variation, and increase the precision of cell counts as compared with manual methods (see Automated Cell Counting Methods, in Chapter 11).

Automated Differential Counters

Automated differential counters utilize the impedance method to construct a size-distributed histogram of white blood cells. In most of these instruments, three subpopulations of white cells are counted: lymphocytes, other mononuclear cells, and granulocytes. A computer calculates the number of particles in each area as a percentage of the total white blood cell count histogram. Any abnormal histograms are flagged for review.

BIBLIOGRAPHY

Bender GT: *Principles of Clinical Instrumentation.* Philadelphia, WB Saunders Co, 1987.

Kaplan LA, Pesce AJ: *Clinical Chemistry Theory, Analysis, and Correlation,* ed 2. St Louis, Mosby–Year Book, Inc, 1989.

Physician's Office Laboratory Guidelines, Tentative Guidelines, Villanova, Pa, National Committee for Clinical Laboratory Standards, 1989; 9:POL 1-T.

Skeggs LT Jr: An automated method for colorimetric analysis. *Am J Clin Pathol* 1957; 28:311.

9 Introduction to Laboratory Computers

Key Terms

Bar-code reader	Interpretive report
Cathode-ray tube (CRT)	Hospital information system (HIS)
Central memory	Laboratory information systems (LIS)
Central processing unit (CPU)	Laboratory report
Data base	Output devices
Hardware	Program
Input devices	Random access memory (RAM)
	Software

PURPOSE OF THE LABORATORY COMPUTER

Because the number of tests performed in the clinical laboratory has grown so dramatically over the years and because so much analytic information has been produced by these tests, the need to process this information efficiently and accurately has become essential. This information is, of course, utilized for the benefit of the patient. We have seen that the quality assurance process requires the documentation of all work involved in patient care. The laboratory computer provides this service.

The number of laboratory tests has increased in part as a result of the development of new diagnostic tests and also because of the increased use of automated analyzers. Many **laboratory information systems (LIS)** have been developed to assist in the delivery of the data. The laboratory computer system must be capable of delivering this information to the physician, billing department, patient record department, and other administrative support sites, and to ensure that the data are communicated in a timely manner.

FUNCTIONS AND USES OF THE LABORATORY COMPUTER

An important function of the laboratory computer is to organize the various pieces of information and provide ready access to this information when it is needed. The information provided by each laboratory procedure should be maximized so that the patient receives the greatest benefit at the lowest cost.

The Laboratory Report

An important use for the laboratory computer is to provide the physician with one comprehensive **laboratory report** that contains all the test information generated by the various laboratories that have performed analyses for the patient. The format of the report should be such that the test results are clear and unambiguous. Many questions need answering to establish or rule out a particular diagnosis and the report should facilitate this process. The report should indicate any abnormality. It should answer these questions: What is the predictive value of the test for the disease in question? Is the result meaningful? What other factors could produce the result? What should be done next?

If the diagnosis has already been made, other uses can be made for the information on the report form. The physician must know the result of the most recent laboratory test, what clinically significant changes have occurred since the last test, whether changes in therapy are indicated, and when the test should next be performed. This information constitutes what is known as an **interpretive report.**

An interpretive report form should be informative about the range of reference values, flag for abnormal values, and provide these data in a readily accessible format.

Other Uses

The laboratory computer system also provides data for the hospital billing department, sends patient laboratory test data to the record room, and provides lists of available laboratory tests for the physician.

Special reports and lists can be generated by the computer. Lists of samples waiting to be tested, quality control data, lists of abnormal test results, and maintenance records all can be generated by the computer with considerable efficiency. The storage of preexisting data—all available tests, specimen requirements, quality control information (means, standard deviations, information included on report forms), instrument parameters—makes up the **data base.**

Intralaboratory Communication

The computer stores information regarding laboratory policies, mission statements regarding specific objectives for the particular laboratory facility, and statements about laboratory medicine philosophy, in general. Procedure manuals with information about each test procedure, reference range statistics, the quality control systems used, test procedure reference materials, dates of adoption of new test methods, and evidence of other periodic review measures can be stored in the laboratory information system. The College of American Pathologists (CAP) accreditation standards, for example, require that laboratories have methods established for communication of needed information to ensure prompt, reliable reporting of results, and appropriate storage of data and retrieval capacity.

Extralaboratory Communication

Information regarding specimen requirements—procurement, transport, and processing—can be stored in an accessible form. Physicians ordering the test, nurses assisting in specimen collection, and others involved with the transport or handling of the specimen, must have this information readily available.

Laboratory information systems often are interfaced with other information systems, most commonly the **hospital information system (HIS).** HIS manages patient census information and demographics, systems for billing, and the more complex systems process and store patient medical information. The interfacing HIS and the laboratory computer facilitates the exchange of test request orders, information about the patient (patient census), the return of analytic results (the laboratory report), and the charges for the test ordered and reported. When the data are verified, results can be retrieved by nurses or physicians in the patient care areas by use of terminals and printers. This linking of hospital and laboratory computer systems is not easy and totally integrated systems require an institutional commitment to the process. A well-designed easily accessible HIS-LIS data base offers significant improvements in medical record-keeping, patient care planning, budget planning, and general operations management tasks.

MAJOR COMPONENTS OF THE LABORATORY COMPUTER

Electronic computer systems are made up of **hardware,** the physical or "hard" parts of the computer, and **software,** the instructions that tell the computer what to do.

Hardware

Hardware for the computer consists of the physical components of the computer system. Central processing units, printers, and other terminals used for information input and output are examples of computer hardware.

Central Processing Unit

The **central processing unit (CPU)** is the central component of the computer. It functions as the brains of the system. The CPU is made up of a control unit, an arithmetic logic unit (ALU), and the central memory. The CPU carries out the instructions (**program**) given by the user.

Data Storage Devices

An important component is the data, or memory, storage section. This contains all the necessary instructions and data needed to operate the computer system. In addition, any short-term information, such as patient records and laboratory data, may also be stored temporarily in the memory. In addition to **central memory,** magnetic tapes and disks are used to store less frequently accessed data. These require more time for retreival but are considerably less expensive than central memory.

Central Memory, Random Access Memory.—Central memory provides storage and rapid access. **Random access memory (RAM)** is a type of central memory and is commonly used to store data that are frequently altered, changed, or updated.

Magnetic Tapes.—Magnetic tapes are the least expensive form of data storage. Access to information is generally slow. Data stored on tapes are *sequential* and all information, whether it is needed or not, must be serially passed over to find the needed information. Access time can take minutes, not seconds. The use of tapes is very common, however, for archival storage of data no longer needed on-line to the computer. Tapes are also used as a standard method for transporting information between computers.

Hard Disks.—Hard disks are revolving disks, small recordlike plates, with a magnetic surface that can be easily accessed. Data are stored in *tracks,* a series of concentric circles on the disk. Data are retrieved by positioning the reading head over the desired portion of the track, allowing a given piece of information to rotate under the head. Accessing information from disks takes milliseconds, not minutes. The transfer of information stored on a hard disk to another computer is usually not possible and the cost of the disks and associated hardware is usually considerably higher than that of magnetic tape.

Floppy Disks.—These are also called *diskettes* and are used in many microcomputer-based instruments and word processors because of their low cost.

Input Devices

Input devices allow communication between the user and the CPU. There are several peripheral devices which allow this communication to take place. Some of these also function as output devices. The exchange of information between the computer and user is called *interfacing*. Interfacing is accomplished through one of several kinds of devices. Most often the computer information is displayed on a video screen—the *display screen*.

Data input and output can be accomplished either by *command line entry* (string entry) or *by menu selection*. Command line entry is a series of individual commands or pieces of information that the user inputs in a single step to instruct the computer about the task to be done. An example of string entry is information about a patient identification number and a specific piece of information about a test result for that patient. Instead of entering each piece of information separately, the data are entered together ("strung" together). Individual command lines are separated from each other by commas. By entering a series of related commands, or inputs, as a single command, the user spends less time at the keyboard, the usual input device.

Menus are programs or functions or other options offered by the system. A cursor is moved to the point on the list that is the option of choice (e.g., a list of tests) and placed on the test desired. The use of a menu for data input is best when there are a limited number of choices to be made and also for persons new to the use of the computer.

Keyboard.—Standardized codes called *ASCII* (American Standard Code for Information Interchange) allow the entire keyboard to be used to enter alphanumeric (letters and numerical symbols) as well as numerical data into the computer. More complex systems use function keys, which enter a series of commands, reducing the number of keystrokes required to carry out a function such as returning to a previous screen or terminating the data entry.

Cathode-Ray Tube.—The **cathode-ray tube (CRT)** allows exchange of information between the user and the CPU on a specially designed television tube. The user can view on the display screen the commands given as well as the data exchanged.

Bar-code Reader.—**Bar-code readers** read a series of black lines (bars) on a label and convert these data to a sequence of numbers representing specific information. This information can be patient identification, tests requested, or identification of a reagent for a test. Bar codes are being used on identification wristbands and hopefully will allow for better control of accuracy for patient identification purposes, as for labels for specimen containers and test requests.

Interfacing.—Much laboratory time has been saved by the use of interfacing the laboratory computer with the analytic testing instrument so that the test result can be entered directly into the computer information system. A *port* is used to permit the main computer to interface with the computer of the analytic instrument. The test results data are transferred directly over a single wire. The port is a memory location in the CPU that is connected to a series of wires. The wires are, in turn, connected to the instrument computer.

Other Input Devices.—Additional input devices can enhance the exchange of information between user and computer. *Touch screens* allow interaction with the CPU through a menu. The position of touch on the screen determines the choice. A *light pen* (stylus) can be used to interact with a light-sensitive screen to indicate a menu choice. A *mouse* is a manual device that moves a cursor when the device is rolled along a flat surface. It also interacts with the computer through a menu.

Output Devices

Output is any information that the computer generates as a result of its calculations or processing. The CRT, printers, and instrument computers all can function as **output devices.** The computer directs the needed data from its central memory or from a storage device (magnetic tape or disk) to the specific output device. For the CRT, the output of the data generated is displayed on the screen. The *printer* is the usual output device of the computer system, and produces a paper copy.

As laboratory results are entered and verified, a documented trail can be produced by the computer system. The computer has stored the data on when the test was ordered, when the specimen was collected, when the test was done in the laboratory, and when the test result was entered and verified. In addition, data are available about who ordered the test, who collected the specimen, and who ran the test in the laboratory. The names of the persons involved in the process are stored in the data base of the computer. This documentation of data is an important part of quality assurance.

Printers.—When the computer-generated data are printed on paper, they are called *hard copy*. The printed output data are placed on the patient's chart and added to the official (legal) medical record of the patient. The format or style of the printed report is determined by the kind of software program used. This allows for changes when needed.

A specific output function utilizing the printer is the generating of printed labels for specimen containers at the time of order entry for the test. Another use for printed output is the generation of a printed list of test requests along with their accession numbers. This list defines the workload for the laboratory for a given time period and thus is called a *work list*. This work list can be used in planning the day's work for specific areas within the laboratory. Computer-generated lists identifying test results flagged for critical values or abnormal results can alert the laboratorian to transmit critical results to the physician or ask to have a test repeated. Some computer systems will compare a patient result with a previous result on that patient. This is called a *difference check* and serves to alert the laboratorian to an otherwise undetected error in analysis. This difference check can also signify a change in the condition of the patient and can alert the physician to this change.

Software

Instructions which direct the computer to perform its specific tasks are called the *software* or *program*. These instructions direct the various tasks to be done, using a predetermined order. Instructions that direct the collection of the data, their assimilation, the various tasks using the data, and the transfer of data are all included in the software program. The program also contains the information needed to communicate with the input and output devices being used.

Software programs are written in a specific language so that the computer can understand or accept it. Only by changing the program can any modification be made in the predetermined instructions for the operation of the laboratory information system.

BIBLIOGRAPHY

Aller RD, Elevitch FR (eds): *Clinics in Laboratory Medicine Symposium on Computers in the Clinical Laboratory,* vol 3. Philadelphia, WB Saunders Co, 1983.

College of American Pathologists: Standards for laboratory accreditation. *Pathologist* 1982; 36:641.

Henry JB (ed): *Clinical Diagnosis and Management by Laboratory Methods,* ed 18. Philadelphia, WB Saunders Co, 1991.

Kaplan LA, Pesce AJ: *Clinical Chemistry Theory, Analysis, and Correlation,* ed 2. St Louis, Mosby–Year Book, Inc, 1989.

PART *II*

DIVISIONS OF THE CLINICAL LABORATORY

10 Chemistry

Key Terms

Acid-base balance	Hyperglycemia
Anion gap	Immunoassays
Chromatography	Ion-selective electrodes
Conjugated bilirubin	Ketoacidosis
Coulometry	Potentiometry
Creatinine clearance	Quality control program
Diabetes mellitus	Renal threshold
Electrolyte battery	Spectrophotometry
Electrophoresis	Standard curve
Enzymology	Therapeutic drug monitoring
Enzyme-linked immunosorbent assay (ELISA)	Thin-layer chromatography
Gestational diabetes	Toxicology
Glucose tolerance test	Unconjugated bilirubin
Glycosuria	

The field of laboratory medicine continues to expand rapidly, and with it the specialty of clinical chemistry. Perhaps chemistry is one area in which changes are occurring most rapidly, because of the variety of automated instrumentation available. For this reason there is an increased demand for well-trained, qualified laboratory personnel to perform the routine chemistry determinations. The uses and general principles of some of the automated methods and apparatus found in the clinical chemistry laboratory are discussed in this chapter (see also Chapter 8).

The techniques of most chemical procedures performed in the laboratory are not in themselves difficult, but their proper execution requires genuine interest, reliability, and a good basic knowledge of the principles involved. It is essential, therefore, that the basic principles as well as the techniques used in clinical chemistry be mastered by the laboratorian. This includes the basic theory of chemical determinations, use and care of laboratory equipment and apparatus, application of quantitative measurement, proper preparation of reagents, recognition of problems when they arise, proper collection and handling of laboratory specimens, reporting of results obtained, and, perhaps most important, the use of quality assurance protocol when performing any procedure in the laboratory.

If one's basic knowledge is adequate, other, more complicated chemistry determinations can be learned more easily. The methods described in this chapter illustrate a few of the procedures used in the clinical chemistry laboratory today. There are many procedures that are not covered, but other methods and procedures for the analysis of different constituents use many of these same basic techniques. In the methods illustrated, principles involved in other laboratory assays are also described. It is inevitable that the medical laboratorian will be called on to perform chemistry tests other than those described in this textbook. One should be able to apply the basic knowledge to new laboratory tests.

Each new manual procedure should be approached in a systematic manner. The laboratorian should be aware of the type of specimen required for the test and should make certain that it is collected, prepared, and preserved properly. Any reagents needed for the procedure must be prepared by following the directions carefully. The procedure should be reviewed beforehand, and it is worthwhile to consult textbooks for the clinical implications and background material for the determination. The principle of the test, why the reagents are used and what they do in the reactions that occur, the stepwise method to be followed, technical factors and sources of error for the particular method, calculations, reporting of results to the physician, and reference values for the substance to be measured are all essential information for the person performing the test.

Specific directions are necessary in performing any laboratory determination, but there is so much to know about even the simplest procedure that the directions alone are not enough. It is the job of well-trained laboratory personnel to do some additional research to gain as much knowledge as possible about the laboratory tests that are performed.

To attain any degree of proficiency, practice and experience are necessary. Repeated practice with the laboratory tools discussed in this chapter and in preceding chapters will result in a much better understanding of clinical chemistry and, eventually, a keen appreciation of honest and accurate performance in the chemistry laboratory.

Clinical applications are discussed throughout this chapter. In this way it is hoped that the laboratorian will not lose sight of the most important aspect of the chemistry determinations performed and the reason for doing them in the first place—for the benefit of the patient.

INSTRUMENTATION IN THE CHEMISTRY LABORATORY

The clinical chemistry laboratory is based on quantitative analytic procedures or analytic chemistry. The kinds of analytic methods and some general types of instruments used to carry out these procedures have been discussed in Chapters 4, 5, and 8. Because there have been such great strides in technology, there have been equally rapid changes in the evolution of equipment used in the clinical chemistry laboratory. Changes have also taken place because of improvement in chemistry methodologies, changes in location of health care facilities—a movement toward more clinic-based and physician office-based laboratories—and the increasing awareness of the need for cost-effectiveness in the use of clinical laboratory tests.

Even with the advent of technologically sophisticated laboratory instruments, these instruments still employ traditional technologies and methodologies. General methods for most assays in the chemistry laboratory include the use of **spectrophotometry,** flame emission (or ionization) photometry, atomic absorption spectrometry, fluorometry, **ion-selective electrodes, electrophoresis,** nephelometry or light scattering, and **immunoassays** utilizing radionuclides, enzymes, or fluorescing materials as markers or tags. Some of these methods are discussed in the following section and others are discussed later under specific chemistry assays.

General Methods Used for Chemistry Assays

Spectrophotometry

In spectrophotometry, the concentration of an unknown sample is determined by measuring its absorption of light at a particular wavelength and comparing it with the absorption of light by known standard solutions measured at the same time and with the same wavelength. The instrument used to perform this measurement is the spectrophotometer. The application of this kind of analysis is dependent on Beer's law which states that the concentration of a solution at a constant light path length and at a constant wavelength and temperature is directly proportional to the amount of light absorbed (see also Absorbance Spectrophotometry, in Chapter 5).

Ultraviolet and Visible Spectrophotometry.—If the wavelength of light absorbed is in the ultraviolet part of the spectrum (nonvisible), short wavelengths of between 200 to 400 nm, the analysis is called ultraviolet (UV) spectrophotometry. If the wavelength of light absorbed is in the visible part of the spectrum, wavelengths of between 400 and 600 nm, the analysis is called visible (VIS) spectrophotometry. The wavelength used for the analysis depends on the wavelength at which there is significant absorption by the substance to be measured.

Flame Photometry

When some elements are heated, e.g., sprayed into a flame, the atoms of the element become excited and re-emit their energy at wavelengths characteristic of the element. The excited elements produce their characteristic flame colors at an intensity which is directly proportional to the concentration of atoms in the solution. The elements which are most often measured in this way are sodium (giving a yellow emission in a flame), potassium (red-violet), and lithium (red). Flame emission photometers are used for this determination (see also Flame Emission Photometry, in Chapter 5).

Fluorescence Spectrophotometry

Upon receiving UV radiation, the electrons of some substances absorb the radiation and become excited. After about 7 to 10 seconds (the electron has returned to its ground state), this energy is given up as a photon of light. Fluorescent light is the result of the absorbance of a photon of radiant energy by a molecule. Once the photon is absorbed by the molecule, the molecule has an increased level of energy. It will seek to eject this excess energy because the energy of the molecule is greater than the energy of its environment. When this excess energy is ejected as a photon, the result is fluorescence emission. Generally, this emitted light is in the visible part of the spectrum. The intensity of the fluorescence is determined using a fluorometer, sometimes called a spectrofluorometer or fluorescence spectrophotometer. This measurement is governed by the same factors that affect the absorption of light (i.e., the light path through the solution, the concentration of the solution, the wavelength of light being used) and also by the intensity of the UV exciting light. Only a few compounds can fluoresce and of those that do, not all photons absorbed will be converted to fluorescent light.

Light Scattering and Nephelometry

Light can either be absorbed, reflected, scattered, or transmitted when it strikes a particle in a liquid. Nephelometry is the measurement of light that has been scattered. Turbidimetry is the measurement of a loss in the intensity of light transmitted through a solution because of the light being scattered (the solution becomes turbid). Turbidimetry will measure light that is scattered, not absorbed or reflected by the particles in the suspension. Nephelometers are used to detect the amount of light scattered.

Electrophoresis

When charged particles are made to move, differences in molecular structure can be seen because different molecules have different velocities in an electric field. The assay utilizing electrophoresis involves the movement of charged particles when an external electrical current is produced in a liquid environment. The electric field is applied to the solution through oppositely charged electrodes placed in the solution. Specific ions then travel through the solution toward the electrode of the opposite charge. Cations (positively charged particles) move toward the negatively charged electrode (cathode) and anions (negatively charged particles) move toward the positively charged electrode (anode). Electrophoresis is a technique for separation and purification of ions, proteins, and other molecules of biochemical interest. It is used frequently in the clinical chemistry laboratory to separate serum proteins.

The equipment needed for electrophoresis generally consists of a sample applicator; a solid medium (such as an agar gel); a buffer system; an electrophoresis chamber which houses the solid medium and the sample; electrodes and wicks; a timer; and a power supply. Additional supplies might be stains for proteins or other substances being assayed and reagents used to remove the stains and to transform the solid media into a stable carrier for further densitometry studies or for preservation needs, depending on the requirements of the laboratory.

Immunoassays

Immunoassays utilize antigen-antibody reactions. When foreign material (called *antigens* or immunogens) are introduced into the body, protein molecules called *antibodies* are formed in response. An example is that of certain bacteria, which, when introduced into the body, elicit the production of specific antibodies. These antibodies combine specifically with the substance that stimulated the body to produce them in the first place, producing an antigen-antibody complex. In the laboratory, an antigen may be used as a reagent to detect the presence of antibodies in the serum of a patient. If the antibody is present, it shows that the person's body has responded to that specific antigen before. This response can be elicited by exposure to a specific microorganism or by the presence of a drug or medication in the patient's serum. Antigens and antibodies are used as very specific reagents. In the clinical chemistry laboratory, antibodies are used to detect and measure an antigen, such as a drug or medication, present in the serum of the patient.

Antibodies are immunoglobulins (Ig) which occur in one of five groups: IgA, IgD, IgM, IgG, and IgE. These immunoglobulins are proteins with antibody activity and are synthesized by certain types of lymphocytes (see also Chapters 17 and 18). IgG is the immunoglobulin that is most often used in immunoassays. In the serum there are many different immunoglobulins which are directed to different antigens. Immunoglobulins with this diversity are called *polyclonal antibodies*. An antibody that results in response to one type of antigen, from one plasma cell clone and its offspring, is called a *monoclonal antibody*.

The number of attachment sites on the antibody var-

ies according to the type of immunoglobulin. IgG antibodies have two sites for attachment to antigens. The number of attachment sites on the antigen available to the antibody also vary. The type of antigen-antibody complex that forms is dependent on the proportion of antibody to antigen in the immunochemical reaction. The size and nature of the complex is dependent on this proportion. When an antigen and antibody form a complex under optimal proportions, a precipitate forms because a critical mass has been reached by these complexes. Precipitation is one means of detecting the formation of an antigen-antibody complex. The complex precipitates out of solution. The term *flocculation* is used to describe a precipitation reaction that produces large, loosely bound precipitate. When antibodies react with large, particulate multivalent antigens, the antigen is said to agglutinate.

There are several quantitative immunoassays that involve specific additional techniques for their use in the laboratory. Some of these are quantitative radial immunodiffusion, electroimmunoassay (rocket electrophoresis), the **enzyme-linked immunosorbent assay (ELISA),** the enzyme-multiplied immunoassay technique (EMIT), radioimmunoassay (RIA), immunoradiometric assay (IRMA), and the substrate-labeled fluorescent immunoassay (SLFIA).

Chromatography

The word **chromatography** comes from the Greek words *chromatos,* color, and *graphein,* to write. In chromatography, mixtures of solutes dissolved in a common solvent are separated from one another by a differential distribution of the solutes between two phases. The solvent is one phase, is mobile, and carries the mixture of solutes through the second phase. The second phase is a fixed or stationary phase. There are a number of variations in chromatographic techniques in which the mobile phase ranges from liquids to gases and the stationary phase from sheets of cellulose paper to internally coated fine capillary glass tubes. The varieties of chromatographic techniques as well as their applications to clinical assays have grown rapidly.

Chromatographic methods are usually classified according to the physical state of the solute carrier phase. The two main categories of chromatography are gas chromatography, in which the solute phase is in a gaseous state, and liquid chromatography, in which the solute phase is a solution or liquid. The methods are further classified according to how the stationary phase matrix is contained. For example, liquid chromatography is subdivided into flat and column methods. In flat chromatography, the stationary phase is supported on a flat sheet such as cellulose paper (paper chromatography) or in a thin layer on a mechanical backing such as glass or plastic (thin-layer chromatography). Column methods are classically liquid chromatography. Gas chromatography is done by a column method.

The chromatographic method is used to separate the components of a given sample within a reasonable amount of time. The purpose of this separation technique is to detect or quantitate the particular component or group of components to be assayed in a pure form. By convention, the concentrations of solutes in a chromatographic system are plotted out vs. time or distance. The bands or zones of the various analytes separated in the technique are usually termed a *peak*.

Electrochemical Methods

When chemical energy is converted to an electrical current (a flow of electrons) in a galvanic cell, the term *electrochemistry* is used. Electrochemical reactions are characterized by a loss of electrons (oxidation) at the positive pole (anode) and a simultaneous gain of electrons (reduction) at the negative pole (cathode). The galvanic cell is made up of two parts called *half-cells,* each containing a metal in a solution of one of its salts. These methods involve the measurement of electrical signals associated with chemical systems that are within an electrochemical cell. Electroanalytic chemistry uses electrochemistry for analysis purposes. The magnitude of the voltage or signal current originating from an electrochemical cell is related to the activity or concentration of the particular chemical constituent being assayed. Measurements can usually be done on very small amounts of sample.

In the clinical laboratory, electroanalytic methods are used to measure ions, drugs, hormones, metals, and gases. Methods are available for the rapid analysis of analytes such as blood electrolytes (Na^+ K^+ Cl^- HCO_3^-) present in relatively high concentrations and other analytes such as heavy metals and drug metabolites that are present in very low concentrations in blood and urine. There are three general electrochemical techniques used in the clinical laboratory: potentiometric, voltametric, and coulometric.

Potentiometry.—**Potentiometry** measures the potential of an electrode compared with the potential of another electrode. The method is based on the measurement of a voltage potential difference between two electrodes immersed in a solution under zero current conditions. This difference in voltage between the two electrodes is usually measured on a pH or voltage meter. One electrode is called the indicator electrode, the other is the reference electrode. The reference electrode is an electrochemical half-cell that is used as a fixed reference for the cell potential measurements. One of the most common reference electrodes used for potentiometry is the silver or silver chloride electrode. The indicator electrode is the main component of potentiometric techniques. It is important that the indicator electrode be able to respond selectively to analyte species. The most commonly used indicator electrode in clinical chemistry is the ion-selective electrode. The use of the ion-selective electrode is based on the measurement of a potential that develops across a selective membrane. The electrochemical cell response is based on an interaction between the membrane and the analyte being measured that alters the potential across the membrane. The specificity of the membrane interaction for the analyte determines the selectivity of the potential response to an analyte.

Coulometry.—**Coulometry** measures the amount of current passing between two electrodes in an electrochemical cell. The principle of coulometry involves the application of a constant current to generate a titrating agent; the time required to titrate a sample at constant current is measured and is related to the amount of analyte in the sample. The amount of current is directly proportional to the amount of substance produced or consumed by the electrode. The most common clinical application of coulometry is in the determination of chloride ions in serum, plasma, urine, and other body fluids (see Chloride under Electrolytes, below).

SPECIMENS: GENERAL PREPARATION

Accurate chemical analysis of biological fluids depends on proper collection, preservation, and preparation of the sample, in addition to the technique and method of analysis used. The most quantitatively perfect determination is of no use if the specimen is not properly handled in the initial steps of the procedure. Each chemical method has unique problems of its own, but in general the collection, means of preservation, and initial preparation or processing of samples follow a similar pattern, regardless of what the final analysis is to be (see Chapter 2). The majority of chemistry tests are done on serum or plasma, processed from whole blood obtained by venipuncture. Occasionally microsamples must be collected.

Collecting Microspecimens for Chemistry

There are instances when only small amounts of blood can be collected, and many laboratory determinations have been devised for very small amounts of sample. In general, the same procedure is followed as for any other drawing of capillary blood (see under Peripheral or Capillary Blood, in Chapter 2). For chemistry procedures, blood can be collected in a capillary tube by touching the tip of the tube to a large drop of blood while the tube is held in a slightly downward position. The blood enters the tube by capillary action. Several tubes (approximately 4 × 75 mm) can be filled from a single skin puncture. Tubes are capped and placed in a test tube to be transported and centrifuged. Careful centrifugation technique must be used because capillary tubes tend to break easily. When the analysis is delayed, the tube is scratched with a file and broken just above the junction of serum and cells. The serum portion of the tube is then recapped and refrigerated. Special microcontainers are also generally available for micro blood collections. (Figs 10–1 and 10–2).

Processing the Specimens

Once the blood has been collected and brought to the laboratory, a series of steps is carried out before the analysis is done. Ideally, all laboratory measurements should be performed within 1 hour after collection. When this is not practical, and often it is not, the specimens should be processed to the point where they can be properly stored so that the constituents to be measured will not be altered. There are two additional reasons for storing specimens: each sample should be retained long enough after analysis to permit a repeat analysis if necessary, and specimens collected in a timed sequence should be stored until they can be analyzed at the same time.

Processing includes separation of cells from serum or plasma, observation of specimen color, refrigeration, and freezing if necessary.

Most chemical determinations are done on venous whole blood, plasma, or serum. Arterial blood is primarily used for blood gas determinations. Plasma is the liq-

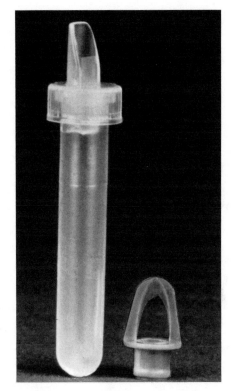

FIG 10–1.
Microtainer tube system. (Courtesy of Becton-Dickinson Vacutainer Systems, Rutherford, N.J.) (From Becan-McBride K, Ross DL: *Essentials for the Small Laboratory and Physician's Office.* St Louis, Mosby–Year Book, Inc, 1988, p 54. Used by permission.)

uid portion of the circulating blood and it contains fibrinogen. Serum is plasma with the fibrinogen removed, which is usually accomplished by the clotting mechanism. To obtain serum, the blood is collected in a plain tube, using no anticoagulant, and allowed to clot for at least 15 to 20 minutes at room temperature. Vacuum tubes used to collect the blood are usually siliconized to minimize hemolysis and to prevent the clot from adhering to the wall of the tube. By allowing the clot to retract for longer than 20 minutes, hemolysis is minimized and the yield of serum is greater. However, if the serum remains on the clot for too long, glycolysis can occur and other constituents are altered—there can be a shift of substances from the cells to the serum, for instance. Therefore, the time to allow for clot retraction depends on the determination to be done. Serum separator tubes

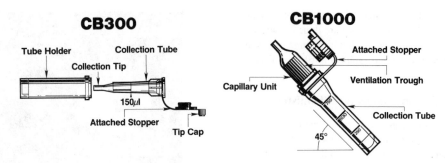

FIG 10–2.
Microvette capillary blood collection system. (Courtesy of Sarstedt Inc, Princeton, N.J.) (From Becan-McBride K, Ross DL: *Essentials for the Small Laboratory and Physician's Office.* St Louis, Mosby–Year Book, Inc, 1988, p 55. Used by permission.)

are commonly used to assist in procurement of a serum sample (see Serum Separator Devices, in Chapter 2). After clotting has taken place, the tube is centrifuged and the supernatant serum is removed. It is important to remind those handling blood specimens in all steps of the laboratory analysis to handle the specimens using universal blood and body substance technique. Universal precautions require all persons handling specimens to wear gloves. Stoppers must be carefully removed from blood specimens after centrifugation, centrifuges must be covered and placed in a shielded area, all serum and plasma samples must be pipetted by mechanical suction, and all specimen tubes and supplies must be discarded properly in biohazard containers.

With so many automated methods, processing the blood often takes longer than the actual analysis. A fast, efficient way of separating serum from cells is needed. Several systems have been devised for this purpose. In one, regular vacuum serum tubes are used for collecting the blood, and then a special unit is placed on the tube of blood before centrifugation. This unit dispenses a silicone mixture during centrifugation that forms an inert barrier between the serum and the cells. The serum can easily be transferred into another container for analysis without having to worry about contamination with cells. With another system, it is necessary to purchase special blood-collecting tubes, which resemble ordinary vacuum tubes but contain inert silicone gel. The gel is displaced up inside the tube during centrifugation and forms a barrier between the serum and the cells. The serum can easily be removed to the appropriate container for testing (see Laboratory Processing of Blood Specimens, in Chapter 2). These products are all designed to save time

and to provide a safer mechanism for processing blood specimens.

Hemolyzed Specimens

Hemolyzed serum or plasma is unfit as a specimen for several chemistry determinations. Hemolyzed serum appears red, usually clear red. Several constituents, such as potassium and the enzymes acid phosphatase, lactate dehydrogenase (LDH), and aspartate amino transferase (AST, GOT) are present in large amounts in red blood cells, so that hemolysis of red cells will significantly elevate the value obtained for red substances in serum. Hemoglobin is released during hemolysis and may directly interfere with a reaction or its color may interfere with photometric analysis of the specimen. The procedure to be done should always be checked to see whether abnormal-looking specimens can be used. A determination of whether the hemolysis is in vitro or in vivo is also useful. Although relatively rare, the recognition of in vivo hemolysis is a significant finding.

Jaundiced Specimens

Jaundiced serum or plasma takes on a brownish-yellow or "vivid" yellow color. One should be especially careful in handling such a specimen. Gloves must be worn and the hands should be washed frequently. Jaundiced serum is a good indication of the presence of hepatitis, which is very infectious. The abnormal color of the serum can interfere with photometric measurements. The use of universal precautions has significantly reduced the incidence of hepatitis B infections in laboratory workers.

Lipemic Specimens

Lipemic serum takes on a milky white color. The presence of lipids in serum or plasma can cause this abnormal appearance. Often, however, the lipemia results from collecting the blood from the patient too soon after a meal. Lipemic serum interferes with photometric readings for some tests.

Drug Effect on Specimens

Blood drawn from patients on certain types of medication can give invalid chemistry results for some constituents. Drugs can alter several chemical reactions. Drugs can affect laboratory results in two general ways: some action of the drug or its metabolite can cause an alteration (in vivo) in the concentration of the substance being measured, or some physical or chemical property of the drug can alter the analysis directly (in vitro). The number of drugs that affect laboratory measurements is increasing.

Logging and Reporting Processes

As part of the processing and handling of laboratory specimens, a careful, accurate logging and recording process must be in place in the laboratory regardless of the size of the facility. A log sheet and a written report form are vital to the operation of any laboratory. The log sheet documents on a daily basis the various patient specimens received in the laboratory.

Items to be listed on the log sheet are the patient's name, identification number, kind of specimen collected (description of the specimen and its source), date and time of specimen collection, and laboratory tests to be done. The log sheet should also indicate the time when the specimen arrived in the laboratory. The log sheet can also include a column for test results and the date when the tests are completed. Results can be documented by hand, by use of laboratory instrument printed reports, or by computer printouts. The log sheet data are part of the permanent record of the laboratory and must be stored and available for future reference.

A written report must be sent to the physician with the vital data pertaining to the test results. The following information should be included in the report: patient's name, identification number, date and time of specimen collection, description and source of specimen, the initials of the person who collected the specimen, tests requested, the name of the physician requesting the tests, the test results, and the initials or signature of the person who performed the test. Much of this documentation of data is being done with the use of laboratory computerized information systems. Copies of this laboratory report may be sent to the medical records department and to the accounting office for patient billing purposes (see also Chapter 9).

Preserving the Specimens

Some chemical constituents change rapidly after the blood is removed from the vein. The best policy is to perform tests on fresh specimens. When the specimen must be preserved until the test can be done, there are ways to retard alteration. For example, sodium fluoride can be used to preserve blood glucose specimens, since it prevents glycolysis.

With few exceptions, the lower the temperature, the greater the stability of the chemical constituents. Furthermore, the growth of bacteria is considerably inhibited by refrigeration and is completely inhibited by freezing. Room temperature is generally considered to be 18 to 30°C, the refrigerator temperature about 4°C, and freezing about −5°C or less. Refrigeration is a simple and reliable means of retarding alterations, including bacteriologic action and glycolysis, although some changes still take place. Refrigerated specimens must be brought to room temperature before chemical analysis. Removing cells from plasma and serum is another means of preventing some changes. Some specimens needed for certain assays, such as bilirubin, must be shielded from the light or tested immediately. Bilirubin is a light-sensitive substance.

Serum or plasma may be preserved by freezing. Whole blood cannot be frozen satisfactorily because freezing ruptures the red cells (hemolysis). Freezing preserves enzyme activities in serum and plasma. Serum and plasma freeze in layers with different concentrations, and for this reason these specimens must be well mixed before they are used in a chemical determination.

Every precaution must be taken to preserve the chemical constituents in the specimen from the time of collection to the time of testing in the laboratory if the results are to be meaningful to the physician. In general, tubes for collecting blood for chemical determinations do not have to be sterile, but they should be chemically clean. Serum is usually preferred to whole blood or plasma when the constituents to be measured are relatively evenly distributed between the intracellular and extracellular portions of the blood.

Removing Interfering Substances

Biological fluids are very complex in their composition. There are hundreds of detectable substances in urine and blood, for instance. Chemical analysis would be impossible if it were necessary to completely isolate each substance before it could be measured. An optimal method is one that can test for a specific substance while the other substances remain. A test is said to be specific when none of the other substances interfere. In chemical analysis, however, almost all determinations are subject to some interference. Sometimes the interference is small enough or constant enough that it does not significantly alter the accuracy or precision of the test results. Sometimes the interference does affect the results, and in such cases the specimen must be specially treated before the analysis can take place. That is, the substances causing the interference must be isolated, or removed, from the specimen.

Removing Protein

Whole blood is made up of cells and plasma. The red cells are largely composed of protein and the plasma also contains a significant amount of protein. Protein molecules tend to have many electrically charged areas, and since chemical reactions involve the transfer of charges, the presence of so many charged protein molecules may interfere with reactions. It therefore may be necessary to remove the proteins before continuing with the determination. Removing proteins also has the effect of preserving the specimen since it removes enzymes, which are proteins.

If proteins are left in the specimen, they can interfere with the determination by causing turbidity, foaming, or precipitation, or by directly interfering with color reactions. Any of these effects can lead to errors in many clinical determinations. Therefore many determinations require preliminary treatment to remove proteins. Proteins may be removed by precipitation with chemicals (acids or salts of heavy metals) or by passing the serum through a dialyzing membrane that allows only the smaller particles to pass through. Acids often used to precipitate proteins are trichloroacetic, tungstic, and picric. Salts of heavy metals that can be used to precipitate

proteins are sodium sulfate, ammonium sulfate, and zinc sulfate. Ethyl alcohol and methyl alcohol are two organic chemicals used in protein precipitation. The dialyzing membrane is used in many automated methods, but the chemical filtrate methods are used for most determinations done manually in the laboratory. Chemistry procedures requiring initial removal of protein will specify how it should be done.

The term *protein-free filtrate* or *protein-free supernatant* is used to describe the solution left after treatment of a specimen to remove the protein. Many separations of protein are accomplished by means of precipitation. Either the substance being determined is removed by precipitation, or the interfering materials are precipitated. The precipitate is isolated by filtration or centrifugation. Chemical precipitation of serum, plasma, whole blood, urine, or cerebrospinal fluid is thus followed by either filtration or centrifugation and subsequent decantation of the crystal-clear protein-free filtrate. Proteins are easily precipitated, and the techniques used include the use of heat, acids, bases, organic solvents, alcohols, salts, metal ions, or a combination of these. Specific methodologies can be found in a basic clinical chemistry textbook.

It is important in all methods for protein precipitation that the filtrate or supernate not show any foaming or cloudiness, which would indicate incomplete removal of protein. Two variables are important for maximal precipitation: the pH of the reaction mixture, and the concentration of the precipitant. There must be sufficient reagent to combine with the protein in the blood. Ordinarily a safe excess is used.

GENERAL TECHNICAL FACTORS AND SOURCES OF ERROR USING NONAUTOMATED METHODS

When performing manual chemistry determinations, there are many causes of poor agreement between duplicates or of inaccurate results. Pipetting errors in preparing the filtrates; in transferring the standards, controls, and filtrates; or in preparing the reagents are one major cause of inaccurate results. Pipetting errors are greater with whole blood than with serum or plasma. Adequate mixing is important, and insufficient mixing can lead to difficulties. Whenever a reagent is added to another mixture, adequate mixing of the contents of the tube is essential. If the photometer is not used correctly or if the blank tube is not adjusted properly at the beginning of the readings, the end results will be inaccurate.

If incubation steps are employed, especially by use of a boiling water bath, it is important that the timing be watched carefully. It is also important that the water be actually boiling to ensure complete reactions. Cold water baths are also essential, for they stop the reaction.

The standards used for the procedure must be in good condition. They must be analyzed at the same time as the rest of the batch, and if another batch is analyzed later in the day, new standards must be included.

STANDARDIZATION OF A PROCEDURE AND USE OF A STANDARD CURVE

The preparation of a **standard curve** is an important component of examining laboratory data for validity. It can indicate abnormalities or variations in the analytic systems being used by the laboratory (see also Ensuring Reliable Results: The Quality Control Program, in Chapter 7).

Once a series of standard tubes have been read in the photometer, the galvanometer readings and standard concentrations are plotted on graph paper. This is the first step in the use of a standard curve, an essential tool in most chemistry determinations.

"Precalibrated" test procedures are commercially available and are used in many automated instruments. They should *not* be used for patient assays unless they have been checked out for accuracy first. Each laboratory must include standards for each batch of determinations whenever possible. Failure to do so can result in errors resulting from the use of new reagents, deterioration or contamination of old reagents, the use of incorrect filters, and changes in instruments.

Types of Graph Paper

Semilogarithmic graph paper is the type most commonly used to plot the percent transmittance or absorbance readings from the photometer. The horizontal axis of this graph paper is a linear scale, and the vertical axis is a logarithmic scale. The concentration in the standard cuvettes is plotted on the horizontal axis. The transmittance or absorbance readings from the photometer are plotted along the vertical axis. In most cases the percent transmittance readings are used (as opposed to optical density or absorbance readings). These readings can be plotted directly on the logarithmic scale, as the concentration is proportional to the logarithm of the galvanometer reading. In this way percent transmittance readings are converted to the appropriate numbers on the logarithmic scale. Using semilogarithmic graph paper is simple and convenient for most laboratory purposes. When percentages are plotted against concentrations on semilogarithmic graph paper, the proportional relationship is direct, and a straight-line graph is obtained when the individual standard points are connected. The criteria for a good standard curve are that the line is straight, that the line connects all points, and that the line goes through the origin, or intersect, of the two axes. The origin of the graph paper is the point on the vertical and horizontal axes where there is $100\%T$ and zero concentration.

Another type of graph paper, called *linear* graph paper, is available for plotting standard curves. This graph paper has both horizontal and vertical linear scales. If linear graph paper is used to construct a standard curve, the percent transmittance readings must first be converted to logarithmic values and the logarithmic values plotted on the vertical axis. If percent transmittance readings are converted to absorbance units, or if the galvanometer scale is calibrated in absorbance units, the readings can be plotted directly against the concentration on the linear graph paper. Again, a straight-line graph must be obtained. To eliminate the conversion of percent transmittance to absorbance in order to obtain the necessary straight-line graph, the use of semilogarithmic graph paper is suggested.

Plotting a Standard Curve

When plotting points on graph paper, whether they represent concentrations or galvanometer readings, care must be taken to note the intervals on the graph paper. Many errors result from carelessness in the initial plotting of points on the graph paper.

When a standard curve is prepared, the axes must also be properly labeled. Additional information usually recorded on the paper includes the name of the person constructing the graph, the procedure for which the graph was prepared, the date, the photometer used, and the wavelength setting used.

Using a Standard Curve

Once the standard curve has been plotted, it is used to calculate the concentrations of any unknowns that were included in the same batch as the standards used to make the graph. To find the concentration of a solution, there must be some way of comparing it with a solution of known concentration. An example of the construction and use of a standard curve is given in Figure 10–3.

In the example shown, three standard solutions are prepared with the following concentrations: standard 1 (S_1), 0.02 mg; standard 2 (S_2), 0.04 mg; and standard 3 (S_3), 0.06 mg. These concentrations are plotted on the linear, horizontal scale of the graph paper. The three standard tubes are read in a photometer, giving the following readings in percent transmittance: S_1, 76^2; S_2, 58^3, and S_3, $45^1\%T$. The percent transmittance readings are plotted under their respective concentrations on the logarithmic, vertical scale of the paper. The points are connected, using a

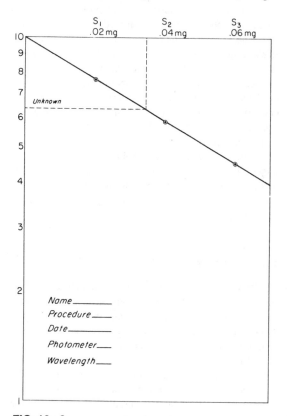

FIG 10–3.
Construction of a standard *(S)* curve.

ruler. An undetermined substance gives a reading of $63^2\%T$. Using the graph in Figure 10–3, the $63^2\%T$ point on the vertical scale is found, followed horizontally to the graph line just drawn, and then followed vertically to the concentration scale. The degree of accuracy with which an unknown concentration can be read depends on the concentrations of the standards used. The accuracy of the unknown can be no more accurate than the standard solutions used. Standard solutions are usually weighed to the fourth decimal place. In this example, the unknown concentration is 0.0343 mg (the figure in the fourth decimal place is approximate).

Using standard solutions to standardize the analyses of each batch, rather than relying on a permanently established calibration curve, allows the clinical laboratory to produce more reliable results. It compensates for variables such as time, temperature, the age of the reagents, and the condition of the instruments. It is always best to use several different concentrations of the standard solution, not just one. To obtain reliable photometric information about the concentration of a substance, standards must be used as the basis for comparison.

Standard solutions are also used in quantitative analytic procedures in which the photometer is not employed. For example, whenever titration is used to measure concentration, a standard solution must be employed. There must be some basis for comparison in this technique also (see Titration under Measurement of Volume, in Chapter 4).

QUALITY CONTROL IN THE CHEMISTRY LABORATORY

The purpose of quality control of analytic testing is to ensure the reliability of the measurements performed on the samples for each patient. A **quality control program** is useful and effective if it can be used to ascertain that the biochemical data generated are consistently precise and accurate. The data can then be used in the medical decision-making process on both a short-term and long-term basis. Quality control is part of the comprehensive set of policies, procedures, and practices that makes up the quality assurance program for the facility (see Chapter 7).

Both control samples and patient samples must be assayed using the same testing system so that results of both reflect changes occurring in the system itself. Quality control specimens are also run to assure the physician that the usefulness of the test result has not been compromised by any changes occurring in the test system. The use of controls and the recording of their values each time they are used is documentation for regulatory agencies that the laboratory routinely performs at a suitable level of competence. The assay results of the control specimen must be recorded or logged (the documentation needed for accreditation agencies), along with dates. If the values are out of control, action must be taken to remedy the problem. Results for the patient assays are also logged, along with the dates. This provides the necessary link between the control assay and patient's assay. It is assumed that when the control values are within the established limits at the time of the patient's assay, the patient results are reliable, valid, and reportable. Results for patient samples are not reported if the control values are out of the acceptable range established for the assay. All data are retained in the laboratory's records, whether the data be out-of-control or within the acceptable range. The length of time for retaining these data varies from laboratory to laboratory. This documentation is part of the quality assurance record of the laboratory.

REPORTING RESULTS AND RECORDING LABORATORY DATA

Results are reported to the physician only when values for the quality control specimens or measures correspond. It is important that all testing be done using the quality control protocol established by the individual laboratory. The use of control specimens is included in all testing assays. A control specimen is handled in the assay exactly the same way as any unknown specimen. When the control value is within the established range for that assay, it is an indication of the overall reliability of the assay values for the unknown specimen (see Chapter 7). The laboratory retains for some time the standard graphs, the galvanometer readings obtained for a particular procedure using manual methods, the results generated by the automated instruments, and all quality control records for the assay. The results themselves are retained by the laboratory indefinitely (see above). The reporting process is done with the use of computer systems in many laboratories.

With the use of computerized information systems,

the information generated from the multitude of laboratory tests can be processed and used efficiently. Utilization of laboratory data for the benefit of the patient is the prime goal of the clinical laboratory in the health care facility (see also Chapter 9).

The laboratory may include not only the specific assay value for the test in question but also information as to whether the test result is abnormal and any other pertinent information of interpretive value. Reference ranges are of interest to the physician in interpreting the result. Reference ranges are available from the traditional clinical chemistry textbooks, from manufacturers of the various laboratory instruments and products used in the laboratory, and from in-house laboratory procedure manuals.

GLUCOSE

One of the most commonly performed procedures in the clinical chemistry laboratory is the determination of blood glucose. Blood glucose tests are performed in all types of clinical laboratories, in hospitals, independent laboratories, clinics, and private physicians' offices. They are used primarily for the diagnosis and treatment (or control) of **diabetes mellitus.** Although several different methods are used to quantitatively measure the amount of glucose in a blood specimen, most methods depend on the formation or disappearance of color in a solution and employ a photometer for this measurement. Most of the methods have been automated, but the same principles apply as for the nonautomated methods. Self-tests for blood glucose are also being done routinely by many diabetics to better manage their disease.

Glucose determinations may be performed on specimens taken from patients in a fasting state, on specimens taken 2 hours after the patient has consumed a high glucose drink or meal (postprandial), or as part of a **glucose tolerance test,** depending on the physician's instructions. The methods used for glucose determinations can be divided into three categories: the classic oxidation methods, which depend on the reducing ability of glucose; aromatic amine methods, which involve a reaction between the aldehyde group of glucose and the amino group of *o*-toluidine, an aromatic amine; and enzymatic methods, which are based on the enzymes glucose oxidase and hexokinase. Since many additional substances that normally occur in the blood can be measured as glucose or interfere with various tests, the term *true blood glucose* is often encountered when tests of blood glucose are described. The enzyme methods are more specific for glucose and are widely used for that reason.

Clinical Significance

Glucose is one of the few chemical constituents of the blood that can change rapidly and dramatically in concentration. Many diseases cause a change in glucose metabolism, but the most frequent cause of an increase in blood glucose is diabetes mellitus.

Diabetes Mellitus

Diabetes mellitus is associated with a relative or absolute deficiency of insulin. This deficiency results in an inability of the body to handle glucose. Diabetes mellitus is a chronic metabolic disorder with deficiencies in carbohydrate, lipid, and protein metabolism. Changes in fat metabolism resulting from diabetes mellitus can be life-threatening when they result in **ketoacidosis,** a condition in which there is an increased concentration of ketone bodies (which are derived from fat catabolism) in the blood and an accompanying decrease in blood pH, or acidosis. Other complications include increased cholesterol in the blood; atherosclerosis, a vascular disease with deposits of fat in the blood vessels; and kidney disease. A person with diabetes has a twofold greater risk of myocardial infarction compared with a nondiabetic person of the same age and sex. There are approximately 8 million recognized diabetes patients in the United States, which is probably only half of the overall incidence, or a prevalence of about 6.6%.* There is a strong family tendency to the disease, although the exact mechanism of acquisition is unknown.

Research has shown that a complex interaction between genetic and environmental factors affects the development of diabetes mellitus. There have been some animal studies that have shown a link between viruses and the development of diabetes.

Of the 8 million Americans with diagnosed diabetes mellitus, type I or insulin-dependent diabetes (IDDM) afflicts more than 2 million. Insulin injection is required to control this disease. This type of diabetes mellitus is caused by insufficient secretion of insulin by the pan-

*Harris MR, Hadden WC, Knowler WC et al: Prevalence of diabetes and impaired glucose tolerance and plasma levels in the U.S. population aged 20–74 yr. *Diabetes* 1987; 36:523.

creas. The remaining diabetes patients are afflicted with type II or non–insulin-dependent diabetes mellitus (NIDDM) which has less correlation with blood insulin levels and more correlation with insulin activity and is not usually dependent on insulin injections. Early diagnosis is important, as proper treatment may delay or minimize the complications of the disease.

The primary symptoms of diabetes mellitus are polyuria, abnormally high blood and urine glucose levels (**hyperglycemia** and **glycosuria,** respectively), excessive thirst (polydipsia), constant hunger (polyphagia), sudden weight loss, and, during acute episodes of the disease, excessive blood and urinary ketones (ketonemia and ketonuria, respectively). These symptoms result from the body's inability to metabolize glucose and the resulting consequences of the presence of high glucose levels.

Diabetes mellitus is controlled clinically through a number of factors. These include various dosages of insulin, oral drugs, and the composition of the diet. The result of uncontrolled diabetes mellitus is a high blood glucose level, with glucose subsequently appearing in the urine.

In a diabetes patient the glucose concentration can be very high or very low. At either extreme the patient may be in a state of unconsciousness. It is therefore necessary for the physician to know whether the unconsciousness results from a high glucose concentration (*diabetic coma*) or a low glucose concentration (*insulin shock*). It is often not obvious from the physical appearance of the patient which condition exists; however, prompt and appropriate treatment is mandatory. It is the responsibility of the laboratory to get the result of the glucose determination to the physician as soon as possible, so that the correct treatment can be started. In this type of emergency glucose determination, the test must be done rapidly but with the utmost accuracy, as an error or delay may have a serious effect.

Other Causes of Altered Glucose Metabolism

In many cases high blood glucose values are caused by conditions other than diabetes mellitus. Some of these are traumatic injury to the brain; febrile disease; certain liver diseases; overactivity of the adrenal, pituitary, and thyroid glands, which produce hormones that increase blood glucose levels; or the ingestion of a heavy meal.

A significant number of people have impaired glucose tolerance. These persons have an abnormal glucose tolerance test but no measured hyperglycemia. **Gesta-**

tional diabetes occurs with some pregnancies. Studies have shown that a significant number of these women will go on to a type II diabetes mellitus 20 years after delivery. It is important to screen pregnant women for gestational diabetes to prevent perinatal complications associated with the hyperglycemia of the mother.

There are also conditions that cause low blood sugar, or *hypoglycemia.* These include liver disease in which the metabolism of glycogen is impaired, and conditions that result in an increased concentration of insulin in the blood *(hyperinsulinemia).* A decrease in blood glucose is life-threatening because the brain and cardiac cells are dependent on glucose in the blood and interstitial fluids. Hypoglycemia may result in muscle spasms, unconsciousness, and death. High concentrations of insulin can result from an overdose of insulin or from certain pancreatic tumors.

Glucose Concentration in the Body

Under ordinary conditions, the concentration of glucose in the blood is kept within a narrow range by an elaborate system of mechanisms collectively called *carbohydrate metabolism.* Some of the mechanisms used by the body to keep the glucose within this range are absorption of glucose by the intestine, storage and breakdown of glycogen (the form in which glucose is stored in the body) by the liver, storage of glucose as glycogen by the mass of skeletal muscles, and production and release of the hormone insulin by the pancreas. Other hormones that affect the blood glucose level are produced by the adrenal cortex, and by the pituitary and thyroid glands.

Glucose is the ultimate source of energy for all body cells. Energy is provided by the oxidation of glucose, ultimately to carbon dioxide and water, through the process called *glycolysis.* Glycolysis, or glucose oxidation, depends on the presence of *insulin.* Therefore the absence of insulin will result in an increased concentration of glucose in the blood (clinically, the condition diabetes mellitus). Insulin is responsible for maintaining a healthy level of glucose in the blood. This is done in a variety of ways, including the processes of glycogenesis and glycolysis. *Glycolysis* is the breakdown or oxidation of glucose. Other forms of glucose utilization, or breakdown, that are also dependent on insulin are the synthesis of fatty acids and amino acids (the building blocks of protein). *Glycogenesis* is the formation of glycogen from glucose. Glycogen is the form in which glucose is stored

in the body, primarily in the liver. Thus, insulin regulates the concentration of blood glucose by either oxidation (glycolysis) or storage (glycogenesis). The secretion of insulin is stimulated by increased blood glucose concentrations.

Glucose can also be provided to the blood by the process of *gluconeogenesis,* the production of glucose from fat and protein. This takes place in the liver, where glucose is derived from certain amino acids (protein) and glycerol (from fat) by glucocorticoid hormones produced by the adrenal cortex. Decreased blood glucose and decreased glycogen storage in cells stimulate this process.

Only a certain amount of glucose can be stored as glycogen. The excess glucose is converted to fatty acids and stored as triglycerides in body fat. Insulin is also necessary for the formation of fat *(lipogenesis)* in the liver and the *adipose tissue* or body fat.

After a period of fasting, the usual amount of glucose in the blood is between 70 and 105 mg/dL of blood, depending on the method of analysis. The blood glucose level usually increases rapidly after carbohydrates are ingested, but returns to normal in 1.5 to 2.0 hours. Aside from this increase after eating, the level of glucose in the blood is kept within a remarkably narrow range. This regulation of the blood glucose level is largely dependent on the activity of the liver. After a heavy meal, the glucose produced from digested carbohydrates is absorbed and the blood sugar rises. Some of this glucose may be oxidized at once for energy. However, the liver removes a large portion and stores it as glycogen, while some is carried to muscles, where it is also stored as glycogen for later use for immediate energy by the muscles. Some of the glucose diffuses into the tissue fluids and provides a direct source of energy for cell activity. After these immediate needs of the body have been supplied, the remainder is converted to fat and stored in the adipose tissue of the body. If the blood glucose level is so great that these control mechanisms cannot remove the excess glucose, the kidneys exert a regulating effect by excreting sugar in the urine. The blood glucose concentration above which glucose is excreted in the urine is called the **renal threshold.** For most persons the renal threshold for glucose is 160 to 170 mg/dL.

As a result of these metabolic processes, the blood glucose gradually returns to its fasting level. Since the body continues to utilize glucose for energy during normal activity, the blood glucose has a tendency to drop. This stimulates the liver to convert stored glycogen to glucose *(glycogenolysis)*, maintaining the normal level of blood glucose.

Several hormones have the effect of raising the blood glucose concentration. The actions of *growth hormone* and *adrenocorticotropic hormone (ACTH)*, which are secreted by the anterior pituitary, are opposite (antagonistic) to that of insulin and tend to raise the blood glucose level. *Hydrocortisone* and other steroids produced by the adrenal cortex stimulate gluconeogenesis. *Epinephrine*, which is secreted by the adrenal medulla, stimulates glycogenolysis. *Glucagon* is secreted by the alpha cells of the pancreas, and acts to increase blood glucose by stimulating glycogenolysis in the liver. Finally, *thyroxine*, which is secreted by the thyroid, also stimulates glycogenolysis and contributes to an increased blood glucose level, besides increasing the rate of absorption of glucose from the intestine.

Specimens

Glucose determinations may be performed on specimens of whole blood, plasma, or serum, but serum or plasma, free of hemolysis, is the preferred choice. The specimen should be centrifuged and separated from the clot or cells as soon as possible. Glucose testing may be requested on other body fluids, especially urine and cerebrospinal fluid. In the past, glucose determinations were usually performed on whole blood; however, for several reasons plasma or serum is now preferred. The glucose concentration in whole blood is not identical to that in plasma or serum. There is a uniform concentration of glucose throughout the water portion of plasma and red blood cells, but there is more water in the plasma than in the red cells, which also contain hemoglobin. Since plasma (or serum) contains approximately 10% to 15% more water than whole blood, the total glucose in plasma (or serum) is about 10% to 15% greater than in whole blood. The exact value can be calculated for any specimen; however, it is dependent on the method of analysis used and the hematocrit, or percentage of packed red blood cells per unit volume of blood.

There are other reasons for using plasma (or serum) rather than whole blood. It is easier to interpret values obtained from a single-component system such as plasma than from a two-component system such as whole blood. It is necessary to mix whole blood thoroughly before sampling. This is a particular problem with automated methods, where samples stand in the sample tray for a period of time before being tested. There are several substances in blood that interfere with tests for blood glucose, either because they are measured as glucose or because they interfere in enzyme procedures. These substances are more concentrated within red blood cells, so tests on plasma tend to be more specific for glucose. As indicated above, values on whole blood tend to vary with the hematocrit. Glucose is more stable in plasma than in whole blood, as many glycolytic enzymes are present in the red blood cell. Finally, plasma or serum is easier to handle, to pipette precisely, and to store than whole blood.

Because the amount of glucose in the blood increases after a meal, it is important that the principle tests to monitor glucose metabolism be done on fasting blood specimens or on specimens drawn 2 hours after a meal (postprandial). A random sample of blood is of little value for a glucose determination.

Fasting Blood Specimen

The blood should be drawn long enough after the last meal that the food has been completely digested and absorbed and any excess has been stored. The specimen for a blood glucose test is usually drawn in the morning before breakfast and is called a *fasting blood sugar*. The term *fasting* in this case means that the patient has had no breakfast, no cream or sugar, no coffee, tea or, other caffeinated drink, no drugs that might affect the blood glucose level, and no emotional disturbances that might cause liberation of glucose into the blood.

Two-hour (Postprandial) Specimen

To more completely detect diabetes mellitus, carbohydrate metabolic capacity is tested by stressing the system with a defined glucose load. To do this, a high carbohydrate drink or meal is given to the patient, blood is collected 2 hours after ingestion, and the glucose concentration is determined. A blood specimen drawn 2 hours after breakfast or lunch is also known as a *postprandial specimen*.

Capillary Blood Specimens

An advantage of using whole blood is the convenience of measuring glucose directly on capillary blood, such as that taken from infants, in mass screening programs for the detection of diabetes mellitus, or in the home monitoring being done by so many diabetes patients. Capillary blood must be thought of as essentially arterial rather than venous. In the fasting state the arterial (capillary) blood glucose concentration is 5 mg/dL higher than the venous concentration.

Effects of Glycolysis

Another factor that must be taken into account in considering specimens for glucose determinations is the *stability of glucose in body fluids*. Many enzymes present in the blood, particularly in the red cells, affect glucose. As whole blood is allowed to stand at room temperature in a test tube, these enzymes destroy glucose. This action is called glycolysis, and it occurs at an average rate of approximately 10 mg/dL/hr, or 5% per hour. Plasma that is removed from the red cells after moderate centrifugation contains leukocytes, which also metabolize glucose. However, cell-free plasma, prepared by adequate centrifugation, shows no glycolytic activity. When unhemolyzed serum or plasma is separated from the cells, the glucose concentration is generally stable for up to 8 hours at room temperature, and up to 72 hours at 4°C. Cerebrospinal fluids are frequently contaminated with bacteria or other cellular constituents such as leukocytes that may cause the breakdown of glucose. Thus, cerebrospinal fluids should be analyzed for glucose without delay. Refrigeration or the addition of a small amount of sodium fluoride to the fluid may retard glycolysis for a few hours.

Keeping these considerations in mind, there are several ways to prevent or retard glycolysis in a specimen to be analyzed. Samples for glucose analysis should be delivered to the laboratory as soon as possible after being drawn from the patient. If plasma or serum is to be used for the glucose determination, it must be separated from the cells or clot within 30 minutes after the blood is drawn unless a specific additive is used (such as flouride).

Using a special anticoagulant, usually sodium fluoride, seems to be the best way to preserve blood glucose specimens. Sodium fluoride acts in two ways to preserve glucose: as an anticoagulant by tying up calcium and thus preventing clotting, and as an enzyme inhibitor that prevents glycolytic enzymes from destroying the glucose. However, clotting may occur after several hours, so it is advisable to use a combined fluoride-oxalate mixture. When the blood sample is placed in fluoride-oxalate tubes, it must be thoroughly mixed to ensure the proper effect. When using some enzymatic glucose methods, fluoride-anticoagulated blood should not be used, as the enzyme might be inhibited by the fluoride. Serum separated gel tubes, processed within 30 minutes, are preferred for these methods.

Measurements of Glucose Metabolism

Fasting and Two-hour Postprandial Tests

Glucose is commonly determined on fasting blood specimens and on 2-hour postprandial specimens when glucose metabolism is being monitored. The fasting blood glucose concentration should normally be less than 105 mg/dL and the blood glucose taken 2 hours after a meal should normally be less than 120 mg/dL. Fasting blood glucose levels equal to or greater than 140 mg/dL on more than one occasion are diagnostic for diabetes mellitus. A fasting blood glucose > 140 mg/dL and an elevated glucose level 2-hours postprandially >200 mg/dL on two occasions are an indication of diabetes mellitus. Impaired glucose tolerance (IGT) is indicated if the fasting blood glucose is between 115–140 mg/dL and one postprandial glucose level is >200 mg/dL. Values other than these may indicate diabetes, but only after other factors have also been evaluated.

Glucose Tolerance Tests

In the detection and treatment of diabetes it is often necessary to have more information than can be obtained from only testing the fasting specimen for glucose. Patients with mild or diet-controlled diabetes may have fasting blood glucose levels within the normal range, but they may be unable to produce sufficient insulin for prompt metabolism of ingested carbohydrates. As a result, the blood glucose rises to abnormally high levels and the return to normal levels is delayed. One glucose tolerance test commonly done employs a 100-g glucose drink to be consumed within a 5-minute time period. The timing begins when the drink has been consumed. This test is known as the oral *glucose tolerance test*.

The glucose tolerance test is usually performed when a person has been found to have a fasting blood glucose concentration above that of most nondiabetic persons (about 105 mg/dL). It can also be done to determine hypoglycemia, an abnormal response to a glucose load that results in a blood glucose concentration much below the normally accepted range. Since early detection and management of diabetes is important to avoid the many complications of the disease, it is desirable to detect these early cases of diabetes or prediabetes. For these reasons, the physician may request a glucose tolerance test.

The glucose tolerance test measures the ability of a person to respond appropriately to a heavy load of glucose. Normally, when such a dose is received by the body, the pancreas responds by excreting insulin in the amount necessary for metabolism of the glucose. The degree and timing of the rising and falling of the blood glucose concentration after administration of glucose indicates how well the person can respond. The test has been standardized by the Committee on Statistics of the American Diabetes Association.

There are many glucose tolerance tests, but all are based on the same basic principles. The test begins with the patient in a fasting state, and blood is sampled and tested as a baseline control. Glucose is then administered, by either ingestion or injection and samples are obtained at timed intervals. The amount of glucose administered and the collection intervals depend on the tolerance test used. Urine specimens may also be tested at fasting and timed intervals coinciding with the blood sampling. In most tolerance tests samples are taken at intervals of 30, 60, 120, and 180 minutes. See Figure 10–4 for oral glucose tolerance test results for normal persons and for diabetes and other disorders.

Glucose Reagent Strips

The use of semiquantitative reagent strips for assessing control of blood glucose in management of diabetes is becoming widespread. These systems are used in emergency units of hospitals, at the hospital bedside, and also by patients for home monitoring purposes. When reagent strips are used for blood glucose measurements, it is essential that the user be trained to properly calibrate

and read the strips. The use of reflectance meters to replace visual readings can minimize errors due to poor lighting or color bias. Variations in the amounts of blood used, in the time allowed for the reaction, in the washing and wiping of the strips, and in the calibration of the reflectance meter can be minimized only through proper and sufficient training programs and by encouraging motivation of the operators, whether they be nurses, physicians, laboratorians, or the patients themselves.

Home Monitoring of Glucose.—Many patients (especially those with type I insulin-dependent diabetes mellitus) now monitor their own blood glucose concentrations on the advice of their physicians, using reagent test strips and reflectance meters. Several companies manufacture reagent test strips for monitoring blood glucose and most of these companies market reflectance meters to be used to electronically read the test results.

The enzyme glucose oxidase is impregnated on these strips. Any glucose present in the blood is converted to gluconic acid and hydrogen peroxide using the glucose oxidase to catalyze the reaction (see discussion of glucose oxidase below). There is a second enzyme, peroxidase, also present on the strip. The peroxidase uses the hydrogen peroxide formed in the first reaction to oxidize an indicator also present on the strip to give a color change which is detectable. This color change can be read visually by comparing the color to the color on a

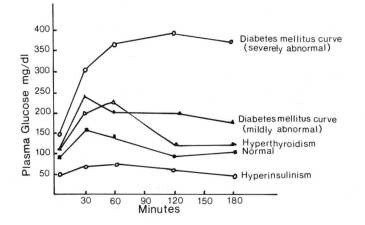

FIG 10–4.
Oral glucose tolerance test results. (From Becan-McBride K, Ross DL: *Essentials for the Small Laboratory and Physician's Office.* St Louis, Mosby–Year Book, Inc, 1988, p 250. Used by permission.)

chart provided with the strip. Alternatively and preferably, the color change can be read in a reflectance meter on which the result (in mg/dL) is visualized.

It is important that the users of these home monitoring techniques be fully instructed and informed about their proper use. The meters must be calibrated with solutions of glucose of a known concentration or with a calibration strip supplied with each lot of reagent strips. The procedure supplied by the manufacturer must always be followed when using any of these products.

The specimens used for these reagent strips are generally capillary blood obtained by finger puncture (see Peripheral or Capillary Blood, in Chapter 2).

Glycated Hemoglobin

When glucose in the blood plasma reaches abnormally high concentrations, glycosylation of many proteins occurs. Two types of tests for these proteins, hemoglobin and serum protein, are used to monitor long-term blood glucose concentration in patients with diabetes. Glycated hemoglobin in the blood indicates long-term hyperglycemia—a high glucose concentration over the previous 4 to 8 weeks. For this reason, this test is considered a better measure of diabetes control than a single blood glucose measurement.

A hemoglobin derivative, hemoglobin A_{1c} or glycated hemoglobin, is formed when glucose and hemoglobin combine. Glycated hemoglobin methods include electrophoresis, ion-exchange chromatography, and high-pressure liquid chromatography. One commercially available product employs a boronate affinity column to separate the various proteins that are glycated from those that are not.

Methods for Quantitative Determination of Glucose

The various methods for the quantitative determination of glucose can be divided into three general categories: oxidation-reduction methods, aromatic amine methods, and enzymatic methods.

Oxidation-Reduction Methods

Oxidation methods for blood glucose depend on the fact that glucose contains an aldehyde group as part of its chemical structure. The presence of this aldehyde gives glucose its reducing properties (Fig 10–5).

Other substances in blood also have reducing prop-

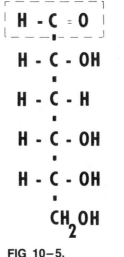

aldehyde group

FIG 10–5.
Glucose molecule.

erties. Some of these *nonglucose reducing substances* are glutathione and ergothioneine, which are found within red blood cells, and other materials such as uric acid, creatinine, ascorbic acid, certain amino acids, homogentisic acid, creatine, phenols, glucuronic acid, and sugar phosphates. These nonglucose reducing substances are also referred to as *saccharoids*. The methods for determining blood glucose differ primarily in the way they handle the nonglucose reducing substances. When the nonglucose reducing substances are removed as part of a glucose determination, the resulting value is called the *true glucose* value.

Nonglucose reducing substances are removed in glucose determinations both by improvements in methodology and by precipitation of protein, which removes other interfering substances by coprecipitation. In the Folin-Wu method, which is a classic copper reduction method, the protein is removed with tungstic acid. This is not recommended because it gives a filtrate that contains significant amounts of nonglucose reducing substances, especially glutathione. The barium hydroxide and zinc sulfate method of removing protein, utilized in the Nelson-Somogyi method, is preferred. It removes most of the nonglucose reducing substances and gives values only slightly higher than those obtained with the glucose oxidase and hexokinase techniques, which are specific for glucose. When glucose is analyzed with automated devices such as the AutoAnalyzer (Technicon Instruments Corp., Tarrytown, NY), the protein is separated from the specimen by means of a dialyzer. Of the many methods available for the determination of blood glucose, one reduction method employs potassium ferricyanide and another uses alkaline copper solutions. In either case, the glucose acts to reduce the reagent to a lower oxidation product. This product is then analyzed photometrically.

Alkaline copper reduction methods for glucose depend on the reduction of copper(II) [Cu(II)] to copper(I) [Cu(I)] while the aldehyde group of glucose is oxidized to gluconic acid.

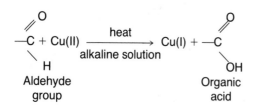

These were among the original methods of testing for glucose. Two classic examples of alkaline copper reduction methods are the Folin-Wu method and the Nelson-Somogyi method. With the older Folin-Wu method, an alkaline copper solution is added to a tungstic acid protein-free filtrate and heated. The copper(II) ion is reduced to copper(I). The copper(I) ion so formed then reduces a solution of phosphomolybdic acid to form a blue solution, which is measured photometrically. The Folin-Wu method is rather nonspecific for glucose, however, as it measures both glucose and nonglucose reducing substances. In the Nelson-Somogyi method, barium hydroxide and zinc sulfate are used for the precipitation of proteins. This is a significant improvement, as the filtrate is virtually free of all nonglucose reducing substances. A disadvantage of all copper reduction methods is the reoxidation of copper(I) ions to copper(II) ions by air. Therefore, steps must be taken to minimize reoxidation in the procedure.

Other procedures that make use of the reducing ability of glucose are the *alkaline ferricyanide methods*. In these methods, a hot alkaline ferricyanide solution, which is yellow, is reduced by glucose to a ferrocyanide solution, which is colorless. The decrease in the yellow color is proportional to the glucose concentration. The reaction may be followed by measuring the loss of yellow color, or by adding ferric ions, which react with ferrocyanide to form Prussian blue. In this case the forma-

tion of a blue color is measured. An advantage of ferricyanide methods is that they are not as subject to reoxidation by air as the copper reduction methods. The ferricyanide method has been automated for use on the AutoAnalyzer. (For specific manual procedures for these oxidation-reduction methods, consult a basic clinical chemistry textbook.)

Aromatic Amine Methods (the O-Toluidine Test)

These methods depend on the fact that various aromatic amines react with glucose in hot acetic acid to form colored derivatives. The aromatic amine commonly used is *ortho*-toluidine (o-toluidine). The methods involve a reaction between the aldehyde group of glucose (see Fig 10–5) and the amino group (—NH$_2$) of the aromatic amine. A green-colored complex is formed which is measured spectrophotometrically. The o-toluidine method, a nonenzymatic method, is highly specific for glucose, is easily performed, and can be adapted to serum or plasma without deproteinization. The manual procedures have been adapted for automated techniques. One automated instrument to which the o-toluidine method has been applied is the AutoAnalyzer continuous-flow system. This system is not used as much today, however, and has been replaced by enzymatic automated methods.

The o-toluidine method makes use of the fact that glucose (an aldohexose) reacts specifically with o-toluidine in glacial acetic acid in the presence of heat to produce a blue-green color. Because aldohexoses other than glucose are usually present in very small concentrations in body fluids, results obtained by this method approach the true value for glucose. The o-toluidine method has the additional advantage that it can be performed directly on serum, plasma, cerebrospinal fluid, or urine without deproteinization. When whole blood is used, or when the specimen is moderately hemolyzed, it must be deproteinized. The procedure can be used on capillary blood. When a nonautomated glucose method is needed, the o-toluidine method is usually employed. The o-toluidine method is not widely used today, however, because o-toluidine is believed to be a carcinogen.

Enzymatic Methods

The use of enzymes is a means of achieving absolute specificity in the determination of glucose concentration. The two most widely used enzyme methods are based on the enzymes glucose oxidase and hexokinase.

$$\beta\text{-D-glucose} + H_2O \xrightarrow{\text{glucose oxidase}} \text{D-gluconic acid} + H_2O_2$$

$$2\,H_2O_2 + 4\,\text{aminopyrine} + 1,7\text{-dehydroxynapthylene} \xrightarrow{\text{peroxidase}} \text{a red dye}$$

Glucose Oxidase Reaction

Glucose Oxidase.—Glucose oxidase catalyzes the oxidation of glucose to gluconic acid and hydrogen peroxide. In some methods the amount of hydrogen peroxide produced or oxygen used is measured by an electrode process. In others a second enzyme, peroxidase, catalyzes the oxidation of a chromogen such as *o*-toluidine to a colored product; in this case the color that is formed is proportional to the amount of glucose present. When peroxidase is used in these procedures, the test is subject to interference from reducing agents such as ascorbic acid, which react with hydrogen peroxide, resulting in falsely low results. The glucose oxidase procedure has been adapted to a wide range of various automated products. These include instruments that employ dry chemistry reagents, either in a strip or film form.

Reagent strips for testing glucose concentration in urine employ the oxidation of iodine to monitor the peroxidase reaction, or use different compounds whose oxidized forms are colored. The strips can be read visually or by using reflectance photometry and can be used for urine or serum to give a semiquantitative measurement of glucose concentration.

The oxidation of an indicator dye is used to form a colored compound used in the automated method using the Ektachem instrument (Eastman Kodak Co., Rochester, N.Y.). The specimen is deposited on the Ektachem slide and is evenly distributed by the spreading layer. Water and any nonprotein components of the serum move to the underlying reagent layer. After the reaction has occurred and after a fixed incubation period, the reflectance density of the red dye formed in the reaction is measured by the spectrophotometer through the transparent polyester support. The result is obtained in about 5 minutes. See glucose oxidase reaction above.

Hexokinase.—Another enzyme used in glucose tests is hexokinase. These methods are less subject to interference than the glucose oxidase-peroxidase methods. The hexokinase method is the one used most often in automated instruments. The DuPont ACA (DuPont Co., Wilmington, DE.) is one instrument utilizing the hexokinase method. This method employs the enzyme hexokinase to catalyze the formation of glucose-6-phosphate from glucose. In the reaction, adenosine triphosphate (ATP) is simultaneously converted to adenosine diphosphate (ADP). The glucose-6-phosphate formed becomes the substrate for a second enzymatic reaction where the coenzyme NADP is reduced to NADPH with 6-phosphogluconate being formed (see also under Clinical Enzymology). See hexakinase reaction below. As seen in the above reaction, for each mole of NADPH formed, 1 mol of glucose has been reacted upon. There is a change in absorbance at 340 nm, and this change is used to measure the concentration of glucose. NADPH is formed in direct proportion to the amount of glucose present in the original specimen.

Although other hexoses can react also in the hexokinase procedure, normal serum concentrations of these other sugars do not usually cause significant interference. No interference is observed with fluoride, heparin, oxalate, and ethylenediamine tetraacetic acid (EDTA) anticoagulants at the usual concentrations. Ascorbic acid does not cause interference in this test.

A set of standards must routinely be included to correct for background absorption. Quality control specimens are run with each batch of tests and their values must be within the established acceptable range for unknown results to be reported out. Daily control charts are maintained and saved to document any trends or problems that may occur.

$$\text{Glucose} + \text{ATP} \xrightarrow{\text{hexokinase}} \text{glucose-6-phosphate} + \text{ADP}$$

$$\text{Glucose-6-phosphate} + \text{NADP} \xrightarrow{\text{glucose-6-phosphate dehydrogenase}} \text{6-phosphogluconate} + \text{NADPH} + H^+$$

Hexokinase Reaction

The hexokinase method is also an excellent method to determine glucose in urine and other biological fluids. This method has been proposed as a basis of reference method because of its accuracy and precision.

Reference Values*

Reference values for the individual glucose methods can vary significantly. Each laboratory must therefore determine and evaluate the reference range for its particular facility.

In the fasting state, the glucose concentration of serum or plasma, as determined by a highly specific method such as the hexokinase method, ranges from 70 to 105 mg/dL. The glucose value in whole blood is less, ranging from 65 to 95 mg/dL. There is no significant difference in glucose concentration between males and females or between races.

In normal cerebrospinal fluid (CSF), the glucose concentration is about 60% to 70% of the plasma level and ranges from 40 to 70 mg/dL. It is therefore important to also measure the blood glucose concentration when a spinal fluid glucose is assayed so that spinal fluid glucose results can be evaluated appropriately.

There is normally no glucose detectable in urine.

Glucose, serum:

Child	60–100 mg/dL (3.33–5.55 mmol/L)
Adult	70–105 mg/dL (3.89–5.83 mmol/L)

Glucose, CSF

Infant, child	60–80 mg/dL (3.33–4.44 mmol/L)
Adult	40–70 mg/dL (2.22–3.89 mmol/L)

ELECTROLYTES

As used in the traditional clinical chemistry laboratory, the term *electrolytes* refers primarily to sodium, potassium, chloride, and bicarbonate, because these substances are the major ions in the body. These four electrolytes are often discussed together because changes in the concentration of one of them are almost always accompanied by changes in the concentration of one or

*Tietz NW (ed): *Fundamentals of Clinical Chemistry*, ed 3. Philadelphia, WB Saunders Co, 1987, p 954.

more of the others. Electrolytes are substances that form or exist as ions or charged particles when dissolved in water. Other electrolytes include calcium, magnesium, sulfate, and phosphate.

One example of an electrolyte is sodium chloride, which forms Na^+ and Cl^- in water. The sodium and chloride ions are also called electrolytes. The sodium ion is called a *cation* because it is attracted by a negatively charged electrode or cathode, and the chloride ion is called an *anion* because it is attracted by a positively charged electrode or anode. All charged particles are either anions (negatively charged) or cations (positively charged). These ions are found throughout the body, but their concentrations or activities vary from one body compartment to another. Assays are usually done on plasma or serum.

The electrolytes are the major charged particles present in the extracellular fluid. The chief negatively charged constituents are chloride (Cl^-) and bicarbonate (HCO_3^-). The chief positively charged constituents are sodium (Na^+) and potassium (K^+). There are other electrolytes, but sodium, potassium, chloride, and bicarbonate are the ones most likely to show variation in electrolyte problems. Collectively, the four charged particles—chloride, bicarbonate, sodium, and potassium—make up a group of laboratory tests referred to as the **electrolyte battery.** It is essential that the positively charged particles balance, or electrically neutralize, the negatively charged particles. When this balance is not achieved, electrolyte imbalance occurs; this is extremely dangerous for the patient and can be fatal. Therefore, to assess electrolyte balance, the laboratory must often perform electrolyte determinations. A set of electrolyte determinations consists of tests for chloride, bicarbonate, sodium, and potassium. These determinations are often done as emergency procedures, for electrolyte imbalance cannot be tolerated by the patient for long. Treatment to remedy the imbalance must be started as quickly as possible. Assay of electrolytes in general is done because many important body functions depend on the maintenance of their proper concentrations. Some of these functions are maintenance of water in the various body compartments, maintenance of pH, activity of blood coagulation and enzyme cofactors, control of neuromuscular excitability, and involvement in oxidation-reduction reactions.

When the body is unable to maintain a normal control over the concentration of the electrolytes, either by excretion or conservation, one or more of the electrolyte constituents will have an abnormal concentration. The kidneys and the lungs are the organs which furnish most control over electrolyte concentration.

Clinical Significance

Sodium

Sodium (Na^+) is the cation, or positively charged particle, found in the highest concentration in extracellular fluid. It is important in maintaining the osmotic pressure and in electrolyte balance. Sodium is associated with the levels of chloride and bicarbonate ion, and for this reason it has a major role in maintaining the **acid-base balance** of the body cells. A low serum sodium level is called *hyponatremia* and a high one is called *hypernatremia*. Low sodium levels are found in a variety of conditions, including severe polyuria (as in diabetes insipidus), metabolic acidosis (as in diabetic acidosis), Addison's disease (where the supply of adrenocortical hormones is inadequate—these hormones have a strong influence on the level of sodium), diarrhea, and some renal tubular diseases. An increased sodium level is found in Cushing's syndrome (where there is hyperactivity of the adrenal cortex and more hormones than normal are produced), severe dehydration caused by primary water loss, certain types of brain injury, diabetic coma after therapy with insulin, and after excess treatment with sodium salts.

Potassium

Potassium ($K+$) is the chief intracellular cation, but it is also found extracellularly. It has an important influence on the muscle activity of the heart. Since potassium is largely excreted by the kidney, it becomes elevated in kidney failure and shock. Like sodium, potassium is influenced by the presence of the adrenocortical hormones and is associated with acid-base balance. An elevated potassium level in serum is called *hyperkalemia* and a decreased level is called *hypokalemia*. High serum potassium levels are generally seen in cases of oliguria, anuria, or urinary obstruction. In renal tubular acidosis, there is increased retention of potassium in the serum. One important purpose of renal dialysis is the removal of accumulated potassium from the plasma. Low serum potassium levels can result from prolonged diarrhea or vomiting, or from inadequate intake of dietary potassium. Even in potassium deficiency, the kidney continues to excrete potassium. The body has no effective mechanism to protect itself from excessive loss of potassium, so a regular daily intake of potassium is essential.

Chloride

The *chloride* ion (Cl^-) is the most important anion of the extracellular fluids in the body. It is the major anion that counterbalances the major cation, sodium, to maintain the electrical neutrality of the body fluids. Electrical neutrality is maintained at all times in the body fluids. This means that the sum of all the cations (positively charged particles) equals the sum of all the anions (negatively charged particles).

Chloride has two main functions in the body: it is important in determining the osmotic pressure, which controls the distribution of water between cells, plasma, and interstitial fluid, and it is important in maintaining the acid-base balance. Chloride also plays an important role in the buffering action when oxygen and carbon dioxide exchange in the red blood cells. This activity is known as the *chloride shift*. When blood is oxygenated, chloride travels from the red blood cells to the plasma, and at the same time bicarbonate leaves the plasma and enters the red cells. Water travels in the same direction as chloride, and the red blood cells become dehydrated when the blood is oxygenated. Whenever bicarbonate goes from the red blood cells to the plasma, as it must during carbon dioxide transport, the bicarbonate anions are replaced by an equivalent amount of chloride anions.

An example of the chloride shift in the laboratory is the replacement action that occurs when a specimen for a chloride determination is allowed to stand for a while before the cells and plasma are separated. When whole blood comes into contact with air, carbon dioxide (and thus bicarbonate) escapes from the blood. As carbon dioxide leaves the plasma, chloride diffuses (or shifts) out of the red cells to replace it. The contact between whole blood and air, therefore, has the effect of lowering the plasma carbon dioxide and raising the plasma chloride. Specimens of whole blood left in contact with air may therefore give falsely high plasma or serum chloride values. The proper general handling of blood specimens is discussed in Chapter 2. The cells must be removed from the plasma by centrifugation as quickly as possible. Once separated from the cells, the serum or plasma has a very stable chloride concentration.

The other important function of chloride is to regulate the fluid content of the body and its influence on the kidney. The kidney maintains the electrolyte concentration of the plasma within very narrow limits. This regulation is necessary for life. Renal function is set to regulate the composition of the extracellular fluid first and then the volume. Consequently, if the body loses salt (sodium chloride), it loses water.

Low serum or plasma chloride values may be seen in nephritis where salt is lost, as in chronic pyelonephritis. A low chloride value may also be seen in the types of metabolic acidotic conditions that are caused by excessive production or diminished excretion of acids, as in diabetic acidosis and renal failure. Prolonged vomiting, from any cause, may ultimately result in a decrease in serum and body chloride.

High serum or plasma chloride values are seen in dehydration and in conditions that cause decreased renal blood flow, such as congestive heart failure. Excessive treatment with or dietary intake of chloride ions also results in high serum levels.

Chloride is found in serum, plasma, cerebrospinal fluid, tissue fluid, and urine. There is very little chloride inside the cells of the body, with the exception of the red cells, which contain some chloride. The chief extracellular anions are chloride and bicarbonate, and there is a reciprocal relationship between them; that is, when there is a decrease in the amount of one, there is an increase in the amount of the other. In the blood, two-thirds of the chloride is found in the plasma and only one-third in the red cells. Because of the difference in chloride concentration between the red cells and the plasma, the test for chloride is routinely performed on plasma (or serum) and not on whole blood. Physiologically, only the concentration of chloride in the extracellular fluid is important. This is another reason why plasma or serum is chosen as the specimen for this determination.

Bicarbonate

Bicarbonate (HCO_3^-), along with chloride, is one of the major extracellular anions in body fluids. As the blood perfuses the lungs, carbon dioxide (CO_2) and H_2O are formed. During the metabolic processes, carbonic acid (H_2CO_3) dissociates and forms bicarbonate. This is reconverted to carbonic acid, followed by the formation of H_2O and CO_2. These reactions are as follows:

Bicarbonate is filtered by the kidney and little or no bicarbonate is found in the urine. The proximal tubules reabsorb 85% of these ions and the remaining 15% are reabsorbed by the distal tubules. Bicarbonate is most commonly measured with other combined forms of CO_2 (CO_2, H_2CO_3, carbamino groups) as total CO_2. Since about 90% of all the CO_2 in serum is in the form of bicarbonate, this combined form approximates the actual bicarbonate very closely. Total carbon dioxide is the total of carbonic acid and bicarbonate. Bicarbonate is usually reported rather than total CO_2 due to potential sample-handling errors with a possible loss of carbonic acid as a result.

Along with pH and carbon dioxide pressure (Pco_2) determinations, the total carbon dioxide concentration is a useful measurement in evaluating acid-base disorders. The importance of the bicarbonate or carbon dioxide value in itself is not as significant as is its value in the context of the other electrolytes assayed. Total carbon dioxide assays are performed volumetrically, manometrically, or colorimetrically, or by using a Pco_2 electrode to measure the rate of released carbon dioxide being formed. Most assays are now performed using automated instruments.

Anion Gap

The calculation of the mathematical difference between the anions (Cl^- and HCO_3^-) and cations (Na^+ and K^+) is known as the **anion gap.** If the Cl^- and bicarbonate are summed and subtracted from the sum of the Na^+ and K^+ concentrations, the difference should be less than 17 mmol/L. If the anion gap exceeds 17 mmol/L, this is usually an indication of increased concentrations of the unmeasured anions (PO_4^{3-}, SO_4^{2-}, protein ions). Increased anion gaps can result from ketotic states, lactic acidosis, toxin ingestion, uremia, or increased plasma proteins. Decreased anion gaps of less than 10 mmol/L can result from either an increase in unmeasured cations (Ca^{2+}, Mg^{2+}) or a decrease in the unmeasured anions.

The anion gap is also useful as a quality control measure for electrolyte results. If an increased anion gap is found for electrolytes in a healthy person, there is reason to suspect that one or more of the test results is erroneous, and the tests should be repeated.

$$CO_2 \text{ (gas)} \rightleftarrows CO_2 \text{ (dissolved)} \underset{H_2O}{\overset{+H_2O}{\rightleftarrows}} H_2CO_3 \rightleftarrows H^+ + HCO_3^-$$

Specimens

Electrolyte testing is usually done on serum processed from a venous blood collection into an evacuated nonadditive tube. Capillary samples can be collected into microcontainers or capillary tubes. Plasma can also be assayed using lithium heparin as the anticoagulant. When plasma is used, the assay can be expedited and the result reported out more quickly for emergency situations. Centrifugation should be done in unopened tubes and the serum or plasma removed promptly. Each assay has specific concerns to note regarding specimen requirements and technical factors relating to the specimen collection and handling.

Sodium

Serum, heparinized plasma, heparinized whole blood, urine, and other body fluids are suitable specimens. Sodium heparin should not be used because the presence of sodium will interfere with the assay. Cells must be separated from serum or plasma within 3 hours to avoid shifts in equilibrium of constituents between cells and serum or plasma.

Sodium is stable in serum for at least 2 weeks at room temperature or in the refrigerator. If flame photometry is used to analyze sodium levels, scrupulous care is necessary. The slightest contamination of specimens or equipment will drastically alter the results. Glassware used for sodium determinations must be clean and free from sodium contamination; when possible, plastic containers should be used to avoid contamination. Sodium can be measured in 24-hour urine specimens and in cerebrospinal fluid.

Potassium

The collection of blood for potassium studies requires special attention and technique. If plasma is used, an anticoagulant containing potassium cannot be used. Lithium heparin is preferred. Since the concentration of potassium in the red blood cell is about 20 times that in serum or plasma, it is imperative that hemolysis be avoided. To avoid a shift of potassium from the red cells to the plasma or serum, it is important to separate the cells from the plasma or serum as quickly as possible. When blood is collected for a potassium test, opening and closing of the fist before venipuncture should be avoided, since this muscle action may result in an increase in plasma potassium levels of 10% to 20%. Potassium levels in plasma are about 0.1 to 0.7 mmol/L lower than those in serum because of the release of potassium from ruptured platelets during the coagulation process. Potassium in serum is stable for at least 2 weeks at room or refrigerator temperature. Potassium levels in urine vary with dietary intake and are measured in a 24-hour collection.

Chloride

Chloride is commonly assayed in serum, plasma, urine, or sweat. Because two-thirds of the chloride in blood is found in the plasma, plasma or serum is routinely used for analysis of chloride. Blood should be collected for a chloride determination in tubes that are free of even trace contamination. There are many sources of chloride in the laboratory, and even tap water may contain a significant amount of chloride. Glassware and pipettes used for the chloride determination must also be free from any contamination with chloride. Serum separator gel tubes are commonly used for collecting blood specimens for chloride tests. The anticoagulant used most frequently is lithium or sodium heparin. Sodium fluoride cannot be used for the chloride determination, because the fluoride is a halogen (as is chloride), and both react in the same way in the assays. If sodium fluoride were used, a falsely high chloride value would be obtained because the fluoride would also be measured. The serum or plasma should be removed from the red cells as soon as possible after the blood is drawn to prevent the chloride shift from occurring. Loss of gaseous carbon dioxide alters the distribution of cloride ions between the cells and plasma (see also under Clinical Significance). Moderate hemolysis does not significantly affect the concentration of chloride in the serum.

Urine and Cerebrospinal Fluid.—Chloride may be measured in other body fluids, such as urine or cerebrospinal fluid. The chloride content in urine can be quite variable, and an amount of specimen should be used in the procedure that will give a suitable titration reading. Urine and cerebrospinal fluid can be used in the Cotlove Chloridometer (Buchler Instruments, Fort Lee, NJ) with good results.

Sweat Chloride.—The chloride content of sweat is useful in diagnosing cystic fibrosis, a disease of the exocrine glands. Affected infants usually have concentrations of sweat chloride greater than 60 mmol/L (normal is 5–45 mmol/L in children). When the disease is mild, it may not be diagnosed until adulthood. In 98% of patients with cystic fibrosis, the secretion of chloride in sweat is two to five times normal. The determination of chloride in sweat, as well as other electrolytes, is considered the most reliable single test in the diagnosis of cystic fibrosis. The chloride content of normal sweat varies with age. To collect the sample, the patient is induced to sweat and the sweat is measured directly by use of ion-specific electrodes.

Bicarbonate

Either serum or heparinized plasma may be used for the bicarbonate assay. Other anticoagulants disturb the balance between red cell and plasma CO_2. Venous blood is generally collected in an evacuated tube, but capillary blood collected in microcontainers or capillary tubes may also be used for this assay. The bicaronate concentration is most accurately determined immediately when the tube is opened and as quickly as possible after collection and centrifugation of the unopened tube has taken place. A specimen to be assayed for total CO_2 must be handled anaerobically to minimize losses of CO_2 and HCO_3^- (converted to CO_2) into the atmosphere. A falsely low total CO_2 would result if this loss has occurred. In the laboratory, the specimen can be protected by covering the specimen container with plastic wrap.

Methods for Quantitative Measurement

The four main electrolytes, sodium, potassium, chloride, and bicarbonate (as total CO_2), are generally grouped together for testing and called, as mentioned above, an electrolyte profile or electrolyte battery. The determination of electrolyte battery concentrations is an important function of the clinical chemistry laboratory. Most electrolyte testing today is done by use of automatic assay instrumentation. Results are reported only when quality control measures meet the established criteria for the laboratory.

Sodium and Potassium

There are two usual methods for determination of sodium and potassium levels in serum or plasma, flame emission photometry or ion-selective electrode potentiometry. An automated flame photometry method is used in some laboratories, in which the sample is automati-

cally diluted and presented to a flame photometer equipped with a recorder or readout device. Since the details of the analyses for potassium and sodium vary with the flame photometer used, they are not included in this discussion. The instruction manual provided with the instrument should be consulted. Basic information on flame photometry as a quantitative technique in the laboratory may be found under Flame Emission Photometry in Chapter 5. The accuracy of the results depends on following the manufacturer's instructions explicitly.

Flame Emission Photometry.—Flame emission photometry is based on the principle that when atoms of many metallic elements, especially sodium and potassium, are given sufficient energy in one form or another, they will emit this energy at wavelengths that are characteristic for the element. Dilute solutions of serum or another biological fluid (such as urine) are atomized into a flame and burned. The elements in these solutions are excited by the flame and emit characteristic spectra. With the use of appropriate filters, the emission from potassium or sodium may be isolated and focused on a photocell, which responds linearly to the light energy directed on it. Since light is emitted in direct proportion to the concentration of sodium or potassium in the unknown fluid, the response of the photocell is directly related to the concentration, and unknowns may be determined by comparing the response with those of known standard solutions.

Sodium always produces a yellow color in a flame and potassium produces a violet color. The amount of color is measured with a detector and read with a meter (see Fig 5–3). In most cases, the internal standard method of flame photometry is used: an exact amount of lithium is added to each sample, and the intensity of the sodium or potassium color in the flame is compared by the instrument with the intensity of the red color from the lithium internal standard. The use of an internal standard (lithium) helps to compensate for changes in the condition of the flame and in the levels of interfering substances in the sample being measured.

It is necessary to dilute samples to be measured in a flame photometer. The extent of dilution depends on the type of instrument used, the type of specimen, and the concentrations of the ions to be measured. Dilution also decreases or eliminates interference by other constituents in the sample. The usual dilution is 1:100 or 1:200.

Standard solutions should be analyzed with the unknown samples. These standards are usually prepared from the chloride salt of sodium or potassium, depending on the element to be measured. Standard solutions should be stored in polyethylene containers to avoid contamination from the sodium that is found in many glass containers.

Water used in preparing reagents should be pure and free from sodium contamination. To check for contamination, water may be aspirated into the flame photometer and any appearance of a yellow color noted. A yellow color would suggest sodium contamination.

The flow of fuel into the flame must be strictly controlled. A change in the rate of flow of fuel or oxidant changes the flame temperature and flame size and thus affects the sensitivity of the test procedure. The use of combustible gases for fuel requires special handling and precautions in the laboratory. Work areas should be well ventilated.

Ion-Selective Electrode Potentiometry.—Ion-selective electrode methods use a glass ion-exchange membrane for sodium assay and a valinomycin neutral-carrier membrane for potassium assay. These methods are used frequently in smaller chemistry analyzers. Ion-selective electrode methods measure the activity of an ion in the water-volume fraction in which it is dissolved. A smaller model of the Kodak Ektachem uses this method. This instrument uses a dry, multilayered slide with a self-contained analytic element coated on a polyester support. Each slide contains a pair of ion-selective electrodes—one being used as a reference electrode and the other as a measuring electrode. Depending upon which slide-electrode is selected, the instrument can assay sodium or potassium. Another ion-selective electrode is also available for chloride assay using this same instrument.

In this method, 10 μL of specimen and reference standard is applied to the appropriate Ektachem slide and the slide introduced into the instrument. An electrometer in the instrument measures the potential difference between the two half-cells of the reference and the sample. The assay is completed in about 3 minutes. When calibrated properly, the instrument automatically calculates the concentration of the specimens being assayed.

Chloride

Many analyses for chloride employ some type of titration procedure. The titrations can be carried out manually or potentiometrically. Manual titration methods for the detection of chloride have generally been replaced by coulometry, the use of chloridometers, or titrators. Chlo-

ride is also measured colorimetrically by automated analyzer methods in many laboratories.

All reagents used in chloride determinations must be free from any outside chloride contamination. No anticoagulant containing a halogen (chloride, bromide, fluoride, or iodide) can be used in the determination because it would give falsely high results. Glassware and pipettes must be chemically clean. Sources of chloride contamination in the laboratory are many (including tap water, which contains significant amounts).

Manual Titration: Schales and Schales Method*.—The interfering proteins are first removed by precipitation with tungstic acid (the modified Folin-Wu filtrate method). Proteins, if present, will interfere with color detection and with the reaction. Titration is the next step. The chloride in the protein-free filtrate is titrated with mercuric nitrate [$Hg(NO_3)_2$], using diphenylcarbazone to indicate when the end point has been reached. When all the chloride in the filtrate has reacted with the mercuric nitrate, the diphenylcarbazone indicator changes color from orange-red to faint blue-violet.

In the titration with mercuric nitrate, the reaction taking place is

$$2NaCl + Hg(NO_3)_2 \longrightarrow 2NaNO_3 + HgCl_2$$

When all the chloride ions have reacted with the mercuric nitrate, the first excess of mercuric ions react with the indicator to form a faint blue-violet complex salt. The reaction is complete when the end point is reached—that is, when the first blue-violet color is produced by the addition of a drop or a split drop of mercuric nitrate. The first, faintest, permanent blue-violet is the end point. It is most important to use caution in titrating, as even a fraction of a milliliter of overtitration will result in grossly inaccurate results. The amount of standard mercuric nitrate used in the titration is an index of the chloride content.

When the titration has been completed, the results are calculated. Chloride results are usually reported in units of millimoles per liter (mmol/L). These units are used because the major functions of chloride in the body are associated with osmotic pressure regulation and acid-base balance.

---

*Schales O, Schales SS: Simple and accurate method for determination of chloride in biological fluids. *J Biol Chem* 1949; 140:879.

Coulometric Titration.—A common assay method measures chloride by coulometric titration with silver ions. Coulometry measures the amount of electricity passing between two electrodes in an electrochemical cell. The amount of electricity is directly proportional to the amount of substance produced or consumed by the process at the electrode.

With the use of a chloridometer, silver ions are generated at a constant voltage from a silver electrode. These silver ions react with chloride ions in the specimen being analyzed to form insoluble silver chloride. The end point is detected amperometrically by a second pair of electrodes. These electrodes can specifically measure the free silver ions that result when all the chloride ions are consumed. In using this method, the time required to titrate a chloride standard solution or the unknown sample, using a constant current, is measured. The unknown concentration is calculated by the following proportion formula:

$$\frac{\text{Chloride concentration (standard)}}{\text{Titration time (standard)}} = \frac{\text{chloride concentration (unknown)}}{\text{titration time (unknown)}}$$

The accuracy of the manual titration methods, such as the Schales and Schales method, depends on a visual end point of the titration reaction. The factor of human judgment, is eliminated with coulometry.

Using the Cotlove Chloridometer* or titrator, silver ions are released from a silver wire when a current is generated in an electrode. The silver ions combine with chloride in the specimen to form insoluble silver chloride. The potential of the solution being titrated changes at the equivalence point, since the solution goes from having an excess of chloride ions to having an excess of silver ions. There must be a sufficient volume of sample that the electrodes are fully immersed in the solution. A small stirrer attached to the electrode assembly thoroughly mixes the specimen as it is being analyzed.

When all the chloride is used, the change in potential is used to shut off the instrument. In this way the end point is detected automatically. The lapsed time for each titration is automatically recorded on a timer. Since the

---

*Cotlove E, Trantham HV, Bowman RL: An instrument and method for automatic, rapid, accurate and sensitive titration of chloride in biological samples. *J Lab Clin Med* 1958; 50:461.

rate of release of silver ions is constant, the amount of time during which they are released is directly proportional to the amount of chloride in the sample. That is, the more chloride present in the sample, the longer it takes to generate enough silver ions to combine with all of it. In the calculations the titration time for the unknown is compared with the titration time for a standard sodium chloride solution. Modern instruments read directly in millimoles per liter.

The chloridometer method is one of the most accurate methods available for determining chloride. Other halogens interfere with this method, just as they do with other methods for chloride. The chloridometer can be used with plasma, serum, cerebrospinal fluid, sweat, and urine specimens. Specimens are diluted in a mixture of acetic and nitric acids containing a small amount of gelatin. The nitric acid provides good electrolytic conductivity and the acetic acid provides a sharper end point. All reagents must be prepared with chloride-free water (distilled or deionized). An automatic diluter is convenient for delivering the acid reagent and the standard or unknown samples into the titration vials. The electrodes of the machine must be rinsed well after each analysis.

Ion-selective Electrode Potentiometry.—Ion-selective electrodes, (ISE), usually with silver chloride–silver sulfide sensing elements, can also be used to assay chloride concentration. The Kodak Ektachem method utilizes these (see above under Methods for Quantitative Measurement).

For chloride measurement in urine and sweat, since there is potentially such a wide variation in possible concentration, a coulometric or ion-selective electrode method is usually used.

Colorimetric Method.—Another common method for chloride assay employs a quantitative displacement of thiocyanate by chloride from mercuric thiocyanate and formation of a red ferric thiocyanate complex. This colored compound is measured with a spectrophotometer. In this method, chloride first combines with free mercury ions to form a colorless compound; it then displaces any thiocyanate from mercuric thiocyanate. The free thiocyanate ions react with iron to produce the red-colored end product.

In this method, the specimen being analyzed for chloride is diluted with a solution of mercuric thiocyanate after being dialyzed to remove the proteins. Ferric nitrate reagent is also added. Mercuric thiocyanate, like mercuric chloride, is undissociated. The chloride ions compete successfully with thiocyanate ions for mercuric ions. The resulting free thiocyanate ions combine with ferric ions to produce a red complex, $Fe(SCN)_3$. This color is measured colorimetrically in the automated analyzer. The amount of color is proportional to the amount of chloride present in the specimen.

Bicarbonate

The routine bicarbonate (reported rather than total CO_2) assay is automated and the first step in automated methods in general is the acidification of the sample to convert the various forms of bicarbonate present to gaseous CO_2. Another important consideration for automated procedures for bicarbonate assays is the need to include several standard solutions with the assay of the unknowns to keep the automated methods in control.

One common automated bicarbonate assay is that utilizing the continuous flow procedure of the Technicon AutoAnalyzer (Technicon Instruments Corp., Tarrytown, N.Y.). The gas formed in the acidification step is quantitatively converted to HCO_3^- and H^+. A change in pH results in a change in the color intensity of the phenolphthalein indicator. This is detected quantitatively with a spectrophotometer. The use of standard solutions is vital to keep the instrument in control.

The ASTRA method (Beckman Instruments, Brea, Calif.) uses a Pco_2 electrode to quantitate the gaseous CO_2 produced in the first acidification step. The CO_2 gas diffuses across a silicon-rubber membrane and this changes the pH of a bicarbonate electrode buffer. The rate of change of pH of the buffer inside the membrane of the measuring electrode indicates the concentration of CO_2 in the sample.

Discrete analyzers such as the DuPont ACA (Du Pont, Wilmington, DE) convert all CO_2 forms to HCO_3^- by addition of alkali to the serum specimen. The HCO_3^- formed is then converted enzymatically to oxaloacetic acid. This is measured by an NADH consumption reaction and quantified spectrophotometrically.

The reference method is manometric. A disadvantage of this method is that it uses metallic mercury in the apparatus and seals. Mercury is toxic. Using the manometric microgasometer, the result for carbon dioxide is calculated from physical properties of gases. It is a time-consuming method and is used for a reference procedure only.

Reference Values*

Sodium:

136–146 mmol/L	serum (infancy through adulthood)
40–220 mmol/24 hr	urine (varies with dietary intake)
138–150 mmol/L	CSF (for person on an average diet)
10–40 mmol/L	sweat
>70 mmol/L	sweat (suggests cystic fibrosis)

Potassium:

3.5–5.1 mmol/L	serum, adults (serum values for newborns are higher)
3.5–4.5 mmol/L	plasma, adults

Chloride:

98–106 mmol/L	serum or plasma (upper limit to 110 mmol/L for both full-term and premature neonates)
118–132 mmol/L	CSF
110–250 mmol/24 hr	urine (varies with dietary intake)
<30 mmol/L	sweat
>60 mmol/L	sweat (in 98% of persons with cystic fibrosis)

Bicarbonate:†

Children:
 18-27 mmol/L
Adults:
 21-31 mmol/L

Differences for the reference values for serum vs. plasma bicarbonate and for CO_2 concentration in arterial blood vs. venous blood have been documented in traditional clinical chemistry textbooks. Each different instrument used to perform the assay will have slightly different reference values. Manufacturer's manuals must be consulted for specific reference values for a particular instrument and specimen type. Based on the use of the manometric reference method, the reference values for total CO_2 are reported on the left.

*Tietz NW (ed): *Fundamentals of Clinical Chemistry,* ed 3. Philadelphia, WB Saunders Co, 1987, pp 948, 963–965.

†Kaplan LA, Pesce AJ: *Clinical Chemistry, Theory, Analysis and Correlation,* ed 2. St Louis, Mosby–Year Book, Inc, 1989, p 872.

NONPROTEIN NITROGEN COMPOUNDS

Nitrogen (N) exists in the body in many forms, mostly in components of complex substances. Nitrogen-containing substances are classified into two main groups: protein nitrogen (protein substances containing nitrogen) and nonprotein nitrogen (NPN). The substances are not removed by the usual protein-precipitating reagents; they remain in the filtrate or supernatant after the protein has been removed.

There are more than 15 different NPN compounds in plasma. Urea is the major NPN constituent and makes up about 45% of the total NPN. Other major compounds (known collectively as NPN) are amino acids, uric acid, creatinine, creatine, and ammonia, listed in the order of their quantitative importance. NPN is most commonly measured in serum. The value of the measurement of total NPN concentration is nonspecific and for this reason the test is not often performed. Increased concentrations of several of the major constituents of NPN are widely used as indicators of diminished renal function, however. Urea, uric acid, and creatinine occur in increased levels as a consequence of decreased renal function. Most laboratories perform serum urea nitrogen and creatinine tests when tests for renal function are needed as they are more specific indicators of renal function disorders. Tests for uric acid, creatine, and ammonia give specific indices for renal function. In a healthy person, in addition to urea of about 45%, amino acids constitute about 20%, uric acid about 20%, creatinine about 5%, and creatine about 5% of the total NPN.

Urea Nitrogen

Urea is the chief component of the NPN material in the blood, is distributed throughout the body water, and is equal in concentration in the intracellular and extracellular fluid. Plasma or serum may be used for urea nitrogen determinations. Gross alterations in NPN usually reflect a change in the concentration of urea. Urea is, in general, a waste product of protein metabolism, being removed from the blood in the kidneys. Accumulation of urea in the blood above a certain amount may indicate a flaw in the filtering system of the kidneys. The chemical formula for urea is NH_2CONH_2. It is sometimes difficult to determine urea in the laboratory, but it is relatively simple to analyze for the nitrogen in the urea. It is common practice, therefore, to determine urea nitrogen in the chemistry laboratory.

Since urea nitrogen is a measure of nitrogen and not of urea, one can convert milligrams of urea nitrogen to milligrams of urea, by multiplying the urea nitrogen value by 2.14, or 60/28. The molecular weight of urea is 60, and it contains two nitrogen atoms with a combined weight of 28.

The liver is the sole site of urea formation; it is the only organ that contains all the enzymes needed. As protein breakdown occurs (as amino acids undergo deamination, for example), ammonia is formed in increased amounts. This potentially toxic substance is removed in the liver, where the ammonia combines with other amino acids and is finally converted to urea. The amount of urea in the blood is determined by the amount of dietary protein and by the kidney's ability to excrete urea. If the kidney is impaired, the urea is not removed from the blood, and as it accumulates, the urea nitrogen level increases. Since the urea concentration is also influenced by diet, people who are undernourished or who are on low protein diets may have urea nitrogen levels that are not accurate indications of kidney function. Because of this problem, the test for creatinine is sometimes considered a better test for kidney function.

Urea nitrogen may be determined in plasma, serum, whole blood, urine, and most other biological fluids. This test is performed routinely in most laboratories.

Clinical Significance

The assay for urea nitrogen is only a rough estimate of renal function. The urea nitrogen will not show any significant level of increased concentration until the glomerular filtration is decreased by at least 50%. As mentioned, a more reliable index of renal function is the test for serum creatinine. Contrary to urea nitrogen concentration, creatinine concentration is relatively independent of protein intake (from the diet), degree of hydration, and protein metabolism.

Because the concentration of urea is directly related to protein metabolism, the protein content of the diet will affect the amount of urea in the blood. The ability of the kidneys to remove urea from the blood will also affect the urea content. However, the urea concentration is primarily influenced by the protein intake. In the normal kidney, urea is removed from the blood and excreted in the urine. If kidney function is impaired, urea will not be removed from the blood and the result will be a high urea concentration in the blood. Considerable deterioration must usually be present before the blood urea nitrogen (BUN) level rises above the reference range. The condition of abnormally high urea nitrogen is called *ure-*

mia. Decreased levels are usually not clinically significant, unless liver damage is suspected. During pregnancy, lower than normal urea nitrogen is often seen.

A significant increase in the plasma concentration of NPN, principally due to urea and creatinine in a kidney insufficiency, is known as azotemia. Azotemia can result from prerenal, renal, or postrenal causes. Prerenal azotemia is the result of poor perfusion of the kidneys and, therefore, diminished glomerular filtration. The kidneys are otherwise normal in their functioning capabilities. Poor perfusion can result from dehydration, shock, diminished blood volume, or congestive heart failure. Another cause of prerenal azotemia is increased protein breakdown, as in fever, stress, or severe burns. Renal azotemia is due primarily to diminished glomerular filtration where urea is retained as a consequence of acute or chronic renal disease. These diseases include acute glomerulonephritis, chronic glomerulonephritis, polycystic kidney, and nephrosclerosis. Postrenal azotemia is usually the result of all types of obstruction where the urea is reabsorbed into the circulation. Obstruction can be caused by stones, an enlarged prostate gland, or tumors.

Specimens

Urea nitrogen may be determined directly in serum, plasma, urine, or other biological specimens. If plasma is used, the sample of blood must be properly anticoagulated. The choice of anticoagulant is very important. An anticoagulant containing nitrogen (such as ammonium salts of heparin) must not be used for a urea nitrogen assay as it would give falsely high results (the nitrogen in the ammonium salt would be measured along with the urea nitrogen). Direct measurement of ammonia is involved in some methods for urea nitrogen measurement. If the method involves an enzymatic reaction—for example, using the enzyme urease to convert urea to ammonium carbonate—sodium fluoride cannot be used as the anticoagulant. Fluoride is an enzyme inhibitor and actually destroys some enzymes.

Since urea can be lost through bacterial action, the specimen should be analyzed within a few hours after collection or should be preserved by refrigeration. Refrigeration preserves the urea nitrogen without measurable change for up to 72 hours.

Urine urea is particularly susceptible to bacterial action, so in addition to refrigeration of the urine specimen at 4 to 8° C, the pH can be maintained at less than 4 to help reduce the loss of urea. Protein-free filtrates are stable for long periods of time, so if a manual test is to be done, the protein-free filtrate can be prepared and stored indefinitely until the analysis is done.

Methods for Quantitative Determination

A wide variety of methods have been devised for the determination of urea nitrogen. Some of them may be performed directly on whole blood, serum, or plasma, while others require a protein-free filtrate.

A group of manual methods used to determine the urea nitrogen concentration, which are very reliable, require the addition of the enzyme urease to whole blood, serum, or plasma. During incubation, urea is converted to ammonium carbonate [$(NH_4)_2CO_3$] by urease. The ammonia in the ammonium carbonate is analyzed in one of several ways.

The enzyme urease is obtained from jack beans, sword beans, or soybeans. It can be purchased in tablet or powder form. At a certain pH and temperature, urease hydrolyzes urea to ammonium carbonate according to the reaction:

$$CO(NH_2)_2 + 2H_2O \xrightarrow{\text{urease}} (NH_4)_2CO_3$$
$$\text{Urea} \qquad\qquad\qquad\qquad \text{Ammonium carbonate}$$

This reaction is complete and highly specific. The amount of urease recommended in the procedure used, along with the incubation times and temperature, is adequate to deal with any concentration of urea that may occur in human blood. Urease obeys the general laws of most enzymes (see under Clinical Enzymology). Enzymes are proteins; therefore, urease is a protein. Any of the urease that is not used in the hydrolysis is removed in the protein-precipitation step. In the urea nitrogen procedure that utilizes an enzyme reaction, the substrate is urea, and the end product is ammonium carbonate.

Use of Recovery for Enzyme Methods.—Since there are many variables in methods utilizing enzymes as reagents, it is advisable to periodically check the accuracy of the method through the use of a recovery solution. An accurately measured amount of recovery solution is added to one of the samples in a batch. It is best to choose a sample that is known to be in the normal range for the substance being assayed. The recovery solution is a quantitatively prepared solution of the substance that is being measured in the unknown patient samples. For example, the recovery solution for a urea nitrogen determination is a solution of urea. Theoretically, the amount of nitrogen in the recovery solution added to the sample should be recovered at the end of the procedure. That is, none should be lost or gained along the way. The use of a recovery solution checks the accuracy of the method. The acceptable recovery range is 90% to 110%. If the recovery is outside these limits, the procedure must be repeated and the results must not be given out until the recovery is within the limits established. The use of a recovery solution tells just how good the method really is.

Bertholet Enzyme Method.—The method of Bertholet, modified by Chaney and Marbach,* measures the amount of ammonium carbonate formed by reacting it with a phenol-hypochlorite solution to yield a deep blue color which can be measured colorimetrically. The intensity of the blue color is proportional to the quantity of urea in the specimen. Sodium nitroprusside acts as a catalyst in the reaction. The urease solution used is buffered with EDTA, which complexes any metal ions that might interfere with the enzymatic reaction. In this method, because a high dilution of sample is used, it is not necessary to precipitate and remove the proteins before measurement. Protein-free filtrates may be used, however.

Gentzkow Enzyme Method.—Another method, devised by Gentzkow,† measures the amount of ammonium carbonate formed by reacting it with Nessler's solution. Before nesslerization, a protein-free filtrate is prepared by the modified Folin-Wu method. Nessler's reagent converts the ammonium carbonate to ammonia and carbon dioxide. The reagent then reacts with the ammonia to produce a yellow color, which can be measured colorimetrically. The intensity of the yellow color is di-rectly proportional to the amount of urea present in the specimen.

Diacetylmonoxime Nonenzyme Method.—One commonly used method for urea nitrogen involves a nonenzymatic reaction. Urea will react directly with diacetylmonoxime to produce a yellow compound that can be measured colorimetrically. This method has been adapted for both manual and automated continuous-flow analyzers; both yield comparable results and use essentially the same reagents.

The diacetylmonoxime method is a direct assay and does not require the removal of protein from the sample before testing because of the specificity of the reagents.‡ Serum is the specimen of choice for this method, but plasma may be used if properly anticoagulated. Cells or clot must be removed from the serum or plasma within 1 hour after collection. The method is based on the direct reaction of urea (not ammonia) with diacetyl to form a yellow compound (a diazine derivative). Because diacetyl is unstable, it is replaced by the reagent diacetyl-monoxime, which is more stable. The color is intensified by the presence of thiosemicarbazide, which is added to the diacetylmonoxime reagent when it is prepared. Ferric ions increase the rate of the reaction. Since diacetyl reacts directly with urea and not with ammonia, the ammonia does not have to be removed from urine specimens for this method to be used with urine. The same reagents and reactions are used in automatic analyzer methods; hence this manual method is used as a back-up procedure in many laboratories. The intensity of the yellow color in the unknowns is compared colorimetrically to that in the standards. The reactions that take place in this method are outlined below:

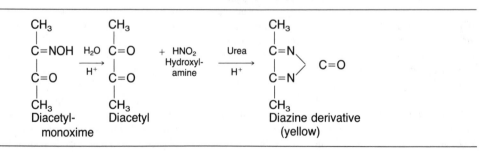

Diacetyl-monoxime · Diacetyl · Diazine derivative (yellow)

*Chaney AL, Marbach EP: Modified reagents for determination of urea and ammonia. *Clin Chem* 1962; 8:131.

†Gentzkow CJ: Accurate Method for Determination of blood urea nitrogen by direct nesslerization. *J Biol Chem* 1942; 143:531.

‡Evans RT: Manual and automated methods for measuring urea based on a modification of its reaction with diacetyl monoxime and thiosemicarbazide. *J Clin Pathol* 1968; 21:527.

Reference Values*

Urea nitrogen, serum:

Adult	7–18 mg/dL (1.2–3.0 mmol urea/L)
>60 yr	8–21 mg/dL (1.3–3.5 mmol urea/L)
Infant/child	5–18 mg/dL (0.8–3.0 mmol urea/L)

Urea nitrogen, urine: 12–20 g/24 hr (200–333 mmol urea/24 hr)

Creatinine

Creatinine in the blood is a product of creatine metabolism in the muscles. Its formation is constant and has a direct relationship to muscle mass. Its concentration varies, therefore, with age and sex.

Serum or plasma specimens are preferred over whole blood as there are considerable noncreatinine chromogens present in red cells which can cause falsely elevated creatinine assay results.

Most methods for creatinine employ the Jaffé reaction (first described in 1886). Creatinine in this reaction reacts with alkaline picrate to form an orange-red–colored solution that is measured in the spectrophotometer. To improve the specificity of the reaction and to eliminate interference from the many pseudocreatinine substances in blood that can also react with the alkaline picrate solution, an acidification step is added. The color from true creatinine is less resistant to acidification than the color from the pseudocreatinine substances. The difference in the two colors is measured.

Clinical Significance

Creatinine in the blood results from the metabolism of creatine in the muscles of the body. Creatinine is freely filtered by the glomeruli of the kidney and is not reabsorbed under normal circumstances. There is a relatively constant excretion of creatinine in the urine which parallels creatinine production. In renal disease, the creatinine excretion is altered and this is reflected in an increase in creatinine in the blood.

The serum creatinine concentration is relatively constant and is somewhat higher in males than in females. The constancy of concentration and excretion makes creatinine a good measure of renal function, especially of glomerular filtration. The concentration of creatinine is not affected by dietary intake, amount of dehydration in

Tietz NW (ed): Fundamentals of Clinical Chemistry, ed 3. Philadelphia, WB Saunders Co, 1987, p 967.

the body, or protein metabolism, which makes the assay a more reliable screening index of renal function than the BUN assay.

A useful index relates creatinine excretion to muscle mass or lean body weight, taking into consideration variables in individual body sizes. This index is known as the **creatinine clearance.**

Creatinine Clearance.—The *creatinine clearance* is defined as the milliliters of plasma which are cleared of creatinine by the kidneys per minute. The result is normalized to a standard person's surface area by using the height and weight of the patient. The creatinine clearance is used to assess the glomerular filtration functioning capabilities of the kidneys.

To perform this test for creatinine clearance, timed specimens of both blood and urine must be collected (see Collection Procedure for Timed Urine Specimens, in Chapter 2). Urine must be carefully collected for 24 hours. The urine specimen is preserved by refrigeration between collections. Blood is collected at about 12 hours into the urine collection period. Creatinine is measured in the blood and in the timed urine specimen (24-hour). The creatinine clearance is calculated as follows:

$$U/P \times V \times 1.73/A = \text{mL plasma cleared/min}$$

where U is the urine creatinine concentration (mg/dL), P is the plasma creatinine concentration (mg/dL), V is the volume in milliliters of urine excreted per minute, A is the patient's body surface area in square meters, and 1.73 is the standard body surface area in square meters. A nomogram is used to find the patient's body surface area (see Fig 10–6). Most automated analyzers have calculating capabilities for this value if the specific patient height and weight data are entered into the system.

Reference values for creatinine clearance are:
male—97–137 mL/min/1.73 m^2
female—88–128 mL/min/1.73 m^2

Specimens

Serum, plasma, or diluted urine can be assayed for creatinine. Usually urine is diluted 1:100 or 1:200. Only thymol or toluene should be used if a preservative is needed for the urine specimen. The creatinine can be assayed on urine stored in the refrigerator for up to 5 days and still give acceptable results. Creatinine is stable in serum or plasma for up to 1 week if the specimen has

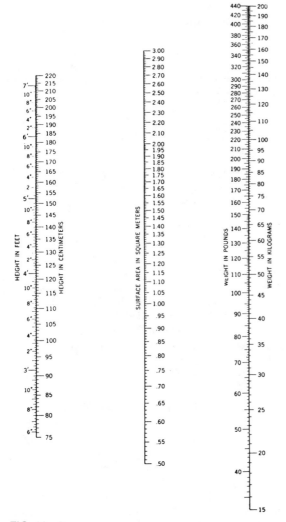

FIG 10–6.
Body surface area nomogram. (From Boothby W, Sandford RB: *N Engl J Med* 1921; 185:337. Used by permission.)

been refrigerated. It is important to separate the cells promptly to prevent hemolysis. Hemolysis causes falsely elevated creatinine values. Common fluoride and heparin anticoagulants can be used if plasma is to be tested. If enzymatic methods are used which measure ammonia production, ammonium heparin should not be used. Another consideration when performing these enzymatic determinations is that the serum should be removed from the clot and the assay done promptly to minimize ammonia production.

Methods for Quantitative Determination

Most of the commonly used methods for creatinine assay are based on the Jaffé reaction where the creatinine present in the specimen is treated with an alkaline picrate reagent to yield a bright orange-red–colored complex. Noncreatinine chromogens (nonspecific) in the specimen can also react, which results in falsely elevated values. There are various modifications which have been developed to give a more specific test for creatinine. One modification uses aluminum silicate to separate creatinine from the noncreatinine chromogens prior to using the Jaffé reaction. This modification is often used as the reference method for "true" creatinine. Another modification involves an acidification step. The color resulting from true creatinine is less resistant to acid than the color from noncreatinine chromogens. In using this modification, the impact of acidification on color development is measured and the difference noted. The Jaffé reaction has been adapted for use with the AutoAnalyzer. Enzymatic procedures for creatinine have also been developed which are more specific and sensitive than the Jaffé reaction.

The Jaffé Method (Manual)

Principle.—Creatinine reacts with picrate under alkaline conditions to give an orange-red color which is quantitated in the spectrophotometer (Procedure 10–1.)

Reagents

1. *Stock creatinine standard (20 mmol/L).* Dissolve 0.226 g creatinine, reagent grade, in 100 mL hydrochloric acid (0.1 mol/L). The hydrochloric acid may be purchased or prepared by diluting 4.15 mL of concentrated hydrochloric acid (specific gravity of 1.19, 37% by weight) to 500 mL with deionized water.

2. *Working creatinine standards.* Standards ranging from 100 μmol/L to 1,200 μmol/L are prepared by diluting volumetrically the following amounts to 50 mL with HCl (0.1 mol/L):

Stock Standard (mL)	Creatinine Concentration
0.25	1.1 mg/dL (100 μmol/L)
0.50	2.3 mg/dL (200 μmol/L)
1.00	4.5 mg/dL (400 μmol/L)
1.50	6.8 mg/dL (600 μmol/L)
2.0	9.0 mg/dL (800 μmol/L)
3.0	13.6 mg/dL (1200 μmol/L)

Procedure 10–1. Creatinine Assay—Jaffé Method

1. Prepare a protein-free solution for each serum or plasma specimen: Into 16- × 125-mm test tubes, pipette 0.5 mL of the patient's serum or plasma (or control specimen). To this add 4.5 mL of tungstic acid reagent. Mix well for 10 seconds. This step has diluted the specimen 1:10 (0.5 mL to 5.0 mL total).
2. Centrifuge at 1,500 rpm for 10 minutes. Use the supernatant solution from these tubes for the following Jaffé reaction.
3. Label photometer cuvettes for a reagent blank, standards, control, control duplicate, and unknowns.
4. Pipette 3 mL of deionized water to the blank cuvette.
5. Pipette 3 mL of prepared working creatinine standard solutions to each of the labeled standard cuvettes.
6. Pipette 3 mL of protein-free supernatant for controls and unknowns to the labeled cuvettes.
7. Add 1 mL of picric acid reagent to all cuvettes. Mix thoroughly and set a timer.
8. At 30-second intervals, add 0.5 mL of sodium hydroxide reagent to the tubes. Mix the contents of the tube after each addition of sodium hydroxide.
9. Exactly 15 seconds after sodium hydroxide has been added, read each tube in the spectropho-

tometer at 500 nm, setting the blank tube to read 0 absorbance (or 100% transmittance). Maintain 30-second intervals between reading each tube. Record all absorbance (A) readings or percent transmittance readings, if these are used.
10. Plot the absorbance (or percent transmittance) vs. the concentration of the standards and construct a standard line. Use semilogarithmic graph paper if percent transmittance readings are used.
11. Read the controls and unknowns from the standard line plotted. Record these values.

$$\frac{A_u}{A_s} \times concentration\ of\ standard$$
$$= mg/dL\ creatinine$$

A_u = absorbance of unknown
A_s = absorbance of standard

Note: If diluted urine specimens are assayed, the dilution factor must be considered in the final calculation. If a urine specimen has been diluted 1:200, the final result must be multiplied by 20 to account for the dilution (no protein removal step has been needed for the urine specimens).

---

3. *Picric acid (0.036 mol/L).* Dissolve 9.6 g reagent-grade picric acid in 500 mL of warm deionized water. Cool and dilute to 1 L with water. Protect this solution from light.

4. *Sodium hydroxide (1.4 mol/L).* Dissolve 54 g reagent sodium hydroxide pellets in 500 mL water. Cool and dilute to 1 L with water. Store in a polyethylene bottle.

5. *Tungstic acid (0.035 mol/L).* Dissolve 1 g polyvinyl alcohol in 100 mL warm water (do not boil). Cool and add to a 1-L volumetric flask containing 11.1 g reagent-grade sodium tungstate dihydrate which has been dissolved in 300 mL water. In another container, add 2.1 mL concentrated sulfuric acid slowly to 300 mL water. Add this to the 1-L volumetric flask containing the sodium tungstate. Dilute the reagent mixture to 1 L with

water. The solution is stable for about 12 months at room temperature. Do not refrigerate.

6. *Aluminum silicate (Lloyd's reagent).* For more accurate results, pretreatment of the deproteinized supernatant using an aluminum silicate clay, purified fuller's earth, is recommended. The specificity of the reaction is improved. Other products can also be used for this step.

Reference Values*
Creatinine, serum (Jaffé manual method):

Adult men	0.9–1.5 mg/dL	(88–133 μmol/L)
Adult women	0.7–1.3 mg/dL	(62–115 μmol/L)

*Tietz NW (ed): *Fundamentals of Clinical Chemistry,* ed 3. Philadelphia, 1987, WB Saunders Co, pp 683, 950.

Creatinine, urine:

Adult men   14–26 mg/kg/24 hr (124–230 μmol/kg/24 hr)

Adult women   11–20 mg/kg/24 hr (97–177 μmol/kg/24 hr)

Creatinine excretion decreases with age.

Creatinine clearance:

Men   97–137 mL/min/1.73 m^2

Women   88–128 mL/min/1.73 m^2

BILIRUBIN

Bilirubin is derived from the heme of hemoglobin, arising from the breakdown of aged red cells. It is transported to the liver complexed to albumin. This bilirubin is called **unconjugated bilirubin** and it is not water-soluble. In the liver cells, this bilirubin is conjugated with glucuronide and is made water-soluble. This bilirubin is thus called **conjugated bilirubin** and it is in this form that it enters the bile fluid for transport to the small intestine. In the small intestine, most of the conjugated bilirubin is converted to urobilinogens (see also Bilirubin in Chapter 13).

One of the most frequently used assays for assessment of the excretory function of the liver is the measurement of the serum bilirubin concentration. The classic clinical manifestation of liver disease is jaundice, the yellow discoloration of the plasma, skin, and mucous membranes, specifically the sclera of the eye. Jaundice, or icterus, is caused by the abnormal metabolism, accumulation, or retention of bilirubin. There are three types of jaundice: prehepatic, hepatic, and posthepatic. Initial evaluation of hyperbilirubinemia depends, in part, on whether there is a predominance of the unconjugated form of bilirubin or whether there is a significant increase in the conjugated form of bilirubin in the blood.

Clinical Significance of Bilirubin

The clinical finding of jaundice is not specific and can be caused by a variety of diseases. Specific diseases involving bilirubin metabolism each represent a defect in the way the liver processes the bilirubin. These can be transport defects of getting the bilirubin from the plasma albumin to the liver cell, impairment in the conjugation step in the liver itself, or a defect in the excretory function of getting the conjugated bilirubin-glucuronide from the liver cells into the canaliculi of the liver and into the bile fluid. Hepatitis and cirrhosis of the liver can result in hepatic jaundice. Obstruction in the biliary tract caused by strictures, neoplasms, or stones can result in posthepatic jaundice.

An increased serum bilirubin concentration may indicate increased destruction (hemolysis) of red blood cells, impaired excretory function of liver cells, or obstruction of the bile flow. In obstructive jaundice there is an increase in total bilirubin; however, this is primarily in the form of conjugated bilirubin—measured as "direct" billirubin—giving an increased value for direct bilirubin. In hemolytic jaundice there is an increase in total bilirubin, primarily unconjugated bilirubin;—measured as "indirect" billirubin (the indirect fraction is increased). With liver damage such as viral hepatitis, both the unconjugated and conjugated bilirubin increase, and total, direct, and indirect fractions are elevated.

Elevations in serum bilirubin occur in some infants in the first few days of life. This is especially true of premature infants. Such neonatal physiologic jaundice may involve either a deficiency of the enzyme that transfers glucuronate groups onto bilirubin, or liver immaturity. In some premature births, infants are born without the necessary enzyme activity of glucuronosyltransferase. This enzyme normally assists in the conjugation of bilirubin glucuronide and when it is not present, bilirubin will not be conjugated and there will be a rapid build-up of the unconjugated bilirubin. This can be life-threatening to the newborn. The unconjugated bilirubin readily passes into the brain and nerve cells and is deposited in the nuclei of these cells. The result is called kernicterus and can result in cell damage and death. Neonatal jaundice can persist until the enzyme glucuronosyltransferase is produced by the liver of the newborn. The blood of the newborn must be monitored frequently to detect any dangerously high levels of unconjugated bilirubin.

Neonatal jaundice is generally a temporary deficiency, which lasts only a few days, until bilirubin metabolism matures. If toxic levels do occur, exceeding 20 mg/dL, which is most likely to happen in cases of incompatibility between the blood groups of the mother and the infant and which has been largely alleviated through the use of Rh immune globulin, treatment must be initiated. Treatment of infants with enzyme deficiency involves phototherapy. Blood incompatibility or bilirubin levels approaching 20 mg/dL may require exchange transfusion.

Specimens

Determinations may be done on serum or plasma, although serum is preferred. The blood should be drawn when the patient is in a fasting state to avoid alimentary lipemia. Exposure of serum to heat and light, especially that of wavelengths at the lower end of the visible region, results in oxidation of bilirubin. For this reason, specimens for bilirubin assays must be protected from the light. The procedure should be carried out as soon as possible, at least within 2 or 3 hours after the blood has clotted. Specimens can be stored in the dark in a refrigerator for up to 1 week or in the freezer for 3 months without significant loss of bilirubin. The presence of hemoglobin results in the measurement of an erroneously low value for bilirubin by a diazo method. However, it must be kept in mind that it is difficult to see hemoglobin in the presence of increased amounts of bilirubin. Carotenemia, the presence of carotene or vitamin A in the specimen, does not interfere with the determination of bilirubin by most methods.

Methods for Quantitative Determination of Bilirubin

Tests for serum bilirubin used in the clinical laboratory are based on the reaction of bilirubin with diazotized sulfanilic acid to form azobilirubin, which has a red-purple color. This reaction was first described by Ehrlich in 1883, and the diazo reagent is also referred to as *Ehrlich's reagent*. The basic reaction has been modified by the addition of alcohol, usually methanol. Azobilirubin has indicator properties in strongly acid or strongly alkaline solutions. Thus, some modifications of the diazo reaction measure the amount of red dye in an acid medium, while others measure the blue color in a strongly alkaline medium. Many procedures involve a modification of the Malloy-Evelyn technique, carried out in an acid solution, which utilizes a diazo reaction with methanol added.* Another commonly used procedure is the Jendrassik-Grof modification.† This is car-

ried out in an alkaline solution. Both the Malloy-Evelyn and Jendrassik-Grof modifications have been automated and are currently the most frequently used bilirubin assays.

As described earlier, bilirubin is present in serum in two forms: unconjugated and conjugated to glucuronic acid. Since the glucuronide form of billirubin is freely soluble in water, it reacts rapidly with Ehrlich's reagent. A reading made at a specific time (usually 1 minute) after the addition of Ehrlich's reagent is generally taken as a measure of the bilirubin glucuronide (conjugated bilirubin or direct bilirubin) concentration. Unconjugated bilirubin is not soluble in water and reacts with Ehrlich's reagent only after the addition of methanol. A reading made after the addition of methanol and a sufficient waiting period, usually 10 or 20 minutes, is a measure of the concentration of the two forms of bilirubin combined. The concentration of unconjugated bilirubin (also referred to as *indirect* bilirubin) is the difference between the total concentration of bilirubin and the concentration of *direct* or 1-minute bilirubin.

Conjugated and unconjugated bilirubin are differentiated by the amount of time needed for the reaction and the solubility of the various fractions of bilirubin. Bilirubin that reacts quickly, in the absence of a solvent, is called direct or conjugated bilirubin. It is also known that a portion of the unconjugated bilirubin is also available to react in the absence of a solvent. The extent of this reaction is determined by the time and temperature of the reaction and the final concentration of the reagents used. The extent of the reaction of the unconjugated bilirubin, or indirect bilirubin, in the presence of a solvent is also dependent on the final concentration of the solvent used.

Chromatography, open column and high-performance liquid chromatography (HPLC), have shown that there is a third fraction of bilirubin called *delta bilirubin*.* The delta bilirubin fraction reacts like conjugated bilirubin and is normally found in very small amounts in serum. When the levels of unconjugated bilirubin are increased, the levels of delta bilirubin are also increased, resulting in an apparent increase in the conjugated bilirubin fraction when using most bilirubin assay methods.

---

*Malloy HT, Evelyn KA: The determination of bilirubin with the photoelectric colorimeter. *J Biol Chem* 1937; 119:461.
†Koch TR, Doumas DT, Elser RC, et al: Bilirubin, total and conjugated, modified Jendrassik-Grof method, in Faulkner, WR, Meites S (eds): *Selected Methods of Clinical Chemistry*, vol 9. Washington, DC, American Association for Clinical Chemistry Press, 1982, pp 113–118.

*Doumas BT, Wu TW, Jendrzejczak B: The reaction of bilirubin firmly bound to protein (δ-bilirubin) with the diazo reagent, *Clin Chem* 1984; 30:971.

Manual Method of Malloy and Evelyn (Modified)*

Principle.—Bilirubin reacts with Ehrlich's reagent (diazotized sulfanilic acid plus nitrous acid) to form the red-purple dye azobilirubin. The intensity of the purple color that is formed is proportional to the bilirubin concentration in the serum. Since bilirubin that has been conjugated with glucuronic acid is soluble in water, it reacts with the diazo reagent in aqueous solution to form a color within 1 minute. This conjugated bilirubin is thus referred to as direct bilirubin. Alcohol (methanol) is added to the test solution for the Total Bilirubin Assay. This accelerates the reaction of all forms of bilirubin in the serum—especially the unconjugated bilirubin that did not react in the aqueous solution and—is therefore referred to as indirect bilirubin. A value for total bilirubin is obtained after letting the color reaction take place for 10 minutes. The concentration of unconjugated bilirubin is the difference between the concentrations of total bilirubin and conjugated bilirubin.

Results for this bilirubin procedure are calculated from a standard graph prepared at the time of the assay. To standardize the procedure, pure bilirubin standards must be used. Commercially available bilirubin varies in purity. Pure crystalline bilirubin is available as a standard reference material from the National Bureau of Standards. Freeze-dried serum controls containing elevated bilirubin levels are also commercially available. The appropriate control specimens or reference samples must be included with each set of determinations to ensure the accuracy and reliability of the procedure. Actual procedures are described as Procedures 10–2 and 10–3.

Reagents

1. *Sulfanilic acid (26.2 mmol/L in 0.702 mol/L HCl).* Add 5.0 g of sulfanilic acid to 60 mL of concentrated hydrochloric acid (approximately 12 mol/L), mix, and dilute to 1 L with distilled water. The solution is stable for up to 6 months at ambient temperature.

2. *Sodium nitrite stock (2.9 mol/L).* Place 20 g of sodium nitrite ($NaNO_2$) in a 100 mL volumetric flask, dissolve in 80 mL of distilled water, and dilute to 100 mL. Store at 4 to 8°C in a brown glass-stoppered bottle.

*Meites S, Cheng MH, Arnold LH, et al: Bilirubin, direct reacting and total, modified Malloy-Evelyn method, in Faulkner WR, Meites S (eds): *Selected Methods of Clinical Chemistry,* vol 9. Washington, DC, American Association of Clinical Chemists Press, 1982, pp 119–125.

Discard when the reagent becomes discolored with yellow nitrate, after several weeks.

3. *Working sodium nitrite solution (290 mmol/L).* Dilute the stock sodium nitrite tenfold with distilled water to prepare a 0.29-mol/L solution. This reagent is unstable and should be prepared daily.

4. *Diazo blank.* Dilute 60 mL of concentrated HCl to 1 L with distilled water. This reagent can be kept at room temperature for at least 1 year.

5. *Diazo reagent.* Add 0.3 mL of working sodium nitrite solution to 10 mL of sulfanilic acid reagent, and mix. This reagent is unstable and should be used within a few hours of preparation.

Procedure 10–2. Conjugated Bilirubin Assay (Direct Test)

Diazotized sulfanilic acid and bilirubin glucoronide couple to form an azobilirubin pigment. This is a 1-minute test, giving the concentration of conjugated bilirubin. No methanol is added and the time shortened to minimize the reaction of unconjugated bilirubin. See Procedure 10–3. For accurate results, the analysis should be performed in subdued light.

1. Dilute serum samples, standards, and control specimens 1:20 by pipetting 1.9 mL of distilled water into a 12- × 75-mm test tube and adding 100 μL of sample. Mix. This can be done accurately with an automatic pipettor.

2. Add 0.5 mL of distilled water to a cuvette labeled *B* (for blank) and 0.5 mL of water to a cuvette labeled *C* (for conjugated).

3. Add 100 μL of diazo reagent to each *C* cuvette and 100 μL of diazo blank reagent to each *B* cuvette.

4. Add 400 μL of diluted serum, standard, or control specimen (see total bilirubin procedure) to the respective *B* and *C* cuvettes. Mix.

5. Exactly 1 minute after the addition of diazo reagent in step 3, read the absorbance of cuvettes *B* and *C* at 450 nm against water set at zero absorbance. Subtract the blank absorbance for each sample from the test absorbance to obtain the net reaction absorbance. Add the samples at 30-second intervals so that absorbance of each reaction tube (*B* and *C*) can be measured within 60 seconds of the sample addition.

6. Record all absorbance readings.

Procedure 10–3. Total Bilirubin Assay (Indirect Test)

This is a 10-minute test, utilizing the addition of methanol to the same reagents and specimens as used for the conjugated bilirubin assay. Methanol accelerates the coupling of the unconjugated bilirubin with diazotized sufanilic acid. See Procedure 10–2. For accurate results, the analysis should be performed in subdued light.

1. Add 0.5 mL of methanol to cuvettes labeled T (for total) and B (for blank) for each patient, standard, and control.
2. Add 100 μL of fresh diazo reagent to the cuvette labeled T, and mix.
3. Add 100 μL of diazo blank reagent to the cuvette labeled B, and mix.
4. Add 0.5 mL of diluted serum, standard, or control to cuvettes T and B. Mix thoroughly.
5. Allow reaction to proceed for 10 minutes in covered tubes at room temperature. Read the absorbance of cuvette T at 560 nm against water set at zero absorbance. Read B reaction vs. water, and subtract this reading from that of the sample to obtain corrected absorbance.
6. Record all absorbance readings.

6. *Methanol (absolute)*. Follow American Chemical Society specifications for purity, that is, at least 99.5% pure. This must be stored in a glass container.

7. *Serum-based calibrating standard*. Bilirubin concentration should be approximately 30 to 50 mg/L. Also, serum-based controls, preferably one at elevated levels, are available commercially.

Calculations.—The blank-corrected absorbance of cuvettes T and C in Procedures 10–2 and 10–3 is compared to the absorbance of the bilirubin calibrator standard to determine the concentration of total and conjugated bilirubin in the samples. The calculation is as follows:

$$\frac{A_s}{C_s} = \frac{A_u}{C_u} \quad C_u = \frac{A_u}{A_s} \times C_s$$

where A_s = absorbance of calibrator standard, A_u = absorbance of unknown, C_s = concentration of standard (mg/L), and C_u = concentration of unknown (mg/L).

If a standard graph has been prepared, unknown values may be read directly from the graph.

Values for unconjugated (indirect) bilirubin are obtained by subtracting the conjugated (direct) value from the total bilirubin value.

Technical Factors.—It is essential that all reagents be added in the specific proportion and order stated in the procedure to avoid turbidity. Any turbidity will invalidate test results. To avoid lipemic specimens, collect the blood from patients in a fasting state. Hemolysis in specimens will give decreased bilirubin values when using diazo methods.

The diazo reagent is unstable and must be used within 30 minutes after preparation. It is therefore prepared fresh with each set of determinations. The instability is caused by the formation of very unstable nitrous acid when the sulfanilic acid solution (solution A) is added to the sodium nitrite solution (solution B).

The amount of time required for full color development in the total bilirubin reaction varies. Procedures have been described with intervals ranging from 10 to 30 minutes. It is important to consistently use the time specified in a procedure; in this example, 10 minutes was chosen.

Since serum bilirubin is relatively unstable, determinations should be made as soon as possible after the specimen is collected and the serum is separated from the clot. The primary source of instability is exposure to light, so specimens should be kept out of the light until the determination is performed. In the frozen state bilirubin in *serum* is stable for several months. However, most prepared bilirubin standards do not appear to have such stability.

Biliverdin (a green-colored oxidation product of bilirubin) does not interfere with the diazo reaction for bilirubin because it does not react with the diazo reagent. However, bilirubin will convert to biliverdin on standing, giving falsely low results.

Beer's law does not apply when concentrations of over 300 mg/dL of bilirubin are present. If a specimen is more concentrated than 300 mg/dL, it must be diluted, or a smaller volume of the serum must be retested, with corresponding corrections for the volume change in the calculations.

Since bilirubin concentrations must be closely followed in infants with jaundice, many microtechniques have been described for the determination of bilirubin. Most of the micromethods proposed are modifications of the Malloy and Evelyn procedure described earlier.

Automated Bilirubin Assays

In the Ektachem analyzers, bilirubin is separated from the protein matrix using its thin-film technology.* Dry reagents are within the multilayered slides and the reaction occurs within the layers as the serum passes through. Total bilirubin is determined by diazotization after unconjugated and conjugated bilirubin have been disassociated from albumin. The bilirubin diffuses into a polymer layer that complexes with the bilirubin. The reaction that occurs is monitored with a reflectance spectrophotometer. The results are available in about 5 minutes and use 10 μL of serum for the assay.

In the Ames Seralyzer (Ames Division, Miles Laboratories, Inc., Elkhart, Ind), plastic strips with a matrix of reagents at one end are used. For the bilirubin assay, the van den Bergh diazo reaction is employed. Results are read using reflectance photometry which give a good correlation coefficient with the manual Jendrassik-Grof method. The results are available in 75 seconds.

Reference Method for Bilirubin

The method used as a reference method for total bilirubin is a modified Jendrassik-Grof procedure.[†] The American Association for Clinical Chemistry (AACC) and the National Bureau of Standards have both published this as the recommended reference method. A modified Jendrassik-Grof procedure utilizing caffeine-benzoate reagent as a solvent for the various bilirubin fractions is recommended when a reference method is needed.

---

*Wu TW, Dapper GM, Powers DM, et al: The Kodak Ektachem clinical chemistry slide for measurement of bilirubin in newborns: principles and performance. *Clin Chem* 1982; 28:2366–2372.

†Doumas BT, Kwok-Cheung PP, Perry BW, et al: Candidate reference method for determination of total bilirubin in serum: Development and validation. *Clin Chem* 1985; 31:1779–1789.

Reference Values[‡]

	Age	Premature	Full Term
Total serum bilirubin in infants:	Cord	<2.0 mg/dL	<2.0 mg/dL
	0–1 day	<8.0 mg/dL	<6.0 mg/dL
	1–2 days	<12.0 mg/dL	<8.0 mg/dL
	3–5 days	<16.0 mg/dL	<12.0 mg/dL
	>5 days	<2.0 mg/dL	0.2–1.0 mg/dL

Direct (conjugated) serum bilirubin: 0–0.2 mg/dL
Conjugated bilirubin levels up to 2 mg/dL are found in infants by 1 month of age and this level remains through adulthood.

Other Liver Function Tests

There are several serum enzymes which are used in the differential diagnosis of liver diseases. These are alkaline phosphatase, γ-glutamyltransferase, lactate dehydrogenase, aspartate aminotransferase and alanine aminotransferase, and 5'-nucleotidase (see also Clinical Enzymology below). Bile acids, triglycerides, cholesterol, serum proteins, coagulation proteins, and urea and ammonia assays are also used in the diagnosis of liver disease. Results from several laboratory procedures must be evaluated by the physician before an accurate diagnosis can be made. The physician or institution may have a preferred battery of tests to determine liver function. A brief description of some of the tests most often included in such a liver profile follows.

Aspartate Aminotransferase (AST)

Aspartate aminotransferase (AST) is found primarily in the liver, heart, kidney, and muscle tissue. Acute destruction of tissue in any of these areas results in rapid release of the enzyme into the serum. AST is therefore elevated in all forms of hepatitis.

Alkaline Phosphatase

This enzyme may be produced in many tissues. It is normally produced in the liver by the bile duct epithelium and in the bone by osteoblasts. The enzyme appears to facilitate the transfer of metabolites across cell membranes and is associated with lipid transport and with the

---

‡Tietz NW (ed): *Fundamentals of Clinical Chemistry,* ed 3. Philadelphia, WB Saunders Co, 1987. p 947.

calcification process in bone synthesis. Serum alkaline phosphatase is particularly useful in the diagnosis of hepatobiliary disease and bone disease associated with increased osteoblastic activity.

Protein Electrophoresis

In normal healthy individuals, the various plasma proteins are present in delicately balanced concentrations with a normal ratio of albumin to globulin. In liver disease this ratio may be altered. A number of tests for liver function are therefore based on the albumin-globulin ratio. Protein electrophoresis is the most effective way to demonstrate significant alterations in the protein fractions. Electrophoretic separation of serum proteins is also of value in following the course of liver disease after diagnosis.

Coagulation Proteins

Another protein formed in the liver is prothrombin. It is necessary for the normal coagulation of blood. If liver function is impaired, less than normal amounts of prothrombin are formed and blood clotting is delayed. A determination of the prothrombin time can be used to test for abnormal liver function. Other coagulation proteins are also synthesized in the liver and can be affected if the liver is diseased.

CLINICAL ENZYMOLOGY

Clinical **enzymology** is a complex and very important area in clinical chemistry. It is necessary to be introduced to the field of clinical enzymology when discussing clinical chemistry in general. Procedures involving enzyme determinations or involving the use of enzymes as reagents are performed under highly controlled conditions.

Enzymes are the catalysts that accompany all biological processes in living organisms. Organisms must carry out most of these processes at a moderate temperature and usually at a nearly neutral pH. Enzymes make this possible by modifying the speed of the reactions without being used up themselves. The organic enzyme catalysts are produced by living cells, but they act independently of the cells that produce them. There are hundreds of enzymes in the human body, and in larger hospital laboratories today enzyme assays may account for as much as 20% to 25% of the workload. As many as 15 enzymes are measured routinely in many clinical laboratories.

Enzymes increase the speed of biochemical reactions without themselves undergoing any permanent change: they are neither used up in the reaction nor do they appear as a reaction product. They greatly accelerate a chemical reaction by lowering the activation energy needed of the reaction. Enzymes are proteins and are therefore susceptible to denaturation by heat or chemical agents. Like other catalysts, enzymes are needed in very small amounts, and their activity is usually specific.

In the clinical laboratory enzymes are utilized in two different ways. They may be employed as analytic tools. That is, an enzyme may be used as a reagent to bring about some desired chemical reaction. The enzymes hexokinase and glucose oxidase are used in this way in two methods for glucose determination (see under Glucose above). Enzymes may also be analyzed for diagnostic purposes (see under Measurement of Enzyme Activity). The measurement of enzymes present in serum and body fluids is expressed in terms of *activity units*, not concentration units. The activity of an enzyme can be described as the amount of substrate it converts to reaction product per unit of time.

The particular substances on which enzymes act are called *substrates*. In the hexokinase glucose procedure utilizing hexokinase, the substrate is the glucose. The new substance formed as a result of the enzyme activity is called the *end product*. The end product formed by the action of hexokinase on glucose is glucose-6-phosphate. Each enzyme catalyzes a special reaction for only a certain type of substrate.

Nomenclature

At one time enzymes were usually named by adding the ending *-ase* to the substrate. As more enzymes became known and more information about them became available, this system became inadequate and a more detailed nomenclature was devised. Often the old names for the enzymes are still used, such as urease, amylase, and lipase. The new nomenclature system provides a practical basis for identifying all enzymes now known as well as enzymes that have yet to be discovered. The International Union of Biochemistry studied systems for identifying enzymes beginning in 1955, and the results of their studies, including a new system of nomenclature, were published in 1964 and revised in 1972.* Their proposals have been accepted by all laboratorians in the field and provide a systematic classification for all enzymes.

Two names are provided for each enzyme, a systematic name, which clearly describes the nature of the catalyzed reaction, and a working or practical name, which may be the same as the systematic name or may be a modification of that name for everyday use. Each enzyme is designated by a numerical code consisting of four numbers separated by periods, such as 1.3.2.4. The first of the four numbers defines the class to which the enzyme belongs. All enzymes belong to one of six classes, characterized by the type of reaction they catalyze:

1. *Oxidoreductases* catalyze oxidation-reduction reactions.
2. *Transferases* catalyze transfer of a group other than hydrogen.
3. *Hydrolases* catalyze the hydrolysis of esters, ethers, peptides, and so on.
4. *Lyases* catalyze removal of a group from a substrate by mechanisms other than hydrolysis, leaving double bonds.
5. *Isomerases* catalyze interconversion of optical, geometric, or positional isomers.
6. *Ligases* catalyze the linkage of two compounds while breaking a pyrophosphate bond.

These six major classes are divided into subclasses. The second and third numbers in the enzyme code indicate the subclass and sub-subclass to which the enzyme is assigned. The last number is the specific serial number given to each enzyme in its sub-subclass.

The systematic name for each enzyme consists of two parts: the first gives the name of the substrate or substrates acted on, and the second, a word ending in *-ase*, indicates the type of reaction catalyzed by all enzymes in the group. Because of the rules governing the terminology of enzymes, an enzyme can be identified by both its code number and its systematic name. This nomenclature for enzymes will appear complicated to the novice, but it becomes understandable with use. The important thing to

*Commission on Biochemical Nomenclature, International Union of Pure and Applied Chemistry and International Union of Biochemistry: *Enzyme Nomenclature (1972).* New York, American Elsevier Publishing Company, Inc, 1973.

remember about the naming of enzymes is that enzyme names end in *-ase* (except for an occasional historical name still in use), the part of the name before the *-ase* gives the type of reaction catalyzed by the enzyme, and the part before that gives the name of the substrate acted on (examples are lactate dehydrogenase and aspartate aminotransferase).

In some laboratories it has become a common and convenient practice to use capital letter abbreviations for the names of certain enzymes. This practice has not been universally standardized, however, and can be confusing when these abbreviations are not used consistently.

Factors Affecting Enzymes

Concentration of Substrate

Many chemical and physical factors affect the action of enzymes. The *concentration of the substrate* is one factor that can affect the action of the enzyme. If the concentration of the substrate is gradually increased in an enzyme reaction system, keeping all other factors constant, the rate of reaction will increase until a maximum value is reached. After this point, an increase in substrate concentration has no further effect on the reaction rate.

Concentration of Enzyme

The *concentration of the enzyme* is very important. The speed of the reaction is proportional to the concentration of the enzyme. Therefore, in a clinical laboratory procedure employing enzyme reactions, the concentration of the enzyme must be constant.

pH

The *pH* is also important. Every enzyme has an optimal pH, at which it is most efficient. Extremely high or low pH values generally result in complete loss of activity for most enzymes. For this reason, it is important to always control the pH by means of an adequate buffer solution or by use of a pH meter. The sensitivity of the enzyme measurement is maximal at the pH of optimal enzyme activity and for this reason, enzyme assays should be carried out at that optimal pH. The buffer system used must be capable of counteracting any potential effect on pH that is caused by adding the enzyme sample (in the serum to be assayed) to the assay system, as well as the effects of any other chemical reactions that occur in the process.

Temperature

The *temperature* used for the enzyme reaction is another important factor. There is a definite relation between temperature and enzyme activity—that is, the speed of enzyme reactions is increased two to three times for each 10°C rise in temperature. This rate of increase is known as the Q_{10}. Each enzyme has its own particular Q_{10}, but the value is around 2 for most enzymes. A Q_{10} of 2 means that for each 10°C rise in temperature the activity of the enzyme is doubled. A Q_{10} of 3 means that for each 10°C rise in temperature the activity of the enzyme is tripled. Each enzyme also has its optimal temperature—the temperature at which the greatest amount of substrate is changed per unit time. In other words, the highest temperature at which the enzyme will react without danger of being inactivated is its optimal temperature. Of the many factors affecting the activity of enzymes, temperature is one of the most critical. Increasing the temperature beyond the optimal temperature for a particular enzyme may result in denaturation of the enzyme. Over a period of time, enzymes will be deactivated or denatured at even moderate temperatures. Enzymes should generally be stored at or below 5°C to maintain their activity. Individual enzymes vary in their stability characteristics and consequently their individual storage requirements will also vary. A few enzymes are inactivated at refrigerator temperatures. Specimen handling requirements for each enzyme to be assayed must be considered.

The choice of temperature for the enzyme assay is of clinical importance. There remains considerable debate on this subject. Whatever temperature is selected, it must be maintained during the assay reaction for the enzyme in question. Because each laboratory has unique practical considerations, it is unlikely that a universal single enzyme temperature will be achieved.

Time

There is a definite relation between *time* and enzyme activity. A particular amount of enzyme will decompose a particular amount of substrate per minute. Therefore, the enzyme reaction must be stopped at a definite time.

Inhibitors

The presence of *enzyme poisons* or *inhibitors* must be avoided in any procedure employing enzyme reactions. If such an inhibitor is present, the reaction will not take place satisfactorily. One enzyme inhibitor already discussed is fluoride, which is present in the anticoagulant sodium fluoride used in some glucose procedures. Other enzyme inhibitors are heavy metals such as mercury, gold, and silver. Even a trace of these heavy metals will make the enzyme assay invalid, because the activity of the enzyme is inhibited. Denaturation of enzymes can also be caused by vigorous shaking or by ultraviolet radiation, as in sunlight. Any substance that precipitates protein would also stop an enzyme reaction.

Conditions for Enzyme Tests in General

All serum enzymes originate in the cells. Some enzymes are found in many tissues while others are unique to specific organs or tissues. It is these differences that enable differential testing to indicate the presence of some enzymes that are specific to certain tissues. Testing for enzymes that are present in all body tissues does not yield as much useful information. Testing for isoenzymes, enzymes with a different molecular form to be found in different tissues, utilizes the diagnostic value of clinical enzymology tests. Only certain isoenzymes have been found to be clinically useful, however. These are the isoenzymes of lactate dehydrogenase, creatine kinase, and alkaline phosphatase.

The increased enzyme value is related to an increased rate of release of the enzyme from the tissues. In diseases where there is increased necrosis of the tissues, as in liver, heart and pancreatic diseases, clinical enzyme tests are of diagnostic value. The pattern of abnormality of the enzyme values determined depends on the normal level of enzyme for the tissue in question and on the type and extent of necrosis, in addition to other less well-understood factors.

Day-to-day consistency should be checked by including a lyophilized or pooled serum control specimen in each batch of enzyme assays performed. It has been difficult to adequately standardize many enzyme tests because of the lack of primary reference standards. For spectrophotometric assays, it is important to use calibrator solutions to at least eliminate any possible error due to differences between photometric instruments. Many of the colorimetric procedures have been adapted for automated measurement of serum enzymes.

As the demand for more enzyme testing has increased, automated methods of assay have been introduced. One method used is that of continuous flow exemplified by the AutoAnalyzer. With this type of analysis, reproducibility of measurements of sample and reagent volumes has been greatly improved. These methods are valid only over a limited range of enzyme activity. In the AutoAnalyzer, enzyme reactions do not go to completion and calibrator solutions must be used. These are solutions with assigned values of enzyme activity.

Since there are so many factors which influence an enzyme assay (e.g., time, temperature, pH, concentration of enzyme activators and inhibitors), methods that control these variables will provide a better-designed enzyme assay. To be used as a valid enzyme assay, the concentration of the enzyme in the specimen must be the only limiting factor. The result should reflect the amount of the enzyme present and should not be influenced by the presence of any other substances. Enzymes are proteins and exist in very small volumes in biological fluids. They are also very similar chemically. For these reasons, many of the enzyme assays measure the activity of the enzyme rather than its concentration. This is not always the best indicator of the enzyme's concentration. This approach to assays for enzymes is called the *kinetic* or *rate method* and it is utilized in many clinical laboratory enzyme tests. Enzymes show specificity with regard to substrate (the substance that is acted upon) and effect (the chemical reaction that occurs). The enzyme-substrate complex forms enzyme and end product, the enzyme not being altered in the reaction. Often the end product or substrate may be colored and if this is the case, it can be quantitated by use of spectrophotometry or colorimetry. Most of the usual enzymes that are determined are measured by using the rate method and most of these procedures employ the NAD, NADH coenzyme system.

NAD, NADH Coenzyme System

Many of the tests for serum enzymes use nicotine adenine dinucleotide (NAD) as a coenzyme in the reaction. NAD has virtually zero absorbance at 340 nm (ultraviolet range) and NADH (the reduced form of NAD) has maximal absorbance at 340 nm and can be used as a coenzyme participant so the reaction can be measured with spectrophotometry. Because NAD can be reduced to NADH and because this change increases absorbance at 340 nm, the reaction can easily be read in the spectrophotometer. The use of a spectrophotometer which measures accurately in the ultraviolet range is essential for clinical enzymology tests. Since in this reaction the absorbance of 1 mol of NADH is known, the amount of NADH can be calculated and related to the number of

moles of substrate altered. Frequently, NAD or NADH is not required for the specific reaction being performed, but the reaction is coupled to one which does require NAD or NADH so the reaction can be more easily followed. These methods all measure the NADH at 340 nm.

Measurement of Enzyme Activity

Enzymes are essential to life and health, and abnormal enzyme activity may be a sign of disease. Measurements of the activity of digestive enzymes in body fluids as an aid to diagnosis date back to the early 1900s, and some of the earliest observations are still useful. One of these early observations was made on amylase in urine, first studied by Wohlgemuth in 1908. Measurements of enzyme activity in serum began in the 1920s and 1930s with studies on alkaline phosphatase in bone and liver disease.

All the factors that influence enzymes in vivo—the concentrations of the substrate and the enzyme, pH, temperature, and the presence of inhibitors—must be considered when enzyme determinations are performed in vitro. Since enzyme activity is easily influenced by changes in the environment, laboratory determinations must be carried out under carefully controlled conditions.

Concentrations of enzymes are measured in the laboratory in terms of activity units in a convenient volume or mass of the specimen analyzed. Since enzymes are active in all parts of the body, determination of enzyme activity is important in the diagnosis and treatment of certain diseases. Some of the more common enzyme determinations that are valuable diagnostic tools are described below.

Choice of Enzymes to Assay

Not all intracellular enzymes are equally valuable as indicators of cellular damage or disease. Another consideration in the selection process for enzymes to assay is the rate at which a particular enzyme will disappear from the blood. An enzyme with a very short half-life in blood has little or no diagnostic value. The most commonly assayed enzymes have a half-life of 6 hours or greater. It is important to use the laboratory findings for enzymes along with the patient's history, the results of the physical examination of the patient, and the other laboratory findings. Some enzymes are used to diagnose diseases of several different organs. There is considerable overlap.

Serum enzymes are reported in international units (IU). This unit is the amount of the enzyme that will catalyze the reaction of 1 mmol of substrate per minute. The SI unit for enzyme activity is the katal (kat) which is the amount of enzyme that will catalyze the reaction of 1 mol of substrate per second.

Methods for enzyme assay commonly measure the end product or substrate concentration by colorimetry or spectrophotometry. Some enzyme assays use ultraviolet wavelengths and require spectrophotometers capable of readings in that range of the spectrum. Other methods for enzyme assay include radioimmunoassay and other immunoassays. Specific methods can be found in clinical chemistry textbooks. Any method selected must include the use of a quality control program.

Lactate Dehydrogenase (LDH)

Lactate dehydrogenase is present in all cells of the body. The most accurate levels are obtained from serum rather than plasma. The assay should be performed on fresh serum, as storage in the refrigerator will result in loss of some of the enzyme activity. Frozen specimens are totally unacceptable. Serum must be removed from the clot as soon as possible. Hemolyzed specimens should not be used, for hemolysis results in the release of LDH from red cells into the body fluid, giving falsely high results.

Lactate dehydrogenase catalyzes the reversible reaction of pyruvate to lactate. Pyruvate is then reduced to form lactate and NADH is oxidized to NAD.

Serum LDH is increased in liver, heart, skeletal, and kidney disease and in some hematopoietic and neoplastic diseases. The total LDH activity is actually the result of the activity of several enzymes. These enzymes have similar structures and work on the same substrates. These are called isoenzymes. A better evaluation of the cause of an elevated LDH can be ascertained by evaluating the isoenzymes separately. There are five well-defined LDH isoenzymes.

LDH Isoenzymes.—The five LDH fractions are labeled LDH_1, LDH_2, LDH_3, LDH_4, and LDH_5. The means of identification of these isoenzymes is usually by serum electrophoresis.

Aspartate Aminotransferase (AST)

Aspartate aminotransferase catalyzes the transfer of an amino group from a specific amino acid to a specific keto acid. Serum or plasma may be used in the determi-

nation. Hemolyzed samples are not acceptable, as there is a high level of AST in red cells.

In viral hepatitis and other forms of liver disease associated with necrosis of the liver tissue, serum AST and alanine aminotransferase (ALT) levels are elevated even before clinical symptoms and signs of the disease appear. Levels for both enzymes may reach 100 times the upper reference limit although 20- to 50-fold elevations are more usual. Alcoholic hepatitis has elevations which are more moderate. Other disorders which give high AST levels are other inflammatory conditions of the liver, infectious mononucleosis with liver involvement, and metastatic carcinoma of the liver. Elevations probably indicate a cellular necrosis process that is continuing.

AST levels rise after a myocardial infarction. There is a relatively high concentration of AST in heart muscle. These AST levels do not usually rise until 6 to 8 hours after the onset of chest pain. For this reason, the collection of timed blood specimens is important for evaluation of the AST concentration results. The peak values are reached after 18 to 24 hours and the activity is roughly proportional to the extent of the cardiac damage.

Alanine Aminotransferase (ALT)

Alanine aminotransferase catalyzes the transfer of an amino group between L-alanine and L-glutamate; the corresponding keto acids in the process are α-ketoglutarate and pyruvate. High levels are seen in the disorders described under AST, although ALT is a more liver-specific enzyme. ALT increases are rarely seen unless the liver parenchyma is diseased.

Creatine Kinase (CK)

Creatine kinase has a wide distribution in many tissues. It is a cytoplasmic mitochondrial enzyme. CK catalyzes the formation of ATP, a nucleotide that is necessary for contractile or transport systems. It is found in very high concentrations in skeletal and heart muscle and appreciable amounts are found in the brain. Very small amounts are found in other organs. CK assays are most useful in the diagnosis of myocardial infarction and muscle disease. Serum, amniotic fluid, and cerebrospinal fluid can be assayed for CK. Serum is the blood specimen of choice; the clot should be removed as soon as possible after processing of the specimen. Heparin can be used if plasma is needed. Anticoagulants other than heparin should not be used, as they can inhibit the CK enzyme activity. The timing of the collection is important because the total CK concentration can be significantly elevated after increased exercise, surgery, intramuscular injection, or acute psychotic reactions. The CK in the serum is light-sensitive so the specimen should be stored in the dark. Specificity of the CK assay is improved by measuring the CK isoenzymes. CK isoenzymes are also assayed using serum. These specimens must be handled carefully and all specimens separated from the cells as quickly as possible.

In diseases affecting skeletal muscle, serum CK is greatly increased. In muscular dystrophy, especially in the Duchenne type, levels of up to 50 times the upper reference value can be seen. In viral myositis and polymyositis the CK values are elevated. Following a myocardial infarction, total CK begins to rise within 4 to 6 hours and peaks within 18 to 30 hours. It rapidly returns to normal by the third day.

CK Isoenzymes.—The CK enzymes found in heart, brain, and skeletal muscle differ in their physicochemical properties. The presence of CK_2 (MB) indicates damage to the heart muscle. It is found in all patients during the 48-hour period following an acute myocardial infarction. It appears within 4 to 8 hours and peaks at 12 to 24 hours after the infarct. CK_3 (MM) is found in patients with muscle trauma, after major surgery, intramuscular injection, or shock. The brain fraction is CK_1 (BB). It is usually not measured in serum even after cerebrovascular accidents because the enzyme does not cross the blood-brain barrier. The various CK isoenzymes are separated and identified by serum electrophoresis.

Alkaline Phosphatase

Alkaline phosphatase hydrolyzes phosphate esters into inorganic phosphorus. Alkaline phosphatase is present in high concentration in the bone and in somewhat lower concentration in the liver, but is found in all body fluids and tissues. Serum or heparinized plasma can be tested; gross hemolysis should be avoided. Serum alkaline phosphatase activity is increased in bone and liver disease.

Acid Phosphatase

Acid phosphatase also hydrolyzes phosphate esters, but is active at a pH of about 5. The largest source of acid phosphatase is the prostatic tissue of the male. Metastatic carcinoma of the prostate gland produces very high serum acid phosphatase levels.

Amylase

Amylase is formed in the pancreas and is found in increased amounts in the serum and urine in varying degrees of pancreatic disturbance. Normally only small amounts of amylase are found in the blood. Increased amounts of pancreatic amylase are found in the blood during the early stage of acute pancreatitis. Amylase catalyzes the hydrolysis of starch into simpler molecules, with maltose as the end product. The measurement of serum amylase is a common laboratory test for enzyme activity and is sometimes done on an emergency basis to detect pancreatitis.

In the body, amylase is present in a number of organs and tissues. The greatest concentration of amylase is in the pancreas, where the enzyme is synthesized and secreted into the intestinal tract for digestion of starches. Amylase is also secreted by the salivary glands and is present in saliva, where it initiates hydrolysis of starches while the food is still in the mouth and esophagus. The enzyme found in normal serum is predominantly of pancreatic and salivary origin. To eliminate the possibility of confusing salivary amylase with that from the pancreas, a test for lipase is often done instead. (See Lipase.)

Amylase is quite stable. The loss of activity is negligible at room temperature for 1 week and at refrigerator temperatures for 2 months. All the common anticoagulants, except heparin, inhibit the activity of this enzyme. The test for amylase activity should therefore be performed only on serum or on heparinized plasma.

Lipase

Lipase, which is found in the pancreas, hydrolyzes fats into fatty acids and glycerol. Increased amounts of this enzyme indicate disease and inflammation of the pancreas (pancreatitis). Lipase is not present in salivary glands so this test is more specific for pancreatic involvement than the amylase test described above. The development of rate reflectance spectrophotometry makes measurement of serum lipsase practical.

Specimens for Enzyme Tests

Serum rather than plasma is the specimen used for most enzyme testing owing to the adverse effects of many anticoagulants on the activity of enzymes in general. Hemolysis is to be avoided because hemolysis may be associated with the release of enzymes from the red blood cells into the serum causing falsely high serum enzyme values. Most enzymes are stable in serum that has been refrigerated for at least 24 hours and are stable at room temperature for less hours. Temperature requirements for specimens must be a consideration for each specific assay, however.

Reference Values*

Lactate dehydrogenase, total, serum,
  Adult 45–90 U/L
  Infant 100–250 U/L
Aspartate aminotransferase, serum,
  Adult 8–20 U/L
  Newborn, infant 25–75 U/L
Alanine aminotransferase:
  Adult 8–20 U/L
  Newborn, infant 5–28 U/L
Creatine kinase, total, serum:
  Adult, male 25–130 U/L
  Adult, female 10–115 U/L
Amylase, serum:
  Adult 25–125 U/L
Lipase, serum:
  Adult 20–208 U/L

DRUG TESTING

In the clinical laboratory, drug testing falls into two major categories: (1) **therapeutic drug monitoring**—the testing of drugs to monitor their medical effectiveness in the treatment of the patient, and (2) the testing of drugs in regard to their possible toxicity, overdose, or abuse. A single drug may fall into both categories. The field of **toxicology** involves the study of poisons or toxicants, especially their chemical and physical properties and their subsequent physiologic or behavioral effects on living organisms. A *poison* is a substance which, when taken in sufficient quantities, will cause an adverse effect, as sickness or death. There is often no difference between

*Tietz NW (ed): *Fundamentals of Clinical Chemistry,* ed 3. Philadelphia, WB Saunders Co, 1987, pp 945, 946, 949, 958–959.

the mechanism of a substance called a drug as compared with one that is considered a poison. A *drug* is defined as a substance that is administered in doses that alter physiologic function to produce a desired therapeutic effect. If a drug is given in doses greater than in the therapeutic range, it may produce toxic effects instead of the beneficial effects desired. The toxicology laboratory serves to identify the amount of substance which, in particular exposure situations, will have an adverse effect on the patient. As stated previously, toxicology or drug testing functions in the clinical laboratory have been subdivided into two major categories: clinical toxicology, or therapeutic drug monitoring, and testing for drugs of abuse (sometimes called *forensic toxicology*). A third category is also included in the discipline of toxicology and that is the specialized branch of environmental toxicology.

Therapeutic Drug Monitoring

When a drug is used for therapeutic purposes, a designated drug effect is desired. The therapeutic range for a drug usually describes the range of doses in which the desired effect occurs. Not all patients will react in the same way to the same dose of the drug. For a single dosage, one person may not receive any benefit while another will have a toxic reaction. Individual variability accounts for the wide response to a particular drug—variations in age, sex, race, health status, and genetic factors.

Many drugs have narrow ranges in which they exert their therapeutic effect. When this therapeutic range is narrow, close therapeutic drug monitoring is required. Since normal liver function is required for the metabolism of many drugs, patients with liver disease require close monitoring. The serum creatinine level or clearance is an important laboratory finding when determining drug dosages, and dysfunctional kidney disease can be a cause of increased drug toxicity effects. It is important that the drug be administered in the correct dose to promote the desired effect—not below the range of medical effectiveness or above the range where toxicity can occur. Toxic effects can include loss of hearing, damage to the liver, or death. Several categories of drugs are monitored in the clinical laboratory. These drugs include cardiac medications, antibiotics, anticonvulsants, antidepressants, analgesics, antineoplastic drugs, immunosuppressant drugs, and antiasthmatic drugs.

Samples

Blood is usually the specimen of choice for therapeutic drug monitoring tests. It is important to note the time as well as the date of the collection. The time of the last drug dose administered is also required. Blood is drawn into tubes that contain no interfering substances. The specific procedure being employed must be reviewed carefully prior to collecting the sample to ascertain any unique collection requirements. Some drug assays require blood that is collected in EDTA or sodium fluoride and potassium oxalate anticoagulants. Some drug assays will give erroneously low results when collected in tubes with serum separator gels in them. Blood for drug testing should be processed immediately—centrifuged as quickly as possible with the removal of serum or plasma from the cells. If testing cannot be done immediately, the specimen of serum or plasma must be refrigerated or frozen until the assay can be done.

Methods of Assay

Many assays done for therapeutic drug monitoring are performed by the use of gas-liquid or high-pressure chromatography. When using chromatographic methods, several families of drugs can be separated, identified, and quantified at once. For small laboratories, the availability of immunoassays has made the testing rapid and accurate. When immunoassays are used, only one specific drug can be quantified. Some immunoassays have been devised for screening purposes and contain antibodies that cross-react with several drugs. Other procedures utilize enzyme immunoassays, fluorescent and fluorescent polarization immunoassays, light-scattering immunoassays, and dry chemistry systems for therapeutic drug monitoring.

Forensic Toxicology and Drugs of Abuse

Whenever drug testing is done, the results must be considered in conjunction with the clinical assessment of the patient being tested. The test must not be an end in itself but used along with other available medical information. There are a large number of potentially toxic substances which can cause acute and chronic illness and it is important that only experienced and well-qualified laboratorians do the testing procedures. Laboratories performing reliable drug testing procedures must employ thorough quality control measures, must participate in a proficiency testing program, and generally must be en-

gaged in an ongoing program of quality assurance at all times. Screening tests are used to detect a toxic substance, and to confirm the clinical assessment. The screening test selected must have a low incidence of false-negatives and false-positives. A positive result is usually confirmed by another assay.

If the physician suspects the presence of one or more drugs of potential abuse, laboratory tests may be done to confirm the drug's presence and to determine the amount present. The data produced by the laboratory can assist the physician in choices for therapy. If the identity of the drug or drugs is completely unknown, the laboratory can perform general drug screening tests. The drug screen can rapidly test for the presence of the major drug groups. A positive result is confirmed by an alternative procedure, along with other general chemistry procedures such as electrolyte, urea nitrogen, and glucose determinations to rule out renal or diabetic conditions.

Samples

Urine is the specimen usually employed for drug screening assays because of the ease of obtaining it and because of the concentration of the drug in the urine. It is important to keep good records of sample collection, noting the time and date of collection, along with making certain that the sample is obtained from the correct person. This chain-of-custody documentation is important, especially if there is a potential for legal action. In some instances it is recommended that the urine collection be witnessed to ascertain its proper collection from the person to be tested. Urine that is not assayed immediately should be refrigerated or frozen. Any positive specimens are stored in the freezer indefinitely.

Methods of Assay

Methods used for this type of drug testing vary with the substance being assayed. Thin-layer chromatography is useful in screening for drugs of abuse. Gas-liquid chromatography and immunoassays are also frequently employed.

Usually at least two types of methods must be available—one for the screening process and another for the definitive or quantitative assay. Thin-layer chromatography is a common screening method. Other screening methods utilize enzyme immunoassay and radioimmunoassay. Thin-layer chromatography methods are useful because they can detect one or more drugs from a large number of possible drugs. It is not as sensitive a method as some other assays, however. One commercial assay employing thin-layer chromatography is the Toxi-Lab (Analytical Systems Division of Marion Laboratories, Kansas City, MO).

Enzyme immunoassay tests are known to be sensitive screening tests for drugs. There are commercial kits that will detect specific drugs or drugs in a family of drugs. The EMIT (enzyme-mediated immunologic technique) kit (Syva Corp., Palo Alto, CA) is an example of a sensitive enzyme immunoassay.

Tests used for confirmatory drug testing are gas chromatography, high-pressure liquid chromatography, or gas chromatography in combination with mass spectrophotometry.

BIBLIOGRAPHY

Becan-McBride K, Ross D: *Essentials for the Small Laboratory and Physician's Office*. St Louis, Mosby– Year Book, Inc, 1988.

Henry JB (ed): *Clinical Diagnosis and Management by Laboratory Methods,* ed 18. Philadelphia, WB Saunders Co, 1991.

Kaplan LA, Pesce AJ: *Clinical Chemistry, Theory, Analysis, and Correlation,* ed 2. St Louis, Mosby– Year Book, Inc, 1989.

Physician's Office Laboratory Procedure Manual, Tentative Guidelines. Villanova, Pa, National Committee for Clinical Laboratory Standards, 1989; 9 POL1-T.

Tietz, NW (ed): *Fundamentals of Clinical Chemistry,* ed 3. Philadelphia, WB Saunders Co, 1987.

Tietz NW (ed): *Textbook of Clinical Chemistry*. Philadelphia, WB Saunders Co, 1986.

11 Hematology

Key Terms

Absolute cell count	Hemoglobin
Anemia	Leukemia
B lymphocytes	Leukocytes
Cell differential	Leukocyte differential
Complete blood count (CBC)	Microsampling
Coulter principle	Osmotic fragility
Erythrocyte sedimentation rate (ESR)	Peripheral blood film
Erythrocytes	Plasma cells
Electronic cell counting device	Pluripotential stem cell (PSC)
Flow cytometer	Red blood cell indices
Enumeration of formed elements	Reticulocyte
Granulocytes	T lymphocytes
Hematocrit	Thrombocytes
Hematopoiesis	Unopette
Hemocytometer	Wright-Glemsa stain

The word *hematology* comes from the Greek *haima,* blood, and *logos,* discourse; hence, study of. Hematology is therefore the science, or study, of blood. In a hematology course, one is concerned with the main constituents of the blood. Blood is composed of plasma and cells; the plasma is the fluid portion of the blood.

The total volume of blood in an average adult is about 6 L, or 7% to 8% of the body weight. About 45% of this amount is composed of the formed elements of the blood and the remaining 55% is the plasma. Approximately 90% of the plasma is water; the remaining 10% are proteins (albumin, globulin, fibrinogen), carbohydrates, vitamins, hormones, enzymes, lipids, and salts.

Blood is part of the circulatory system of the body and has several functions. It carries nutrients to the tissues, the most important nutrient being oxygen, which is carried by the red cells. Waste products (end products of metabolism) are carried by the blood to the organs of excretion. Many natural defense agents circulate continuously with the blood supply. Much valuable information can be readily obtained from hematologic tests, and certain routine measurements and examinations are now a part of virtually every hospital admission.

The blood cells, or formed elements, to be discussed in this chapter are the red blood cells (**erythrocytes**), the white blood cells (**leukocytes**), and the platelets (**thrombocytes**). The laboratory tests performed in the area of hematology center around the cells and some of their constituents: their number or concentration, the relative distribution of various types of cells, and their structural or biochemical abnormalities that contribute to disease. The entire range of types of disease is seen: hereditary, immunologic, nutritional, metabolic, traumatic, and inflammatory (including infectious, hormonal, and neoplastic). In many instances the hematologic examination is virtually diagnostic, and in many instances it is a major contribution to the eventual solution of a diagnostic problem.

Diseases with a primary hematologic cause are not common, but hematologic manifestations secondary to other diseases are quite common. A wide variety of diseases may show signs or symptoms of a hematologic nature. Many diseases produce anemia, and others produce enlarged lymph nodes. Additional examination will usually indicate the primary involvement of some system besides the blood and lymph nodes.

The major source of the blood cells is the bone marrow, although the lymph nodes and spleen contribute some of the white blood cells. Many other sources make contributions to the blood.

Several hematologic tests are required as part of every patient's initial hospital admission report and are also a part of the physical examination in a physician's office. Many of these tests are considered routine and can be done by a laboratorian with limited training. The routine admission and office examination tests include **hemoglobin, hematocrit, white blood cell count,** and **cell differential.** The differential is a classification of the white blood cells (WBCs) and usually includes an examination of the red blood cells (RBCs) and platelets. These tests are referred to as the **complete blood count (CBC).** With the prevalence of electronic cell counters, other values or tests are also considered routine. The meaning of CBC will vary depending on the institution. It may refer to the complete hematology profile generated by the instrument. The RBC count and calculated RBC indices are a part of the routine CBC in many laboratories. In addition to their use for screening, the CBC results are helpful in the diagnosis of many diseases. They can reflect the body's ability to fight disease and may be used to determine how the patient is progressing in certain disease states such as infection or **anemia.** That these tests are done frequently does not mean that they are unimportant. The physician can obtain valuable information about a patient's physical condition from accurately performed routine hematologic determinations.

In this chapter, the student should gain enough basic knowledge about the formed elements of the blood, their enumeration, and their characteristics to perform routine tests accurately and conscientiously in the clinical laboratory. This knowledge should include the basic theory of the determinations, use and care of the equipment used to perform the tests, proper preparation of the reagents, ability to recognize problems when encountered, proper handling of the specimens, calculation of the results, and an appreciation of the need for accuracy and care in performing hematologic determinations. (See Chapter 2 for a detailed account of the collection of blood for hematologic studies.)

Performing accurate hematologic determinations requires repeated practice. Many of the techniques call for manual dexterity and experience in the manipulation of equipment and instruments. Because the techniques in hematology have greatly expanded in recent years, there has been increased use of automated equipment, which can accurately handle large volumes of work. Some of the automated devices and methods are discussed in this chapter.

Clinical applications of the hematologic tests are also discussed. Again, it is important that anyone performing the tests remember the reason why the laboratory determination was ordered in the first place. The patient's welfare is the ultimate concern of the laboratory and of the physician who uses the information provided by the laboratory, as quality assurance policies demand.

Procedures performed in the hematology laboratory require microscopic observation, macroscopic observation, and, in some instances, a combination of both. In certain of the routine procedures, spectrophotometry is used.

SPECIMENS

Since samples for hematologic study are usually obtained by finger puncture or venipuncture, the student should review the collection of specimens and the approach to the patient in general (see under Types of Specimens Collected in Chapter 2).

Capillary Blood

Capillary blood can be used with good results for morphologic studies in hematology. For doing differential blood counts and for enumerating cellular elements, capillary or peripheral blood can be obtained from the fingertip, earlobe, heel, or big toe. This kind of sampling is sometimes called microsampling. In newborn infants, blood is generally obtained from the plantar surface of the big toe or heel, since these areas are more accessible than the fingertip. Newborns have a small blood supply, and removing blood by venipuncture would deplete too much of their blood. If blood is needed from very young children, the third or fourth fingertip is generally punctured. In adults that have very poor veins or whose veins cannot be used because intravenous solutions are being administered, the tip of the third or fourth finger is punctured to obtain the blood sample. A free flow of blood is needed for the results obtained with capillary blood to agree with those from venous blood.

Tests Using Capillary Blood

For the hematology laboratory, when capillary blood is used for manual blood cell counts and hemoglobin determinations the tip of the pipette is placed in the drop of blood. The pipette is not touched to the skin. Special disposable micropipettes are available, especially for some of the routine hematologic determinations. This system uses a self-filling pipette and a polyethylene reagent reservoir for dilution of the blood. This unit is called a Unopette (Becton, Dickinson & Co.). Usually, blood for the hemoglobin test is taken first. The blood measured in the hemoglobin pipette must be put into the diluent immediately and mixed well. It can be read in the spectrophotometer later.

White cell counts are done next. Blood measured in the white cell pipettes must be diluted immediately with the proper diluting fluid. After dilution, the mixture must be immediately mixed. If blood and diluent are not shaken immediately, proper mixing will not occur and clots may form. Remixing is done prior to cell counting.

Venous Blood

Because it is not always practical to obtain capillary blood for hematology, venous blood is often used. More tests can be done with a tube of venous blood, including the measurement of sedimentation rate, which requires more blood than some of the other hematology determinations. There must be some means of preventing coagulation, as clotted blood cannot be used. The types of anticoagulants available and their use are discussed under Additives and Anticoagulants in Chapter 2. For most hematologic studies the anticoagulant used is ethylenediamine tetraacetic acid (EDTA). This preserves the morphology of the cellular elements and prevents coagulation. It is important that the blood be mixed well with the

anticoagulant immediately after it is collected to ensure proper anticoagulation. Not even small clots are acceptable for hematology. When refrigerated properly, EDTA specimens can be preserved for several hours until the work can be done. White cell counts, microhematocrit, platelet counts, and sedimentation rates can be measured up to 24 hours after blood is collected in EDTA if it is refrigerated at 4° C. The EDTA binds the calcium ions in the blood and thus inhibits coagulation.

In addition to keeping the blood in a liquid form (preventing clotting), the anticoagulant must maintain the natural appearance of the RBCs, WBCs, and platelets. EDTA is the anticoagulant in general use that can do all these things.

Immediately after the blood has been properly drawn and placed in the tube containing the anticoagulant, it should be gently mixed by repeated inversion. This is necessary to ensure thorough contact with the anticoagulant. Clotted specimens are absolutely unacceptable for most tests done in the hematology laboratory, especially cell counts. If there is even a tiny clot in a specimen, the cell count will be grossly inaccurate.

Processing and Testing the Specimen

After the blood specimen has been collected from the patient, it must be transported to the laboratory for analysis. Assuming that the specimen was properly labeled when it was drawn and that it has been handled properly, it is examined in the laboratory as quickly as possible to prevent deterioration. Laboratory tests are done on fresh specimens whenever possible. Special handling of specimens for the various hematologic determinations is discussed later in this chapter in connection with specific tests.

To comply with universal precautions, gloves must be worn during all laboratory handling and testing using blood specimens. All samples are to be considered as potentially infectious and the proper use of barrier-protective apparel and devices is essential.

Immediately before a test is performed on a blood specimen, the blood sample must be mixed by repeated inversion 15 times. This can be accomplished by hand or with a mechanical tube inverter. If the blood sample has stood for a few minutes, it should be mixed again.

When a preserved blood specimen is allowed to stand for a period of time, the components will settle into three distinct layers: (1) the plasma, or top layer, (2) the buffy coat, a grayish-white cellular layer composed of

WBCs and platelets, and (3) the RBCs, the bottom layer. Some hematologic procedures are based on the ability of the blood specimen to settle into layers when it has been preserved by use of an anticoagulant.

Appearance of Specimens

When the blood specimen has been properly drawn and preserved in the prescribed manner, the plasma will have its natural color, a very light yellow or straw hue. There are occasions when the plasma may have an altered color because of a disease process, but color changes can also result from improper handling of the specimen by the laboratory worker.

Hemolysis

The color change most often seen is the appearance of red in the plasma caused by the release of hemoglobin into the solution when the RBCs are broken up. This breakup, or rupturing, of red cells is called *hemolysis*. Hemolysis is one of the changes resulting from alterations in osmotic pressure in the solution surrounding the red cells. It can also occur when the membrane surrounding the red cells has been mechanically ruptured.

Unsuitable Hematologic Specimens

Two types of blood samples are unsuitable for hematology tests: clotted samples and samples that are hemolyzed in the process of collection or handling. Clotted specimens are not suitable for cell counts because the cells are trapped in the clot and are therefore not counted. A cell count on a clotted sample will be falsely low. In hemolyzed specimens the red cells are no longer intact, and red cell counts on hemolyzed samples will also give falsely low results.

Homeostasis

If blood is collected, anticoagulated, and allowed to settle, or be centrifuged, three layers will separate and be observed (Fig 11–1).

The bottom layer will consist of packed red blood cells and will normally make up 40% to 47% of the total blood volume (the percentage differs in males and females). On top of this layer a thin whitish layer called the *buffy coat* will be seen. This consists of the leukocytes and platelets and normally makes up about 1% of

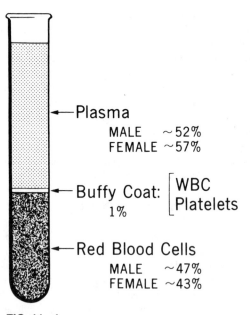

FIG 11–1.
Layers of normal blood (after centrifugation).

the total blood volume. The uppermost layer is a colloidal liquid called plasma. The plasma layer normally represents 52% to 57% of the total blood volume.

All of the fluid and cellular elements that make up the blood are in a constant state of exchange. The overall effect is a state of equilibrium in which the supply is equal to the demand for normal body function. This state of equilibrium is termed *homeostasis,* and various tests that are done on blood measure the overall state of homeostasis within the body. Many of the constituents of plasma (or serum, if the blood is allowed to clot) are measured in the clinical chemistry laboratory.

Principle of Osmotic Pressure

The principle of osmotic pressure and osmosis is very important whenever a solution or diluent is used as part of a procedure. In many hematologic procedures, diluents are used. In simple terms, *osmosis* is the passage of a solvent through a membrane from a dilute solution into a more concentrated one. The difference in concentration between the solutions on either side of the membrane causes the phenomenon called *osmotic pressure*. If the concentrations of these solutions are the same, there will not be any pressure.

Isotonic, Hypotonic, and Hypertonic Solutions

When the concentration is the same in the diluent solution as it is inside the RBC, the diluent is called an *isotonic* solution. If the diluent is less concentrated than the inside of the RBC, the solution is called *hypotonic*. From the definition of osmosis it can be seen that in the case of a hypotonic solution (dilute), the passage of diluent will be from outside the red cell into the red cell, causing the cell to swell and eventually to rupture, or hemolyze. If the solution outside the RBC is more concentrated than that inside it, the outside solution is called *hypertonic*. In the case of a hypertonic solution, the osmosis of the solvent is from the inside of the red cell to the surrounding solution. When this happens, the red cell will shrink from loss of liquid and will become crenated.

When red cells are in plasma, they are in an isotonic solution. For this reason, any diluent used to dilute blood for hematology tests must have the same concentration as plasma. When a solution has the same concentration as, or is isotonic with, plasma, it is called a *physiologic solution*. One very common physiologic solution used in hospitals is isotonic saline solution, a 0.85 g/dL solution of sodium chloride (NaCl). If RBCs are placed in an isotonic saline solution, their size is preserved. Hypotonic and hypertonic solutions are unsatisfactory for hematologic studies.

FORMATION AND FUNCTION OF BLOOD CELLS AND COMPONENTS

Hematopoiesis

During early fetal life, blood cells are formed in many of the body tissues. During this period, the liver and spleen are the most active sites of blood cell production, or **hematopoiesis.** At about the fourth month of fetal life, the bone marrow begins functioning as a blood cell producer. Shortly after birth, under normal conditions, the marrow is the only tissue that continues to produce red cells, granular leukocytes (granulocytes), monocytes, and platelets. Until the age of 5 years, the marrow in all the bones is red and cellular, and actively produces cells. Between 5 and 7 years, the long bones become inactive and fat cells appear to replace the active marrow. Red marrow is gradually displaced by fat cells in the other bones through the maturing years. In other

words, red marrow is transformed to yellow marrow. After age 18 to 20 years, red marrow remains only in the vertebrae, the ribs, the sternum, the skull, and partially in the femur and the humerus.

However, the marrow is able to become active again when necessary, as in hemolytic anemias or chronic hemorrhage, when there is an increased loss of RBCs from the body and a demand for increased RBC production. Such increased marrow activity is helpful to normal body function. This is not the case in other instances, as in **leukemia** or other malignancies, where increased marrow activity of one cell type is detrimental to the body as a whole. Another situation that is incompatible with life occurs when the marrow is suppressed or unable to function normally in cell production. In this case the marrow is said to be *aplastic*. Bone marrow aspirations may therefore be necessary to detect abnormal changes in the newly formed cells or in their quantity. Early blood disease may be detected by an examination of the bone marrow.

The leukocytes found in normal circulating peripheral blood consist of the granulocytes (neutrophils, eosinophils, and basophils), monocytes, and lymphocytes. The bone marrow produces the erythrocytes, granulocytes, monocytes, and platelets. Lymphocytes are produced primarily by the lymphoid tissue (lymph nodes and nodules, thymus, and spleen); some are also produced in the bone marrow.

These formed elements of the blood go through a normal series of developmental steps or stages in the marrow or lymphoid tissue and are found in the general peripheral blood circulation only when they are sufficiently developed or mature. However, immature cells, or cells in early developmental stages, may appear in the peripheral blood in certain disease states. Each cell type has a normal life span and function. When their normal life span is complete, the formed elements are eliminated from the body by processes in which parts of the cells are reused and parts are eliminated from the body.

When the body is functioning normally, the production and destruction of the formed elements of the blood are balanced so that a constant supply is available. When one of the steps in these processes is not functioning properly or is occurring too rapidly, a blood disorder will result, and this will cause alterations in the other steps as well, since they are all closely related. These alterations might reflect diseases of the blood formation system or diseases of nonhematologic origin. For example, chronic bleeding resulting from a nonhematologic cause such as gastric ulcer or carcinoma results in hypochromic anemia. A similar condition of hematologic origin results from simple dietary iron deficiency. When tests are performed in the hematology laboratory, changes in the appearance of the red blood cells or other formed elements, or changes in the manner in which whole blood or various components react under certain test conditions, are noted to determine whether alterations in function have occurred.

Normal Red Blood Cells (Erythrocytes)

Formation of Red Blood Cells

In adults, erythrocytes are formed in the bone marrow. The mature RBC is often described as a biconcave disk—that is, it is doughnut-shaped, with a depressed area rather than a hole in the center, as shown in Figure 11–2. It does not contain a nucleus (it is nonnucleated) and is about 7 to 8 μm in diameter.

The RBC begins as a nucleated cell within the bone marrow. As the cell matures in the bone marrow, its diameter decreases and the nucleus becomes denser, smaller, and is finally released from the cell (extruded). While this occurs the concentration of hemoglobin increases and the cytoplasm (cell material other than the nucleus) progressively changes from blue to orange in appearance on a stained blood film. The whole sequence of maturation from an early cell precursor to a circulating red cell takes 3 to 5 days.

Reticulocytes.—The young RBC that has just extruded its nucleus is referred to as a **reticulocyte.** It is about the same size as or slightly larger than a mature RBC. Reticulocytes differ from mature RBCs morphologically because they contain a fine basophilic reticulum or network of RNA (ribonucleic acid), a cytoplasmic remnant that decreases as the cell matures. When stained with Wright's stain, the reticulocyte appears pinkish-gray or has a slight bluish tinge. This *polychromasia* (many colors) represents the presence of RNA within the cell. With a special stain, such as brilliant cresyl blue or new methylene blue, the basophilic reticulum of RNA appears blue (see under Counting Reticulocytes). Under normal conditions, reticulocytes remain and mature further in the bone marrow for a day or two before they are released into the peripheral blood. RBCs are released into the peripheral blood as reticulocytes by squeezing (or insinuating) through openings in the endothelial cells lining the marrow cavity. These reticulocytes become fully mature—that is, they lose all RNA—within a day or two. Therefore, the number of reticulocytes in the peripheral blood is an indication of the degree of RBC production by the marrow. Normally about 1% of the circulating RBCs are reticulocytes.

Function of Red Blood Cells

The main function of the RBC is to carry oxygen to the cells of the body. The oxygen is transported in a chemical combination with hemoglobin. Thus, the concentration of hemoglobin in the blood is a measure of its capacity to carry oxygen, on which all cells are absolutely dependent for energy and therefore life. To combine with and therefore transport oxygen, the hemoglobin molecule must have a certain combination of substances, namely heme (which contains iron) and globin. Deficiencies in the presence or metabolism of any of these substances will result in a decrease in hemoglobin and oxygen-carrying capacity.

Elimination by Reticuloendothelial System

Red blood cells have a total life span of about 120 days, and the body releases new red cells into the circulatory system every day. When red cells are worn out, the body stores the cell components that are reusable, including protein from the globin portion of the hemoglobin molecule, and iron, and eliminates the nonreusable components. The heme portion of the hemoglobin molecule is such a waste product. It is converted to bilirubin, concentrated in the bile, and eliminated from the body by way of the feces, and to a much smaller extent the urine, as urobilin and urobilinogen. The metabolism and elimi-

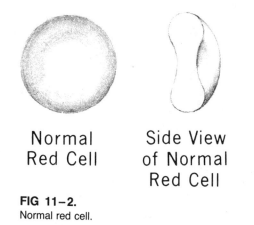

Normal
Red Cell

Side View
of Normal
Red Cell

FIG 11–2.
Normal red cell.

nation of bilirubin are described in Chapters 10 and 13. A schematic representation of the blood formation and destruction process is shown in Figure 11–3.

Dead red cells are broken down by the reticuloendothelial system (RES). The RES is composed of connective tissue cells that carry on *phagocytosis,* a process in which a cell engulfs, or eats, foreign material. The RES cells are located in the blood sinusoids (tiny blood vessels) in the liver, spleen, and bone marrow, and lining of the lymph channels in the lymph nodes. They are important in the body's defense mechanism and in the breakdown of globin to amino acids, which are returned to the protein storage pool of the body. They are also essential for the retention and reuse or storage of iron, which is needed for the formation of hemoglobin and transport of oxygen. A deficiency of iron results in anemia, a condition in which the oxygen-carrying capacity of blood is decreased. Iron deficiency anemia, one of the more common types of anemia, may result from a dietary deficiency of iron or from loss of iron from the body through bleeding.

Normal White Blood Cells (Leukocytes)

The leukocytes are nucleated and are part of the defense mechanism of the body. Unlike the red cells, white cells use the bloodstream primarily for transportation to their place of function in the body tissues.

Function of White Blood Cells

The neutrophils, eosinophils, and monocytes act as phagocytic scavengers—they engulf and destroy invading microorganisms and clear the body of unwanted particulate material such as dead or injured tissue cells. This is the first step in the repair of injured tissue. The lymphocytes and **plasma cells** act as immunocytes, inactivating foreign antigens by antibody production and by delayed hypersensitivity reactions. Plasma cells are not normally found in the peripheral blood. Lymphocytes and plasma cells are produced primarily in the lymphoid tissue (lymph nodes, nodules, and spleen) and secondarily in the marrow.

Types of Normal White Blood Cells

Under normal conditions, five types of leukocytes are found in the blood: lymphocytes, neutrophils, monocytes, eosinophils, and basophils. When a blood film is stained with Wright's stain and examined with the microscope, the majority of the cells seen will be RBCs, which appear as small, rounded, pink, or reddish-orange bodies. Scattered among the red-staining cells are the less numerous leukocytes. There are normally 600 to 800

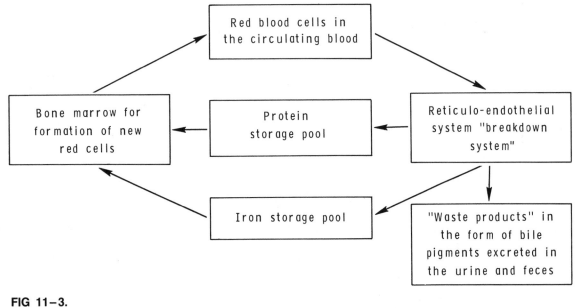

FIG 11–3.
Blood formation and destruction process.

red cells to each leukocyte. The leukocytes are larger and more complex in appearance than the RBCs. They consist of a nucleus surrounded by cytoplasm. Usually the nucleus is in the center of the cell and is a prominent purple-staining body. It can be round or oval (as in the lymphocyte) or lobulated (as in the neutrophil and eosinophil). The cytoplasm, which gives the cell its shape, stains a variety of colors, depending on its contents. The size of the cell, the shape and size of the nucleus, and the staining reactions of the nucleus and the cytoplasm aid in the identification of leukocytes.

Leukocytes are categorized as granulocytes and nongranulocytes. **Granulocytes** are leukocytes that contain specific granulation in their cytoplasm. Granulocytes are neutrophils, eosinophils, and basophils (see also Staining the Blood Film). Nongranulocytes may contain nonspecific granulation, but specific granules are not seen; they include the monocytes and lymphocytes. Granulocytes are cells belonging to the *myeloid* series, but monocytes are also classified as myeloid cells (see also under Origin and Function of Blood Cells Related to Morphologic Examination; and Leukocyte Alterations).

The five types of leukocytes are discussed more thoroughly under Normal Leukocyte Morphology, but a brief description of each follows.

Neutrophil.—This cell is normally the most numerous and most prominent of the white cells seen in an adult blood film. The nucleus is lobulated (with three to five lobes), and the cytoplasm stains pinkish-lavender and contains numerous fine lilac granules.

Lymphocyte.—This cell is the next most numerous in adult blood samples (usually about three neutrophils are seen to each lymphocyte). The nucleus is round or oval, and the cytoplasm stains blue and is usually free from any granules, although nonspecific azurophilic granules may be present. Lymphocytes are further classified as small or large.

Monocyte.—This is the largest white cell and is often confused with the lymphocyte. It usually has a horseshoe- or kidney-shaped nucleus (although it may be round) that stains lavender. The cytoplasm stains slate-gray or muddy blue and can be vacuolated.

Eosinophil.—This cell is easily recognized by the large, red, beadlike granules seen in the cytoplasm. Nor-

mally, few eosinophils are present (only about 3 per 100 total white cells counted).

Basophil.—This cell is the one least likely to be seen (only 1 per 100 total white cells counted). It is easily distinguished, however, by the dark purple-blue bead-like granules seen in the cytoplasm.

Normal Platelets (Thrombocytes)

Another formed element of the blood is the platelet, or thrombocyte. Platelets are small colorless bodies 1 to 4 μm in diameter. They are generally round or ovoid, although they may have projections called *pseudopods.* Platelets have a colorless to pale blue background substance containing centrally located, reddish to violet granules.

Formation of Platelets

Platelets are produced in the bone marrow by cells called *megakaryocytes,* which are large and multinucleated. They do not have a nucleus and are not actually cells—they are portions of cytoplasm pinched off from megakaryocytes and released into the bloodstream.

Function of Platelets

In the bloodstream, platelets are an essential part of the blood clotting mechanism. They act to maintain the structure or integrity of the endothelial cells lining the vascular system by plugging any gaps in the lining. They also function in the clotting process by (1) acting as plugs around the opening of a wound, and (2) releasing certain factors that are necessary for the formation of a blood clot.

Plasma Portion of Blood

The formed elements of blood are suspended in a fluid called *blood plasma.* Plasma is the protein fraction of the blood, and it contains in solution many substances that are necessary for maintenance of the body. It is a complex mixture including water, proteins, carbohydrates, lipids, electrolytes, and clotting factors, plus enzymes, vitamins, hormones, and trace metals.

CLINICAL HEMATOLOGY

Clinical hematology is primarily concerned with testing the formed elements within the blood. The oxygen-carrying capacity of the blood is routinely measured by measuring the hemoglobin concentration and the hematocrit (percentage of total blood volume occupied by the RBCs), counting the RBCs, and observing the morphology or appearance of the RBCs on a peripheral blood film. RBC production by the marrow is assessed by means of a reticulocyte count, and examination of the bone marrow may be necessary in certain disease states.

The leukocytes in the blood are routinely assessed by counting the number of cells present in a particular volume, and observing the morphology and determining the percentage of each cell type present in a peripheral blood film. This is referred to as a white blood cell *differential*. Here again, examination of the bone marrow may be necessary in certain cases; however, this is not a routine procedure.

Platelets are also routinely assessed in clinical hematologic studies by observing their number and morphology in the peripheral blood film. If certain disorders are suspected, they may also be counted. The blood clotting mechanism may also be checked, when necessary, by testing for the clotting factors that are present within the plasma.

Since the equilibrium of the blood is affected by a great many factors, hematology tests are useful in the study of all sorts of disease states, of hematologic or nonhematologic origin. Thus, hereditary, nutritional, metabolic, traumatic, inflammatory and infectious, hormonal, immunologic, neoplastic, drug-induced, and other disease states can be assessed by hematologic studies. The physician will depend on such laboratory results, in combination with the clinical history and physical examination, to determine the state of health or disease of the patient.

HEMOGLOBIN

The determination of hemoglobin (Hb) is the test ordered most frequently in the clinical hematology laboratory. It is included in the routine CBC for most new hospital admissions. With the use of automated cell counters, the meaning of CBC will vary from institution to institution. The measurement of hemoglobin is relatively simple and can be done quickly by the laboratory. Along with the hematocrit measurement, the hemoglobin value is used to follow many disease states, especially the anemias. The measurement of the concentration of hemoglobin in the blood is called *hemoglobinometry*.

Synthesis and Structure

Hemoglobin synthesis is a complex process, starting in the bone marrow with the production of the erythrocytes. The heme (iron-containing) portion of the molecule combines with globin (the protein portion) and forms an activated form of hemoglobin that is ready to transport oxygen. Each hemoglobin molecule consists of four heme groups and a globin moiety, which is composed of four polypeptide chains (Fig 11–4).

Heme

The heme group is an iron complex containing one iron atom. Iron is essential for the primary function of the hemoglobin molecule—carrying oxygen to the tissues. If iron is lacking, because of either inadequate intake or increased loss from the body, anemia results, since hemoglobin is not formed in sufficient quantity. When reduced hemoglobin is exposed to oxygen at increased pressure, oxygen is taken up at the iron atom until each molecule of hemoglobin has bound four oxygen molecules, one molecule at each iron atom. Since this is not a true oxidation-reduction reaction, the hemoglobin molecule carrying oxygen is said to be oxygenated. The molecule fully saturated with oxygen (four oxygen molecules per hemoglobin) is called *oxyhemoglobin*. It contains 1.34 mL of oxygen per gram of hemoglobin. Oxyhemoglobin carries oxygen from the lungs to the tissues of the body. Hemoglobin returning with carbon dioxide from the tissues is known as *reduced hemoglobin*.

Heme is itself a complex molecule. It is made up of a series of tetrapyrrole rings, terminating in *protoporphyrin*, with a central iron, as shown in Figure 11–4. Since the heme molecule is a porphyrin, a group of diseases called the *porphyrias* result from certain disorders of heme synthesis. Normally heme is excreted from the body as bilirubin, which is eventually converted to the various bile salts and pigments. The iron is normally removed and retained by the RES, stored, and reused in the production of new hemoglobin.

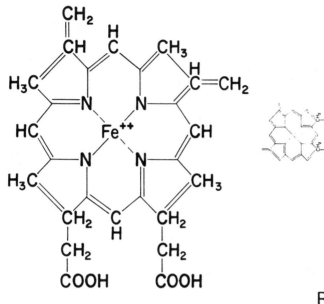

A. Heme Moiety

B. Hemoglobin A Molecule

FIG 11–4.
Hemoglobin molecules. **A,** heme molecule (one protoporphyrin ring with a single iron atom). **B,** hemoglobin A molecule (made up of four heme groups with their appropriate globin chains—two alpha and two beta).

Globin

The globin portion of the hemoglobin molecule is a protein substance that consists of four chains of amino acids (polypeptides). Each of the four globin chains is attached to a heme portion to form a single hemoglobin molecule.

Forms of Hemoglobin

Different forms of hemoglobin may occur in the red cells. These forms differ in the content and sequence of amino acids in the globin chains.

Hemoglobin A

The principal adult hemoglobin, Hb A, contains two α and two β globin chains, as shown in Figure 11–4. In another form of adult hemoglobin (Hb A$_2$), the α chains are paired with two δ polypeptide chains. These are the major normal forms of adult hemoglobin. Other genetically determined forms of hemoglobin may be demonstrated by means of electrophoresis. Many abnormal

forms of hemoglobin lead to clinical illness because they interfere with the oxygen-carrying capacity of the blood.

The combination of Hb A and Hb A$_2$ should normally make up 95% of the hemoglobin in an adult, with Hb F making up 5% or less.

Hemoglobin F

Hemoglobin F is the major form found during intra-uterine life and at birth. In fetal hemoglobin (Hb F), the two α globin chains are paired with two γ chains. Adult hemoglobin (Hb A) is formed in small amounts by the fetus and rapidly increases after birth. Screening for abnormal hemoglobins should be postponed until several months after birth, because only at the age of 6 months does the proportion of adult hemoglobin forms become definitive.

Structurally Abnormal Hemoglobin

Disorders in which the presence of a structurally abnormal hemoglobin is considered to play an important role pathologically are called *hemoglobinopathies*. In some hemoglobinopathies, all the hemoglobin is in one abnormal form. In others, two abnormal forms may be present. In still others, some normal forms and some abnormal forms are present.

One fairly common abnormal hemoglobin is Hb S. It occurs almost exclusively in the black population and is responsible for the disease sickle cell anemia. The four clinically important abnormal hemoglobins are Hb S, Hb C, Hb D, and Hb E. These are all hereditary, and the disorders affect the protein portion of the hemoglobin molecule, altering the structure of the polypeptide chain. These abnormal hemoglobins, as well as the normal ones, can be distinguished from one another by electrophoresis.

Hemoglobin Derivatives and Complexes Formed

The circulating blood carries a composite of hemoglobin, oxyhemoglobin, carboxyhemoglobin, (hemoglobin combined with carbon monoxide), methemoglobin, and minor amounts of other forms of this pigment. Hemoglobin can combine with other substances besides oxygen, some normally and some abnormally. If hemoglobin is converted to an abnormal hemoglobin pigment, it is no longer capable of oxygen transport, and if this impairment is severe, a condition of *hypoxia*, or *cyanosis,* will occur.

Carboxyhemoglobin

The hemoglobin molecule has a much greater affinity for carbon monoxide than for oxygen and will readily combine with carbon monoxide if it is present even in low concentration. The formation of *carboxyhemoglobin* is reversible, and if carbon monoxide is removed the hemoglobin will once again combine with oxygen. Carboxyhemoglobin is found normally in small amounts, especially in the blood of smokers; concentrations range from 1 to 10 g/dL.

Methemoglobin

Methemoglobin is a type of abnormal hemoglobin in which the iron has been oxidized from the ferrous to the ferric state and is therefore incapable of carrying oxygen, which is replaced by a hydroxyl radical. The formation of methemoglobin results from the presence of certain chemicals or drugs, and is reversible. Methemoglobin is

normally present in the blood in concentrations of 1 to 2 g/dL.

Sulfhemoglobin

Another abnormal hemoglobin derivative is *sulfhemoglobin*. Sulfhemoglobin is formed irreversibly and remains for the life of the carrier RBC. Its exact nature is not clear, but it is thought to be formed by the action of some drugs and chemicals such as sulfonamides. Sulfhemoglobin is not capable of transporting oxygen.

Hemiglobincyanide (Cyanmethemoglobin)

To measure hemoglobin accurately in the blood, it is necessary to prepare a stable derivative containing all the hemoglobin forms that are present. All forms of circulating hemoglobin are readily converted to hemiglobincyanide, except for sulfhemoglobin, which is rarely present in significant amounts. For this reason, the *hemiglobincyanide*, or *cyanmethemoglobin* method, is used in most laboratories for the determination of hemoglobin. Another procedure called the *oxyhemoglobin* method has been used, but it does not detect sulfhemoglobin or methemoglobin, and it has been largely replaced by the cyanmethemoglobin method.

Variations in Reference Values

The reference (or normal) values for hemoglobin in the peripheral blood vary with the age and sex of the individual. Altitude also affects the hemoglobin measurement, in that the normal hemoglobin concentration is higher at high altitudes than at sea level. At birth, the hemoglobin concentration is normally 17 to 23 g/dL. It decreases to 9 to 14 g/dL by about 2 months of age. By 10 years of age, the normal hemoglobin will be 12 to 14 g/dL. Normal adult values range from 12 to 15 g/dL in women and 14 to 17 g/dL in men. There may be a slight decrease in the hemoglobin level after 50 years of age.*

When the hemoglobin value is below normal, the patient is said to be *anemic*. Anemia is a very common condition and is frequently a complication of other diseases (see under Erythrocyte Alterations in this chapter). In this condition the circulating erythrocytes may be deficient in number, deficient in total hemoglobin content per unit of blood volume, or both. A decrease in hemo-

---

*Brown B: *Hematology Principles and Procedures*. Philadelphia, Lea & Febiger, 1988, p 79.

globin can result from bleeding conditions, in which the patient loses erythrocytes. An increase in hemoglobin, usually as a result of an increase in the number of erythrocytes *(erythrocytosis),* is seen in polycythemia and newborn infants.

Specimens

The test for hemoglobin can be done on free-flowing capillary blood obtained from a finger puncture, or on venous blood preserved with an anticoagulant. The anticoagulant of choice for hematologic studies, including hemoglobin determinations, is EDTA. The hemoglobin content of blood remains unchanged for several days when properly anticoagulated and refrigerated at 4° C.

Methods for Measurement of Hemoglobin

Hemoglobin is determined as grams of hemoglobin per 100 mL of blood, or grams per deciliter. Reporting hemoglobin as a percentage of a normal value is not satisfactory because there are so many different methods and each method has its own normal value. For example, 80% of normal for one method may be the same as 98% of normal for another. The values for 100% hemoglobin in five different testing methods are listed below.

Sahli   17.3 g/dL
Dare   16.0 g/dL
Haden   15.6 g/dL
Wintrobe   14.5 g/dL
Haldane   13.8 g/dL

Visual Hemoglobin Methods, Historical Perspective

Some methods for determining the amount of hemoglobin present in a blood specimen are much more commonly used than others. Many years ago, before the use of the photometer, most hemoglobin methods depended on the human eye to determine the changes in color intensity caused by hemoglobin concentration differences; these methods were not very accurate. Some of the visual methods are the Tallquist, Dare, Haden, Haldane, and Sahli methods. Visual methods are limited to use in areas of the world where electricity is not available.

In the Sahli method, the hemoglobin in the blood sample is converted to acid hematin by the addition of 0.1N hydrochloric acid (HCl). The addition of acid to

blood converts the red hemoglobin to a brown color. Since brown is more easily matched by the human eye than red, Sahli's method for testing hemoglobin is one of the more acceptable visual methods. The error in a visual method is great, however, and these methods are certainly not recommended.

Gasometric Methods

Gasometric analysis with the Van Slyke apparatus is the most accurate method for determining hemoglobin, but it is not used routinely in the clinical laboratory because it is time-consuming and complicated. It is used as a reference method to obtain the hemoglobin concentration in blood samples used for standardization of hemoglobin procedures.

Quantitative Spectrophotometric Methods

A method for measuring hemoglobin must be chosen that will detect all forms of hemoglobin. The one used by most laboratories is the cyanmethemoglobin, or hemiglobincyanide, method. This is now the internationally recognized method of choice. Another method used by some is the oxyhemoglobin method. Both methods utilize spectrophotometry (see Chapter 5).

Spectrophotometric hemoglobin determinations are rapid and can give accurate results. The degree of accuracy will also depend on the basic technique used and the accuracy of the equipment, stability of the reagents, and cleanliness of the glassware.

Oxyhemoglobin Method.—The oxyhemoglobin method uses 0.04 ml/dL ammonium hydroxide (NH_4OH) solution to hemolyze the RBCs and convert the hemoglobin to oxyhemoglobin for measurement in the spectrophotometer. This conversion is complete and immediate and the resulting color is stable. Reference standards are not available for this method.

Hemiglobincyanide (Cyanmethemoglobin) Method.—The hemiglobincyanide (cyanmethemoglobin) method uses a modified Drabkin's reagent. The original Drabkin's reagent combined three chemicals: sodium bicarbonate ($NaHCO_3$), potassium cyanide (KCN), and potassium ferricyanide [$K_3Fe(CN)_6$] This original Drabkin's reagent required at least 10 minutes for color conversion of hemoglobin to hemiglobincyanide and also sometimes produced turbid solutions caused by protein precipitation or incomplete lysis of red blood cells. This reagent is no longer recommended. Alternative modifications are used with two main differences from the original Drabkin's: another buffering system (other than $NaHCO_3$) is used, such as monobasic potassium phosphate (KH_2PO_4), which shortens the conversion time from 10 minutes to 3 minutes; and a nonionic detergent is added, which minimizes turbidity and enhances red cell lysis.

When the modified hemiglobulincyanide (cyanmethemoglobin) reagent is mixed with the blood specimen, the stable pigment hemiglobincyanide is formed. This pigment can be measured quantitatively in the spectrophotometer.

Automated Hemoglobinometry

Various automated and semiautomated techniques have been employed to measure hemoglobin. Automatic pipettors and dilutors are used for portions of the measuring and diluting steps in many procedures. A special flow-through apparatus attached to the Coleman Junior Spectrophotometer enables a faster, more efficient spectrophotometric measurement of the unknown hemoglobin solution (see under Procedure for Operation of the Coleman Junior Spectrophotometer in Chapter 5). This apparatus is designed to increase the speed with which samples can be introduced and discharged from the spectrophotometer. One automatic apparatus, the model S Coulter counter (Coulter Electronics, Hialeah, Fla.), measures hemoglobin as well as the white cell count, red cell count, hematocrit, and red cell indices. Automation has made a significant contribution to the efficiency of the hematology laboratory (see under Counting the Formed Elements of the Blood).

Hemoglobin determination done by an automated instrument applies the same principle as that described for the manual method. The sample is lysed using the modified Drabkin's reagent and light absorbance is measured at 540 nm.

Equipment for Nonautomated Hemoglobinometry

Disposable, self-filling, self-measuring dilution micropipettes are commercially available for determination of hemoglobin. One such system is the Unopette (Fig 11–5; see also Chapter 2). These systems are easy to use and are available with a series of different diluting fluids for different purposes. The **Unopette System** for hemoglobin determination consists of a self-filling, self-measuring pipette attached to a plastic holder; the pipette fills with blood automatically by capillary action. A plas-

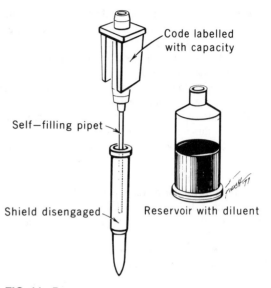

FIG 11–5.
Self-filling disposable pipette and diluent reservoir.

tic reagent container, called the reservoir, is filled with modified Drabkin's reagent (hemiglobincyanide) in the hemoglobin Unopette system. The pipette containing the blood is inserted into the reagent reservoir, emptied, and rinsed according to the manufacturer's instructions. The blood is mixed well with the reagent and is then ready to be read in the spectrophotometer.

A special pipette called a *Sahli pipette* can also be used for hemoglobin determinations. The Sahli pipette is calibrated to contain 20 μL (or 0.02 mL) of blood. Since it is a to-contain pipette, it must be rinsed with the diluent to ensure proper measurement of the blood sample. The accuracy of hemoglobin pipettes must be checked before the pipettes can be used for hematologic determinations. This can be done simply by comparing the new pipette with US Bureau of Standards pipettes, which have been very carefully calibrated.

When Sahli pipettes are used, special rubber tubing with an aspirating device must be attached to the pipette for suction. It is difficult to use this type of pipette with mechanical suction devices. Because of the universal precautionary policies used in all laboratories (and the use of barriers between blood and laboratorian), use of Sahli pipettes has all but been replaced by the disposable pipetting systems described.

Since most hemoglobin determinations employ photometry, a spectrophotometer of good quality and in good working order is essential. Most brands of spectrophotometers give good results if certain precautions are taken. Before a spectrophotometer can be used to determine the hemoglobin concentration, it must be standardized. Since the Coleman Junior Spectrophotometer is in general use and has been discussed in some detail in Chapter 5, the procedure presented in this section for standardization of the spectrophotometer will deal specifically with this instrument. However, the same general procedure can be followed for any type of spectrophotometer.

Standardization of the Coleman Junior Spectrophotometer.—Before any unknown solution can be measured with a spectrophotometer, the instrument must be standardized, that is, a standard curve must be prepared from which to read the unknowns. To do this, samples of known concentration of the substance to be measured (the standard solutions) must be read in the spectrophotometer. The principles of Beer's law are applied (see under Absorbance and Transmittance of Light—Beer's Law, in Chapter 5). When the wavelength of light and its path length are a constant (K factor) for the procedure, the concentration (C) of hemiglobincyanide in each sample is directly proportional to the absorbance (A) obtained.

Procedure Using Commercial Certified Standards.—Stable standard hemiglobincyanide solutions representing 1:250 dilutions of whole blood containing

---

Procedure 11–1. Standardization of the Coleman Junior Spectrophotometer Using Commercial Certified Hemoglobin Standards

1. Label 11 cuvettes (test tubes may be used if the flow-through type of apparatus is available for the spectrophotometer) as follows: blank, 1, 1 duplicate; 2, 2 duplicate; 3, 3 duplicate; 4, 4 duplicate; and 5, 5 duplicate. High quality disposable glass tubes also may be satisfactory for use in the spectrophotometer in place of calibrated cuvettes.
2. Using volumetric pipettes, pipette the following amounts into the cuvettes:

Tube	Standard (mL)	Hemiglobincyanide Reagent (mL)
Blank	0	5
1	1	4
1 duplicate		
2	2	3
2 duplicate		
3	3	2
3 duplicate		
4	4	1
4 duplicate		
5	5	0
5 duplicate		

3. Mix the contents of the cuvettes well.
4. Read in the spectrophotometer, using a wavelength setting of 540 nm.
5. Record absorbance (A) readings directly or record percent transmittance $(\%T)$ readings and convert to absorbance.
6. Calculate the concentration (C) of hemoglobin (mg/dL) for each of the standard cuvettes (see the original concentration of standard solution used).
7. Calculate the concentration of hemoglobin (g/dL) for each of the standard dilutions.
8. Calculate the K value for each standard ($K = A/C$) and calculate the average K value for the spectrophotometer.
9. Plot the standard line on semilogarithmic graph paper with percent transmittance readings (use linear graph paper for absorbance readings). Draw the straight line through the points that gives the best fit for the graph. Subsequent hemoglobin concentrations can then be read directly from this straight line. Generally, readings between $20\%T$ and $80\%T$ are more accurate than readings at either end of the scale. If a patient sample gives a reading greater than $80\%T$, the test is repeated with twice as much blood. If a patient sample gives a reading less than $20\%T$, the blood sample is diluted with twice as much diluent and the test is repeated. Volumes must be taken into account in the calculations.

5, 10, and 15 g of hemoglobin per 100 mL of blood are available commercially and are certified by the College of American Pathologists (CAP). This type of hemoglobin standard is commonly used by all clinical laboratories. When a certified standard (CAP) is used, the following procedure may be followed in setting up the cuvettes for reading in the spectrophotometer (Procedure 11–1):

An alternative method is to calculate the constant factor K ($= A/C$) for the instrument (see step 8 above). By using the average K value, hemoglobin concentrations corresponding to all the potential galvanometer readings may be calculated and a standard chart may be prepared.

The standard chart will show the range of hemoglobin concentrations that can be accurately determined with a particular spectrophotometer. Only hemoglobin values obtained from the linear portion of the graph may be used to prepare the standard chart. The chart prepared from data obtained with one spectrophotometer cannot be used with any other spectrophotometer.

Using Laboratory-Prepared Standards.—For
the hemiglobincyanide (cyanmethemoglobin) method, standards can be prepared in the laboratory by obtaining a sample of blood on which the hemoglobin has already been determined by the oxygen capacity or iron content. The oxygen capacity determination is the reference method most frequently used for hemoglobin standardization. It is based on the assumption that 1 g of hemoglobin will combine with 1.34 mL of oxygen. The following formula can be used to find the hemoglobin (Hb) concentration:

$$\text{Hemoglobin (g/dL)} = \frac{\text{oxygen capacity (mL/dL)}}{1.34 \text{ (mL/g)}}$$

This blood sample is used for the stock standard solution. For the hemiglobincyanide method, the sample is diluted in a volumetric flask with hemiglobincyanide reagent so that the hemoglobin concentration is approximately 25 to 30 g/dL. This standard should be stored in a refrigerator until ready for use. From the stock standard, a series of working standards are prepared, including duplicate sets for each of ten dilutions having a total volume in each cuvette of 10 mL. The first cuvette should contain 10 mL of stock standard only, the second cuvette 9 mL of stock standard and 1 mL of reagent, the third cuvette 8 mL of stock standard and 2 mL of reagent, and

so on, ending with the tenth cuvette containing 1 mL of stock standard and 9 mL of reagent.

A blank tube containing 5 mL of reagent is placed in the cuvette well, and the galvanometer beam is adjusted to read $100\%T$ with the wavelength scale set at 540 nm. The percent transmittance for each of the standards is obtained by reading the samples in the spectrophotometer, reinserting and reading the blank tube between samples. The readings for the standards are recorded and transcribed on semilogarithmic graph paper as percent transmittance (ordinate) vs. concentration of hemoglobin in grams per 100 mL (abscissa). A line is drawn through the plotted points, and a table is prepared from this graph showing the concentration of hemoglobin corresponding to each percent transmittance reading. This table is used to obtain subsequent hemoglobin values for that machine.

Manual Method—Hemiglobincyanide (Procedure 11–2)

Principle.—A 20-µL portion of blood is diluted and hemolyzed in hemiglobincyanide reagent, which contains potassium ferricyanide and potassium cyanide. The ferricyanide converts the hemoglobin iron from the ferrous state (Fe^{2+}) to the ferric state (Fe^{3+}) to form hemiglobin or methemoglobin (Hi). This combines with potassium cyanide to form the stable pigment hemiglobincyanide (HiCN). The chemical reaction which occurs is, briefly:

$$Hb + K_3Fe(CN)_6 \rightarrow Hi$$

$$Hi + KCN \rightarrow HiCN$$

Hemiglobin is hemoglobin in which the iron has been oxidized to the ferric state. Hemiglobincyanide is methemoglobin banded to cyanide ions. The hemiglobincyanide reagent has three primary purposes: to dilute the blood, to lyse the red cells, and to convert hemoglobin to hemiglobincyanide.

The color reaction takes 3 minutes to reach completion if the reagent contains KH_2PO_4 as a buffer, 10 minutes if $Na\ HCO_3$ is used. All derivatives of hemoglobin, except sulfhemoglobin, are measured using this method. The color intensity of this mixture is measured in a spectrophotometer at a wavelength of 540 nm (corresponding to a yellow-green filter). Absorbance is directly proportional to the concentration of hemoglobin. The concentration (C) of hemoglobin (g/dL) can be calculated from $C = A/K$, where K is the constant for the spectrophotometer used in the standardization and *A* is absorbance. The concentration can also be read directly from a standard line or from a hemoglobin table prepared from a standard line.

Reagents.—A Unopette reservoir with 5 mL of hemiglobincyanide reagent already in it is supplied by the manufacturer. The manufacturer's directions must be followed carefully.

If the laboratory prepares its own reagent for hemoglobins, hemiglobincyanide reagent contains KH_2PO_4, KCN, and $K_3Fe(CN)_6$. It should be prepared fresh at least once a month and should be stored in a brown bottle to prevent deterioration; it is unstable in light. Hemiglobincyanide reagent is a clear, pale yellow solution. It should be discarded if it becomes turbid. Although the reagent contains only a small amount of cyanide, it is still regarded as a poison and must be treated with caution.

Quality Control Solution.—A control solution should be used for every hemoglobin determination. Daily controls should be run using either a commercial control specimen or one prepared by the laboratory.

A control sample is run in duplicate with each batch of hemoglobins or for the first batch run by each new shift on duty in the laboratory. Controls must be assayed in exactly the same manner as the unknown samples. Control values are plotted on a quality control chart. This chart indicates the previously established acceptable range or limits for the hemoglobin values in grams per deciliter. Each laboratory establishes its own acceptable quality control limits. One acceptability criterion includes: replicate hemoglobin values on the same specimen agree within 0.4 g/dL of each other; if a "true" value is known for a control or patient sample, results must agree within ±0.4 g/dL of that value; if hemoglobin values do not meet these limits, they will be repeated in duplicate; results will not be reported unless the control values run simultaneously with the unknown batch of patient samples is within the acceptable range.

Daily use of control values gives information about the state of the hemoglobin reagent (whether deterioration has occurred), the accuracy of the pipettes used, the variation and cleanliness of the calibrated photometer cuvettes, and the variation in the photometer used to measure the amount of hemoglobin in the samples. Technical skills are also checked. When the control values for the duplicate control specimens run are not within the ac-

ceptable limits, hemoglobin values for the unknown patient blood specimens being measured should not be reported until the reason for the control error is found, corrected and the sample retested. "Out-of-control" values are seen with deterioration of reagents, faulty equipment (spectrophotometer), dirty glassware, inaccurate standardization of the spectrophotometer, deterioration of the control specimen, inaccurate or broken pipettes, or poor technique (see Chapter 7).

Using 0.02-mL To-Contain Pipettes.—In the instance where Sahli pipettes or other to-contain pipettes are being used to measure the blood sample for hemoglobins, extreme caution is emphasized. Because the possibility of bloodborne infection is always present, any pipetting not done by mechanical means is discouraged. Use of Sahli pipettes requires an aspirating tube and suction and this presents a real biohazard to the person doing the pipetting. *Any* direct contact with blood presents a biohazard, however.

The 0.02-mL measured blood sample is added to 5 mL of hemiglobincyanide reagent in a test tube or cuvette. The pipette must be rinsed several times with the reagent until all blood is removed from the pipette. The reagent and blood sample are mixed well and the necessary conversion time allowed; usually 3 minutes is adequate. The mixture is read in a spectrophotometer at 540 nm and readings in percent transmittance are observed and recorded as described under the procedure for using the Unopette system.

Precautions, Technical Factors, and Sources of Error

Several precautions have already been discussed. Photometric methods for the determination of hemoglobin are rapid and give accurate results only when the equipment is in good working condition. The spectrophotometer must be working well, and the pipettes and calibrated cuvettes must be clean and free from breaks or scratches. Hemiglobincyanide reagent, if prepared by the laboratory, must be prepared fresh each month and stored in a brown bottle to prevent deterioration. Spectrophotometers must be standardized before being used for the hemoglobin determination. They should be restandardized periodically and the calibrated hemoglobin tables redone when changes occur in the values. Each spectrophotometer must have a calibration table.

Before the unknown samples are read in the spectrophotometer, they must be crystal-clear. If there is any

---

Procedure 11–2. Hemoglobin: Hemiglobincyanide Manual Method Using the Unopette System

1. Allow the spectrophotometer to warm up adequately. Set the wavelength scale at 540 nm.
2. Prepare a blank tube with 5 mL of hemiglobincyanide reagent. Use one hemoglobin Unopette reservoir to fill a cuvette.
3. Label cuvettes or tubes for each specimen.
4. Assemble necessary equipment: Unopette 20-μL (0.02 mL) capillary pipette, and reservoir with 5-mL hemiglobincyanide reagent.
5. Puncture the neck of the reservoir with the shielded pipette to make an opening for the blood sample.
6. Obtain blood sample from a free-flowing finger or heel puncture or from a well-mixed venous blood specimen collected in EDTA.
7. Holding the capillary pipette in an almost horizontal position, touch the tip of the pipette to the blood. Capillary action fills the pipette and the blood collection into the pipette stops automatically. Wipe any excess blood off the *outside* of the pipette, making certain to remove no blood from *inside* the capillary bore.
8. Insert the capillary pipette into the reservoir through the open diaphragm (neck) without seating the pipette firmly in the reservoir neck.
9. Squeeze the reservoir. Cover the upper opening of the pipette (overflow chamber) with the index finger and then seat the pipette firmly into the reservoir. Remove the finger from the pipette opening and blood will be drawn into the diluent by suction.
10. Squeeze the reservoir gently two or three times to rinse the capillary bore, forcing diluent up into, but not out of, the overflow chamber, releasing pressure each time to return the mixture to the reservoir.
11. Place the index finger over the upper opening of the pipette and *gently* invert a few times to mix blood and diluent.
12. Wait at least 3 minutes for color development to take place.
13. Invert the reservoir tube over the cuvette used for spectrophotometry and squeeze the entire contents of the reservoir into the cuvette. If a spectrophotometer with a flow-through system is being used, the contents of the reservoir are emptied directly into the flow-through apparatus.
14. Read the blank solution at 540 nm and adjust to 100%*T*. Then read the unknown hemoglobin samples using the same wavelength. Record readings in percent transmittance to the nearest ¼ %T unit.
15. Convert the percent transmittance readings to concentrations by using the calibration curve or table prepared for the photometer (see under Standardization of the Coleman Junior Spectrophotometer).
16. Report hemoglobin results to the first decimal place.
17. Test quality control samples daily and plot the values on the control chart for the machine. Only when the control values check out are the patient values reported out to the physician.
18. Duplicate determinations should agree within 0.4 g/dL or the procedure should be repeated.

---

turbidity, a falsely high result will be read. Turbidity may result from exceptionally high white blood cell counts, the presence of Hb S or Hb C, the presence of abnormal globulins, or lipemic blood specimens. The use of the modified hemiglobincyanide reagents (with detergents added) have eliminated many of these interferences.

Blood containing carbon monoxide requires 3 hours for the formation of hemiglobincyanide from carboxyhemoglobin with hemiglobincyanide reagent.

One of the greatest causes of error is improper pipetting technique. Using precalibrated, self-filling pipettes (such as the Unopette) helps to eliminate some of this error. If the capillary blood flow is slow and the finger is squeezed to obtain the sample, error can result from the introduction of tissue juice into the blood sample. If venous blood is not mixed well before measurement, gross errors result.

Salts and solutions of cyanide are poisonous and care should be taken to avoid getting them into the mouth or inhaling their fumes. Hemiglobincyanide reagent contains 50 mg of potassium cyanide per liter, significantly less than the lethal dose for an average 70-kg person. Nevertheless, this reagent must be handled with great care. Many laboratories obtain the reagent commercially, so that handling KCN is not necessary. The salt is potentially very dangerous and must be kept in a secure place if it is used by the laboratory.

Samples and reagents must be discarded carefully and under no circumstances come in contact with acid. Hydrogen cyanide gas (HCN) is released when the hemiglobincyanide reagent is acidified. Samples and reagents can be poured down a laboratory sink drain while using large amounts of running tap water before, during, and after disposal to eliminate the danger of cyanide fumes.

Because Sahli to-contain pipettes may be less accurate than claimed by the manufacturer, it is wise to set aside several calibrated pipettes for use in hemoglobin tests, if possible. Most Sahli pipettes supplied by reputable companies should be accurate to 1%. They should be cleaned with acid and thoroughly washed with water once a week. They must be washed and dried between measurements.

To eliminate error resulting from poorly calibrated cuvettes or cuvettes that are not matched correctly, many photometric instruments are supplied with a flow-through cuvette system. The solution to be read is poured directly into the system. After each reading, the solution is emptied into a discard container by means of a valve in the bottom of the cuvette. Since all readings, standards, controls, and unknowns are taken through the same flow-through cuvette, errors caused by imperfectly matched cuvettes are eliminated.

Reference Values*

For adult male:
  15.7 (14.0–17.5) g/dL
For adult female:
  13.8 (12.3–15.3) g/dL
For 12-month-old:
  12.6 (11.1–14.1) g/dL
For 10-year-old:
  13.4 (11.8–15.0) g/dL
The mean hemoglobin level of blacks of both sexes and all ages is reported to be 0.5–1.0 g/dL below the mean for comparable whites.

*Williams WJ, Beutler E, Erslev A, et al: *Hematology*, ed 4. New York, McGraw-Hill Book Co, 1990, pp 10, 18.

HEMATOCRIT (PACKED CELL VOLUME)

The hematocrit (Hct) is a macroscopic observation by which the percentage volume of the packed RBCs is measured. Hematocrit is therefore also known as the packed cell volume, or PCV. This test is relatively simple and reliable. It gives useful information about the RBCs which may be correlated with the number of RBCs and their hemoglobin content (see under Counting Erythrocytes and Leukocytes and under Hemoglobin). These measurements together enable the red cell indices to be calculated (see under Red Cell Indices). The hematocrit measurement is more useful and reliable than the red cell count done manually because much less error is associated with it. Most hospital laboratories perform hematocrit determinations along with hemoglobin measurements, and some do the hematocrit even more regularly. A fast quality control check on hemoglobin results (in g/dL) is done by comparing them with the hematocrit results, (in % units) using the following formula:

$$Hb \times 3 = Hct \pm 3 \text{ units}$$

The hematocrit is used in evaluating and classifying the various types of anemias according to red cell indices. There are two manual methods for determining the hematocrit described in this book: the Wintrobe method, a macrohematocrit method, and the microhematocrit method. The microhematocrit method has the advantages that it takes less time and labor and requires a smaller blood sample and has generally replaced the macro method in clinical use. The procedure is well-suited to screen for anemia in certain clinics where actual hemoglobin determinations are impractical, such as for potential blood donors or for children for adequate nutritional status, especially for iron deficiency. The electronic cell counters give a calculated hematocrit value and have generally replaced the manual methods.

When whole blood is centrifuged, the heavier particles fall to the bottom of the tube and the lighter particles settle on top of the heavier cells. The hematocrit is the percentage of red cells in a volume of whole blood. It is expressed as units of percent or as a ratio in the SI system. The value determined in venous blood by the Wintrobe method agrees closely with the value in capillary blood by the microhematocrit method. When reading the hematocrit result, it is important to take the reading *at the top* of the RBC layer, particularly when there is an extremely elevated white cell or platelet count. The buffy coat (WBCs and platelets) should not be included in the measurement of red cell volume for the hematocrit result.

Methods for Quantitative Measurement

The microhematocrit method is used commonly. It can be done with either free-flowing capillary blood from a finger puncture or EDTA-anticoagulated venous blood; a very small amount of blood is needed. The test is also done with a high-speed centrifuge, which means a relatively short centrifugation time. The microhematocrit is therefore a quick test and the results can be ready in a short time.

The Wintrobe method is a macromethod that requires more blood and a longer centrifugation time. Blood must be drawn by venipuncture and properly anticoagulated. This method is not used as much because it is time-consuming.

Both methods provide reliable values and have the same normal values, if the procedures are followed exactly.

An automated hematocrit result is obtained when electronic cell counters are used. This result is computed from individual red cell volumes and is not affected by the trapped plasma left in the red cell column for the manual microhematocrit and Wintrobe methods. Therefore, the hematocrit value obtained with the automated cell counters is lower than the value obtained by the centrifugation methods.

Specimens

Blood for the Wintrobe method must be anticoagulated with EDTA or heparin which do not alter the volume of the RBCs. The blood sample must be well mixed before doing the test.

Capillary blood can be used for the microhematocrit method. Special capillary tubes are filled with the blood directly from the puncture site. These glass tubes are coated with heparin for use with capillary blood and can also be purchased without heparin for use with anticoagulated venous blood. Heparin-lined tubes must always be used with capillary blood but must not be used with anti-

coagulated venous blood as an excess of anticoagulant can cause cell shrinkage resulting in falsely low values. Free-flowing blood must be used for the microhematocrit measurement.

Properly anticoagulated blood using EDTA is used for automated analysis.

Equipment for Nonautomated Methods

For the Wintrobe method, a special hematocrit tube called the *Wintrobe tube* is used. This thick-walled glass tube is specially made with a uniform inner diameter and is graduated from 0 to 105 mm. It has a rubber cap, which prevents evaporation during the long period of centrifugation (30–45 minutes). Disposable tubes may be purchased for this method, and this eliminates washing small-bore glass tubes. The Wintrobe tube is filled with blood by using a *Pasteur pipette*. This is a long-stemmed glass capillary pipette and is usually disposable. A standard laboratory centrifuge capable of generating a relative centrifugal force of 2,300 to 2,500 g (g is the acceleration due to gravity) is needed to pack the RBCs sufficiently in the Wintrobe tube. For Wintrobe hematocrit procedure, see Procedure 11–4.

For the microhematocrit method, special nongraduated glass capillary tubes are used. These tubes are 1 mm in diameter and 7 cm long. They can be purchased lined with dried heparin for use with capillary blood, or plain (without heparin) for use with previously anticoagulated venous blood. Plain capillary tubes may be coated with heparin by filling them with a 1 : 1,000 dilution of heparin and drying in a 56° C oven. Some type of seal is needed for one end of the tube when it contains blood. A special sealing compound (similar to modeling clay) can be used for this purpose, or the end can be heat-sealed with a small gas flame. A special microhematocrit centrifuge is used, capable of producing centrifugal fields up to 10,000 g. The centrifugation time is 5 minutes; this being determined by centrifuging many samples at constant speed for 1 to 10 minutes and observing when the hematocrit measurement leveled off with maximum packing of red cells. Some centrifuges can reach speeds of 12 500 rpm. Because this greater speed leads to a greater relative centrifugal force (RCF), complete cell packing can be reached in 3 minutes with these centrifuges. The head of the microhematocrit centrifuge is made to hold the small capillary tubes. Since the capillary tubes are not graduated, a special reading device is used to measure the percentage of packed red blood cells after centrifugation. For microhematocrit procedure, see Procedure 11–3.

Procedure 11–3. Microhematocrit: Manual Method

1. Well-mixed EDTA-anticoagulated venous blood or blood from a finger puncture (or heel in an infant) from which blood flows freely is used.
2. Two microhematocrit capillary tubes are filled one-half to two-thirds full.
3. The dry end of each tube is sealed with a specially manufactured plastic sealing clay for these tubes. The tubes can also be heat-sealed.
4. The sealed tubes are centrifuged in a microhematocrit centrifuge for 4 to 5 minutes at 10,000 rpm.
5. The microhematocrit result is read with a graphic reading device or some other accurate measuring device. Graphic reading devices give the hematocrit directly as a percentage. Results for duplicate tests should agree within 2%. Alternatively, each result is reported in ratio units using the SI system, read to the nearest 0.005 unit. Duplicates should agree within 0.02 unit. In using these undesignated units, units of liter per liter are implied. This is a more recent reporting method utilizing SI units, of liter per liter as compared with an expression of percent. Using the former, hematocrit results are reported as a decimal fraction. A 45% result is reported as 0.45, for example. *Reference values* are influenced by the age and sex of the individual, as well as by the altitude (see also under Hemoglobin). For normal adults, the usual reference ranges for hematocrit are: females 0.40 ± 0.05; males 0.46 ± 0.05.

Precautions and Technical Factors

The blood sample must be properly collected and preserved. Anticoagulated blood samples using EDTA should be centrifuged within 6 hours of collection. EDTA is the anticoagulant of choice for both the Wintrobe and microhematocrit methods. The blood must not be clotted or hemolyzed for any hematocrit test. If clotted blood is used there will be false packing of the red cells, and the true packing in the tube will not be noted (a falsely high result will be observed). In a hemolyzed specimen some of the red cells have been destroyed, so again the packing of the red cells will not be true (a falsely low result will be observed). Centrifugation must be sufficient to yield maximum packing of the red cells. Preferably the centrifugation should be done with the hematocrit tube in an upright position, because it may be difficult to read the level of the packed cells when the tube is on a slant.

The hematocrit value is frequently accompanied by a hemoglobin determination. There should be a correlation between the two results: the hematocrit result in percent units should be approximately three times the hemoglobin result.

For the microhematocrit method, any capillary blood samples collected should be freely flowing. The capillary tubes must be properly sealed so that no leakage occurs. Since these tubes are not calibrated, the level of packed red cells and the total volume of the cells and plasma must be accurately measured by some convenient reading device. The buffy coat layer is not included in the reading for the hematocrit.

The microhematocrit centrifuge provides a greater relative centrifugal force, and less plasma is trapped in the cell layer. The results are therefore more accurate because the plasma does not interfere with the measurement of the red cell layer.

Even with adequate centrifugation, providing tightly packed red cells, a small amount of plasma remains trapped around the red cells. This is unavoidable and in normal blood, with normally shaped and sized red cells, this trapped plasma accounts for 1.5% to 3.0% of the height of the red cell column in a microhematocrit tube. When the red cells have an irregular shape or size, there will be an increase in the amount of plasma being trapped. When macrohematocrits are being done, the speed of centrifugation is slower and more plasma is trapped. Therefore, macrohematocrit values are consistently higher than microhematocrit values on the same sample. When hematocrits are determined using automated hematology analyzers, the hematocrit is determined indirectly by determining the average size of the

---

Procedure 11–4. Wintrobe Hematocrit: Manual Method*

1. The Pasteur pipette is used to transfer well-mixed venous blood to a clean, dry Wintrobe hematocrit tube. This is properly done by first placing the pipette in the bottom of the tube and gradually withdrawing it while expelling blood using a mechanical suction bulb until the tube is filled to the 100-mm mark. Bubbles in the tube must be avoided.

2. The tube is sealed with a cap and centrifuged at full speed in a suitable centrifuge (2,260 g) for 30 minutes. During centrifugation, the red cells, which have the highest specific gravity of the blood elements, settle to the bottom. The Wintrobe tube is calibrated from 0 to 105 mm (or 0–10.5 cm), and the levels of the various layers may be easily read.

3. After centrifugation, three layers are apparent in the tube (see Fig 11–1). These are, from the bottom: (1) red cells; (2) buffy coat, containing platelets, leukocytes, and other nucleated cells when present; and (3) plasma.

4. The level of the red cell column and the total height of the column of blood are noted. If the tube has been filled to exactly the 100-mm mark, the hematocrit in volume percent is equal to the reading at the top of the layer of packed red blood cells. If the tube is calibrated in centimeters instead of millimeters, the reading is multiplied by 10. When the height of the column of cells and plasma is not exactly 100 mm, a simple calculation can be made to correct for this. The following general formula applies:

$$\text{Hct } (\%) = \frac{packed \text{ RBC } height}{total \text{ blood } height} \times 100$$

This is exactly the same as setting up a proportion, as illustrated below:

$$\frac{Reading \text{ of packed RBC}}{Reading \text{ of plasma level}} = \frac{x}{100}$$

where x = hematocrit (%).

---

red cell population (the mean corpuscular volume, or MCV) and multiplying it by the total red cell count. The hematocrit value as determined by automation is therefore consistently lower than that done by the microhematocrit method, utilizing centrifugation, on the same blood sample.

Unique to the microhematocrit is the error caused by excess EDTA (inadequate blood for the fixed amount of EDTA in the blood collection tube). The microhematocrit will be falsely low because of cell shrinkage. Thus, heparinized capillary tubes must not be used with anticoagulated blood samples.

With good technique, the precision of the hematocrit is ±1%. Inadequate centrifugation will give falsely high results. If the tubes are not sealed properly, falsely low results will be obtained because more RBCs will be lost than plasma.

*Wintrobe M: *Clinical Hematology,* ed 8. Philadelphia, Lea & Febiger, 1981, pp 10–11.

Reference Values†

For adult male:
   Mean 0.46; 0.42–0.50 (42%–50%)
For adult female:
   Mean 0.40; 0.36–0.45 (36%–45%)

RED BLOOD CELL INDICES

In the classification of anemias, quantitative measurements of the average size, hemoglobin content, and hemoglobin concentration of the RBCs are of substantial aid to the physician (see under Erythrocyte Alterations). These can be calculated from the total number of red cells, the hemoglobin content per unit volume, and the hematocrit. The indices are the mean corpuscular (cell)

†Williams WJ, Beutler E, Erslev A, et al: *Hematology,* ed 4. New York, McGraw-Hill Book Co, 1990, p 10.

volume (MCV), mean corpuscular (cell) hemoglobin (MCH), and mean corpuscular (cell) hemoglobin concentration (MCHC).

The MCV defines the volume or size of the average RBC, the MCHC defines the hemoglobin concentration or color of the average RBC, and the MCH defines the weight of hemoglobin in the average RBC.

Another quantitative measurement of the red cells, the mean corpuscular diameter (MCD), is made directly. A derived measurement determined electronically is the red cell distribution width (RDW). This is a measurement of the degree of red cell variability.

Determination of these indices has become routine with the use of the electronic cell counter, such as the model S Coulter counter. This instrument determines the hemoglobin, MCV, and RBC count, and then automatically calculates the hematocrit, MCH, and MCHC.

When the indices are calculated from manually determined values for hemoglobin, hematocrit, and red cell count, the greatest inaccuracy results from errors associated with the red cell count. By electronically counting the number of RBCs, this error is significantly reduced. Indices calculated by electronic methods have been found to be more accurate by several investigators. It is important to verify all indices against observations of stained blood films. When the red cell indices are used in conjunction with an examination of the stained blood film, a clear picture of red cell morphology is obtained.

Since an RBC is very small and the amount of hemoglobin in a single cell is minute, the units in which the red cell indices are measured and recorded are micrometers (μm) and picograms (pg). The values for the red cell indices stay relatively constant and do not vary by more than one unit for any of the three indices. Because of this small variation, even in pathologic conditions (such patients do not show great variation either, unless they have received a blood transfusion), the indices are useful as a measure of quality control.

The red cell indices are part of the routine automated hematology profile performed on most patients and the data are considered highly reliable.

Mean Corpuscular Volume

The MCV is the average volume of an RBC in femtoliters (fL = 10^{-15} L). It is calculated manually by di-

viding the volume of red cells per liter by the number of red cells per liter, using the formula

$$MCV \ (fL) = \frac{Hct \ (\%) \times 10}{RBC \ count \ (\times 10^{12}/L)}$$

where the factor 10 is introduced to convert the hematocrit reading (in %) from volume of packed red cells per 100 mL to volume per liter. For example, if the Hct reading is 40% and the red cell count is 5 million (5 $\times$ 10^{12}/L) cells per liter,

$$MCV = \frac{40 \times 10}{5} = 80 \ fL$$

Another example given when the hematocrit is measured in liter-per-liter units:

$$MCV \ (fL) = \frac{Hct \ (L/L)}{RBC \ count \ (\times 10^{12}/L)} \times 10^3$$

The MCV in normal adults is between 80 and 96 fL.

The MCV indicates whether the RBCs will appear microcytic, normocytic, or macrocytic. If the MCV is less than 80 fL, the red cells will be microcytic. If it is greater than 96 fL, the red cells will be macrocytic. If it is within the normal range, the red cells will be normocytic. In some macrocytic anemias (for instance, pernicious anemia) the MCV may be as high as 150 fL. In microcytic anemia with marked iron deficiency, it may be 60 to 70 fL. The chief source of error in the MCV is the considerable error in the manual red cell count if used.

With the advent of automated cell counters and electronically calculated indices, the MCV has become increasingly valuable. It is now considered the most reliable automated index and is probably the most effective discriminant for the classification of anemias. Previously, the MCHC was the most reliable index, since it was calculated from the two manual measurements that could be done most accurately, the hematocrit and the hemoglobin concentration.

Mean Corpuscular Hemoglobin

The MCH is the average weight of hemoglobin content in an RBC in picograms (pg = 10^{-12} g). It is obtained by dividing the hemoglobin content of 1 L of blood (in g/L) by the number of RBCs in 1 L. A simple formula can be used to calculate this value:

$$MCH\ (pg) = \frac{Hb\ (g/dL) \times 10}{RBC\ count\ (\times 10^{12}/L)}$$

For example, if the hemoglobin content is 15 g/dL and the RBC count is $5 \times 10^{12}/L$

$$MCH = \frac{15 \times 10}{5} = 30\ pg$$

The normal range for the MCH is 27 to 33 pg. It should always correlate with the MCV and MCHC. It may be as high as 50 pg in macrocytic anemias or as low as 20 pg or less in hypochromic microcytic anemias.

The chief source of error is the RBC count if counted manually, which must be accurate if this calculation is to be of use to the physician. This value is calculated electronically by the electronic cell counters.

Mean Corpuscular Hemoglobin Concentration

The MCHC is an expression of the average hemoglobin concentration per unit volume of packed red cells. It is expressed as grams per deciliter. It may be calculated from the MCV and the MCH or from the hemoglobin and hematocrit values by using the following formula:

$$MCHC\ (g/dL) = \frac{MCH}{MCV} \times 100$$

or

$$MCHC\ (g/dL) = \frac{Hb\ (g/dL)}{Hct\ (L/L)}$$

For example, if the hemoglobin concentration is 15 g/dL and the Hct is 0.40 L/L (40%)

$$MCHC = \frac{15}{0.40} = 37.5\ g/dL$$

This measurement tells what percentage of a unit volume (1 dL) of RBCs is hemoglobin. Normal values range from 33 to 36 g/dL, and values below 32 g/dL indicate hypochromia. An MCHC above 40 g/dL would indicate malfunctioning of the instrument or error in the calculation of the manual measurements used, because an MCHC of 37 g/dL is near the upper limits for hemoglobin solubility, thus limiting the physiologic upper limits for the MCHC. In true hypochromic anemias the hemoglobin concentration is reduced, and values as low as 20 to 25 g/dL are not uncommon.

Red Cell Distribution Width

This is a measurement of the degree of anisocytosis present, or the degree of red cell size variability in a blood sample. This measurement is derived by the electronic cell counters that can directly measure the MCV as one of the parameters determined. If anisocytosis is present on the peripheral blood film, and the variation in red cell size is prominent, then there is an increase in the standard deviation of the MCV from the mean.

In the Coulter Model S Plus, for example, a red cell histogram is plotted and the RDW (%) is defined as the coefficient of variation of the MCV:

$$RDW\ (\%) = \frac{SD\ of\ MCV}{mean\ MCV} \times 100$$

The reference range for RDW is from 11% to 15%, but varies with the instrument used.

Indices: Precautions, Technical Factors, and General Comments

Any manual RBC count, hematocrit, and hemoglobin concentration used in the calculations must be accurate. It is also essential to check the appearance of the RBCs in a well-stained blood film against the calculated indices. The calculations must agree with the appearance of the red cells in the blood film. For example, a corresponding decrease in hemoglobin color intensity should be observed on the blood film when there is a low MCHC (an increase in the amount of central pallor in the red cells), but often it is difficult to recognize hypochromasia under these circumstances. The MCHC is often below 30 g/dL before hypochromasia is observed on the blood film.

Reference Values*

Mean corpuscular volume (MCV): mean 88.0 fL (range 80–96.1 fL)
Mean corpuscular hemoglobin (MCH): mean 30.4 pg (range 27.5–33.2 pg)
Mean corpuscular hemoglobin concentration (MCHC): mean 34.4 g/dL (range 33.4–35.5 g/dL)
Red cell distribution width (RDW): mean 13.1% (range 11.5%–14.5%)

ERYTHROCYTE SEDIMENTATION RATE

The erythrocyte sedimentation test is another hematologic determination that employs macroscopic observation. If blood is prevented from clotting (by using a suitable anticoagulant) and allowed to settle, sedimentation of the erythrocytes will occur. The rate at which the red cells fall is known as the **erythrocyte sedimentation rate (ESR).** This rate depends on three main factors: (1) the number and size of erythrocyte particles, (2) plasma factors, and (3) certain technical and mechanical factors.

The most important factor determining the rate of fall of the RBCs is the size or mass of the falling particle: the larger the particle, the faster it falls. The size of the falling particles depends on the formation of red cell aggregates, which in turn depends on the presence of certain factors in the plasma. The rate of sedimentation appears to be dependent on the amount of fibrinogen or globulin present in the plasma. In normal blood, the red cells tend to remain separate from one another because they are negatively charged (zeta potential) and tend to repel one another. In many pathologic conditions the phenomenon of erythrocyte aggregation is caused by alteration of the erythrocyte surface charge by plasma proteins. The protein that is most often involved is fibrinogen, although increases in gamma globulins or abnormal proteins also produce this effect. These factors determine the size of the aggregates of erythrocytes. With increased concentrations of large molecules in the plasma, there is a greater tendency for erythrocytes to pile up in rouleau formation (resembling a stack of coins).

*Williams WJ, Beutler E, Erslev A, et al: *Hematology,* ed 4. New York, McGraw-Hill Book Co, 1990, p 10.

Stages of Erythrocyte Sedimentation

The sedimentation of erythrocytes in a sample of blood may be plotted as a curve on graph paper, with the millimeters of fall as the ordinate and the time in minutes as the abscissa. Such a curve shows at first a variable period of gradual fall during which the aggregates of erythrocytes are forming (rouleau formation). Next, very rapid and marked fall of the aggregates occurs, constituting the main portion of the sedimentation of erythrocytes. The last part of the curve represents a more gradual, but relatively slight, falling off of the sedimentation rate as the erythrocyte aggregates are being packed at the bottom of the sedimentation tube. This packing will be more marked in an anemic patient than in a person with the normal number of erythrocytes. In any event, the effect of anemia on the sedimentation rate will be relatively slight. By far the most important factor in determining the rate of sedimentation is the size of the erythrocyte aggregates, or rouleau.

Clinical Significance of the Erythrocyte Sedimentation Rate

The ESR is a nonspecific screening test for inflammatory activity. In the vast majority of infections there is at least some increase in the ESR; chorea and undulant fever are two exceptions. The ESR also increases in most cases of carcinoma, leukemia and diseases of the bone marrow, degenerative vascular disease, active rheumatic fever, multiple myeloma, systemic lupus, rheumatoid arthritis, and acute gout. As patients recover from infectious diseases, the sedimentation rate slowly returns to normal. It may still be increased long after other clinical manifestations have disappeared, showing that the defense mechanisms of the body continue to be more active than normal. Increased numbers of erythrocytes, as seen in cases of polycythemia and failure of the right side of the heart, tend to cause a marked slowing of sedimentation. When the hematocrit is greater than 48% to 50%, sedimentation is markedly slowed, regardless of any factors present that might otherwise accelerate it.

A decrease in the ESR will result when the plasma fibrinogen level is decreased, as in cases of severe liver disease (e.g., acute yellow atrophy). The ESR is not increased in viral diseases, such as infectious mononucleosis and acute hepatitis, probably because fibrinogen production is not increased in these diseases in spite of a pronounced inflammatory reaction. The ESR is also not usually increased in chronic degenerative joint disease (it is increased, however, in inflammatory joint disease).

Methods for Determination of the Erythrocyte Sedimentation Rate

There are two traditional methods for determining the sedimentation rate: the Westergren method (Procedure 11–5) and the Wintrobe method. Normal values for both methods are sedimentation rates of 0 to 20 mm in 1 hour for women and 0 to 15 mm in 1 hour for men. The normal ESR varies with age, sex, and the specific methodology used.

Both methods use venous blood, which must be properly anticoagulated. EDTA is used as the usual anticoagulant. Heparin is unsatisfactory and should not be used for the ESR test.

Wintrobe Method

For the Wintrobe method, enough blood is drawn into a Pasteur pipette to fill a *Wintrobe hematocrit tube* to the 100-mm mark. Bubbles must be avoided. The tube is placed in the support rack in an exactly vertical position so that the cells will sediment properly, and the time is noted. At the end of 1 hour, the ESR is read as the length of the plasma column above the cells. This method is simple and requires a small amount of blood.

Westergren Method

The Westergren method is the reference method for the ESR.* For this test, the procedure should be carried out within 2 hours after the blood has been drawn. The blood is mixed well with sodium citrate or NaCl and drawn into a *Westergren tube* to the zero mark. The tube is placed in a rack in an exactly vertical position at room temperature. Direct drafts, sunlight, and vibrations must be avoided. In most Westergren methods, a liquid sodium citrate solution is added to the blood before it is drawn into the tube. One modification of this method eliminates the addition of the citrate solution and still gives satisfactory results. The time when the tube is placed in the rack is noted and a reading is taken at 60 minutes. The length of the plasma level above the red cells is measured in millimeters from the markings on the tube. A larger amount of blood is required for the Westergren method. See Procedure 11–5.

One commercial product utilizing the Westergren method for performing the ESR test is the Sediplast System (LP Italiana S.p.a., Acculab, a division of Precision Technology, Norwood, N.J.). This employs a capped vial prefilled with 3.8% sodium citrate. To this vial is added the required amount of blood sample which results in the correct sodium citrate-to-blood ratio of 1:4. This diluted sample is used to fill the Sediplast Autozero tube which is placed in a vertical position in its special rack on a level surface. The ESR is read after 1 hour. See Procedure 11–6.

Equipment for the Westergren Method.—The Westergren tube is really an open-ended pipette. The classic tube is 300 mm long with an inner diameter of 2.5 mm and is graduated in millimeters from 0 at the top of the tube to 200 at the bottom. The graduated volume of the tube is 1.0 mL. A special rack to hold the Westergren pipettes in a vertical position is needed for this test. The Westergren sedimentation rack is constructed so that rubber stoppers attached to springs close the open ends of the tubes when they are placed properly in the rack. Mechanical suction should be used to fill Westergren tubes.

Procedure 11–5. Erythrocyte Sedimentation Rate Using the Modified Westergren Method

1. Five milliliters of venous blood is drawn into EDTA.
2. Two milliliters of well-mixed EDTA blood is diluted with 0.5 mL of 3.8 g/dL sodium citrate or 0.5 mL of 0.85 g/dL NaCl. (The original Westergren method used sodium citrate as the anticoagulant. The modified method employs EDTA blood, but this is diluted to give results consistent with the classic Westergren method.)
3. The diluted blood-citrate mixture is mixed well.
4. A Westergren tube is filled to the zero mark with the diluted blood using mechanical suction and placed vertically in the Westergren rack.
5. The upper level to which the red cells fall is read in millimeters from the graduation marks on the tube at 60 minutes. These readings are recorded.

---

*Westergren A: The techniques of the red cell sedimentation reaction. *Am Rev Tuberc Pulmonary Dis* 1926; 14:94.

Procedure 11–6. Erythrocyte Sedimentation Rate Using Sediplast

1. Remove the cap on the vial containing sodium citrate. Using a disposable pipette, fill the vial to the indicated fill line with the well-mixed EDTA blood sample to be tested (approximately 0.8 mL of blood is required). Mix thoroughly using the pipetting device.
2. Insert the autozero Westergren (Sediplast) tube into the vial using a slight twisting motion, allowing the blood to rise to the zero mark and the excess blood to flow into the reservoir overflow compartment at the top of the tube. Continue inserting the tube until it rests at the bottom of the vial. The tube must completely touch the bottom of the vial to ensure proper results with this system.
3. Allow the sample to stand vertically for exactly 1 hour and then read the numerical results of the erythrocyte sedimentation in millimeters. Record.
4. Discard all supplies after use in a suitable biowaste container.

Precautions and Technical Factors

An anticoagulant that not only prevents clotting but preserves the shape and volume of the red cells must be used. Anticoagulants that prevent erythrocyte sedimentation are unsuitable for this test. Since erythrocyte numbers influence the rate of fall, the specimen must not be hemolyzed. Fibrin clots must not be present. The tube used for the test must be placed vertically in the rack; an angle different from this position can alter the rate of fall significantly. As the blood specimen stands after the venipuncture, the suspension stability of the erythrocytes increases. The test must be set up in the Westergren tube within 2 hours after the blood has been drawn to ensure a reliable sedimentation rate. Preferably the test should be set up within 1 hour. Specimens may be refrigerated for up to 6 hours. Temperature and vibrations can affect the sedimentation rate, and these factors should be taken into consideration.

Reporting of Test Results

The RBCs in the ESR tube are allowed to sediment for 1 hour. The results of the test are expressed in milli-meters, the distance of fall of the top of the red cell column, after 1 hour. Reporting an ESR result in this manner indicates that this test measures a *distance* of fall after a specified time interval. A reference ESR procedure has been devised which uses a standardized hematocrit.[*] The whole blood specimen anticoagulated with EDTA is adjusted to a hematocrit of 0.35 by adding or removing the patient's own plasma. After adjustment to the desired hematocrit, the Westergren ESR is set up. This procedure is for standardization only and is not used for routine laboratory ESR testing.

Reference Values[†]

Erythrocyte sedimentation rate:
  Male: 0–10 mm/hr
  Female: 0–20 mm/hr

COUNTING THE FORMED ELEMENTS OF THE BLOOD (HEMOCYTOMETRY)

Enumeration of the formed elements of the blood is a fundamental measurement in the hematology laboratory. The procedures used for enumeration include manual microscopic observation and the use of electronic counting devices. The cells counted in routine practice are RBCs, WBCs, and platelets. Manual techniques, however, lend themselves to enumeration of all small separate bodies in the field of pathology (such as spermatozoa, eosinophils, and cells in cerebrospinal fluid). The main principles for cell enumeration and examination are (1) selection of a diluting fluid that will dilute the cells so that manageable numbers may be counted and will either identify them in some manner or destroy contaminant cellular elements, and (2) use of a **hemocytometer,** or electronic cell counter, that will present the cells to the laboratorian or to an **electronic counting device** in such a way that the number of cells per unit volume of fluid can be counted. The electronic counting device avoids human error. It is also statistically more accurate because

---

[*]*Reference Procedure for Human Erythrocyte Sedimentation Rate (ESR) Test. Approved Standard.* Villanova, Pa, National Committee for Clinical Laboratory Standards, 1988; 8(August) H2-A2.

[†]Wintrobe MM: Clinical Hematology, ed 8. Philadelphia, Lea & Febiger, 1981, p 1885.

it can count many more cells than can be counted manually.

Since there are a great many formed elements per unit volume of blood, it is necessary to dilute the blood before attempting to count them. Methods for counting the formed elements of the blood are designed to obtain the number of cells in 1 L of whole blood, the unit (SI) of measurement of volume recommended by the International Committee for Standardization in Hematology (ICSH). The units formerly used to record cell counts were cells per cubic millimeter and cells per microliter.

Units Reported

Since the enumerated constituents are to be reported in units per liter of blood, the number of cells or formed elements actually counted (platelets, RBCs, WBCs, eosinophils) must be converted to the number present per liter of blood. The alternative method is units of cells per cubic millimeter (mm^3) or microliter (μL) since 1 μL is essentially equal to 1 mm^3. The reporting unit of choice, however, is cells per liter of blood. Therefore, the following conversion *example* applies:

$$1 \ mm^3 = 1 \ \mu L = 10^{-6} \ L$$

$$1 \times 10^6 \ \mu L = 1 \ L$$

General Methods Used to Count Blood Cells

Whether an electronic cell counter or one of the nonautomated manual methods is used, the steps in the procedure include diluting the blood sample quantitatively by using special measuring devices (pipettes) and diluents, determining the number of cells in the diluted sample, and converting the number of cells in the diluted sample to the final result—the number of cells in 1 L of whole blood.

Blood cell counts are done on minute portions of already small samples of an individual's blood. For this reason, errors are inherent in the best methods, and the steps in the procedure must be performed as carefully as possible to reduce the variation of the final result from the actual or true count.

To provide experience in counting the formed elements, practice is done using preserved blood samples. Before using any blood sample, the laboratorian must make certain that it has been preserved with the proper anticoagulant and has been properly labeled, and that its appearance indicates that a good collection technique was used. Each sample should be checked for hemolysis and small clots (known as fibrin clots) as soon as it is received. Clotted blood or samples with fibrin clots are unacceptable for cell counts. Universal precautions must always be used when handling any blood specimen.

Counting Erythrocytes and Leukocytes

The leukocyte count is routinely included in most initial studies for a new patient. It is a basic procedure in the hematology laboratory. With common use of automated cell counters the erythrocyte count is also considered a routine laboratory examination. Before the advent of automatic cell counting devices, the erythrocyte count had been virtually eliminated from most routine laboratory tests because of the large error ($\pm 20\%$) in the manual methods of counting red cells. White cells are still counted manually in smaller laboratories, and when carefully done, this is an accurate measurement.

Manual cell counting methods are stressed in this chapter. The manufacturers of electronic cell counting devices supply the purchaser with details of the use and care of the instruments. When a new instrument is used, manufacturer's instructions must be followed explicitly.

Clinical Significance of Cell Counts

Leukocyte Counts.—The normal leukocyte count varies from 4.4 to 11.3 $\times 10^9$/L. An increase in the leukocyte count above the normal upper limit is termed *leukocytosis*. A decrease below the normal lower limit is termed *leukopenia*. Leukopenia may occur after x-ray therapy; after the administration of certain drugs; in infections with agents such as the typhoid group, certain viruses, and malaria; and in pernicious anemia. Leukocytosis may occur in many acute infections, in severe malaria, after hemorrhage, during pregnancy, postoperatively, in some forms of anemia, in some carcinomas, and in leukemia. Leukemia is characterized by proliferation of the leukocytes and their precursors in the tissues of the body and is associated with many changes in the circulating cells of the blood. Blood films prepared from leukemia patients should be examined only by qualified persons—a pathologist or an experienced medical technologist. There are two main classifications of leukemia, *lymphocytic* and *nonlymphocytic,* according to the predominant type of leukocyte seen. Leukemias are further divided into the subclassifications *acute* and *chronic*. In the acute condition, the disease progresses rapidly and morphologic changes are marked. In the chronic condition, the changes are neither as rapid nor as marked.

The normal leukocyte count varies with age. The white cell count of a newborn baby is $10-30 \times 10^9/L$ at birth and drops to about $10 \times 10^9/L$ after the first week of life. By about age 4 years, the white cell count reaches the normal level.

As mentioned earlier, the leukocyte count is used by the physician to indicate the presence of infection and to follow the progress of certain diseases. It may be elevated in acute bacterial infections, appendicitis, pregnancy, hemolytic disease of the newborn, uremia, and ulcers, and may be decreased in hepatitis, rheumatoid arthritis, cirrhosis of the liver, and lupus erythematosus. A child's leukocyte count usually shows a much greater variation during disease than an adult's. An individual's leukocyte count is subject to some variation during the course of a normal day, being slightly higher in the afternoon than in the morning. There is also an increase in the leukocyte count after strenuous exercise, emotional stress, and anxiety.

Erythrocyte Counts.—*Anemia* is a term generally applied to a decrease in the number of erythrocytes. There are many types of anemias. Anemia can be caused by excessive blood loss or blood destruction (called *hemolytic anemia*). Anemias caused by decreased blood cell or hemoglobin formation include pernicious anemia, bone marrow failure anemia, and iron deficiency anemia. Polycythemia is a condition in which the number of erythrocytes is increased.

Nonautomated (Manual) Cell Counts

Diluents Used.—Because the blood cells are so numerous, they cannot be counted accurately without dilution.

For Erythrocytes.—When RBCs are counted, we know from the principle of osmosis that the most important characteristic of the diluent is isotonicity. Two other necessary characteristics of a diluent for red cell counts are that it prevents clumping or clotting of the cells and has the proper specific gravity, so that all the cells will settle as evenly as possible. Hayem's solution is a diluent commonly used for manual counting of red cells. It contains mercuric chloride ($HgCl_2$) to prevent clumping of the red cells, and sodium sulfate (Na_2SO_4) and sodium chloride (NaCl) to provide the proper specific gravity and

isotonicity. Other diluents for red cell counts include 0.85 g/dL saline solution, Gowers' solution, Toison's solution, and Rees-Ecker solution.

Directions for Preparation of Hayem's Solution for Red Cell Counts.—Dissolve 15 g of NaCl, 33 g of anhydrous Na_2SO_4, and 7.5 g of $HgCl_2$, and dilute to 3,000 mL with deionized water.

For Leukocytes.—In the methods for leukocyte counts, the diluting fluid must meet a very different requirement—it must destroy the more numerous red cells so that the white cells may be counted more readily. (The white cells need not be eliminated when counting red cells.) The principle of osmotic pressure is again employed, but in a different way. The diluent used most commonly for white cell counts is 2 mL/dL acetic acid, which (1) darkens the nuclei of the white cells so that they are easier to see, and (2) hemolyzes the red cells. When the acetic acid hemolyzes the red cells, it converts the hemoglobin released from the red cells into acid hematin, which gives the resulting solution a brown color. The intensity of the brown color is directly related to the amount of hemoglobin present in the red cells. When using the Unopette system, the reservoir for white cell counts contains 0.475 mL of 3 mL/dL acetic acid. Another diluting fluid used for white cell counts is 0.1N HCl. The principle is the same with either 2 or 3 mL/dL acetic acid or 0.1N HCl.

Directions for Preparation of Acetic Acid for White Cell Counts (2 mL/dL).—Dilute 60 mL of glacial acetic acid to 3,000 mL with deionized water. Any diluent used must be filtered immediately before use to eliminate foreign particles, which might be confused with the cells to be counted.

Unopette System for Cell Counts.—The standard Unopette system is comprised of a self-filling glass pipette available in various sizes depending on the procedure to be performed. Each pipette is color-coded and marked with its measuring capacity. The end opposite the pipette tip is termed the *overflow chamber* (see Fig 11–5). The shield over the pipette tip protects the pipette and is also designed to puncture the diaphragm of the reservoir prior to use.

The reservoir is the other main component of the Unopette system. The reservoir contains a premeasured volume of diluent. The container is sealed with a covering of plastic, the diaphragm, located in the neck of the reservoir. It is this diaphragm that must be opened by puncture with the pipette shield prior to actual use.

The Unopette system is a self-filling, disposable system that has proved extremely useful where manual cell counts must be performed: manual cell counts for eosinophils, platelet counts in thrombocytopenic patients, and leukocyte counts in neutropenic patients.

Special Unopettes are available for platelet counts, leukocyte counts, hemoglobin measurement, erythrocyte counts, reticulocyte counts, eosinophil counts, and erythrocyte fragility tests. Unopette systems are available for various hematologic automated analyzers and for some chemistry determinations (blood lead and sodium and potassium determinations by flame photometry).*

The use of these disposable, self-filling precalibrated glass capillary pipettes for measuring and diluting blood for cell counts has proved extremely helpful. The Unopette system was described previously under Hemoglobin. It consists of a special glass pipette attached to a holder, and a plastic reservoir containing diluent (see Fig 11–5). The pipette fills automatically with blood, either capillary or venous, by means of capillary action, and the blood stops automatically when the pipette is filled (see Procedure 11–2). This avoids the errors inherent in drawing blood into Thoma pipettes. The 25-µL capillary Unopette pipette used for white cell counts is inserted into the reservoir containing 0.475 mL 3 mL/dL acetic acid for dilution of WBCs, emptied carefully, and rinsed, and the resulting solution in the reservoir is mixed well. The Unopette pipette and reservoir system is easily converted to a dropper assembly for charging the counting chamber. The manufacturer's directions must be followed carefully.

Thoma Pipettes for Cell Counts.—To ensure proper dilution of the sample to be used for counting blood cells, the blood measurement and correct dilution can be done with Thoma pipettes (Fig 11–6 and Procedure 11–7).

Thoma pipettes require aspirating tubes and suction. Because of the importance of universal precautionary techniques and the employment of barrier protective devices, the use of the Thoma pipettes has virtually been replaced by automated analyzers and the Unopette, if

*Laboratory Procedures Using the Unopette Brand System. Rutherford, NJ, Becton Dickinson & Co, 1977.

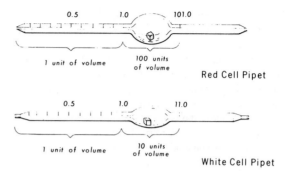

FIG 11–6.
Red cell *(above)* and white cell *(below)* Thoma diluting pipettes.

manual counting must be done. The Thoma pipette is, nevertheless, described for those laboratories where this pipette is still in use.

Laboratories employ various brands of diluting pipettes, all of which are generally of the same structure. The important differences are determined by the grade of glass used in the manufacture of the pipette and the calibration. Precalibration by the manufacturer and calibration checking in the hematology laboratory may appear complex. The procedure is more easily understood if it is compared to a matching process. The pipettes can be matched with National Bureau of Standards pipettes either by comparing the weight of some substance, such as mercury, contained in the unknown pipette with the weight of the same substance contained in the standard pipette, or by actually counting blood cells in equivalent cell samples. The mark (if any) on the pipette indicating that it has been checked will vary from laboratory to laboratory. It is therefore necessary to identify the calibration check mark and use only pipettes that have been properly calibrated. Using matched pipettes reduces the error from one source in blood cell counts by increasing the consistency of the dilution.

Several companies manufacture the type of pipette for white and red blood cell counts known as the *Thoma pipette*. Thoma is not a brand name but a type of pipette used for blood cell dilution. It is important to select only brands of pipettes that are reliable and accurate.

The Thoma pipette does not measure blood or diluent in definite amounts such as milliliters or millimeters, but instead provides the proper dilution in terms of a certain part of its volume to the total volume. It consists of a graduated capillary tube divided into 10 parts and marked 0.5 at the fifth mark and 1.0 at the tenth; a mixing bulb above the capillary tube containing a glass bead (which facilitates mixing of the blood and diluent); and another short capillary tube above the bulb with an engraved graduation mark (11.0 on the white cell pipette and 101.0 on the red cell pipette) (see Fig 11–6). The marks on the Thoma white cell pipette indicate that there are 11 units of volume in the pipette from the tip to the 11.0 mark above the bulb (see Fig 11–6). The 1.0 mark on the stem means that one of the units of volume for that pipette is contained in the stem from the tip of the pipette to the 1.0 mark. The single unit of volume in the stem is divided into 10 equal portions by measuring from the tip. The bulb is defined as extending from the 1.0 mark on the stem to the 11.0 mark on the short stem above the bulb, and it contains 10 units of volume.

Routinely, the dilution made for the white cell count is 1:20. This is accomplished by measuring whole blood from a well-mixed sample to the 0.5 mark and washing the sample into the bulb with the diluent to the 11.0 mark. The mixture in the bulb will contain 0.5 part of blood and 9.5 parts of diluent in the total of 10 units of volume in the bulb. The one unit in the stem contains diluent only and does not enter into the calculation of the dilution. The dilution factor is calculated by dividing 10 by 0.5, which is the same as determining what the total volume would have to be if 1 unit of blood were used with the same relative amount of diluent. The dilution is therefore 1:20.

The same procedure is used for the RBC dilution, except that the red cell pipette allows a ten times greater dilution than the white cell pipette. Rather than 11.0 total units of volume, the red cell pipette has 101.0 units of volume (see Fig 11–6). Therefore, when 0.5 unit of blood is measured and diluted to the 101.0 mark, the dilution is 1:200. There is 0.5 unit of blood and 99.5 units of diluent in the mixture contained in the bulb, which holds a total of 100 units. The 1 unit in the stem of the red cell pipette contains only diluent.

General Precautions for Pipetting With Thoma Pipettes.—Several precautions can be taken to avoid errors when doing a manual red or white blood cell count in the hematology laboratory. Pipettes must be clean, dry, and without chipped or broken tips. Technique must be practiced until completed pipettes are free from bubbles, packing, or clumping of cells. Contaminated diluting fluid must not be used. Periodically check the fluid in the diluting bottle; no blood should be al-

---

Procedure 11–7. Dilution With Thoma Pipettes

1. Filter the appropriate diluting fluid from the stock bottle into a small diluting bottle.
2. Using a properly mixed whole blood sample and the diluting pipette with aspiration tube attached, draw blood into the capillary bore of the pipette to slightly above the 0.5 mark.
3. Wipe off the *outside* of the pipette with gauze, and adjust the blood level to the 0.5 mark *exactly* by tapping the tip of the pipette with a gloved finger or using another nonabsorbent material. Do not use gauze for this adjustment, because the liquid portion of the sample inside the stem will be drawn into the gauze, leaving a higher concentration of cells inside the stem. Hold the pipette in a horizontal position.
4. Maintain the blood level at the 0.5 mark and place the tip of the pipette into the diluting fluid well below the surface of the liquid.
5. Using constant suction, draw the diluent into the pipette while at the same time lightly twirling the pipette between the fingers. Draw the mixture to the top mark above the bulb. While the bulb is being filled, tap the pipette with the finger to knock the bead down below the surface of the solution in the bulb. This will help to prevent bubbles from forming.
6. While removing the pipette from the diluent bottle, maintain the level of the mixture exactly on or slightly (never more than 1 mm) above the top mark by closing the pipette tip with the index finger. Holding the pipette in a horizontal position is also important. Remove the rubber aspirator tubing carefully, continuing to hold the index finger over the pipette tip.
7. As soon as the rubber tubing is removed, hold the pipette horizontally with the thumb and third finger at either end. Shake the pipette vigorously at right angles to its long axis for a few seconds. The glass bead in the pipette should move from one side to the other during the mixing. After shaking, the pipette may be put aside in a horizontal position, preventing any loss of its contents until the cell count is done.

lowed to get into the diluent because this will affect subsequent cell counts with the same diluent.

The upper dilution mark on the pipettes may be exceeded by no more than 1 mm, and the mixture must not be corrected back to the top mark if overdiluted. Adjusting the upper dilution back to the mark forces cells from the bulb into the lower stem of the pipette. The fluid in this stem must be free from cells when dilution has been completed. Absorbent material such as gauze must not be used to adjust the upper blood level to the 0.5 mark. The sample in the stem can be falsely concentrated if gauze or other absorptive materials are used to adjust the blood level.

Preserved blood samples must not be hemolyzed or contain fibrin clots.

Counting Chamber for Red and White Blood Cell Counts.—After proper handling of the blood sample and careful dilution by a known amount to obtain a less concentrated solution, the number of cells in a known volume of the diluted sample is determined. The counting chamber is often called a hemocytometer. Technically, however, a hemocytometer consists of a counting chamber, a coverglass for the counting chamber, and the diluting pipettes. In this section the terms *counting chamber* and *hemocytometer* are used interchangeably. For a routine count by a manual method, the counting chamber used most often is the Levy-Hausser hemocytometer with Neubauer ruling.

To understand how a counting chamber gives the blood cell count in terms of volume when the chamber is a flat surface, we start with a cube and work backward. Picture a cube 1 mm on each side. The counting chamber allows the cube to be divided into equal units that are 0.1 mm in depth. When the counting chamber is viewed from the side, one can see that when the coverglass is placed on the chamber, it rests on supports (Fig 11–7). The space between the bottom of the coverglass and the surface of the counting chamber is 0.1 mm. Essentially, the chamber provides a series of "slices" of the cube that are 1 mm^2 in area and 0.1 mm in depth. The only way to be sure the depth is 0.1 mm is to use plane-ground cover-glasses that have a constant weight and even surface. The 0.1-mm slices are arranged so that one may count the cells in one of the slices or in portions of one slice by varying the area of the ruled surface of the chamber. Each counting chamber has two precision-ruled counting areas 3 mm wide and 3 mm long (Fig 11–8). All hemocytometers used in the hematology laboratory must meet the specifications of the National Bureau of Standards.

When the ruled area of the counting chamber is viewed for the first time under the microscope, it may be difficult to see the nine basic 1-mm squares because each one has been ruled into smaller areas. The 1-mm^2 sections in the four corners are ruled into 16 equal portions (Fig 11–9). The square in the center of the ruled area is divided into 25 equal portions (see Fig 11–9). In turn, each of the $\frac{1}{25}$-mm squares is divided into 16 parts, providing $\frac{1}{400}$-mm squares (see Fig 11–9). With the surface of the counting chamber ruled in this manner, it is possible to measure aliquots of the diluted blood sample that are contained in 1-mm, $\frac{1}{16}$-mm, $\frac{1}{25}$-mm, $\frac{1}{80}$-mm, and $\frac{1}{400}$-mm squares, all of which are 0.1 mm in depth. The area to be counted will depend on the type of count to be done.

Other types of counting chambers can also be used to count blood cells. Some of these are the Spencer

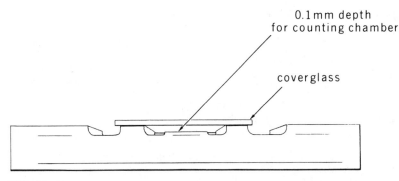

FIG 11–7.
Counting chamber—side view.

(9 square millimeters)

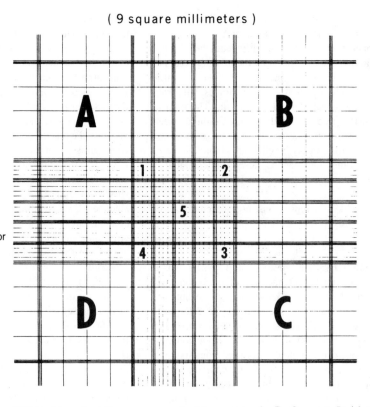

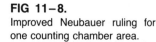

FIG 11–8.
Improved Neubauer ruling for one counting chamber area.

White blood cells are counted in areas A, B, C, and D (4 sq. mm.)
Red blood cells are counted in areas 1, 2, 3, 4, and 5
(80/400 sq. mm.)

Brightline with Neubauer ruling and the Levy chamber with Fuchs-Rosenthal ruling.

Mixing and Mounting Samples in the Counting Chamber.—The diluted blood in the pipette (Unopette or Thoma type) must be mixed before the mixture is placed on the counting chamber. It is important that the hemocytometer and its coverglass be carefully cleaned with alcohol and dried before anything is mounted on it. After cleaning, the coverglass must be centered over the ruled areas of the counting chamber, being careful to touch only the edges of the coverglass.

Using the Unopette System.—For the Unopette system, the equipment for the initial blood measurement and dilution can be converted to a dropper assembly. In this way, the blood-diluent mixture can be easily

mounted on the counting chamber. For doing a white cell count, after the blood has been diluted, a period of about 10 minutes is needed for the red cells to lyse. Diluted samples are stable for 3 hours. The sample must be mixed well just prior to mounting on the counting chamber using the easily converted dropper assembly capability incorporated into the Unopette system.

While the pipette is held at an angle of about 40 degrees, the chamber between the ruled area and the coverglass is filled with a single drop, which should be drawn rapidly into the chamber by capillarity. The pipette is placed at the edge of the coverglass, the reservoir gently squeezed so the diluted blood flows evenly under the coverglass. Do not move the coverglass. Both sides of the hemocytometer must be filled. If the fluid spills into the dividing moats or is otherwise distributed unevenly, mounting must be repeated. Only one drop can be used to fill the chamber. It should not be filled partially with a

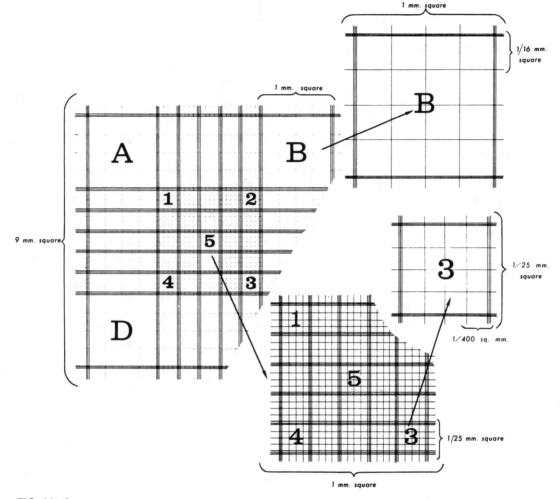

FIG 11–9.
Counting areas of the hemocytometer.

small drop and filled completely with a second drop; this would result in uneven distribution of the cells. The counting chamber is filled in the same manner for both red cell and white cell counts.

Shaking the Unopette and reservoir, discarding three to four drops, and properly filling the counting chamber are important factors in obtaining a good distribution of cells in the counting areas and in obtaining accurate cell counts. The dilution of blood is the same for both the Unopette and Thoma methods, so the calculations for both methods are the same when the Levy-Hausser hemocytometer with Neubauer ruling is used.

Using Thoma Pipettes.—For the Thoma pipette, mixing can be done by hand for a minimum of 5 minutes by holding the pipette so that the mixing bead moves freely and the cells are not pushed into the stem. Usually, a mechanical shaker will be available, and the time will vary according to the type of shaker used. Immediately after shaking the pipette and before placing a small portion of the mixture on the chamber, three drops are expelled from the white cell pipette and five drops from the red cell pipette to discard the cell-free diluent. The tip is wiped and the cells are counted in the next drops, which are mounted on each side of the counting chamber and are representative of the well-mixed cell suspension. Pipettes may vary in size, so discarding three to five drops may not be adequate. In that case, approximately one-third of the mixture in the bulb should be expelled before mounting.

Counting and Calculating Cell Counts.—Before any counting is done, the microscope must be properly adjusted (review Chapter 3). It is necessary to know how to adjust the microscope for proper illumination, and how to focus correctly (avoiding damage to the objectives and the object to be viewed).

The filled counting chambers should be allowed to sit for at least 1 minute before any counting is begun. Place the filled counting chamber on the stage of the microscope and fasten securely. Place one of the ruled counting areas of the chamber in position over the condenser. Using the low-power objective, turn the coarse-adjustment knob until the objective is about 0.25 in. above the coverglass. Adjust the light, so that the field is evenly illuminated and comfortable to view, by moving the condenser down slightly and then adjusting the iris diaphragm and rheostat. Turn the coarse-adjustment knob slowly until the ruled area comes into focus, and use the fine adjustment knob to bring the area into perfect focus. Use the iris diaphragm to adjust the light. If this technique is used, there is little danger of damaging the coverglass with the objective. If the objective touches

the coverglass, the cell distribution is altered and a new mounting must be made. After the ruled area is in focus, scan it quickly to identify the various ruled portions. Approximately 1 mm^2 can be seen in each field with the low-power ($\times 10$) objective.

When the counting chamber is properly in place on the microscope and the various ruled areas are identified and understood, cell counting can begin.

White Blood Cells.—White blood cells are counted under low magnification ($\times 10$ objective) in the four-corner 1-mm squares of the ruled area of the counting chamber. Each square is divided into 16 equal parts. Cells touching the lines on the left side or on the top of the squares are included in the count, but cells touching the lines on the right side or on the bottom of the squares are *not* counted (Fig 11–10). In this way, every cell is assigned to a square and cells are not counted twice or omitted from the count.

The counts obtained in the 1-mm^2 sections in the four corners are tabulated separately in practice laboratories. These values should not differ by more than 10 cells. Tallying the squares separately provides a check of the distribution of the cells and indicates whether mixing and mounting were adequate. When the values do not agree within 10 cells, another pipette must be used, because remounts from the previously used pipette usually result in progressively higher counts.

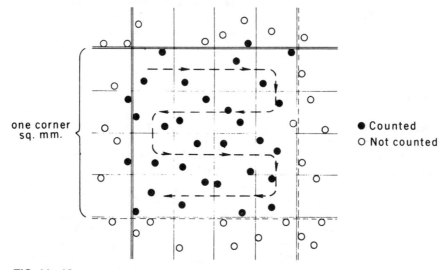

FIG 11–10.
Examples of white blood cells counted in a representative area.

In calculating the total count per unit volume of blood, four important facts must be considered: (1) the total number of cells counted in the four 1-mm squares, (2) the dilution of the blood sample, (3) the square area counted, and (4) the depth of the counting chamber. These four factors are used in the following general formula:

Cells counted in 1-mm² areas × dilution of blood

× area counted × depth of chamber

= white cells per microliter of whole blood (or cells per mm³)

Cells/microliter (μL) × 10⁶ = cells × 10⁹/L

The dilution factor for the blood is 1:20, since 25 μL of blood is diluted in 0.475 mL of 3 mL/dL acetic acid (giving 0.025 mL blood in a total of 0.500 mL of blood and diluent), using the Unopette system, for example. This means that to obtain the white cell count for a unit of undiluted blood, the calculation must be multiplied by 20, the dilution factor.

The square area and depth can be considered together as the volume factor since the volume of any solution is the product of its area times its depth. For the routine white cell count, four 1-mm² corners are counted. The depth of the counting area is 0.1 mm. Therefore the volume of the area counted is 0.4 mm³ or 0.4 μL:

$$4 \text{ mm}^2 \times 0.1 \text{ mm} = 0.4 \text{ μL}$$

To obtain the number of white blood cells in 1 μL of blood, the number of cells counted in 0.4 μL is multiplied by 1/0.4 or 2.5, the volume factor.

For example, the sum of the cells counted in the four 1-mm² corner areas is 33 + 32 + 40 + 35 = 140. In this case, the calculation would be $\frac{140}{1} \times \frac{20}{1} \times \frac{1}{4} \times \frac{1}{0.1}$ = 7,000/μL. If the square areas and the depth are considered as volume, the general formula is

Cells counted in 4 squares × dilution of blood
$$\frac{}{\text{Volume}}$$
$$= \text{white cells/μL}$$

where volume = area × depth

The count when a total of 140 cells are counted in the four squares would be calculated as

$$\frac{140 \times 20}{4 \times 0.1} = 7,000/\text{μL or } 7 \times 10^3/\text{μL}$$

Because the current units of choice for reporting are in cells counted per liter of blood, the WBCs per microliter are multiplied by 10⁶. White cell counts are reported to the nearest 100 cells. Using the example from above, a count of 7,000/μL is the same as 7 × 10³/μL. To report this in cells per liter

$$7 \times 10^3/\text{μL} \times 10^6 = 7 \times 10^9/\text{L}$$

For each white cell count completed in the routine manner, the dilution of the blood and the volume of diluted blood used for counting remain constant. Therefore, the total cells counted may be multiplied by a constant factor to find the final result. Leaving out the number of cells in the last equation, 20/(4 × 0.1) = 50. Any total number of cells counted in 4 square mm can be converted to the number of white cells per microliter of blood by multiplying by 50. Thus, 50 is the constant factor for counting white cells in the routine manner by the manual method presented.

White cells should be counted in duplicate until accuracy is attained, after which duplicate determinations may be done when appropriate (for low counts or counts of grave clinical importance).

The allowable difference between duplicate pipettes for the same blood sample is 500/μL for counts within the normal range (4.4–11 × 10³/μL or 4.4–11 × 10⁹/L) and 10% of the lowest count when the total count is above or below the normal range. The resulting white cell count is rounded off to the nearest 100 cells as results are reported to the first decimal place. For example, a white cell count calculated as 8,050 would be reported as 8,100 μL or 8.1 × 10⁹/L and a count calculated as 7,950 would be reported as 8,000 μL or 8.0 × 10⁹/L. The general rule for rounding off numbers to the next significant figure is used.

Red Blood Cells.—RBCs are counted under high-dry magnification (×40 objective). The central 1-mm² area of the counting chamber is used. It is best to find this area with the low-power objective and then change to the high-dry objective. The cells in 80 of the $\frac{1}{400}$-mm squares are counted. This is equivalent to counting the cells in $\frac{1}{5}$ of 1 mm^2 ($\frac{80}{400}$). The volume is determined by multiplying the depth (0.1 mm) by $\frac{1}{5}$, and is equal to 0.02 μL.

The preferred method for counting the cells in $\frac{1}{5}$ mm^2 is to count the cells in five of the $\frac{1}{25}$-mm squares (Fig 11–11). Since each $\frac{1}{25}$-mm square contains 16 smaller squares, eighty $\frac{1}{400}$-mm squares will have been counted. The distribution is checked by making duplicate mounts.

The calculation of the red cell count is based on the same principles as those used for the white cell count. The usual blood dilution is 1:200, the area counted is $\frac{1}{5}$ mm^2, and the depth is 0.1 mm. For example, if 475 red cells are counted in the proper area, the calculation would be $\frac{475}{1} \times \frac{200}{1} \times \frac{400}{80} \times \frac{10}{1} = 4,750,000/\mu L$ (or 4.75 $\times$ 10^6/μL). If the area and depth are converted to volume first, the general equation would be

$$\frac{\text{Cells counted in } \frac{1}{5} \text{ mm}^2 \times \text{dilution}}{\text{Volume}} = \text{red cells/}\mu L$$

where volume = area × depth.

(Center Square Millimeter)

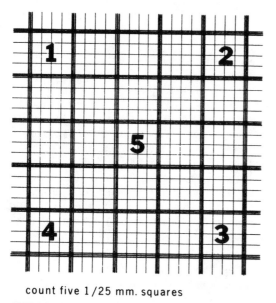

count five 1/25 mm. squares

FIG 11–11.
Red cell counting area.

To report this result in cells counted per liter of blood, multiply the cells per microliter times 10^6, or

$$4.75 \times 10^6/\mu L \times 10^6 = 4.75 \times 10^{12}/L$$

The constant factor for the RBC count is 200(0.2 × 0.1) = 10,000.

The RBC count is one of the least accurate manual procedures done in the hematology laboratory. For this reason, every sample is pipetted in duplicate, and each pipette is mounted on two sides of the counting chamber, giving four possible counting areas. If the counts with the two pipettes do not check within 10%, the determination is repeated. A generally accepted normal range for red cell counts is 4.1 to 5.1 million cells per microliter (4.1–5.1 × 10^{12}/L) for women, and 4.5 to 5.9 million cells per microliter (4.5 5.9 × 10^{12}/L) for men.

The rules for counting the cells touching the top and left lines of a particular area are the same for red cell counts as for white cell counts.

Precautions and Technical Factors for Manual Cell Counts.—Errors in counting white and red blood cells manually are related to the extremely small size of the sample, the nature of the sample, faulty laboratory equipment, faulty technique, and the inherent error of cell distribution in the counting chamber.

The minute size of the blood sample is illustrated by the fact that a variation of even 1 cell in the red cell count changes the final result by 10,000 cells.

Venous blood must be free of clots and mixed well immediately before it is diluted. Peripheral blood or capillary blood must be obtained freely flowing from a puncture and must be diluted rapidly to prevent coagulation.

Thoma pipettes, if used, must be checked against National Bureau of Standards pipettes. Pipettes must be clean and dry and without chipped tips. The counting chamber must be clean and dry. The usual practice is to clean the chamber and coverglass immediately before each use by flooding them with medicated alcohol and wiping them dry with a piece of gauze. Dirt on the chamber can alter the count.

The blood sample must be measured precisely and diluted properly. The counting chamber must be charged with only one drop of the diluted sample—an excess could raise the coverglass and thus change the depth factor.

Even with excellent technique and equipment, the probable error in manual red cell counts can be 20%, because of the chance error in the distribution of the cells in the counting chamber. The same distribution factor can also affect the WBC count, and the error in this count can be 15%.

In certain conditions, such as leukemia, the WBC count may be extremely high. If it is more than 30×10^9/L, a greater dilution of the blood should be used. Using a Thoma red cell diluting pipette, the blood is drawn up to the 1.0 mark and diluted to the 101 mark with the white cell diluting fluid, giving a 1:100 dilution. Other dilutions may be employed when necessary, and are taken into account when the final calculations are made.

When the white cell count drops below 3×10^9/L, a smaller dilution of blood should be used to achieve a more accurate count. In this case, the blood is drawn up to the 1.0 mark in the Thoma white cell diluting pipette, and diluted to the 11 mark for a final dilution of 1:10. The white cell count is determined as usual, using the change in blood dilution in the calculations.

The diluting fluid used for the WBC count destroys or hemolyzes all nonnucleated red cells. In certain disease conditions, nucleated RBCs may be present in the peripheral blood. These cells cannot be distinguished from the white cells and are counted as white cells in the hemocytometer. Therefore, whenever there are 5 or more nucleated red cells per 100 white cells in a differential done on a stained blood film, the white cell count must be corrected as follows:

$$\frac{\text{Uncorrected WBC count} \times 100}{100 + \text{number of nucleated RBCs per 100 WBCs}} = \text{corrected WBC count}$$

The WBC count is then reported as the corrected count.

Use of electronic cell counters does not relieve the laboratory worker of the responsibility for being constantly alert for sources of error. Unless equipment is properly calibrated and fundamental aspects such as the quality of the sample are considered carefully, electronic counters are merely tools for producing inadequate results faster.

Automated Cell Counting Methods

A wide range of automated and semiautomated devices are available for measuring different hematologic parameters. The most useful instruments are those for counting cells. Automated cell counters count larger numbers of cells than manual counting methods and thus allow much greater precision. Thousands of particles pass through the instrument's aperture in a few seconds. The coefficient of variation (CV), or allowable error, in a manual cell counting method varies from 8% to 15%, depending on the type of cell counted. Automated counting methods have been reported as having a CV of 1% to 3%.

There are two general methods used by automated cell counters for hematology. These are optical methods using focused laser beams and impedance methods utilized by the **Coulter principle.** Impedance counting was developed by Coulter in the late 1950s and because it has been used so extensively, it is referred to as the *Coulter principle*.

A commonly used automated system is the model S Coulter counter. This instrument performs WBC, RBC, hemoglobin, and MCV. It also calculates the hematocrit, MCH, and MCHC. It utilizes a voltage pulse counting mechanism with measurable impedance changes indicating cell counts.

Cell Counters Using the Voltage Pulse Counting Principle (Coulter Counters).—In the basic Coulter counter, cells passing through an aperture through which a current is flowing cause changes in electrical resistance that are counted as voltage pulses (Fig 11–12). A reduced pressure system operated by a vacuum unit draws the suspension through the aperture into a system of tubing following a column of mercury. The Coulter counter system is based on the principle that cells are poor electrical conductors, compared with saline or Isoton (Coulter Diagnostics, Hialeah, FL), which are good conductors.

The instrument system has a glass aperture tube that can be filled with the conducting fluid (the suspension of diluted cells, for example) and has an electrode (the internal electrode) and an aperture or small orifice that is 100 μm in diameter. Just outside the glass aperture tube is another electrode (the external electrode). The aperture tube is connected to a U-shaped glass tube that is partly filled with mercury and has two electrical contacts—an activating counter and a deactivating counter. The aperture tube is immersed in the cell suspension, filled with conductive solution, and closed by a stopcock valve. A current now flows through the aperture between the internal and external electrodes. As the vacuum unit draws the mercury up the tube, the cell suspension flows through the aperture into the aperture tube.

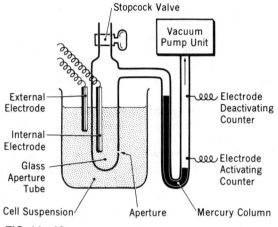

FIG 11–12.
Schematic diagram of a cell counter based on voltage pulse counting (Coulter principle). Cells flow through an aperture that separates two compartments. The electrical potential between electrodes changes as the cells pass. The number of impulses translates to the cell count and the amplitude of the pulse depends on the cell volume that displaces the conductive fluid.

Each cell that passes through the aperture displaces an equal volume of conductive solution, increasing the electrical resistance and creating a voltage pulse, because its resistance is much greater than that of the conductive solution. The pulses, which are proportional in height to the volume of cells, are counted. The section of tubing between the activating and deactivating counters is calibrated to contain 0.5 mL (see Fig 11–12). The counting mechanism is started when the mercury reaches the activating counter and is stopped when it reaches the deactivating counter. During this time the cells are counted in a volume of suspension exactly equal to the volume of glass tubing between the two contact wires in the activating and deactivating electrodes.

If two or more cells enter the aperture at the same time, they will be counted as one cell. This produces a coincidence error for which a correction must be made. The size of the coincidence error may be decreased by decreasing the concentration of the cells and the size of the aperture. However, decreasing the concentration of the cells increases the dilution error and the inherent counting error and makes the error resulting from background "noise" from contaminating particles more critical. When the aperture is decreased, it may become partially or completely plugged with debris. For this reason

a compromise is made, and for a count above a certain critical number, a coincidence correction is made by referring to a chart supplied by the manufacturer of the counting instrument.

Variations of the current measured across the aperture make it possible to determine the particle or cell count, cell volume, and particle size. All the cells in 0.5 mL of suspension are counted and the results are displayed. This pulse or count is amplified, numerically registered by the counter, and visualized on an oscilloscope.

Quality control specimens are run and their results must meet the established values in order to report out any results for patient samples.

Coulter Counter, Model S.—To minimize laboratory error and increase speed and reliability, the model S Coulter counter is used in many hematology laboratories (Procedure 11–8). The model S uses the voltage pulse counting principle described for general basic models of Coulter counters. It provides seven hematologic parameters: the white cell count, red cell count, hemoglobin, hematocrit, MCV, MCH, and MCHC. Hemoglobin is determined photometrically by passing a light beam through the mixture in the white cell aperture bath. The light absorbed by the solution at a specific wavelength is proportional to the hemoglobin concentration and is measured by a photosensitive device. The principle is the same as that of the hemiglobincyanide (cyanmethemoglobin) method (see under Hemoglobin).

The model S Coulter counter (Coulter Diagnostics, Hialeah, Fla.) has a totally automated diluting system which aspirates and pipettes approximately 1 mL of whole blood and carries it through the blood sampling valve where it is diluted. Part of the sample is diluted with Isoton, an isotonic solution which preserves the size and shape of the cells when counting white and red blood cells. A lysing reagent is added causing complete lysis of red cells and a hemoglobin reference reading is made.

For cell counts, a specific amount of diluted blood is passed through the orifice of the glass aperture tube. Each time a cell passes through this orifice, a change in the current flowing between the external and internal apertures is observed. (see Fig 11–12). This change in current produces a voltage pulse, the magnitude of which is proportional to the size of the cell causing the change. Three WBC counts are done simultaneously with an average of the three counts taken and recorded.

Hemoglobin is measured using the diluted sample used for the white cell count. The amount of light passing through the solution is measured with a photosensitive device and this reading is converted into a hemoglobin value.

A separate solution diluted for counting RBCs is passed through the orifice of the aperture tube in a similar manner as for counting WBCs. The changes in current produced by the number of red cells passing through the orifice are similarly recorded as for white cells. In addition, the red cell MCV is electronically derived and recorded.

The hematocrit is calculated from the values for

Procedure 11–8. Cell Counts Using the Model S Coulter Counter*

Note: Specific manufacturer's directions must be followed carefully.

1. Turn on the instrument and allow time for warming up.
2. Place the reporting card in one side of the printer and label with the patient's name and identification data.
3. Mix the blood sample well and check for clots using two wooden applicator sticks.
4. Place the blood tube under the aspirator so the aspirator is at least 1 in. into the sample.
5. Press the touch control bar and allow the aspirator to remain in the specimen until the red light behind the bar comes on. Remove the blood sample tube and when the light turns green, wipe the outside of the aspirator with gauze.
6. The aspirator will draw up approximately 1 mL of blood and carry it through the various sampling steps, including dilution, cell lysing, cell counting, hemoglobin measurement, and other measurements and calculations. Voltage pulsations are observed on the instrument's oscilloscope screen and represent the various cells being enumerated.
7. The final results for the seven parameters are printed out on the special card which has been placed in the printer.

Instruction and Service Manual for the Model S Coulter Counter, Hialeah, Fla, Coulter Electronics, Inc, 1970.

RBCs counted and the derived MCV. The MCH and MCHC are also calculated.

The final results for the seven parameters measured or calculated are printed out on a special card placed in the printer accompanying the analyzer.

Coulter Counter, Model S Plus.—Another Coulter counter is the model S Plus which is more computerized, more compact, and has a less complicated pneumatic system. In addition to the seven parameters reported by the model S, the S Plus also performs a platelet count and tests the degree of anisocytosis by measuring the RDW. This measures the coefficient of variation of the red cell size distribution or shows the degree of variation of the MCV from the mean. The RDW is determined and calculated using the MCV and the red cell count.

Flow Cytometry: Use of a Focused Laser Beam.— Cells or particles passing through a focused beam of a laser can be used for counting blood cells. The blood is diluted in isotonic saline and passed through the laser beam as a stream of single cells. The principle of hydrodynamic focusing allows the focusing of the blood cells with a second fluid, forming an outer sheath of liquid moving in the same direction. The instrument accomplishing this task is known as a **flow cytometer.**

Light is scattered at angles proportional to the structural features of a cell as it passes through the light beam (Fig 11–13) Most laser systems utilize light sensors that detect forward scatter of the beam (180 degrees from the light source) and right-angle (90 degree) scatter. Forward scatter is correlated with cell volume or density, analogous to the impedance counting of the Coulter principle instruments. Right-angle deflection is dependent on cellular contents, mainly the granularity of the cell cytoplasm. Photodetectors convert the light signals to electrical impulses which are processed by a computer. The display of data includes cell counts and MCV, but it also can produce simple cell differential counts (granulocytes as compared with nongranulocytes).

A fluorochrome dye can be employed in the cell suspension to enhance the cell identification. This dye can directly stain or tag certain cell components such as a granule or an enzyme. The dye can be attached to an immunologic component such as an antibody to a lymphocyte surface antigen. Different wavelengths of light excite different types of fluorochrome dyes enabling particular tagged cells to be counted separately. Differential

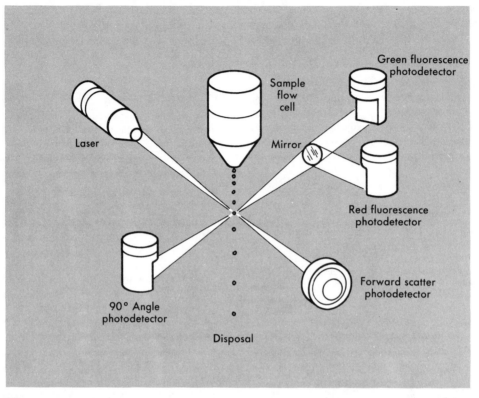

FIG 11–13.
Flow cytometry: optical detection of cells by a laser-based system. Cells are focused by the laminar flow of a sheath fluid. Cells are counted and partly identified by differential light scatter of a laser beam. (From Powers LW: *Diagnostic Hematology.* St Louis, Mosby–Year Book, Inc, 1989, p 452. Used by permission.)

leukocyte counts or reticulocyte counts are done using two or more laser detection systems in sequence.

For specialized testing, the flow cytometry principle is used to separate cells. Positive or negative electrical charges are applied by a charging collar to the labeled cell as it passes through the laser beam (Fig 11–14). The charged cell is sorted into a unique stream obtaining a sample of specific cells that can be identified by specific cell markers.

Reference Values*
For red blood cell count ($\times 10^{12}$/L):
Men: mean 5.2 (range 4.5–5.9)
Women: mean 4.6 (range 4.1–5.1)

*Williams WJ, Beutler E, Erslev A, et al: *Hematology,* ed 4. New York, McGraw-Hill Book Co, 1990, pp 10,18.

For white blood cell count ($\times 10^{9}$/L):
12-mo   mean 11.4; (range 6.0–17.5)
10 yr   mean 8.1 (range 4.5–13.5)
21 yr   mean 7.4 (range 4.5–11.0)
>21 yr   mean 7.8 (range 4.4–11.3)

Counting Platelets

Platelets, or thrombocytes, function in the coagulation of the blood and are therefore associated with the bleeding and clotting, or hemostatic, mechanism of the body. Platelets are formed in the bone marrow from megakaryocytes. They are difficult to count accurately for several reasons: they are small and difficult to discern, they have an adhesive character and become attached readily to glassware or to particles of debris in the diluting fluid, and they clump easily and are probably not

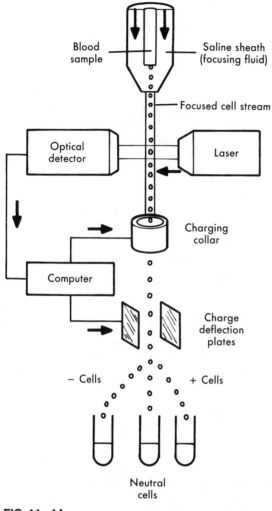

Blood sample

Saline sheath (focusing fluid)

Focused cell stream

Optical detector

Laser

Charging collar

Computer

Charge deflection plates

− Cells

+ Cells

Neutral cells

FIG 11–14.
Flow cytometry: sorting cells. A laser detection system is combined with a computer and a charging collar. Cells of a particular identity (carrying fluorescent tags that react to the laser) are charged and deflected to a collection container. (From Powers LW: *Diagnostic Hematology.* St Louis, Mosby–Year Book, Inc, 1989, p 453. Used by permission.)

Specimens

Capillary blood from a finger puncture can be used, but venous blood generally gives more satisfactory results. Platelet counts on capillary blood are generally lower than those on venous blood because of immediate platelet clumping at the puncture site. EDTA is the anticoagulant of choice for platelet counts as it lessens the tendency for platelet clumping.

Methods Used to Count Platelets

With good technique and experience, platelets can be manually counted accurately. One basic manual method, the Brecher-Cronkite method, utilizes phase-contrast microscopy.* The Brecher-Cronkite method uses a blood diluent, 1 g/dL ammonium oxalate, that completely hemolyzes the red cells. A Unopette system is also available for platelet counts. The platelets are then counted, generally with a phase hemocytometer and a phase-contrast microscope to enhance refractiveness of the platelets. An ordinary light microscope may be used to count the platelets, but the differentiation is not as sharp. Manual methods are time-consuming, cause eyestrain, and are not recommended for large-volume work. A manual platelet count is always done using duplicate pipettes.

In general, the best results are obtained by using some variation of the direct manual methods. Some hospitals have discontinued manual platelet counts altogether because the error involved can be very large and a well-prepared blood smear can be used to estimate platelets. With any direct method, the blood used must be freshly obtained from a finger puncture or it must be preserved with EDTA.

Manual methods to be discussed in this chapter include the Rees-Ecker direct method (Procedure 11–9), and the Unopette method. In the Rees-Ecker method, whole blood is diluted with a solution of brilliant cresyl blue, which stains the platelets a light bluish color. The platelets are then counted with a Spencer Brightline hemocytometer. The metallic surface of this hemocytometer makes the platelets easier to see.

The Unopette system described for platelets utilizes a self-measuring dilution system and enumeration of platelets using a phase hemocytometer and phase microscopy.

Manual methods are time-consuming. Manual

*Brecher G, Cronkite EP: Morphology and enumeration of human blood platelets. *J Appl Physiol* 1950; 3:365.

evenly distributed in the blood in the first place. Platelets disintegrate easily and are difficult to distinguish from debris. Because of their sticky nature, they also tend to adhere to other platelets in clumps. By using EDTA as an anticoagulant, the clumping tendency of platelets can be decreased.

counts are always verified by performing a platelet estimate on a blood film.

An automated method for counting platelets with the model S Plus Coulter counter is used in many laboratories. In the S Plus model, as platelets and red cells pass through the apertures, particles that are between 2 and 20 fL are counted as platelets. A platelet graph is also plotted according to the size distribution of the platelets counted.

It is always necessary to correlate the automated count with that estimated from a stained blood film.

Manual Platelet Counts
Using the Unopette System.—A Unopette diluting system is available for counting platelets. The platelet Unopette capillary pipette measures 20 µL of anticoagulated (EDTA) blood which is diluted in a Unopette reservoir containing 1.98 mL of 1 g/dL ammonium oxalate which hemolyzes the red cells, leaving white cells and platelets intact. Using the method described for manual white cell counts using the Unopette system, the diluted sample is mounted on a hemocytometer after a 10-minute waiting period for complete red cell lysis to take place. The diluted specimen for platelet counts is mounted on both sides of two hemocytometers.

A phase hemocytometer is used preferably to enhance platelet refractiveness for an easier microscopic enumeration. After mounting on the phase hemocytometer, the unit should be placed in a high humidity chamber for at least 15 minutes so the platelets come to rest in the same focal plane. If a phase hemocytometer is not available, the dilution is mounted on a Spencer-Brightline hemocytometer and the platelets are counted using a light microscope remembering to allow the platelets to settle to one focal plane as for the phase hemocytometer.

Using the Rees-Ecker Method and Thoma Pipette (Procedure 11–9)
Diluents for Manual Platelet Count.—The diluent used for counting platelets must meet certain requirements. It must (1) provide fixation to reduce the adhesiveness of the platelets, (2) prevent coagulation, (3) prevent hemolysis (unless the method chosen eliminates the RBCs), and (4) provide a low specific gravity so that the platelets will settle in one plane. A diluent that meets all these requirements is Rees-Ecker solution. Rees-Ecker solution contains sodium citrate, which prevents coagulation, preserves the RBCs, and provides the necessary low specific

gravity; formalin, which is a fixative; and brilliant cresyl blue, which is a dye used for the identification of the diluent. This dye does not stain the platelets, and it is not essential for the counting procedure. All diluents used, including Rees-Ecker, must be stored in the refrigerator and filtered before each use.

Preparation of Rees-Ecker Diluting Fluid.—In a volumetric flask, 3.8 g of sodium citrate and 0.2 mL of formalin is diluted to 100 mL with deionized water. A small amount of brilliant cresyl blue is added to color the solution light blue.

Equipment for Manual Platelet Count.—The pipettes used for platelet dilution must be scrupulously clean; it is preferable to clean them with acid, although a

---

> ### Procedure 11–9. Platelet Count: Rees-Ecker Method (Using the Thoma Pipette)
>
> 1. The capillary bore of a red cell diluting pipette is rinsed with Rees-Ecker diluting fluid. Any excess fluid is thoroughly expelled from the pipette.
> 2. Freely flowing blood from a finger puncture or venous blood preserved with EDTA is drawn rapidly into the pipette to the 0.5 mark.
> 3. The blood is diluted rapidly with Rees-Ecker fluid to the 101 mark on the pipette. Two pipettes and two counting chambers are used for each platelet count; each pipette is mounted on both sides of a counting chamber. Blood films are also made at this time in order to check the platelet count.
> 4. The pipettes are shaken immediately after dilution for a minimum of 1 minute.
> 5. After thorough mixing (for at least 5 minutes) six to eight drops are expelled from each pipette and discarded. The next two drops are mounted, one on each side of one counting chamber. Repeat with the duplicate pipette.
> 6. The platelets are allowed to settle in the chambers for 15 minutes and then counted. The chambers are covered to prevent evaporation—for instance, with a Petri plate containing moistened gauze.

hot detergent appears to give good results. Anything in the pipette to which the platelets could adhere must be removed.

To reduce the error in the initial pipetting and diluting steps, a Unopette system may be used. Unopette pipettes and reservoirs are available for counting platelets. Empty reservoirs can be purchased to which the appropriate diluent is added before use.

The Spencer Brightline chamber, in which the lines appear white against a dark background, appears to have definite advantages over other types of counting chambers for platelets. The platelets seem easier to see against the metal-coated surface of the Spencer Brightline chamber. The cell distribution also seems to be better, since the chamber's surface is smoother. However, this type of chamber is more difficult to mount correctly.

Counting Platelets in the Counting Chamber.

—Place the chamber under the microscope and locate the center ruled area using the low-power objective ($\times 10$). Carefully change to the high-power objective ($\times 40$) and adjust the light for maximum contrast.

Using phase microscopy, platelets should appear as shiny structures with a halolike area of light around them. Focus up and down on the platelets. Fine projections can be seen on the platelet edges with the phase microscope.

With light microscopy, the platelets appear as small, round, refractile bodies. Platelets are counted in the center square millimeter of each of the four counting areas, using the high-power objective ($\times 40$). The cell counts on the four center squares must agree within $25 \times 10^9/L$ for duplicate mounts and within $40 \times 10^9/L$ for duplicate pipettes. When the platelet count is below $200 \times 10^9/L$, replicate counts should agree within $30 \times 10^9/L$. When the platelet count is above $200 \times 10^9/L$, replicate counts should agree within $50 \times 10^9/L$. Manual platelet counts should be done by mounting duplicate Unopettes (or pipettes) on both sides of a chamber and averaging the replicates, if they are within the acceptable range. Platelet counts are reported to the nearest 1,000/μL.

Calculations for Manual Platelet Count.

—The number of platelets per liter of whole blood must be calculated. The important factors are: (1) the average number of platelets counted in 1 mm^2; (2) the dilution of the blood (1:100 using the Unopette system); and (3) the volume of diluted blood counted, which is equal to the depth of the chamber (0.1 mm) times the area in which the cells are counted (1 mm^2), or 0.1 μL. The following general formula applies:

$$\frac{\text{Average no. of platelets in 4 squares} \times 1\ mm^2 \times 100}{0.1\ mm}$$
$$\times 10^6 = \text{platelets} \times 10^9/L$$

In this case, a constant factor of 1,000 can be used. The normal range for the platelet count with Rees-Ecker diluent is 170,000 to 400,000/μL or $170-400 \times 10^9/L$.

Precautions and Technical Factors

Many of the precautions described for manually counting erythrocytes and leukocytes also apply to platelet counts. In platelet counts, however, it is imperative that peripheral blood be freely flowing when obtained from a finger puncture. Pipettes and counting chambers must be clean and free from lint, since platelets may be confused with dirt and debris. Rapid dilution of the blood is essential, or the platelets may form clumps and the blood may clot. If clumps of platelets are noted during the platelet count, the procedure should be repeated. Clumping may result from inadequate mixing of the blood with the diluent or from poor technique in obtaining the blood sample.

To minimize the error for manual platelet counts, duplicates are always prepared and duplicate counts done on both sides of two counting chambers. Duplicate counts of a sample should agree within 10% to be acceptable.

For an extremely low platelet count, the original blood specimen can be diluted with a white cell diluting pipette instead of a red cell pipette. The correct dilution factor must be used in the calculations.

Constant focusing of the microscope is necessary to identify the platelets among the larger, more numerous other cells still present (such as WBCs). A blood film is made, stained, and viewed microscopically to check each platelet count.

If a platelet count is requested in combination with other counts for the same patient and one wishes to utilize the same finger puncture, it is necessary to take the blood for the platelet count first before performing the remaining counts. The finger must not be squeezed excessively when drawing the blood into the pipette.

Clinical Significance of the Platelet Count

The normal number of platelets, depending in part on the method employed for their enumeration, ranges from 172 to 450 $\times$ 10^9/L whole blood. A count lower than normal may be associated with a generalized bleeding tendency and a prolonged bleeding time. A count higher than normal may be associated with a tendency toward thrombosis.

There are several diseases in which a high or low platelet count can result. Thrombocytopenia, or a decrease in platelets, is found in thrombocytopenic purpura, in some infectious diseases, in some acute leukemias, in some anemias (aplastic and pernicious), and when the patient is undergoing x-ray treatment or drug treatment. Thrombocytosis, or an increase in platelets, can be found in rheumatic fever, asphyxiation, following surgical treatment, following splenectomy, with acute blood loss, and with some types of chemotherapy used in the treatment of leukemia.

Reference Values*

Mean 311 $\times$ 10^9/L (range 172–450 $\times$ 10^9/L)

MICROSCOPIC EXAMINATION OF PERIPHERAL BLOOD

Microscopic examination of the peripheral blood is part of the routine hematologic workup for most patients seen by a physician and for most new hospital patients. It is most often done by preparing, staining, and examining a thin film of blood on a glass slide. A **peripheral blood film** (also called a blood smear) is part of the CBC in most hospitals and physicians' offices. The CBC generally includes hemoglobin measurement, the WBC count, the microhematocrit, and a blood film evaluation.

The blood film is the only permanent record of routine hematologic work that can be retained in the laboratory. It may occasionally be necessary to examine a blood film again to check for errors or to evaluate changes in the clinical status of the patient.

More information can be obtained from the examination of a blood film than from any other laboratory test. It is used to study the morphology (form and structure) of the red cells, white cells, and platelets. The various types of white cells are classified and the percentage of each is recorded; this is the **leukocyte differential** count. The blood film can also be used to verify the hemoglobin value, the hematocrit, and the red cell count. It is used to check or estimate the white cell, reticulocyte, and platelet counts and the red cell indices. Because the blood film has so many uses, a well-made smear is essential. Generally, two good films are prepared with each blood count or set of hematologic tests. One of these films is stained and the other is kept in reserve.

Sources of Blood for the Blood Film

The source of blood used for the blood film is an important consideration. Fresh blood from a finger, heel, or big toe puncture can be used for morphologic examination of the white and red cells. The finger must not be squeezed excessively to obtain the drop of blood, and it must not be touched with the glass slide. Only the drop of blood is touched to the glass slide, not the skin. If the slide touches the finger, oils or moisture from the finger will lead to a poorly prepared film. The ear lobe is sometimes used for making blood films if the finger site is unavailable or for special morphologic studies. When the ear lobe is used, it must be wiped thoroughly with alcohol and dried well, for it is waxy and wax may lead to bubbles in the film.

If venous blood rather than capillary blood is drawn, EDTA is the anticoagulant of choice. Most of the work in the hematology laboratory is done on venous blood. EDTA preserves the morphologic features of the white and red cells and gives a more even distribution of the platelets. If blood is collected in EDTA for morphologic studies, the film should be prepared as soon as possible, certainly within 2 hours.

Preparation of the Blood Film

Blood is most often examined under the microscope by preparing a thin film or smear of blood on a glass slide or a coverglass, fixing the blood film, and then staining it with a polychromatic stain (Fig 11–15). Wet films of blood can also be prepared and observed with a phase-contrast microscope or by use of a supravital stain, but these techniques are used less often in the examination of blood. Smears can also be prepared by centrifugation where centrifugal force is used to spread a monolayer of blood cells over the surface of a glass slide (see Fig 11–15).

---

*Williams WJ, Beutler E, Erslev A, et al: *Hematology,* ed 4. New York, McGraw-Hill, Book Co, 1990, p 10.

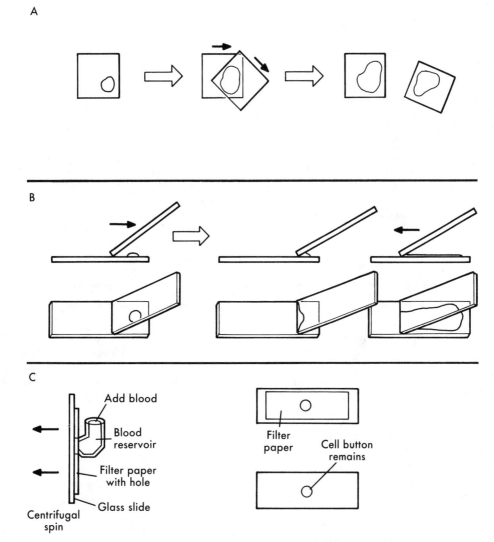

FIG 11–15.
Preparation of blood smears. **A,** coverglass preparation. A drop of blood or marrow is spread between two coverglasses as they are pulled in opposite directions. **B,** wedge smear. A drop of blood is pulled across the slide by another slide at an acute angle, creating a wedge-shaped smear with decreasing cell density. **C,** centrifugal smear. A drop of blood is spun from a central point, creating an evenly dispersed monolayer of cells. (From Powers LW: *Diagnostic Hematology*. St Louis, Mosby–Year Book, Inc, 1989, p 445. Used by permission.)

Cover Glass Blood Films

When a coverglass is used to prepare a blood film, more of the prepared film can be examined, which reduces the sampling error. With a glass slide only a relatively small counting area can be examined. In addition, the leukocytes and platelets are more evenly distributed on a coverglass. The disadvantages of the coverglass method are that it is more time-consuming, more difficult to learn and perform correctly, and requires more care in handling the preparations. Automatic staining devices are available for glass slides, but not for coverglasses.

Wedge Blood Films

Alhough the coverglass method is recommended by many hematologists, the glass slide wedge method is far more commonly used. The glass slide, or wedge, blood film method is described in detail in this text (Procedure 11–10). The directions for the examination of the blood film also can apply to the coverglass method. In either case, for the correct interpretation of a blood film, (1) the film must be prepared in a technically correct manner, (2) it must be stained correctly, and (3) it must be examined correctly. A film that is not prepared and stained correctly is useless for microscopic examination.

The equipment used for making blood films must be meticulously clean. Precleaned glass slides or slides cleaned with alcohol and wiped dry give the best results. Use of a spreading device is recommended—for example, a margin-free spreader slide with ground-glass edges may be used to spread the film of blood on the clean, lint-free slide. The edges of the spreader slide must be clean and free from chips. Coverglasses can also be used as spreading devices (Fig 11–16). The spreading device must be cleaned thoroughly with alcohol and dried between films, and it must be discarded when chipped or broken.

Cytocentrifuged Blood Films

With the use of a cytocentrifuge, a monolayer of cells can be prepared. These centrifuges facilitate rapid spreading of the cells across a slide from a central point by virtue of their high torque and low inertia motors (see Fig 11–15). With a cytocentrifuged preparation, cellular destruction and artifacts present in the glass wedge slide method are eliminated. Only small volumes of a sample are used, and the cells are evenly distributed and less distorted, producing better conditions for critical morphologic studies.

Procedure 11–10. Making a Blood Film (Wedge Slide Method)

1. Place a drop of capillary or well-mixed venous blood preserved with EDTA on one end of a slide, on the midline about 1 cm from the end. The drop should be about 2 mm in diameter (about the size of a match head), as shown in Figure 11–17. Venous blood must be well mixed by gentle inversion at least 15 times; it should also be checked for clots. If capillary blood is used, touch the top of the drop to the slide, being careful not to let the skin touch the slide. Transfer venous blood to the slide with the aid of two wooden applicator sticks or a capillary pipette.

2. Lay the specimen slide on a flat surface and hold it in position at the left end (these directions are for a right-handed person) with the middle finger or thumb and index finger of the left hand (see Fig 11–15).

3. Place the smooth clean edge of the spreader slide on the specimen slide just in front (to the left of) the drop of blood (see Figs 11–15 and 11–17).

4. Using the right hand, balance the spreader slide on one or two fingers (for example, the middle finger or the index and middle fingers) and draw it backward into the drop of blood at an angle of approximately 45 degrees to the specimen slide.

5. Decrease the spreader slide angle to about 25 to 30 degrees and allow the blood to flow evenly across the edge of the spreader slide (see Fig 11–17).

6. When the blood has spread evenly across the edge of the spreader slide, quickly push the spreader slide over the entire length of the specimen slide. As the spreader is moved, a thin film of blood will be deposited behind it. The blood film should take up one-half to three-fourths of the slide when properly prepared (Fig 11–18). The goal is to achieve a wedge-shaped smear with a thin, feathery edge.

7. Turn the spreader slide over (this gives another clean edge) and prepare a second blood film, using the same procedure. Two films should always be prepared for the same blood specimen.

8. Dry the blood film immediately. If not dried quickly, the blood cells will shrink and appear distorted.

9. Label the film by writing the name of the patient and the date in the blood at the thick end of the film, using a lead pencil (see Fig 11–18).

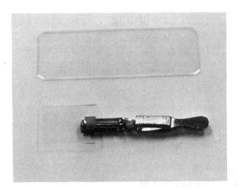

FIG 11–16.
Spreading devices.

Criteria and Precautions for a Good Blood Film

A blood film should satisfy certain criteria when observed macroscopically, as shown in Figure 11–18. The body of the film should be smooth and not interrupted by ridges, waves, or holes. It should be thickest at the origin and gradually thin out, rather than having alternate thick and thin areas. Pushing the spreader slide with an uneven motion results in thicker and thinner areas in the body of the film.

A good blood film should cover one-half to three-fourths of the length of the slide. All of the initial drop of blood should be incorporated in the film, not just part of it.

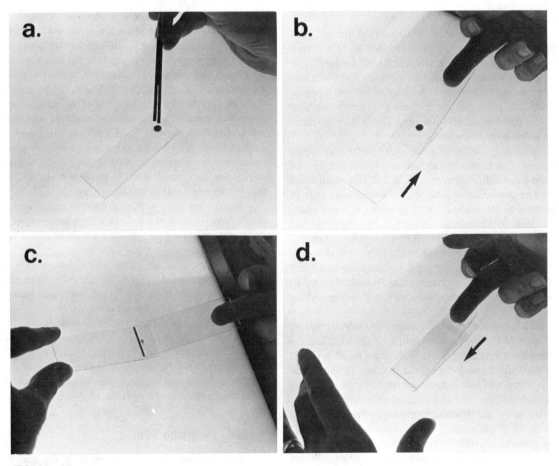

FIG 11–17.
Preparing the blood film.

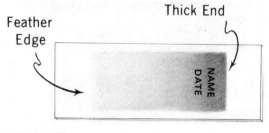

FIG 11–18.
Good blood film.

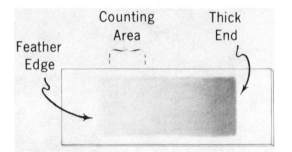

FIG 11–19.
Blood film: counting area.

The thin end of the smear should have a good feather edge; that is, the film should fade away without a defined border on the end. In some institutions a fairly straight feather edge is sought, while others prefer a more tonguelike edge.

A defined border at the end of a blood film indicates that most of the white cells have piled up at the end. When this occurs, the heavier neutrophils accumulate at the end to a greater extent than the other types of white cells, giving an incorrect distribution of the types of white cells in the body of the smear. Platelets also tend to accumulate at the end of a smear, decreasing the number in the body of the smear.

Chipped or dirty spreader slides will cause abrupt endings, thin streaks in the body of the film, or tails of blood beyond the feather edge. This will also result in inaccurate percentages for the cell types within the body of the film, as the relatively stickier neutrophils and platelets tend to concentrate in such tails. Chips in the spreader slide may be detected by running the index finger lightly over the spreading edge. The spreader slide should be cleaned by rubbing it vigorously with a piece of gauze moistened with medicated alcohol. Be sure all the alcohol is evaporated (the edge is dry) before making the film.

Slides should be made in almost one motion; that is, the drop of blood should be placed on the slide and the smear made immediately. As soon as the blood is placed on the slide it should be spread, because drying of the blood drop will lead to an uneven distribution of cells in the body of the film and the larger white cells will accumulate at the end. Rouleau formation by the red cells and clumping of the platelets will also occur if the blood is not spread immediately. Pressing down on the spreader slide will also lead to an accumulation of white cells and platelets at the end. This is why it should be balanced on

the finger as the blood is spread, rather than held between the finger and thumb.

The degree of thickness or thinness of the blood film is also important. When a film is too thick the cells pile up, which makes them difficult to count and obscures their morphology. A very thin film is satisfactory for morphologic studies, but it may be tedious to examine. The thickness of the film is determined by the size of the drop of blood used, the speed of the stroke used to move the spreader slide, and the angle at which the spreader slide is moved. A thick film results when the drop of blood is large, the angle is greater than 45 degrees, and the spreading motion is fast. A thin film results when the drop of blood is small, the angle is less than 30 degrees, and the motion is slow.

Blood films with vacuoles or bubbles result from the use of dirty slides or in some cases from an excess of fat in the specimen (as in a specimen obtained after a fatty meal).

Rapid drying of the blood film is essential. When blood films are not dried rapidly, the red cells become crenated, the white cells shrink, and there is an increase in rouleau formation by the red cells.

Only a small part of a blood film is actually examined microscopically. This part is referred to as the examination or counting area, as shown in Figure 11–19. The counting area must be one where the red and white cells are clearly separated and well distributed. It should be about one cell thick and approximately 6 to 7 mm wide.

Staining the Blood Film

After a blood film has been prepared, the next step is the staining procedure. The blood film should be stained as soon as possible. If it cannot be stained within a few hours it should be fixed by immersion in absolute methyl alcohol (methanol) for 1 or 2 seconds and air-dried. If this is not done, the slides will stain with a pale blue background of dried plasma.

The stain most often used for the examination of blood films is Wright's stain or a variation of it—the **Wright-Giemsa stain** (Procedure 11–11). Both Wright's stain and Wright-Giemsa stain are adaptations of polychrome Romanovsky stains. Such polychrome stains produce multiple colors when applied to cells, since they are made up of both basic and acidic aniline dyes. Romanovsky stains contain methylene blue (a basic dye), eosin (an acidic dye), and methylene azure (an oxidation product of methylene blue also referred to as polychrome methylene blue). Variations of the Romanovsky stains differ in the way the methylene azure is produced or added to the stains.

Polychrome stains produce multiple colors since they dye both acidic and basic cell components in an acid-base reaction. The acidic cell components such as nuclei (nuclear DNA) and cytoplasmic RNA are stained blue-violet by the basic methylene azure. They are called *basophilic* (base-loving) as they stain with the basic dye. The more basic cell components such as hemoglobin and eosinophilic granules are stained orange to pink and are called *acidophilic* (acid-loving) since they stain with the acidic dye. Some structures within cells stain with both components, such as the neutrophilic granules, while the azurophilic granules stain with methylene azure.

The staining method for blood films fixes dead cells, as opposed to supravital staining, which is used with living cells. Fixation is the process by which the blood is made to adhere to the slide and the cellular proteins are coagulated. Wright's stain and Wright-Giemsa stain are used as methanol solutions. The blood cells are fixed by the methanol in the first step of the staining reaction when the Wright's or Wright-Giemsa dye mixture is added to the blood film. Heat can also be used for fixation, but it is not necessary when the stain contains methanol. The actual polychrome staining of the blood film takes place in the second step of the procedure when an aqueous phosphate buffer solution with a pH of 6.4 is added to the Wright-Giemsa dye.

Wright's stain or Wright-Giemsa stain can be purchased as a dry powder, which is diluted in absolute, anhydrous, acetone-free methyl alcohol (CP), or as a prepared methanol solution. Both powders and solutions are certified by the Biological Stain Commission.* The preparation of methylene azure by oxidation of methylene blue and addition of eosin is quite complex, so Wright's stain powder may vary slightly from lot to lot. This necessitates determination of fixing and staining times for each new batch.

Preparation of Wright-Giemsa Stain and Buffer

1. Wright-Giemsa stain. The dye can be purchased as a powder and diluted in methanol.
   a. Dissolve 2.0 g of certified Wright's dye and 0.1 g of Giemsa dye in 800 mL of absolute, anhydrous, acetone-free methyl alcohol (CP).
   b. Mix the reagents in a tightly stoppered brown bottle.
   c. Shake the mixture vigorously at intervals for several days.
   d. Allow the stain to age for about 1 month before use. Incubation of the stain at 37° C will hasten the aging process.
   e. Filter the stain each day before use.
2. Phosphate buffer (pH 6.4).
   a. Dilute 6.63 g of anhydrous monobasic potassium phosphate (KH_2PO_4) and 2.56 g of anhydrous dibasic sodium phosphate (Na_2HPO_4) to 1,000 mL with deionized water. (Some authors say that distilled water may be substituted for the buffer if the pH is approximately 6.4. This is not recommended as the pH of water may vary from day to day.)
   b. Check the pH of the prepared phosphate buffer with a pH meter before use. The resulting solution can be made more alkaline by decreasing the amount of KH_2PO_4 and increasing the amount of Na_2HPO_4.

Rapid Staining Methods Using a Dipping Technique

Modification of Wright's stain has been incorporated into various commercially available quick staining methods. Blood films are prepared in the classic way, usually by the wedge method, and then stained. Each

*Conn HJ, Darrow MS: *Staining Procedures Used by the Biological Stain Commission,* ed 2. Baltimore, Williams & Wilkins Co, 1960.

Procedure 11–11. Staining Blood Films Using Wright-Giemsa Stain

1. Place the dried blood film on a level staining rack, with the film side up and the feather edge away from you. Allow the dried film to set at least 5 minutes before staining is begun.
2. Fix the film by *flooding* the slide with the *filtered* stain. The amount of stain is important. There must be enough to avoid excessive evaporation, which would result in precipitation of stain on the slide.
3. Allow the stain to remain on the slide for 3 to 5 minutes. This is the fixation period. Determine the exact timing for each batch of stain used.
4. Without removing the Wright-Giemsa stain, add phosphate buffer, using about 1 to $1\frac{1}{2}$ times as much buffer as stain on the slide so that a layer piles up but none spills off. Add the buffer drop-wise, then blow on the surface to mix the stain and buffer. A metallic greenish sheen should form on the surface when the slide is buffered adequately.
5. Allow the stain and buffer mixture to remain on the slide for 10 to 15 minutes. During this time the staining takes place as a result of the combination of dye and buffer at the correct pH.
6. Wash the slide with a steady stream of deionized water. Precipitation of the metallic scum on the film must be avoided. This is done by first flooding the slide with water, then washing and tipping the slide simultaneously. If this is not done and the dye is poured off the slide before it is washed, the insoluble metallic scum will settle on the blood film.
7. Wipe the dye from the back of the slide when it is still wet by rubbing with a piece of moist gauze.
8. Place the slide in a vertical position to air-dry, with the feather edge (thin edge) up. Never blot a blood film dry. The heaviest part of the film is at the bottom to allow precipitated stain to flow away from the thin edge, which will be used for examination of the blood film.
9. Do not use the slide for microscopic examination until it is dry.

---

commercial product is somewhat different so the manufacturer's instructions must be carefully followed. The advantage of these products is that they are faster to use than the traditional Wright's staining method described earlier. Slides are usually dipped into each of the various staining reagents, taking only a few seconds for each step. For critical morphologic studies, the traditional Wright's stain should be used, as some of the morphologic detail is lost when certain of the quick stains are used.

Characteristics of a Properly Stained Blood Film

If the blood film has been stained properly, it will appear pink when observed with the naked eye. When examined microscopically with the low-power ($\times 10$) objective, the film should be thin enough so that the red and white cells are clearly separated. There should not be an excessive accumulation of white cells and platelets at the edge of the film. In addition, there should be no precipitated stain.

The background or space between the cells should be clear. The RBCs should appear red-orange through the microscope. Correctly stained leukocytes should have the following colors under the microscope. The lymphocytes and neutrophils should have dark purple nuclei, while the monocyte nuclei should be a lighter purple. The granules should be bright orange in the eosinophils and dark blue in the basophils. The appearance of the cytoplasm varies with the type of leukocyte. In monocytes, the cytoplasm should be blue-gray or have a faint bluish tinge. The neutrophil cytoplasm should be light pink with lilac granules, and the lymphocyte cytoplasm should be a shade of blue, generally clear blue or robin's-egg blue. The platelets should stain violet to purple. If the blood film does not meet these criteria, it should be discarded and a new film should be stained and examined.

Precautions and Comments on Staining Blood Films

When staining the blood film, it is important that the staining rack be level so that the stain is uniform throughout the film.

It is important that the stain and buffer be made correctly. When prepared in the laboratory, the stain should stand for 1 month before it is used. There are Wright's and Wright-Giemsa stains that can be purchased ready to use. These reagents must be checked out carefully before being used for daily staining needs.

The pH of the buffer must be correct. With every new batch of stain and buffer, the fixing and staining times should be checked by staining a few slides. If staining of the cells is satisfactory, the times used for fixing and staining should be noted and used with that batch of reagents. If the pH is too acid or too alkaline, the stain will give a false color and appearance to the cells.

Adequate fixing time must be allowed. A minimum of 3 minutes is recommended for the initial reaction of the blood film and Wright-Giemsa stain. Since inadequate fixation allows dissolution of the nuclear chromatin, overfixation is preferable. To achieve the proper staining reactions in the cells, the stain and buffer must be prepared correctly, the correct timing must be determined for each batch of stain and buffer, and the correct staining technique must be used.

Properly applied Wright-Giemsa stain dyes both acidic and basic components of the blood cells. The phosphate buffer controls the pH of the staining system. If the pH is too acid, the parts of the cell taking up acidic dye will be overstained and will appear too red, while the parts of the cells taking up basic dye will appear pale. If the pH of the staining system is too alkaline, the parts of the cells taking up basic dye will be overstained, giving an overall blue effect, with very dark blue to black nuclear chromatin and bluish red cells. The following situations will indicate *staining errors.*

A faded or washed-out appearance of all the cells is caused by overwashing, understaining, or underfixing, leaving water on the slide, or by using improperly made stain. When the slide has an *excessively blue appearance* on gross examination, the red cells will appear blue-red and the white cells will be darker and more granular microscopically. This may result from overfixing or overstaining, inadequate washing, using a stain or buffer that is too alkaline, or using too thick a film. It may be corrected by decreasing the fixation time (the time before the buffer is added to the dye), or increasing the time during which the buffer and stain mixture stands on the slide. Alternatively, the amount of stain used may be decreased and the amount of buffer increased. Finally, the pH of the buffer may be checked with a pH meter and readjusted to 6.4, or a new Wright-Giemsa stain may be tried. When the slide has an *excessively red*

appearance to the naked eye, the red cells will appear bright red, the white cells will appear indistinct with pale blue rather than purple nuclei, and brilliant red eosinophilic granules will be seen microscopically. This may be caused by understaining; overwashing; or use of stain, buffer, or wash water that is too acid. To correct this situation the following measures may be tried. The fixation or staining time may be increased. The washing technique may be corrected so that it is adequate but not excessive. The pH of the buffer and water may be checked with a pH meter and adjusted, or a new stain or buffer may be used. *Large amounts of precipitated stain* on the film result from either improper washing (not washing enough to remove the metallic scum) or using an old stain that has started to precipitate. This may be corrected by using the proper washing technique—first flooding the slide with water and then tipping and washing the slide simultaneously—and making sure the stain is filtered daily.

Examination of the Blood Film

Since accurate examination of the blood film depends on proper use of the microscope, a general review of the procedure to be used is presented for the student viewing a blood film for the first time (see Chapter 3). The film is first examined with the low-power ($\times 10$) objective, moving the slide with the mechanical stage to get different areas into the field of view. The difference in appearance of the various areas results from the technique used in preparing the film: the film is relatively thick at the beginning and gradually thins out to a feather edge. Most of the cells seen under the low-power objective are RBCs, which appear as small, round, reddish-orange bodies.

Scattered among the red-staining cells are the less numerous WBCs, which are larger and more complex in appearance than the RBCs. The white cells consist of nuclei surrounded by cytoplasm. The nuclei stain purple, and the cytoplasms stain different colors, depending on their contents. The size of the cell; the shape, size, and chromatin pattern of the nucleus; the presence of nucleoli in the nucleus; and the contents, staining reaction, and relative size of the cytoplasm are used in the identification of WBCs.

With the low-power objective, an area of the film is found where the red cells are just touching and are not overlapping or piled on top of one another. This area will be found near the feather edge of the film (see Fig 11–19). The color of the cells should be examined at this magnification. When this area has been found, the oil-immersion (×100) objective should be used next. The high-dry (×40) objective is not suitable for examination of blood films, as important morphologic changes cannot be seen at this magnification. To change to the oil-immersion lens, the low-power objective is moved out of position and a drop of immersion oil is placed on the selected site (where the red cells are just touching one another). The oil-immersion lens is moved into the oil while looking at it from the side. The oil must be in direct contact with the lens. If necessary, it can be focused with the fine adjustment. If the slide has been placed upside down on the microscope stage, it will be impossible to bring the blood cells into focus. More light will be needed with the oil-immersion lens. It can be obtained by repositioning the condenser (which should be all the way up for maximum resolution under oil immersion), opening the iris diaphragm, and turning up the light source rheostat.

Under the oil-immersion objective, red cells appear as round, structureless bodies containing no nuclei, granules, or discrete material. The red color is darker at the edge of the cell than in the center. This variation is caused by the biconcave shape of the red cell, which contains less pigment (hemoglobin) in its thinner center. With oil immersion, most of the red cells in a normal blood film are about the same size, averaging 7.2 μm in diameter. A normal red cell is uniformly round on a dry film, although variations in shape can be produced by poor spreading technique in the preparation of the blood film.

When experience has been gained in using the microscope to view blood films, a more specific technique is used to observe the morphologic features of the blood cells.

Certain things must be done whenever peripheral blood films are examined. The blood film must first be evaluated for acceptable gross appearance and staining, as previously described. It must be evaluated for acceptable white cell distribution by observing the feather edge under low power. The numbers of erythrocytes, leukocytes, and platelets should be estimated, and the erythrocyte and platelet morphology should be described. Finally, the percentage of each type of leukocyte should be estimated.

Microscopic Examination of the Blood Film

After the initial preparations manipulations of the microscope and the observations described above, the following steps are taken in the examination of every blood film. These steps will be described in detail; however, in more general terms the blood film will be examined under low power and oil immersion. The *low-power examination* of the blood film should include (1) an evaluation of the quality of the blood film, and (2) an estimate of the red cell count and the leukocyte count, and a scan of the blood film. The *oil-immersion examination* of the blood film should include (1) an examination of the erythrocytes for alterations and variations in morphology, (2) an evaluation of platelet numbers and morphology, and (3) the differential count of the leukocytes and examination of the leukocytes for morphologic alterations. Detailed descriptions of these steps follow.

1. *Evaluate the quality of the blood film, using the low-power objective.* The film should be thin enough that the red and white cells are clearly separated. The space between the cells should be clear. There should be no precipitated dye. The red and white cells should be properly stained, and there should not be a large accumulation of white cells at the feather edge of the blood film. If the blood film does not meet these criteria, it should not be examined further; a new film must be made.

2. *Estimate the red and white cell counts and scan for abnormal cells and clumps of platelets, using the low-power objective.* A rough estimate of the red cell count can be made by noting the number of cells and the space between them. Normally, fewer and fewer intercellular spaces will be seen as one moves into the thicker portion of the blood film. In the optimal counting area, there should be no agglutination (clumping) or rouleaux (cells stacked like coins).

A blood film should be used to check every white cell count. The number of white cells is estimated in the counting area of the film (the area where the red cells lie side by side with no overlapping) with the low-power objective. With the low-power objective (×10) and the usual eyepiece (×10)—a total magnification of ×100— approximately 20 to 30 white cells per field are equivalent to a white cell count of approximately 5×10^9/L. Under the same magnification, 40 to 60 white cells per field are equivalent to a white cell count of approximately 10×10^9/L. In other words, 5 white blood cells in one low-power field are equal to approximately $1 \times 10^9/L$. Five low-power fields should be counted and the number of white cells averaged to estimate the white cell count.

The slide should also be examined under low power for the presence of immature or abnormal cells. With experience, the cells may be recognizable under low power; however, they are positively identified under oil immersion. If very few such abnormal cells are present they may be overlooked if the slide is examined under oil immersion alone, where the examination area is much smaller. Such abnormal cells should be looked for especially in the feather edge and along the sides of the slide.

The optimal counting area, sides, and feather edge should also be scanned for clumps of platelets. Clumps of platelets should not be seen normally; however, when the platelet count is increased they may be found along the sides and in the feather edge.

3. *Examine red cells for alterations and variations in morphologic features under oil immersion.* The normal red cell is a nonnucleated biconcave disk containing hemoglobin. Most red cells measure 7.2 to 7.9 μm on a stained blood film. The normal red cell is approximately 2 μm thick; values of 2.14, 2.05, 1.84, and 1.64 μm have been reported as the normal mean thickness. Its mean volume, calculated from the hematocrit and the red cell count, is 87 fL. In estimating the diameters of WBCs or other structures, it is often advantageous to use the red cell as a 7-μm measuring stick.

When normal red cells are studied on dried and stained blood films, they are nearly uniform in size, shape, and color. Such normal-appearing cells are referred to as *normocytic*. A tool that may be used in evaluating red cell size is a micrometer disk, which is inserted into the microscope; however, this is not necessary with experience. The normal red cell appears as a disk with a rim of hemoglobin and a clear central area, referred to as *central pallor*. The area of central pallor is normally less than one-third the diameter of a red cell, although there is some variation within the film. The amount of color in the cell (the staining reaction) and the corresponding amount of central pallor reflect the amount of hemoglobin in the cell. Normal red cells are pink. The staining reaction is referred to in terms of chromasia, and red cells with a normal amount of color are referred to as *normochromic* or, less frequently, *orthochromatic*. Normochromic, normocytic red cells are shown in Figure 11–20.

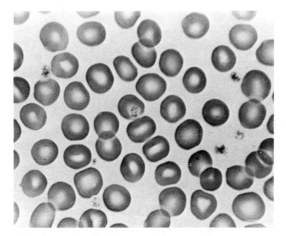

FIG 11–20.
Normal red blood cells (oil-immersion objective).

It is important to observe red cell morphology only in the optimal counting area. In the thick end of the film the morphologic characteristics of the cell are difficult to distinguish, and at the very thin edge of the film the red cells flatten out, appear completely filled with hemoglobin (showing no area of central pallor), and are generally distorted.

When red cells are examined morphologically, the following characteristics must be observed and noted: (1) variations in color, (2) variations in size, (3) variations in shape, (4) variations in structure and inclusions, (5) the presence of artifacts and abnormal distribution patterns, and (6) the presence of nucleated red cells. These changes are thoroughly described under Erythrocyte Alterations. A brief summary follows.

Various terms are used to describe changes in the red cell shape, size, and staining reaction. Alterations in size are described by the terms *anisocytosis,* excessive variation in cell size; *macrocytosis,* predominance of large red cells, with a mean corpuscular diameter (MCD) greater than 9 μm; and *microcytosis,* predominance of small red cells, with an MCD less than 6.5 μm. Alterations in shape are described in terms of *poikilocytes,* red cells with markedly irregular shapes; *sickle cells,* red cells that are sickle-shaped or long and clublike in appearance; *spherocytes,* small, spherical red cells that appear round and completely filled with hemoglobin; and *ovalocytes,* red cells that are oval. Variations in the staining reaction are described by terms such as *hy-*

pochromasia, lack of color (pale-staining cells with very pale central areas); *anochromasia,* concentration of pale-staining hemoglobin around the periphery of the cells, with the center pale; *orthochromasia* or *normochromasia,* the normal amount of hemoglobin and normal staining; and *polychromasia,* mixed staining because of the presence of RNA and hemoglobin (polychromatic "red" cells vary in color from muddy blue to a grayish red-orange and appear as reticulocytes when stained supravitally). The degree of the observed red cell alteration is noted as slight, moderate, or marked.

Several inclusions are also seen under certain conditions in the red cells, and they must be identified. *Basophilic stippling* is seen as pinpoint to granular particles stained blue-green to blue-black. These particles consist of precipitated RNA. Some red cells that show basophilic stippling with Wright's stain will prove to be siderocytes. *Siderocytes* (siderosomes) are red cells that contain particulate iron, which stains bright blue-green after staining with ferric ferrocyanide (Prussian blue). *Howell-Jolly bodies* are spherical particles 1 to 2 μm in diameter that stain purple to black. These particles are also nuclear remnants, and one or more may be present within an RBC.

Rouleaux formation by the red cells is also to be noted. It is seen in certain disease conditions, but more often is caused by poor technique in the slide preparation. When the blood film is not dried immediately after it is spread on the slide, rouleaux can result.

4. *Correct white cell count for nucleated red cells, when present.* When nucleated red cells *(normoblasts)* are seen on the blood film, the number of these cells per 100 white cells is reported. It is necessary to correct the total white cell count when normoblasts are present, since they are not destroyed by the acetic acid diluents used for the white cell count and will be counted along with the white cells. The total white cell count can be corrected in the following way:

Corrected white cell count

$$= \frac{\text{uncorrected white cell count} \times 100}{100 + \text{number of nucleated RBCs per 100 WBCs}}$$

5. *Evaluate the platelet count and morphologic changes with the oil-immersion objective.* The blood film is examined with the oil-immersion objective to estimate the number of platelets and to detect morphologic alterations. The platelet count is estimated as adequate, decreased, or increased.

Platelets generally vary from 2 to 5 μm in diameter. They are ovoid structures having a colorless to pale-blue background (hyalomere) containing centrally located, reddish to violet granules (chromomere). Platelets are not cells, but portions of cytoplasm pinched off from megakaryocytes, giant cells of the bone marrow. Platelets are often increased in size when the blood is being actively regenerated; their size is also a function of age, with younger cells being generally larger. Bizarre forms are also noted after splenectomy and in myelofibrosis, hemorrhagic thrombocytosis, and polycythemia vera. Giant platelets are characteristic of platelet disorders associated with thrombocytopenia.

Normally, 6 to 20 platelets should be seen in each oil-immersion field, representing a normal platelet count of $172-450 \times 10^9/L$. A rough estimate of the platelet count can be made by letting each platelet seen in an oil-immersion field equal approximately $20 \times 10^9/L$. Values as low as 3 to 5 platelets per oil-immersion field have been considered to represent a normal platelet count. The difference in normal values is probably a result of the use of specimens from different sources: the lower value is more consistent with capillary blood, where some of the platelets are utilized in the clotting mechanism, while the higher value is consistent with anticoagulated venous blood.

One system for estimating platelet counts follows. The platelet estimate is reported as adequate if 6 to 20 platelets are seen per oil-immersion field. Several fields should be checked, and the platelets should be kept in mind while doing the white cell differential. If the average number of platelets is less than 6, the estimate should be reported as a *slight, moderate,* or *marked decrease,* depending on the magnitude of the decrease. Before this is done, however, the slide should be scanned for clumps of platelets with the low-power objective, especially at the feather edge. If the blood film is well made, without aggregates at the feather edge, and platelets can be found only with great difficulty, the platelet count is below $20 \times 10^9/L$. In addition, the tube of blood should be rechecked for the presence of clots, as platelets would be utilized in the clots and the blood film value artificially decreased. If there are more than 20 platelets per oil-immersion field, the estimate should be reported as a *slight, moderate,* or *marked increase,* depending on the magnitude of the increase. If there are many masses of platelets at the feather edge and platelets are sufficiently abundant to attract the attention of the observer, it is reasonable to assume almost automatically that the platelet count is increased.

The platelet morphology should be observed and the presence of large, bizarre, or atypical forms should be reported. These should also be observed while doing the white cell differential (Fig 11–21).

6. *Perform the differential count of white cells and examine for morphologic alterations, using the oil-immersion objective.* The differential count consists of identifying and counting a minimum of 100 white cells. After the red cells and platelets have been examined, the white cells are classified and counted in the optimal counting area of the blood film under oil immersion. The slide should be moved in a way that will allow continuous counting and classification of white cells from margin to margin of the film. When a margin is reached, the slide should be moved toward the thicker end (a distance of one or two microscope fields) and the white cells counted and classified from margin to margin again (Fig 11–22). When exactly 100 white cells have been counted, the numbers of the different types of white cells recorded are estimates of the percentages of these types making up the total white cell count. For example, if 3 of the 100 cells counted are eosinophils, then 3% of the circulating white cells are assumed to be eosinophils. This is of relative value.

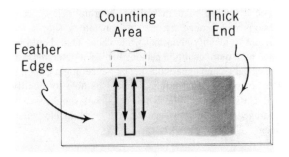

FIG 11–22.
Pathway for differential cell count.

If any nucleated red cells are encountered in the white cell differential, they should be counted separately; they should not be included in the 100 cells counted. However, the white cell count must be corrected when nucleated red cell forms are noted. This correction was described in step 4 above.

In certain situations it may be necessary to count more or fewer than 100 cells. If the relative numbers of specific types of white cells differ markedly from the accepted normal values, it is advisable to count 200 cells or more before recording percentages. Specifically, 200 cells should be counted if more than 5% of the cells are eosinophils, if more than 2% are basophils, if more than 10% are monocytes, or if the percentage of lymphocytes is greater than that of neutrophils (except in children). If the differential for an adult with a normal white cell count shows fewer than 15 or more than 40 lymphocytes, an additional 100 cells should be counted on another blood film to rule out distribution errors. In cases of leukopenia, if the white cell count is less than $1 \times 10^9/L$, only 50 cells should be counted in the white cell differential. When such changes are made, the percentages of the different cell types must be calculated, and the number of cells actually counted in the differential must be noted on the report form; for example, 3% basophils— 200 cells counted. Occasionally, the absolute number of cells of each type is of interest, although values are usually reported as percentages. To calculate the absolute value, multiply the percentage of each cell type, expressed as a decimal, by the total white cell count.

As the cells are being classified and counted, any morphologic alterations or abnormalities should be noted, as described later in this section. A white cell cannot be skipped because it cannot be identified. Experience is necessary for morphologic studies of white cells,

Normal Platelets

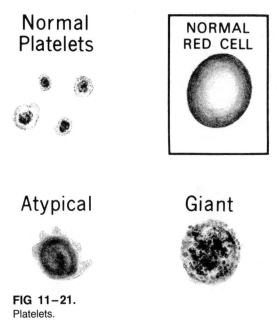

Atypical

Giant

FIG 11–21.
Platelets.

NORMAL RED CELL

especially when an immature or abnormal cell is seen. Persons with limited training in hematology should not attempt to identify abnormal white cells. This should be done by a more qualified person, such as a pathologist or a medical technologist with special hematologic training. Persons with limited training should be able to identify and classify the normal white cells, but should be encouraged to seek assistance when a questionable cell is seen.

Leukocyte Differentials Provided by Hematology Analyzers

Many of the automated hematology analyzers provide some degree of differentiation of leukocytes. Techniques used by these instruments employ either image analysis or flow cytometry (see also Flow Cytometry—Use of a Focused Laser Beam, under Automated Cell Counting Methods in this chapter). The major advantage of automated differentiation of leukocytes is that many thousands of cells are analyzed rapidly. The major disadvantage is that these cells are not actually "seen" by anyone (when compared with the microscopic examination of blood films). Automated differentials can provide a great amount of useful information when interpreted by an experienced laboratorian and can be used as a

complement to the microscopic differential. Different cellular characteristics are measured by each method and comparison of results between automated and microscopic differentials is not always easy to do.

In most automated analyzers, three subpopulations of leukocytes are identifiable: lymphocytes, other mononuclear cells, and granulocytes. The Coulter principle is utilized to construct a size-distributed histogram of leukocytes. A computer in the analyzer calculates the number of particles in each as a percentage of the total WBC count. For routine screening, the calculated values are useful to approximate a three-cell differential.

Leukocyte Differential Reporting Methods: Relative vs. Absolute Numbers

The numbers and types of leukocytes counted are traditionally reported in percent numbers—cells identified while examining and counting 100 WBCs in a systematic fashion. These results are reported in *relative numbers, or percent*. The alternative method is to report the differentials in terms of *absolute numbers*. In using this method, the numbers and types of cells counted are reported in number of cells $\times$ 10^9/L. Increases or decreases of individual cell lines are reported separately

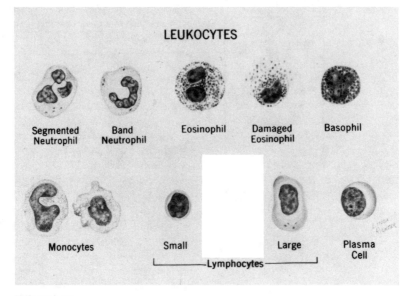

FIG 11–23.
Leukocytes.

and give more meaningful information to the physician regarding the status of the blood leukocytes.

The **absolute cell count** by cell type is obtained by multiplying the relative number of white cells (in decimal units) by the total white cell count per liter. For example, if a patient's WBC count is 7.5×10^9/L and 68% neutrophils are identified while doing the leukocyte differential, the *relative neutrophil count is 68%*. The *absolute neutrophil count is: 0.68 $\times$ 7.5 $\times$ 10^9/L = 5.1 $\times$ 10^9/L*. The absolute count should be reported to the nearest 0.1×10^9/L cells. Many laboratories report both the relative and absolute values for leukocyte differentials.

Normal Leukocyte Morphology

The five types of WBCs encountered in normal peripheral blood are shown in Figure 11–23. Certain characteristics should be kept in mind when cells are to be classified; these are related to size, the nucleus, and the cytoplasm. Whether the cell is small, medium, or large and how it compares to a normal red blood cell, which is approximately 7 μm in diameter, should be noted. Characteristics of the nucleus that should be considered are the shape, the size compared to the rest of the cell, the chromatin pattern (smooth or coarse), and the presence of nucleoli. Characteristics of the cytoplasm that should be considered include the presence or absence of granules, their staining characteristics, and whether they are specific or nonspecific, as well as the staining properties and relative amount of the cytoplasm. These properties should be noted for all types of cells that may be encountered in the peripheral blood or bone marrow, whether they are of the granulocyte, lymphocyte, erythrocyte, or megakaryocyte series.

Segmented Neutrophils

The most numerous of the granulocytes are the polymorphonuclear neutrophilic (PMN) leukocytes or segmented neutrophilic granulocytes ranging from 10 to 14 μm in diameter. The mean relative total neutrophil count for adults is 59% with a range of 35% to 71%. The mean relative adult value for segmented neutrophils is 56%.* Infants and children have fewer neutrophils and more lymphocytes (see Reference Values for Routine Hematologic Procedures at the end of this chapter). Neutrophils vary in diameter from about 10 to 14 μm, and

the nucleus forms a relatively small part of the cell. The nucleus can assume various shapes, but its usual configuration is lobular—that is, the elongated nucleus is usually constricted in one to four places, forming a series of bulges or lobes connected by narrow strands of chromatin or narrow filaments; it may have two to five lobes. The chromatin is irregularly arranged in fairly compact masses, and it stains deep reddish-purple. These chromatin masses are distinct and clearly distinguishable from the lighter-staining (generally pink-staining) parachromatin (nucleoplasm or karyoplasm). The nuclear membrane is distinct and no nucleoli are visible. The abundant cytoplasm has a faint pink color and contains a large number of very small, often indiscrete granules distributed irregularly throughout it. These granules are usually light pink or very light violet. A few darker granules may be present. About two thirds of the granules are specific neutrophilic granules, while the remaining one third are azurophilic.

Band Neutrophils

The band neutrophil is a younger form of the mature neutrophil. Both segmented and band neutrophils should be classified separately in the white cell differential. The mean relative band neutrophil count for adults is 3%.† Morphologically, band neutrophils are like segmented cells except for the shape of the nucleus. In band neutrophils the nucleus may be rod- or band-shaped, when distinct lobes have not yet formed, or it may have begun to form lobes. In the latter case, the lobes are connected by wide strips or bands rather than narrow threads or filaments as in segmented neutrophils. The College of American Pathologists defines a band as a connecting strip or isthmus that is wide enough to show two distinct margins with nuclear material in between. A filament, on the other hand, is so narrow that there is no visible nuclear material between the two sides. The differentiation between band and segmented neutrophils may be difficult; if there is doubt, the cell should be classified as segmented. (see Fig 11–23).

Generally, an increased white cell count (leukocytosis) results from an increase in the absolute number of neutrophils present in the blood; in this case it is called *neutrophilia*. Neutrophilia is found in acute infections; metabolic, chemical, and drug intoxications; acute hem-

---

*Williams WW, Beutler E, Ersley A, et al: *Hematology*, ed 4. New York, McGraw-Hill Book Co, 1990, p 18.

†*CAP Surveys Manual*. Section 2, Appendix 1: *Glossary of Terms, Hematology—Coagulation/Clinical Microscopy*. Northfield, Ill, College of American Pathologists, 1990.

orrhage; postoperative states; certain noninflammatory conditions such as coronary thrombosis; malignant neoplasms; and after acute hemolytic episodes. It is usually accompanied by a *shift to the left,* or an increase in the number of immature cells, and by toxic changes in the cytoplasm. An increase in the number of band forms, which may be accompanied by the presence of more immature neutrophils, is significant. The presence of forms more immature than bands is also termed a *leukoblastotic reaction.* Toxic changes in the neutrophil cytoplasm are indicated by the presence of deeply stained basophilic (or toxic) granules, pale-blue Döhle bodies, and vacuolization. Toxic changes in the nucleus include hypersegmentation (more than five lobes) and degeneration, or pyknosis. The cell size may be increased or decreased.

Eosinophils

Eosinophilic granular leukocytes, or eosinophils, make up a mean of 3% of the total number of leukocytes.* They are slightly larger than neutrophils, and the nucleus occupies a relatively small part of the cell. The nucleus is also polymorphic, but it usually has fewer lobes than do neutrophil nuclei. Usually two and occasionally three lobes are seen. The nuclear structure is much like that of the neutrophil, but the lobes are plumper and the chromatin often stains lighter purple. The nuclear membrane is distinct, and no nucleoli are visible. The cytoplasm is usually colorless, but it may be faintly basophilic; it is crowded with spherical acidophilic granules, which stain red-orange with eosin and are larger and more distinct than neutrophilic granules. The eosinophilic granules are hard, firm bodies that are not easily damaged; they remain intact when pressed into the nucleus or even when the whole cell is damaged and the cell membrane is broken. Eosinophilic granules are also highly refractive, a feature that is often a valuable distinguishing characteristic.

If more than 5 eosinophils are encountered in the 100-cell differential, 200 cells should be counted. The percentage of each cell type present should then be calculated and the number of cells counted noted on the report form.

Eosinophilia, an increase in the number of eosinophils above normal, is associated with allergic reactions, certain skin disorders, parasitic infections, and other infections such as brucellosis, Hodgkin's disease, and certain leukemias.

Basophils

Basophilic granular leukocytes, or basophils, constitute 0.5% of the total leukocytes.* They are about the same size as neutrophils, but their nuclei usually occupy a relatively greater portion of the cell. The nucleus is often extremely irregular in shape, varying from a lobular form to a form showing indentations that are not deep enough to divide it into definite lobes. The nuclear pattern is indistinct; there appears to be a mixture of chromatin and parachromatin, and this mixture stains purple or blue and shows little structure. The nuclear membrane is fairly distinct and no nucleoli are visible. The cytoplasm is usually colorless; it contains a variable number of deeply stained, coarse, round, or angular basophilic granules. The granules (metachromatic) stain deep purple or black; occasionally a few smaller, brownish granules may be present. Since the granules are soluble in water, occasionally a few or even most of them may be dissolved during the staining procedure. When this occurs, the cell will contain vacuoles in place of granules, and the cytoplasm may appear grayish or brownish in their vicinity. The cytoplasm of a mature basophil is colorless. An immature basophil has a pale blue cytoplasm and is seen only in myelogenous or nonlymphocytic leukemia.

If more than two basophils are encountered in the 100-cell differential, 200 cells should be counted. *Basophilia,* an increase in the number of basophils, is associated with chronic myelogenous or nonlymphocytic leukemia. It is also seen in allergic reactions, myeloid metaplasia, and polycythemia vera. The basophil number may increase temporarily after irradiation, and basophilia may be present in chronic hemolytic anemia and after splenectomy.

Tissue basophils, also called *mast cells,* are similar but not identical to basophilic granulocytes. They are larger and differ somewhat in their chemical makeup and function.

Monocytes

Monocytes constitute a mean of 4% of the leukocytes in the blood of normal adults.† They are the largest of the normal leukocytes, measuring 15 to 22 μm in diameter. The nucleus is fairly large; it may be oval, lobu-

---

*Williams WW, Beutler E, Erslev A, et al: *Hematology,* ed 4. New York, McGraw-Hill Book Co, 1990, p 18.

†Williams WW, Beutler E, Erslev A, et al: *Hematology,* ed 4. New York, McGraw-Hill Book Co, 1990, p 18.

lar, notched, or polymorphic, but most frequently it is kidney-shaped. It stains faintly, usually with a very characteristic pattern. Chromatin and parachromatin are sharply segregated, and the chromatin is distributed in a linear arrangement of delicate strands, which gives the nucleus a stringy appearance. (Occasionally the nuclear pattern resembles that of a lymphocyte, and the cytoplasmic differences must be relied on for identification.) The nuclear membrane is delicate but not distinct, and nucleoli usually are not seen. The cytoplasm is abundant, slightly basophilic, and often vacuolated, and has a slate-gray or muddy blue color. Extremely fine and abundant azurophilic granules are present; this granulation is called *azure dust* and is seen only in monocytes. The granules vary in color from light pink to bright purplish red.

Lymphocytes

Lymphocytes constitute a mean of 34% of the leukocytes in the normal adult.* Infants and children normally have more lymphocytes and fewer neutrophils than adults. Lymphocytes fall in two general size groups: small (approximately 10 μm), and large (up to 20 μm). There are numerous gradations of size and form from one type to another; some lymphocytes can be as large as monocytes.

The small lymphocyte is composed chiefly of nucleus and is the type of lymphocyte predominating in normal adult blood. The nucleus is round or slightly notched, and the nuclear chromatin is in the form of coarse, dense, deeply staining blocks. There is relatively little parachromatin, and it is not very distinct. Almost the entire nucleus stains deep purple. The nuclear membrane is heavy and distinct, and nucleoli are not usually seen. The cytoplasm appears in the form of a narrow band that stains relatively dark blue, usually free of azure granules.

The large lymphocyte shows a further increase in the size of the nucleus and an increase in the relative amount of cytoplasm. The nucleus contains more parachromatin, and so stains more lightly than the nuclei of the smaller forms. However, the chromatin is still present in clumps, without distinct outlines because of the blending of chromatin and parachromatin. The nuclear membrane is distinct and nucleoli usually are not seen. The cytoplasm in this form can be abundant and is most frequently smooth; it may, however, be spongy;

*Williams WW, Beutler E, Erslev A, et al: *Hematology,* ed 4. New York, McGraw-Hill Book Co, 1990, p 18.

azure granules are frequently seen. Nucleoli are rarely seen in lymphocytes of normal blood, but they may be seen in cells that have been crushed during the spreading of the film. It is possible that blood lymphocytes contain nucleoli but that they are normally obscured by the coarse nuclear chromatin.

It is sometimes difficult to distinguish between nucleated red cells (normoblasts) and small lymphocytes. The staining reaction of the parachromatin of the two cells is an important diagnostic criterion; the parachromatin of the lymphocyte is pale blue or violet, and that of the normoblast is red or pink. In addition, the cytoplasm of nucleated erythrocytes contains hemoglobin, which stains pink in blood films.

Lymphocytosis, an increase in the number of lymphocytes, is characteristic of certain acute infections (infectious mononucleosis, pertussis, mumps, and rubella, or German measles) and of chronic infections such as tuberculosis, brucellosis, and infectious hepatitis. The toxic changes seen in these diseases are referred to as reactive changes, and are particularly associated with infectious mononucleosis. The cells are called reactive lymphocytes, as the increased amount and apparent activity of the cytoplasm indicate that it may be reacting to some sort of stimulus (see under Leukocyte Alterations).

Plasma Cells

In addition to the five types of white cells that normally appear in the peripheral blood, the *plasma cell (plasmacyte)* can occur in certain blood specimens. The plasma cell is thought to be a derivative of the B lymphocyte. It is large, with a round or oval nucleus that is usually in an eccentric position. The chromatin consists of deeply stained, heavy masses that may be arranged in a radial pattern. The cytoplasm is strongly basophilic. There may be a pale, clear zone in the cytoplasm to one side of the nucleus, referred to as a *hof*. Immature forms may occasionally be seen. Plasma cells function in the synthesis of immunoglobulins. They may be found in the peripheral blood in cases of measles, chickenpox, or scarlet fever and in the malignant conditions multiple myeloma and plasmacytic leukemia.

Blood Cell Alterations

Morphologic changes in the red and white blood cells seen on the stained blood film aid in determining the nature of many blood diseases. Certain diseases produce fairly characteristic alterations of red cells, white cells, and platelets, in addition to other clinical signs. It is important that the laboratory personnel be well acquainted with the appearance of normal blood cells, so that abnormal or immature cell forms will be recognized immediately. Abnormal or immature cells should be identified by someone experienced in cell morphology. The general laboratorian should screen the films and give questionable ones to a pathologist or an experienced medical technologist for final evaluation.

Most abnormalities found in white cells are related to the age of the cell. All white cells in the circulating blood should be mature, and the presence of immature white cells in the blood is considered abnormal. Immature white cells may be differentiated from mature ones by size, the appearance of intracellular structure (e.g., the presence of granules or changes in the nucleoli, chromatin, or nucleus), the staining properties, and the cell function. There is a progressive decrease in cell size with maturity, with the nucleus becoming smaller and the cytoplasmic ratio correspondingly increasing. In granulocytes, granules appear with maturity. In immature white cells the nucleus is round; with age it becomes lobular or indented. Chromatin is fine and lacy in the young cell and eventually becomes coarse and clumped. Nucleoli may be present in young cells and absent in the mature forms. The cytoplasm is basophilic (stains blue) in young granulocytes, and eventually turns pink with maturity. The young nucleus stains reddish violet and becomes strongly basophilic with maturity. The granules in the cytoplasm assume specific staining qualities with increasing cell maturity.

Certain evidence of cell function is observed that is characteristic of specific developmental stages of the white cells. Examples are the presence of nucleoli, which indicate a young cell; mitotic figures, which indicate a young cell; cytoplasmic inclusions, which are characteristic of a mature cell; phagocytosis, which is seen in mature cells; and hemoglobin, which is seen in mature red cells.

The laboratorian should be able to differentiate an immature cell from a mature one. There are many stages of young cells, and it is not necessary for all levels of laboratory personnel to be able to differentiate among these stages; the trained medical technologist or pathologist makes this evaluation. The general medical laboratorian should be aware of the various developmental stages of the blood cells, however, and for this reason the following material is presented.

Origin and Function of Blood Cells Related to Morphologic Examination

Final agreement on the origin of all types of blood cells and their relationships to one another has not been reached, and several theories have been put forth. Practically speaking, the origin of blood cells is not important for their identification. According to one theory, all blood cells originate from two or more specific primitive cells. According to another theory, all blood cells have a common origin in one type of cell, which is given various names, such as the primitive stem cell, **pluripotential stem cell (PSC),** colony-forming unit (CFU), uncommitted stem cell, undifferentiated mesenchyme or stem cell, and hemocytoblast.

These colony-forming units or pluripotential stem cells may become committed to a lymphoid, myeloid, or erythroid line—all are hemopoietic cells (Fig 11–24). Other body cells may also originate from this original stem cell. Proliferation and maturation processes vary with the cell line to which the stem cell has become "committed." Stimulating factors are produced and regulated, but all mechanisms for these activities are still unclear.

The original hemopoietic stem cell has the following properties that can be considered characteristic of young cells in general: The cell is large, approximately 20 to 40 μm in diameter on films prepared with Wright's stain. It has abundant cytoplasm, which is slightly basophilic or blue and which may contain a few nonspecific azurophilic granules. The margin of the cell is not clearly defined; it is usually indefinite. The nucleus is small in relation to the rest of the cell. The chromatin pattern is fine and open (the term *reticular pattern* is based on the appearance of this nucleus). The nucleus stains pale rose-purple.

Blood cell differentiation and maturation occur primarily in the bone marrow. There the environment is well organized and complex. Mature cells must migrate across the sinusoidal endothelia of the marrow capillaries to enter the peripheral circulation (Fig 11–25). The endothelial membrane allows the passage of the more deformable mature cells and holds back the immature cells which are more rigid and less motile. Pathologic processes can facilitate the release of more immature cells by affecting the cellular composition of the sinusoidal endothelia.

A diagrammatic representation of one blood cell or-

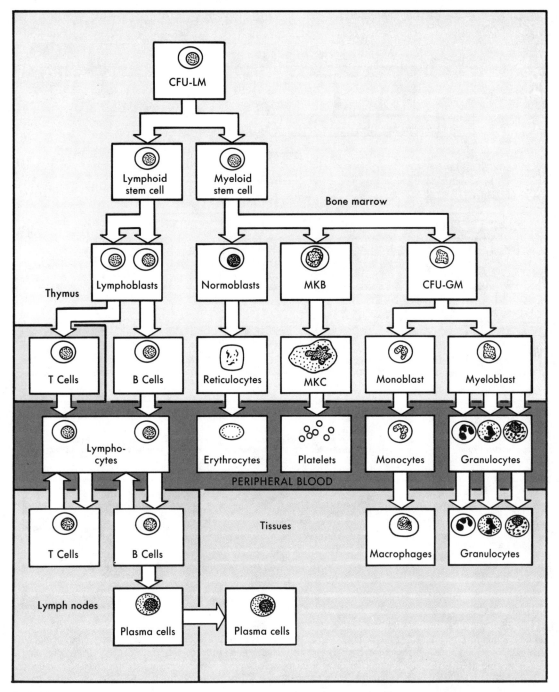

FIG 11–24.
Blood cell differentiation and maturation. A general model of cellular differentiation and maturation shows the relationships of the mature cell lines and stem cells. Intermediate stages are not shown for all cells. *CFU-LM* = colony-forming unit, lymphoid-myeloid; *CFU-GM* = colony-forming unit–granulocyte-monocyte. *MKB* = megakaryoblast; *MKC* = megakaryocyte. (From Powers LW: *Diagnostic Hematology.* St Louis, Mosby–Year Book, Inc, 1989, p 87. Used by permission.)

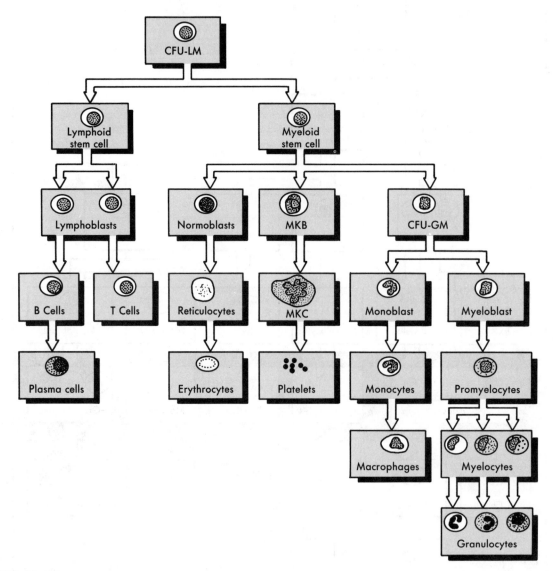

FIG 11–25.

Blood cells in marrow, blood, and tissue compartments. Not all tissue–blood cell relationships are depicted. Lymphocytes, for example, recirculate between various organs, lymphatic vessels, and the bloodstream. *CFU-LM* = Colony-forming unit, lymphoid-myeloid; *CFU-GM* = Colony-forming unit–granulocyte-monocyte. *MKB* = megakaryoblast; *MKC* = megakaryo-cyte. (From Powers LW: *Diagnostic Hematology*. St Louis, Mosby–Year Book, Inc, 1989, p 77. Used by permission.)

igin theory, showing the origin and relationships of all blood cell types, is given in Figure 11–26. It should be remembered that this is theoretical and the actual details are unknown. All stages in the maturation process are gradual, and it is often impossible to identify an exact

stage with certainty. The most immature forms in all se-ries (pronormoblast, myeloblast, lymphoblast, and plas-mablast) appear very similar morphologically, and their identification is often based on surrounding cell types in various stages of development. The origin of the mono-

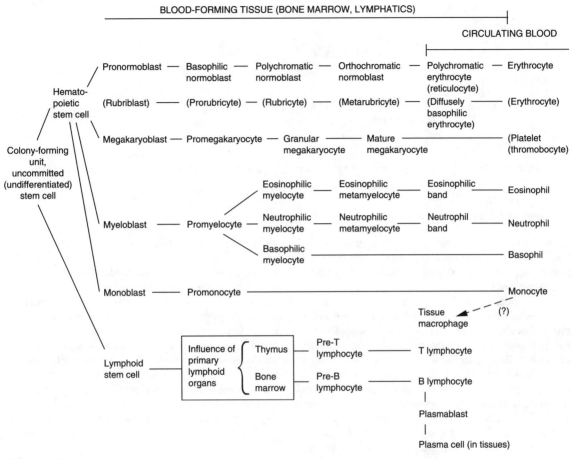

FIG 11–26.
Origin of blood cells. (Adapted from Henry JB: *Clinical Diagnosis and Management by Laboratory Methods,* ed 18. Philadelphia, WB Saunders Co, 1991, p 607; and Diggs LW, Sturm D, Bell A: *The Morphology of Human Blood Cells,* ed 5. Abbott Park, Ill, Abbot Laboratories, 1988, p 1; with permission.)

cyte is still largely unknown, although it is believed to originate in the bone marrow.

Erythrocyte Maturation

Red blood cells are normally produced in the bone marrow. Their maturation takes 3 to 5 days, and six stages of development have been described. Several systems of nomenclature have been used to describe these stages, two of which will be discussed here. The stages of erythrocyte maturation from the youngest to the mature cell are: pronormoblast (rubriblast), basophilic normoblast (prorubricyte), polychromatophilic normoblast

(rubricyte), orthochromic normoblast (metarubricyte), reticulocyte (diffusely basophilic erythrocyte), and mature erythrocyte. These stages are diagrammed in Figure 11–27 (see also Fig 11–26).

Remember that cells do not jump from one stage to another; there is a gradual progression, and exact classification is often very difficult. Rather than learning the characteristics of the specific stages, one should understand certain statements that are applicable in general to explain the maturation of the erythroblast to a nonnucleated erythrocyte.

Concerning the cell size and cytoplasm, there is a progressive decrease in size and there is also a decrease

Pronormoblast	Basophilic Normoblast	Polychroma- tophilic Normoblast	Orthochromic Normoblast	Reticulocyte	Mature Red Cell
(Rubriblast)	(Prorubricyte)	(Rubricyte)	(Metarubricyte)	(Diffusely Basophilic Erythrocyte)	(Erythrocyte)

FIG 11–27.
Maturation of the erythrocyte series.

in the intensity of the blue color because of loss of RNA. There is an increase in red color caused by an increased hemoglobin concentration. Finally, there are no granules in the cytoplasm.

Concerning the nucleus, it is generally round and in the center of the cell. In the early stages the chromatin is fine and lacelike. As the cell matures and the nucleus becomes smaller, the chromatin becomes coarse and more condensed. Finally, the nucleus degenerates into clumps or a solid pyknotic mass, which is eventually released (or extruded) from the cell. At the same time, the color of the nucleus changes from purplish red to dark blue. When the nucleus is extruded, it is phagocytosed and digested by marrow macrophages. The reticulocyte, or early non-nucleated erythrocyte, then squeezes through an opening in the endothelial lining of the marrow cavity and thus enters the peripheral circulatory system.

The earliest normoblast (pronormoblast) appears morphologically very much like the myeloblast or lymphoblast, and it may be impossible to distinguish them. It may be necessary to depend on their association with and transition to hemoglobin-containing cells in the same area of the marrow for identification. Cells of the erythrocyte series tend to stain more intensely than myeloblasts or lymphoblasts because of the combination of hemoglobin and RNA in the cytoplasm. The stages are described in terms of the staining reaction of the cytoplasm as it gains in hemoglobin concentration: basophilic cytoplasm is blue, polychromatic cytoplasm shows shades of blue and gray as hemoglobin increases, and orthochromatic cytoplasm is orange-red.

Another erythrocyte developmental series is that of

the *megaloblastic erythrocytes*. It is similar to the sequence of maturation of the normoblasts, but the cells are larger, as the name implies. Megaloblasts are found in certain anemias, called *megaloblastic anemias,* which are the result of vitamin B_{12} or folic acid deficiency. As they develop, cells of the megaloblastic sequence have a more open chromatin pattern in the nucleus. This is referred to as asynchronous maturation or dyssynchronous development of the nucleus and cytoplasm. In megaloblastic anemia these changes are not limited to the erythrocyte series—all types of cells normally produced in the bone marrow are similarly affected, as evidenced by large hypersegmented neutrophils. This increase in size of all the cells makes it difficult to appreciate the increased red cell volume.

Granulocyte Maturation and Function

Neutrophils normally mature in the bone marrow in the following stages from the youngest to the most mature: myeloblast, promyelocyte (progranulocyte), myelocyte, metamyelocyte, band, and segmented neutrophils. These maturation stages are similar for all granulocytes and are diagrammed in Figure 11–28.

Cells of the neutrophil series are generally round with smooth margins or edges. As the cells mature they become progressively smaller. Most immature cells have cytoplasm that stains dark blue, and becomes light pink as the cells mature. As the cells mature from the myeloblast to the promyelocyte stage, nonspecific granules that stain blue to reddish-purple appear in the cytoplasm. Eventually, these nonspecific granules are replaced by

| Myeloblast | Promyelocyte | Myelocyte | Metamyelocyte | Band Neutrophil | Mature (Segmented) Neutrophil |

FIG 11–28.
Maturation of granulocytes.

specific neutrophilic granules. Both types of granules are not produced at the same time, but they may both be seen in the promyelocyte and myelocyte stages.

Nuclear changes also occur as the cells mature. In the myeloblast the nucleus is round or oval and very large in proportion to the rest of the cell. As the cell matures, the nucleus decreases in relative size and begins to contort or form lobes. At the same time, the nuclear chromatin changes from a fine delicate pattern to the more clumped pattern characteristic of the mature cell. The staining of the nucleus also changes from reddish-purple to bluish-purple as the cell matures. Nucleoli may be apparent in the early forms but gradually disappear as the chromatin thickens and the cell matures.

The term *shift to the left* refers to the release into the peripheral blood of immature cell forms, which are normally present only in the bone marrow. It is derived from the diagrammatic representation of cell maturation, where the more immature forms are shown on the left side (see Fig 11–28).

Neutrophils exist in the peripheral blood for several hours after they are released from the marrow. During this time they move back and forth between the general blood circulation and the walls of the blood vessels, where they accumulate. They also leave the blood and enter the tissues, where they carry out their primary functions. In the tissues, they are utilized to fight bacterial infections and are then destroyed or eliminated from the body by the excretory system (intestinal tract, urine, lungs, or saliva).

Metabolically, neutrophils are very active and can carry out both anaerobic and aerobic glycolysis. The neutrophilic granules contain several digestive enzymes that are able to destroy many kinds of bacteria. The cells are capable of random locomotion and can be directed to an area of infection by the process referred to as *chemo-*

taxis. Once in the tissues, the neutrophils destroy bacteria by engulfing them and releasing digestive enzymes into the phagocytic vacuole thus formed.

Not as much is known about the other granulocytes—the eosinophils and basophils. Eosinophils exist in the peripheral blood for 8 to 12 hours after release from the marrow. Eosinophils are capable of locomotion and phagocytosis; however, they are more active in later stages of inflammation, in which they ingest antigen-antibody complexes. The eosinophilic granules contain histamine, peroxidase, and acid hydroxylases and are active in allergic reactions and certain parasitic infections, especially those involving parasitic invasion of the tissues. The basophils are capable of sluggish locomotion. The granules contain histamine, heparin or a heparin-like substance, and 5-hydroxytryptamine. Functionally, little is known about basophils except that they apparently play a role in allergic reactions.

Monocyte Maturation and Function

Monocytes, like granulocytes, are produced mainly in the bone marrow. The stages of development are myelomonoblast, promonocyte, and monocyte. The myelomonoblast looks very much like the myeloblast or the lymphoblast, and it may be impossible to distinguish them morphologically on films prepared with Wright's stain. In such cases, the term *blast* is used. It may be necessary to classify the type of blast present on the basis of other cell types in the area.

Monocytes remain in the peripheral blood for hours to days after leaving the bone marrow, depending on the reference cited. They are very motile and phagocytic cells. Unlike neutrophils, monocytes do not die after they engage in phagocytic activity. Instead, after 1 to 3 days in the peripheral blood, they move into the body tissues and are transformed into *macrophages*. Macrophages are thought to be derived from both monocytes and histiocytic cells. Cells that have become free are known as *histiocytes,* and a histiocyte that has begun to phagocytose is called a macrophage. The macrophage is the final mature form of the monocyte when it travels through the tissues. Therefore, monohistiocytic cells, histiocytes, monocytes, and macrophages are considered to be related in terms of function and origin. In addition to phagocytosing bacteria, macrophages appear to make antigens and interact with lymphocytes in the synthesis of antibodies.

Lymphocyte Maturation and Function

Lymphocytes are normally produced in the lymphoid tissue (nodes, spleen, and thymus) but may also be produced in the bone marrow. The stages of development are: lymphoid stem cell, lymphoblast, pre-T cell or pre-B cell and T lymphocyte or B lymphocyte. The number of precursor stages that exist from the lymphoid stem cell to the first identifiable **B lymphocytes** and **T lymphocytes** is not known. Lymphoid stem cells are indistinguishable from other undifferentiated stem cells. These stem cells are also called lymphoblasts by many hematologists. Lymphoid stem cells, or lymphoblasts, look very much like myeloblasts and their morphologic differentiation is beyond the scope of this book. When observed microscopically, lymphocytes are described based on their size and cytoplasmic granularity. Small lymphocytes are found in the greatest numbers, ranging in size from 6 to 10 μm. Large granular lymphocytes are also regarded as mature cells. These cells contain additional cytoplasm which appears typically sky-blue as does the cytoplasm of the small lymphocyte. The cytoplasm of the large granular lymphocyte can be deeply basophilic. Mature lymphocytes include different subsets of highly specialized lymphocytes. Morphologically, B and T lymphocytes appear identical on a Wright's stained blood film. Only when immunologic studies are performed can these cells be identified as belonging to specific subsets of lymphocytes. As lymphocytes mature, their identity and function are specified by the antigenic structures on their external membrane surface.

The cell membranes of B lymphocytes contain immunoglobulins which can be identified by immunofluorescent techniques. Characteristic antigens and receptors on the B lymphocyte membranes can also be identified and differentiated from T lymphocytes by the use of cell markers employing monoclonal antibodies. T lymphocytes lack immunoglobulins on their membranes but do contain a receptor for sheep erythrocytes. In a test utilizing sheep erythrocytes, the sheep red cells form rosettes with T lymphocytes, in which the presence of three or more sheep red cells attach to the cell membrane of the T lymphocyte.

The lymphatic system consists of a network of vessels throughout most of the body tissues. The smaller vessels unite to form larger and larger vessels, which finally come together in two main trunks, the right lymphatic duct and the thoracic duct. The ducts empty into the circulatory system through veins in the neck. Lymph nodes are located all along the lymphatic vessels, and the lymph (fluid within the system) circulates through the nodes as it progresses through the lymphatic system. Many of the lymphocytes are formed in the lymph nodes and circulate back and forth between the blood, the organs, and the lymphatic tissues. Functionally there are two types of lymphocytes, *T cells,* or *T lymphocytes,* and *B cells,* or *B lymphocytes.*

B lymphocytes most likely mature in the bone marrow and function primarily in antibody production or the formation of immunoglobulins. They are related to plasma cells and may transform into plasma cells if appropriately stimulated. B lymphocytes have a short life span, measured in days, and constitute about 10% to 30% of the blood lymphocytes.

T lymphocytes mature in the thymus, an organ found in the anterior mediastinum, and function in cell-mediated immune responses such as delayed hypersensitivity, graft-vs.-host reactions, and homograft rejection. They make up the majority of the lymphocytes circulating in the peripheral blood and have a life span of months to years as they continually recirculate from blood to lymph.

Lymphocytes act to direct and effect the immune response system of the body. Maturation of lymphocytes in the bone marrow or thymus results in cells that are immunocompetent. The cells are able to respond to antigenic challenges by directing the immune responses of the host defense. They migrate to various sites in the body to await antigenic stimulus and activation.

After antigenic stimulation, small lymphocytes can undergo transformation. These transformed cells appear large (15–25 μm) on films prepared with Wright's stain, with a relatively large amount of deep blue cytoplasm and are called large granular lymphocytes. The large nucleus has a reticular appearance, with uniform chromatin and prominent nucleoli. Such cells have various names, including *reactive, atypical,* and *reticular* lymphocytes.

Clinical Significance of Blood Cell Alterations

Erythrocyte Alterations

Clinically, alterations in erythrocyte morphology are associated with many diseases and especially with anemia. Anemia is not a specific disease, but a condition in which there is a decrease in the oxygen-carrying capacity of the blood and therefore in the amount of oxygen reaching the tissues and organs. Its causes are many and varied, and the type of anemia present and its underlying cause must be determined by the physician before treatment can be effectively undertaken. It may or may not be the result of a disorder of the blood or blood-forming tissues.

Classification (Types) of Anemia.—Clinically, all patients with anemia have similar symptoms or complaints regardless of the cause of the anemia. The severity is generally dependent on the hemoglobin concentration of the blood, as most symptoms result from the decreased oxygen-carrying capacity. The primary complaints are fatigue and shortness of breath. Other common complaints are faintness, dizziness, heart palpitation, and headache. All of these symptoms are general and can be present without the clinical condition of anemia. Once the existence of anemia has been demonstrated, usually on the basis of the blood hemoglobin concentration, the physician must determine the underlying cause. Besides the case history and physical examination, the physician will rely on various laboratory procedures, including the appearance of the red cells on the peripheral blood film, in establishing this diagnosis.

Generally, anemias are classified according to either the appearance of the red cells (morphologic classification) or the physiologic cause of the anemia (etiologic or pathogenetic classification). A morphologic classification, showing some of the more common types of anemia that result in the alterations in red cell morphology observed on the peripheral blood film is one classification used. Such morphologic classifications fail to deal effectively with the hemolytic anemias, and these are described separately. Although they are helpful to the physician, these observations will be transferred into an etiologic system in determining the appropriate therapy for the patient.

Morphologically, anemias are generally classified as (1) normochromic-normocytic, (2) macrocytic, or (3) hypochromic-microcytic. These types are discussed in terms of common laboratory changes, especially as reflected by the red blood cell indices, and common examples of each type are given. These changes are summarized in Table 11–1.

Normochromic-Normocytic Anemias.—Normochromic-normocytic anemias are characterized by normal-looking red cells on the peripheral blood film and normal red cell index values. The cells produced by the marrow are normal, but the number of cells in circulation is reduced for a variety of reasons. Such anemias may result from acute blood loss resulting from external trauma such as a wound, or internal trauma such as an acute bleeding ulcer or a ruptured organ. Conditions resulting in increased plasma volume, such as pregnancy and overhydration, will also result in normochromic-normocytic anemia. If the bone marrow is suppressed (hypoplastic), as seen in cases of aplastic anemia (a possible result of exposure to various chemicals or drugs), the red cells that remain are normal. Suppressed marrow results in a deficiency of the myeloid series and platelets, seen as decreased leukocyte and platelet counts. Likewise, if the marrow is infiltrated with a neoplasm or malignancy, as in leukemia or multiple myeloma, the remaining red cells appear normal although they are decreased in number. In certain hemolytic diseases and chronic kidney and liver diseases the red cells also appear normal but are reduced in number.

Macrocytic Anemias.—Macrocytic anemias are primarily represented by the megaloblastic anemias resulting from vitamin B_{12} or folic acid deficiency, or a combination of the two. The deficiency may be nutritional or may result from a malabsorption syndrome such as pernicious anemia, where the patient is unable to absorb vitamin B_{12}. In either case, the deficiency leads to a nuclear maturation defect and megaloblastic anemia. The marrow shows certain changes in the red cell, granulocyte (myeloid), and megakaryocyte (platelet) series. Megaloblastic changes are characterized by larger cells having a more open chromatin pattern in the nucleus (asynchronous maturation or dyssynchronous development of nucleus and cytoplasm) and by the presence of larger, hypersegmented neutrophils in the peripheral blood. The enlarged red cells (macrocytes) have MCV

TABLE 11–1.

Morphologic Classification of Anemias

Type of Anemia	Changes in Red Cell Indices			Common Red Cell Alterations*	Common Examples and Causes
	Mean Corpuscular Volume (MCV)	Mean Corpuscular Hemoglobin (MCH)	Mean Corpuscular Hemoglobin Concentration (MCHC)		
Normochromic-normocytic	Normal	Normal	Normal	Normal size, shape, and hemoglobin content; decreased cell count	Acute blood loss; aplastic anemia; increased plasma volume; infiltrated bone marrow; some hemolytic diseases; some chronic renal and liver diseases
Macrocytic	Increased	Increased	Normal	Macrocytosis (elliptocytes, ovalocytes)	Megaloblastic anemias from vitamin B_{12} or folic acid deficiency; chronic liver disease
Hypochromic-microcytic	Decreased	Decreased	Decreased	Microcytosis (cells may appear large because of decreased hemoglobin content and flattening out on the slide); anisocytosis (slight to marked depending on condition and severity); poikilocytosis (changes characteristic of certain diseases); various inclusions, depending on cause	Iron deficiency (from blood loss, dietary deficiency, or iron metabolism error); globulin synthesis disorders (e.g., thalassemia, porphyria); heme synthesis disorders (e.g., sideroblastic anemias, lead poisoning)

*Seen on films of peripheral blood stained with Wright's stain.

values of the order of 120 to 140 fL. Actual hyperchromasia is impossible, but the red cells appear to contain more hemoglobin because of their increased size and therefore thickness. Although the anemia may be severe, the red cell count is decreased more than the hemoglobin concentration, since the cells that are present are large and fairly completely filled with hemoglobin. Other changes seen in the blood film include anisocytosis (erythrocytes varying in size), poikilocytosis (erythrocytes varying in shape), and Howell-Jolly bodies.

Nutritional deficiency of vitamin B_{12} is relatively rare, but nutritional deficiency of folic acid is fairly common. It may be found in chronic alcoholism or other conditions where the diet is not well balanced. Folate deficiency is also observed when the requirement is increased, as in pregnancy, infancy, certain hemolytic ane-

mias, and hyperthyroidism. Celiac disease, tropical sprue, certain drugs, contraceptives, and liver disease may lead to malabsorption and megaloblastic anemia.

Hypochromic-Microcytic Anemias.—Hypochromic-microcytic anemias are probably the most common types encountered, with iron deficiency anemia being the one most frequently seen. However, iron deficiency is not a simple classification, as there are several possible causes of this clinical condition. In simplified terms, iron deficiency anemia may result from decreased iron intake (either from inadequate diet or impaired absorption), increased iron loss (generally from chronic bleeding from a variety of causes), or an error of iron metabolism. In addition, the increased iron requirements in infancy, pregnancy, and lactation may result in iron deficiency anemia. The physician must determine the cause of the anemia in order to treat it. If it results from a dietary deficiency of iron, a relatively simple and effective treatment is to administer iron, usually orally as ferrous sulfate tablets. However, if it is caused by another condition the administration of iron will do no good, and may do harm either of itself or because it delays the use of appropriate therapy.

If the iron deficiency anemia results from chronic bleeding, the cause of the bleeding must be determined. The bleeding is most often gastrointestinal, although women with excessive menstrual flow often develop iron deficiency anemia. Gastrointestinal bleeding leading to iron deficiency anemia may result from such causes as ulcer, carcinoma or other neoplasms, hemorrhoids, hookworm, or even the ingestion of salicylate (usually as aspirin). The treatment is different for each of these.

All iron deficiency anemias produce similar changes in red cell morphology. The cells are smaller than normal (microcytic) and the MCV is decreased. Unfortunately, the decreased size is not always as apparent on the blood film as it is in the MCV value. In iron deficiency anemia the amount of hemoglobin within each red cell is significantly decreased; such cells are *hypochromic* (deficient in color). This shows up in the red cell volume, which is primarily a function of hemoglobin, but may not be evident on the slide because the hypochromic red cell spreads out or flattens and may appear to be of normal size or even larger than normal. The hypochromic cell is extremely pale, showing only a thin rim of color with a significantly increased area of central pallor. The decreased hemoglobin per red cell is measured in the laboratory as decreased MCH and decreased MCHC. Other changes that are characteristic of iron deficiency anemia include anisocytosis and poikilocytosis, which vary in degree with the severity of the disease. Other tests that may be useful in the investigation of iron deficiency anemias include examination of the stool for occult blood, determination of serum iron and total iron-binding capacity, radiographic study of the gastrointestinal tract, and sometimes bone marrow examination.

Another group of anemias that are microcytic and hypochromic are those that result from disorders in the synthesis of globin, another component of the hemoglobin molecule. These are the thalassemias, a group of inherited disorders of hemoglobin synthesis. The microscopic appearance of the red cells varies with and within the various types of thalassemias. However, microcyto-

sis, hypochromasia, and basophilic stippling are general observations. Anisocytosis, poikilocytosis, and target cells may also be present, as well as decreased **osmotic fragility.** Actual differentiation of various forms of thalassemia requires family studies and fairly sophisticated laboratory tests.

The last group of hypochromic-microcytic anemias that will be discussed are those resulting from disorders of porphyrin and heme synthesis. Again, the hemoglobin molecule is malformed. The sideroblastic anemias are a heterogeneous group of disorders that have in common increased storage of iron, especially in the RES. The bone marrow in these conditions shows sideroblasts, nucleated red cells with granules of iron that can be demonstrated with Prussian blue stain. The granules occur characteristically in a full or partial ring around the nucleus. Besides microcytosis and hypochromasia, the peripheral blood from these patients shows siderocytes, non-nucleated red cells with granules of iron (see also under Alterations in Erythrocyte Structure and Inclusions). As the body is already overloaded with iron that is not being utilized appropriately, iron therapy in these anemias would be harmful to the patient.

A number of chemicals cause sideroblastic anemias by inhibiting heme synthesis. Lead poisoning produces an anemia that is characteristically mildly microcytic and hypochromic and is often characterized by basophilic stippling of the red cells. It is most often seen in children who have ingested lead paint chips and may be seen in adults as the result of industrial exposure to lead.

Hemolytic Anemias.—One problem with a morphologic classification of anemias is that it does not deal conveniently with a broad etiologic class of anemias, namely the hemolytic anemias. The hemolytic anemias are generally classified as congenital or acquired. They are characterized by increased destruction or hemolysis of red cells from a variety of causes, accompanied by increased production of red cells by the bone marrow. This is seen as polychromasia and even nucleated forms of red cells on blood films prepared with Wright's stain, and increased reticulocyte counts. Anisocytosis and poikilocytosis are characteristic of hemolytic anemias in general. An inherited form of spherocytic anemia, hereditary spherocytosis, results from an inherited red cell abnormality and is characterized by the presence of spherocytes in the peripheral blood. This condition is indistinguishable morphologically from certain acquired disorders that result in spherocytic anemia. In such cases a useful laboratory test is the direct antiglobulin (Coombs') test which shows antibodies on red cells of a patient with an acquired (or autoimmune) hemolytic spherocytic anemia.

The direct antiglobulin test is used to detect red cells that have been coated, or sensitized, with antibodies. This is one of the most useful procedures for distinguishing immune from nonimmune mechanisms which can underlie hemolytic anemias. When red cells are precoated with an antibody, the direct antiglobulin test usually will be positive. The routine test will not detect the antibody if the amount on the cell membrane is too small. Red cells can become sensitized when an autoimmune process is in effect. In this type of disorder, antibodies are produced by the patient's own immune system that react with specific antigens on the patient's own red cells. These anemias can be temperature-induced or drug-induced.

Other changes of shape (poikilocytosis) characteristic of certain hemolytic anemias include the following: Elliptocytes are characteristic of hereditary elliptocytosis, a red cell membrane disorder. Sickle cells are characteristic of sickle-cell anemia, an inherited hemoglobin abnormality. Schiztocytes or fragmented cells are characteristic of the microangiopathic hemolytic anemias, and may be produced by mechanical fragmentation caused by some sort of intravascular pathologic condition or intravascular coagulation.

The hemolytic anemias are listed below.

1. Congenital (hereditary) hemolytic anemias.
   a. Membrane (shape) abnormalities.
      (1) Hereditary spherocytosis.
      (2) Hereditary elliptocytosis.
   b. Abnormal forms of hemoglobin.
      (1) Sickle cell disease.
      (2) Hemoglobin C disease.
      (3) Congenital Heinz body hemolytic anemia.
      (4) Thalassemias.
   c. Abnormal enzyme content (nonspherocytic hemolytic anemias).
      (1) Glucose-6-phosphate dehydrogenase (G6PD) deficiency.
      (2) Glycolytic enzyme deficiencies.
2. Acquired hemolytic anemias.
   a. Environmentally caused.
      (1) Hypersplenism (from a variety of causes).
      (2) Intravascular pathologic conditions (microangiopathic hemolytic anemias).

(3) Plasma lipid abnormalities.
(4) Parasites (as in malaria or bartonellosis).
(5) Chemical toxins.
(6) Antibodies (immune hemolytic anemias).
   (a) Isoantibodies (incompatible transfusions or hemolytic disease of the newborn.
   (b) Autoantibodies.
   (c) Drug-induced antibodies.
   b. Acquired red cell abnormalities.
      (1) Paroxysmal nocturnal hemoglobinuria.
      (2) Severe vitamin B_{12}, folate, or iron deficiency.

Morphologic Evaluation of Blood Film.—The morphologic examination of red cells is very helpful in evaluating and determining the cause of anemia. Therefore, it is important that the clinical laboratorian recognize and report changes in red cell morphology so that the physician can effectively evaluate and treat the patient. The following must be observed and noted (see under Examination of the Blood Film): (1) color or staining reaction, (2) size, (3) shape, (4) structure and inclusions, (5) artifacts and abnormal distribution pattern, and (6) nucleated red cells. Red cells are described as normocytic when they are of normal size, shape, and color.

Alterations or abnormalities that may be observed are listed below.

1. Color (staining reaction).
   a. Normochromic.
   b. Anisochromic.
      (1) Hypochromic.
      (2) "Hyperchromic."
      (3) Polychromatic.
2. Size.
   a. Anisocytosis.
      (1) Macrocytosis.
      (2) Microcytosis.
3. Shape.
   a. Discocyte (normal RBC).
   b. Poikilocytes.
      (1) Elliptocytes (oval cells).
      (2) Drepanocytes (sickle cells).
      (3) Codocytes (target cells).
      (4) Spherocytes.
      (5) Stomatocytes.
      (6) Schistocytes (fragmented cells).
      (7) Dacryocytes (teardrop cells).

(8) Echinocytes (burr cells, crenated cells).

(9) Acanthocytes (spike cells).

(10) Leptocytes (thin cells).

(11) Keratocytes (horn cells).

4. Structure and inclusions.

  a. Basophilic stippling.

  b. Siderosomes (Pappenheimer bodies).

  c. Howell-Jolly bodies.

  d. Cabot's rings.

  e. Parasitized red cells (malarial).

5. Artifacts and distribution pattern.

  a. Crenation.

  b. Punched-out red cells.

  c. Platelets on top of red cells.

  d. Rouleaux.

  e. Agglutination.

Alterations in Erythrocyte Color or Hemoglobin Content (Fig 11–29)

Normochromic Cells.—Red cells are described as normochromic when they contain the normal amount of hemoglobin. With Wright's stain the cells show a deep orange-red color in the peripheral area, which gradually diminishes toward the center of the cell. The diameter of the pale central area (central pallor) is less than one-third the diameter of a normochromic erythrocyte.

Anisochromic Cells.—These are cells that stain with more than the normal variation in color. They should be described by one of the more specific terms described below.

Hypochromic Cells.—Red cells that are very pale and show an increased area of central pallor (diameter more than one-third that of the cell) are termed *hypochromic.* Hypochromasia is the result of a decrease in the hemoglobin content of the cell and is often accompanied by a decrease in cell size, or microcytosis, evidenced by low MCH and MCHC values. The cells tend to flatten out on the blood film and may appear normal in size. Such cells are particularly characteristic of iron deficiency anemias.

"Hyperchromic" Cells.—True hyperchromasia cannot exist because normal red cells are filled with hemoglobin and cannot be oversaturated as the cell membrane would burst. However, certain red cells appear to have an increased hemoglobin content. For example, cells that are larger than normal (macrocytes) are also thicker, and therefore the color intensity appears greater on the blood film. Another abnormally shaped red cell, the spherocyte, which is a round cell without a depression in the center, also appears hyperchromic because it is thicker and stains equally throughout the cell.

Polychromatic Cells.—These red cells show a faint blue or blue-orange color with Wright's stain. They are young cells that have just extruded their nuclei and stain

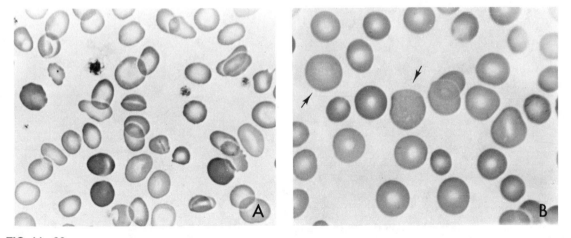

FIG 11–29.
Alterations in erythrocyte color. **A,** hypochromic red blood cells. Compare with the four transfused normal cells (oil-immersion objective). **B,** polychromatic red cells. These cells are reticulocytes when stained with supravital dye (oil-immersion objective).

diffusely basophilic because of the presence of small numbers of ribosomes (or cytoplasmic RNA). When such cells enter the bloodstream they lack 20% of their final hemoglobin content and retain the ribosomes for hemoglobin synthesis. Polychromatic red cells are generally larger than mature red cells. With supravital dyes such as new methylene blue, the RNA reticulum stains blue and the cells are called *reticulocytes*. The presence of polychromasia (or an increased reticulocyte count) is an indication of increased red cell formation by the marrow and is characteristically seen in the various hemolytic anemias.

Alterations in Erythrocyte Size (Fig 11–30)

Anisocytosis.—This is a general term indicating increased variation in the size of red cells in the blood film. It is often accompanied by variations in hemoglobin concentration.

Macrocytosis.—Macrocytes are large red cells. They have a mean cell diameter greater than 9 μm or an MCV greater than 100 fL. They should be differentiated from polychromatic red cells. Macrocytes are characteristic of the megaloblastic anemias of folic acid or vitamin B_{12} deficiency.

Microcytosis.—Microcytes are small red cells, less than 6.5 μm in diameter, with an MCV less than 78 fL. They are often associated with hypochromasia, but their decreased size may not be appreciated on the blood film because they tend to flatten out. Microcytosis is characteristic of iron deficiency anemia, thalassemia, lead poisoning, sideroblastic anemia, idiopathic pulmonary hemosiderosis, and anemias of chronic diseases.

Alterations in Erythrocyte Shape (Fig 11–31)

Discocytes.—When an RBC is not being subjected to an external deforming processes, its normal shape is that of a smooth biconcave disk. One term used to describe a red cell with a normal shape is *discocyte*.

Poikilocytes.—Poikilocytosis, the presence of poikilocytes is a general term indicating an increased variation in the shape of red cells. Many different variations in shape are seen in blood films, and red cells have been described as appearing pear-, oat-, teardrop-, or helmet-shaped, triangular, fragmented, or having various numbers and types of membrane projections. The size and hemoglobin content can vary greatly within poikilocytes. They are found in a variety of anemias and hemolytic states, and a particular shape may or may not indicate a specific type of disease.

Elliptocytes (Oval Cells, Ovalocytes).—These red cells are oval or egg-shaped, showing varying degrees of elliptic shaping from slightly oval to almost a cylindrical form. Large elliptocytes, called *macroovalocytes,* are characteristic of megaloblastic anemias. Because of their

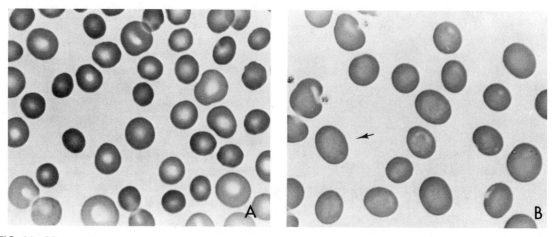

FIG 11–30.
Alterations in erythrocyte size. **A,** anisocytosis (oil-immersion objective). **B,** macrocytosis. Oval macrocytes are also present (oil-immersion objective).

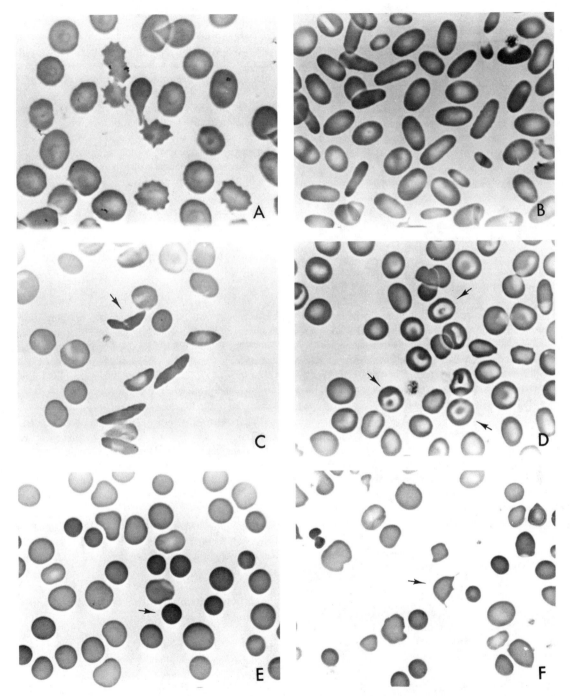

FIG 11–31.
Alterations in erythrocyte shape (photomicrographs taken using the oil-immersion objective). **A,** poikilocytosis. Note the variation in shape of the red blood cells, including crenated cells. **B,** elliptocytes. **C,** drepanocytes (sickle cells). **D,** codocytes (target cells). **E,** spherocytes. **F,** schiztocytes (fragmented cells). The *arrow* indicates a helmet cell.

increased size and thickness, these cells may not show an area of central pallor on the blood film. More elongated forms may occur in a variety of conditions, the most striking and least pathologic being hereditary elliptocytosis.

Drepanocytes (Sickle Cells).—Drepanocytes are sickled cells that are most typically narrow and crescent-shaped, but can vary in shape from bipolar, spiculated forms to cells with long irregular spicules. They have defective membranes and do not function normally. They are the result of a genetic condition in which abnormal hemoglobin is present in the red cells. Sickle cells may be found in sickle cell disease (Hb S) or sickle cell trait (Hb SC or Hb S–thalassemia). Sickling of red cells is enhanced by lack of oxygen.

Codocytes (Target Cells).—Codocytes look like targets, showing a peripheral ring of hemoglobin, an area of pallor or clearing, and then a central area of hemoglobin. This cell circulates as a bell-shaped cell, but takes on the target shape when dried on a slide for morphologic examination. They represent another membrane defect. Target cells have excessive cell membrane in relation to the amount of hemoglobin. They are seen in a variety of clinical conditions, especially in various hemoglobin abnormalities and in chronic liver disease.

Spherocytes.—Spherocytes are red cells that are not biconcave; instead, they appear round or spherical because of the loss of a portion of the cell membrane. As a result, they are small cells, usually less than 6 μm in diameter, and are often called *microspherocytes*. They *appear* hyperchromic, staining a uniform intense orange-red because of the lack of central pallor, a result of the round shape. Spherocytes are characteristic of certain hemolytic anemias, both hereditary (hereditary spherocytosis) and acquired (e.g., drug-induced).

Stomatocytes.—Stomatocytes show a slitlike or mouthlike rather than round area of central pallor on the blood film. They are not biconcave, but are bowl-shaped, or concave on only one side. They are often found in chronic liver disease.

Schiztocytes (Fragmented Cells, Schiztocytes).—Schiztocytes have a variety of names and forms, depending on what is left after the cell is physically fragmented.

Helmet cells are small triangular cells with one or two pointed ends that resemble a helmet. Schiztocytosis is a very serious pathologic condition. It may be the result of mechanical fracture of cells as they pass through the circulatory system, as on filaments of fibrin resulting from intravascular coagulation or on artificial heart valves. They are also seen in cases of severe burns. The fragmentation may also be the result of toxic or metabolic injury, as seen with certain malignancies. Schiztocytes are characteristic of microangiopathic hemolytic anemias and their presence is a danger signal requiring immediate action by the physician.

Dacryocytes (Teardrop Cells).—These are pear-shaped or teardrop-shaped red cells with an elongated point or tail at one end. They may be the result of the cell squeezing and subsequently fracturing as it passes through the spleen.

Echinocytes (Burr Cells, Crenated Cells).—These are red cells with scalloped, spicular, or spiny projections regularly distributed around the cell membrane. They can usually revert back to normal cells. The term *crenated* is sometimes reserved for artifactual spicular cells, such as artifacts that result when the blood film is not adequately waved dry.

Acanthocytes (Spike Cells, Acanthoid Cells).—Acanthocytes are similar to echinocytes, but their spiny projections are irregularly distributed around the cell membrane. They are not artifacts and cannot revert to normal cells. They are related to and may occur with schistocytes, and represent serious pathologic conditions.

Keratocytes (Horn Cells).—Keratocytes are shaped like a half-moon or spindle. They have a relatively normal cell volume but have been deformed so they appear to have two or more spicules.

Alterations in Erythrocyte Structure and Inclusions (Fig 11–32)

Basophilic Stippling.—The presence of dark blue granules evenly distributed throughout the red cell is called basophilic stippling. The stippling may be very fine or dotlike, or it may be coarse and larger. The stippled cell may resemble the polychromatic red cell; however, these are actual granules, not just an overall blueness. Stippling does not exist in the circulating red cell

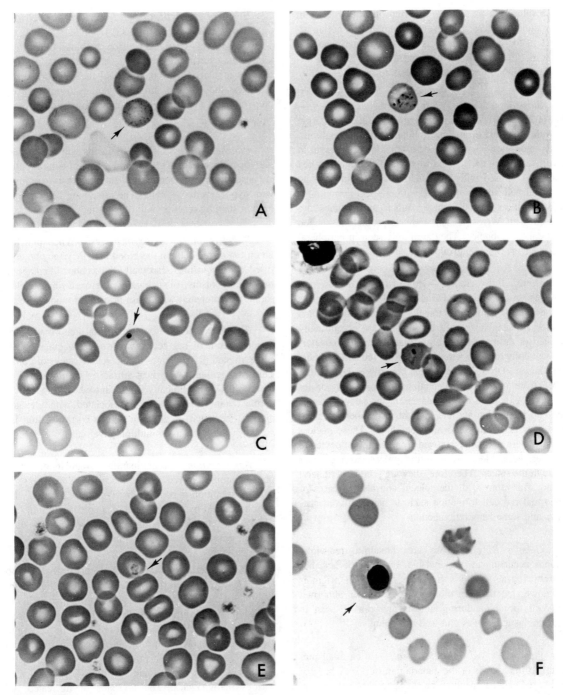

FIG 11–32.
Alterations in erythrocyte structure and inclusions (photomicrographs taken using the oil-immersion objective). **A,** basophilic stippling. **B,** siderosome granules (Pappenheimer bodies). **C,** Howell-Jolly body. **D,** parasitized red cell (malarial). Compare this with **(E),** platelet on top of red cell. **F,** nucleated red cell in peripheral blood.

but results from precipitation of ribosomes and RNA in the staining process. However, the stippling is not an artifact in the clinical sense, as it may indicate abnormal red cell formation in the marrow, as in thalassemia minor, megaloblastic anemia, and lead poisoning.

Siderosomes (Siderocytes, Pappenheimer Bodies).— These are cells containing small, dense, blue-purple granules of free iron, uncombined with hemoglobin. Usually only one or two of these granules are present in a cell, and they are located in the cell periphery. They may be confused with Howell-Jolly bodies and can be distinguished and seen better with a specific stain for iron, such as Prussian blue. When siderosomes are stained with Wright's stain they are sometimes called Pappenheimer bodies. They are rarely seen in peripheral blood except after removal of the spleen.

Howell-Jolly Bodies.—Howell-Jolly bodies are round, densely staining purple granules that stain like dense nuclear chromatin. Usually only one or two such bodies are seen in the red cells. They are eccentrically located in the red cell and less than 1 μm in diameter. Howell-Jolly bodies are remnants of the red cell nucleus, and thus are DNA. Under normal conditions they are derived from nuclear fragmentation *(karyorrhexis)* or incomplete expulsion of the nucleus in the later stages of red cell maturation and are thought to be aberrant chromosomes in certain abnormal conditions. These nuclear remnants are normally removed from the reticulocytes in the peripheral blood by a pitting process as they pass through the spleen. Therefore, they are seen in peripheral blood after removal of the spleen, and also in cases of abnormal red cell formation such as megaloblastic anemias and some hemolytic anemias.

Cabot's Rings.—These are threadlike red-violet strands occurring in ring, twisted, or figure-of-8 shapes in reticulocytes. Cabot's rings are rare. Their origin is unknown, but they are thought to result from abnormal red cell formation during mitosis and can be seen in megaloblastic anemias and lead poisoning.

Parasitized Red Cells (Malarial).—In cases of malaria, various stages of the malaria parasites may be seen in the red cells. Depending on the species of malaria organism present, the parasites may appear as, and be confused with, Cabot's ring bodies, basophilic stippling, or platelets lying on top of red cells.

Erythrocyte Artifacts and Abnormal Distribution Patterns (Fig 11–33)

Crenation.—Crenated cells on the blood film appear like echinocytes, with scalloped, spicular, or spiny projections regularly distributed around the cell surface. In this case they are an artifact resulting from incorrect preparation of the blood film, usually failure to dry it adequately.

Punched-out Red Cells.—Red cells with a punched-out appearance rather than a normal area of central pallor are also drying artifacts. They should not be confused with hypochromic red cells. The remaining cell shows a normal staining reaction with this artifact.

Platelets on Top of Erythrocytes.—When platelets lie on top of red cells in the blood film they may be confused with inclusions, especially the trophozoite stage of malaria organisms. In such cases, the overlying platelets should be compared with those in the surrounding field.

Rouleaux.—Rouleaux represent an abnormal distribution pattern of red cells, which stick together or become aligned in aggregates that look like stacks of coins. This arrangement is a typical artifact in the thick area of blood films. It is clinically significant when found in the normal examination area and associated with elevated plasma fibrinogen or globulin with a corresponding increase in the ESR, as in multiple myeloma.

Agglutination.—Agglutination, irregular or amorphous clumping of red cells in the blood film, represents another alteration in red cell distribution. Clinically, this may be caused by the presence of a cold agglutinin (antibody) in the patient's serum and may indicate an autoimmune hemolytic state or anemia.

Nucleated Red Cells in the Peripheral Blood (Fig 11–32, F).—Normally, red cells do not enter the blood until the reticulocyte stage of maturation, just after extrusion of the shrunken nucleus. Therefore, the presence of earlier nucleated forms of red cells in the peripheral blood is abnormal. It indicates intense marrow stimulation, such as that seen in acute blood loss, megaloblastic anemias, or pathologic conditions associated with various malignancies. The presence of nucleated red cells is termed an *erythroblastotic reaction.*

Cells in the later stages of maturation are most often present, so the cytoplasm is orange-red because the cells

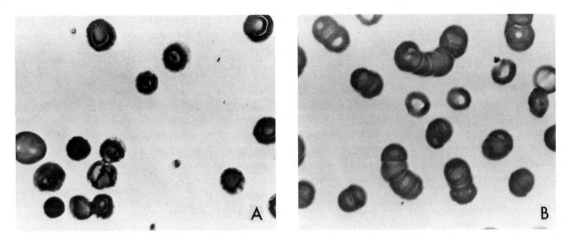

FIG 11–33.
Erythrocyte artifacts and abnormal distribution patterns (photomicrographs taken using the oil-immersion objective). **A,** drying artifact in red cells. **B,** rouleau formation, an abnormal distribution pattern.

contain hemoglobin. However, the nucleus is also present, although shrunken and dark blue in color. Earlier forms may occur and may be difficult to distinguish from small lymphocytes or plasma cells; the presence of pink in the red cell cytoplasm is helpful in such cases. The presence of nucleated red cell forms in the peripheral blood is characteristic of megaloblastic anemias. In these cases the young red cells are larger (macrocytic) and tend to have a more open chromatin pattern than corresponding stages of normocytic red cells (dyssynchrony of nucleus and cytoplasm).

It is important to remember that the white cell count must be corrected when nucleated red cells are observed in the peripheral blood film as these cells are counted as white cells when present.

Leukocyte Alterations

In the examination of peripheral blood, leukocytes are studied for alterations in both quantity, or number, and quality, or morphology.

Quantitative changes in leukocytes are measured by the white cell count—the actual number of leukocytes in a certain volume of blood. A white cell count above normal is leukocytosis; a count below normal is leukopenia. There can also be increases or decreases in number of any of the five types of white cells that are enumerated collectively in the white cell count, and such changes are measured by the white cell differential. Quantitative changes in any of the cell types are described by the fol-

lowing terms: *neutrophilia* (increase), *neutropenia* (decrease); *eosinophilia, eosinopenia; basophilia, basopenia; lymphocytosis, lymphopenia;* and *monocytosis, monocytopenia.*

In addition, these increases or decreases may be *relative* or *absolute.* (See Leukocyte Differential Reporting Methods: Relative vs. Absolute Numbers.) If the change is absolute, the particular cell type shows a numerical increase or decrease from its normal concentration in the blood. If it is relative, there is an alteration (either high or low) of the percentage of the particular cell type as determined in the leukocyte differential, while the numerical concentration is within normal values. Finally, there may be both an absolute and a relative change when both the percentage and the numerical values are above or below normal.

Qualitative or morphologic alterations in circulating leukocytes may be described in terms of a shift to the left, referring to the presence of younger or more immature cell forms than are normally found in the peripheral blood. Such changes may be found within any cell line, including erythrocytes. The presence of younger forms of leukocytes in the blood may be termed a *leukoblastic reaction.* Since they often occur along with younger or nucleated red cell forms, the term *leukoerythroblastic reaction* is also used.

Most alterations in leukocyte morphology can be classified as (1) toxic or reactive changes, (2) anomalous changes, or (3) leukemic or other malignant changes.

Toxic or Reactive Leukocyte Alterations.—Toxic changes in leukocytes are generally associated with a bacterial infection or a toxic reaction. They are seen on a blood film as toxic granulation, vacuolization, hypersegmentation (hyperlobulation) of neutrophils, a shift to the left, the presence of Döhle bodies, increased or decreased cell size, degeneration or pyknosis of the nucleus, and karyolysis (dissolution of the nucleus).

Reactive leukocyte alterations are particularly characteristic of lymphocytes. Reactive lymphocytes can be seen in viral infections and are often associated with infectious mononucleosis, although many other conditions produce reactive cell forms. Changes generally include increased cytoplasmic basophilia with or without radial or peripheral localization, increased or decreased cytoplasmic volume, increased coarse azurophilic granulation, and alterations in the nuclear chromatin, which becomes either loose, delicate, and reticular, or dark, heavy, and clumped. These changes will be defined further later in this section.

Anomalous Changes.—An anomaly is a deviation from the common rule, or an irregularity. Hematologic deviations from normal may be congenital or acquired. Leukocyte anomalies are described later in this section.

Malignant or Leukemic Changes.—Leukemia is a disease of the blood-forming tissues that is an abnormal, uncontrolled proliferation of one or more of the various hematopoietic cells that progressively displaces normal cellular elements. There are usually, but not always, qualitative changes in the affected cells.

The exact cause of leukemia is not known. There is evidence to suggest hereditary factors and genetic predisposition. Environmental causes have also been cited, especially exposure to gamma radiation producing genetic mutations or chromosome damage. Various chemicals and drugs have also been implicated, and viruses have been shown to be related to leukemia in mice and other animals.

Leukemias are classified as acute or chronic on the basis of clinical course (prognosis) and the number of blasts present. *Acute leukemias* usually occur with sudden onset. There is usually anemia, which is normocytic and normochromic and which increases as the disease progresses. The platelet count is low to markedly decreased. The leukocyte count varies but is usually moderately to markedly elevated—with 50,000 to 100,000/µL (50.0 to 100.0 × 10^9/L) being not uncommon—although the count may be normal or decreased. Blast cells are present in the peripheral blood film; generally, more than 60% blasts indicates an acute leukemic process. The bone marrow is hypercellular and consists predominantly of blast cells. Untreated acute leukemias can lead to death within 2 to 3 months. Death is often the result of hemorrhage, which increases in severity as the platelet count falls below 20,000/µL (20.0 × 10^9/L), or infection, which results as the granulocyte count falls below 1,500/µL (1.5 × 10^9/L). Infection is now the primary cause of death, as bleeding has been reduced with prophylactic platelet transfusions and vigorous transfusion therapy when patients are in a bleeding crisis. Treatment includes chemotherapy and bone marrow transplantation.

Chronic leukemias begin slowly and insidiously and may exist for a long time without symptoms. Symptoms develop slowly and include fatigue, night sweats, weight loss, and fever. Anemia usually develops late in the disease, but hemolytic anemia may develop as the disease progresses. The platelet count is usually normal and may even increase in chronic nonlymphocytic leukemia; however, in the later stages both thrombocytopenia and anemia usually occur. The white cell count is usually markedly increased, often higher than 100,000/µL (100.0 × 10^9/L), but it can be normal or even decreased. Morphologically, less than 10% myeloblasts will be seen in the peripheral blood in chronic nonlymphocytic leukemias, and the blood tends to look like bone marrow as it contains all granulocyte developmental stages. In chronic lymphocytic leukemia (CLL), very few to no lymphoblasts are seen in the peripheral blood. The blood characteristically shows a monotonous picture of lymphocytes that are all similar in size and morphology. In addition, many damaged or basket cells may be present, as the lymphocytes tend to be fragile. The average length of survival for patients with chronic nonlymphocytic leukemia is 3 to 4 years. CLL has an average survival of about 10 years, although prolonged survival for up to 35 years is possible, and about 30% of the patients die of causes unrelated to the disease. Infection is the most common cause of death related to CLL. Chronic nonlymphocytic leukemia tends to proceed to an acute or accelerated stage called a *blast crisis,* and patients eventually die of hemorrhage or infection, as in acute leukemia.

Leukemias are classified morphologically according to either (1) the cell type involved, or (2) the number of blasts in the peripheral blood and the corresponding clinical course or prognosis (designated acute, subacute, or chronic). In the first of these systems there are generally two classes of leukemia, *lymphocytic* (or *lymphoid*) and *nonlymphocytic* (*myeloid, myelogenous*). The youngest cell forms or blasts common to these leukemias are the lymphoblast and the myeloblast, respectively. It may be impossible to distinguish between the myeloblast and the lymphoblast morphologically, especially in the most serious or acute forms of the disease, when only blast forms are seen in the blood. The presence of *Auer bodies* (granules or rods of lysosomal material, an azurophilic substance) in the cytoplasm is diagnostic of the myeloblast. However, Auer bodies are not seen in all cases of nonlymphocytic (myelogenous) leukemia. Other considerations in the differentiation of myeloblasts and lymphoblasts are the nucleocytoplasmic ratio, the number of nucleoli, and the nuclear chromatin pattern. However, such differences are often inconclusive and may be misleading. If more mature cells are present, they may aid in the morphologic identification.

Although, traditionally, morphologic criteria are used to classify leukemias, the use of cytochemical and histochemical staining techniques and immunologic markers now makes it possible to identify abnormal hematopoietic precursors with more assurance. A testing battery of special studies using staining and immunologic methods is employed as part of the complete workup for a patient with leukemia. Tests for myeloperoxidase activity using Sudan black stain, leukocyte alkaline phosphatase activity, TdT enzyme activity, nonspecific and specific esterase activity, and the periodic acid–Schiff (PAS) reaction for lymphoblast granules are included in these special studies.

The major symptoms of leukemia are fever, weight loss, and increased sweating, especially night sweats. The liver, spleen, and lymph nodes may be enlarged. There may be a bleeding tendency if the platelet count is decreased (thrombocytopenia).

Leukemia can occur at any age, but certain forms appear to be age-related. CLL is generally a disease of later adult years (generally over 50 years of age). Treatment is usually only for complications of the disease. ALL is generally a disease of children under 10 years of age (seldom over 20 years) and peaks between the ages of 3 and 7. ALL is the most prevalent form of malignancy in children. Despite some progress in the length of remission using chemotherapy, the mortality rate still remains high, depending on the stage of the disease when it is first diagnosed and on other clinical parameters. Bone marrow transplantation with chemotherapy is especially useful in treatment of this type of leukemia. Chronic nonlymphocytic leukemia (CNLL), or chronic myelogenous leukemia (CML), usually occurs between the ages of 20 and 50. Chemotherapy is commonly used to suppress the proliferation of leukemic cells. Other treatment includes symptom-related administration of antibiotics and transfusions. Remissions are usually shorter than in ALL and are more difficult to achieve. Acute nonlymphocytic leukemia (ANLL), or acute myelogenous leukemia (AML), occurs at all ages, but is primarily a disease of middle age. Treatment can include platelet transfusions for thrombocytopenia, antibiotics for infection, and chemotherapy to inhibit the proliferation of the leukemic cells. Survival rates and prognosis are less encouraging than in ALL. Bone marrow transplantation is being used in some patients under 45 years of age in their first remission.

Other Malignant Changes.—Malignant hematologic conditions other than leukemia include plasma cell dyscrasias (multiple myeloma, primary macroglobulinemia, and Fe fragment or heavy chain disease), Hodgkin's disease (or malignant lymphoma, Hodgkin's type), non-Hodgkin's malignant lymphomas, and some unusual tumors closely resembling hematologic malignancies.

The laboratory has a significant role in the diagnosis and management or treatment of patients with these various hematologic diseases. Many laboratory procedures will be requested by the physician, such as cell and platelet counts, tests for the presence of anemia, coagulation studies, white cell differential count, blood film examination, cytochemical and histochemical stains, immunologic tests, and preparation and selection of appropriate blood products for transfusion therapy.

Again, the actual examination of the blood film in cases of such altered and complex morphology is left to the trained hematologist. Such changes should be recognized as abnormal during routine screening of blood films and referred to the pathologist or technologist with special training. To identify changes in leukocyte morphology, the cells should be examined for the following features: (1) nuclear chromatin pattern, (2) nuclear shape, (3) size and number of nucleoli, when present, (4) cytoplasmic inclusions, and (5) nucleocytoplasmic ratio. Various alterations in leukocyte morphology are described below and illustrated in Figure 11–34.

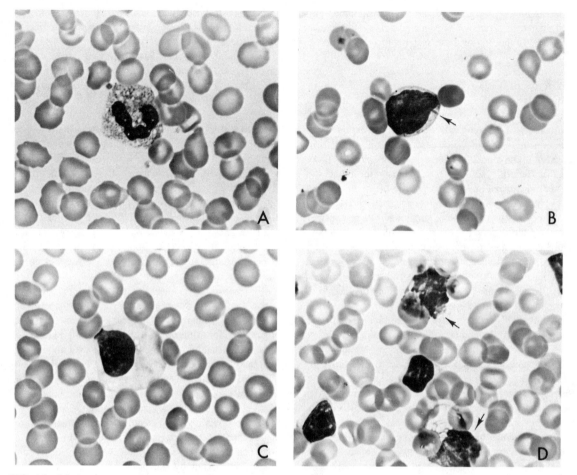

FIG 11–34.
Leukocyte alterations (photomicrographs taken using the oil-immersion objective). **A,** neutrophil showing toxic changes (toxic granules, vacuoles, Döhle bodies). **B,** Auer rod in myeloblast. **C,** reactive lymphocyte. **D,** smudge or basket cells *(arrows)*. Lymphocytes are also present.

Descriptions of Morphologic Alterations in Leukocytes

Toxic Granulation.—Toxic granules are deeply staining basophilic or blue-black larger-than-normal granules found in the cytoplasm of neutrophils. Their presence is associated with acute bacterial infections, drug poisoning, and burns.

Döhle Bodies.—These are round or oval, small, clear light blue staining areas found in the neutrophil cytoplasm. They are remnants of cytoplasmic RNA from an earlier stage of neutrophil development. They are often seen together with toxic granulation in infections,

burns, after administration of toxic agents, and in pregnancy.

Cytoplasmic Vacuolization.—Vacuoles may develop in leukocytes from blood anticoagulated with EDTA. Vacuoles are also signs of toxic change and imply the occurrence of phagocytosis. They may be accompanied by irregular depletion of granules or areas of clearing in the neutrophil cytoplasm and may also be seen in the nucleus.

Hypersegmentation of Nucleus.—Neutrophils that are hypersegmented contain five or more lobes in their nuclei. They are characteristic of the megaloblastic anemias of vitamin B_{12} and folic acid deficiency and are therefore often called pernicious anemia neutrophils. The megaloblastic neutrophil is larger than the normal neutrophil (all cell types are larger in the megaloblastic process).

Barr Bodies.—A Barr body is a small knob attached to or projecting from a lobe of the neutrophil nucleus and consisting of the same nuclear chromatin or substance. It is often referred to as the sex chromatin or sex chromosome, as it is seen in some of the neutrophils of normal females and is thought to be an inactivated X chromosome.

Auer Bodies (Auer Rods).—Auer bodies or rods are slender, rod-shaped or needle-shaped bodies found in the cytoplasm that stain reddish-purple (like azurophilic granules). They are composed of lysosomal material, fused primary granules. They are found only in the cytoplasm of myeloblasts or promyelocytes and are considered diagnostic in distinguishing nonlymphocytic (myeloblastic granulocytic) from lymphocytic leukemias.

Pelger-Huët Anomaly.—This anomaly is seen as a failure of the granulocyte nucleus to segment or form lobes normally. The neutrophil nuclei are band-shaped or at most have two lobes in this condition. In addition, the chromatin is quite coarsely clumped. This is a benign anomaly that can be inherited or acquired. In its acquired form, it is known as pseudo–Pelger-Huët anomaly.

Chédiak-Higashi Anomaly.—Large amorphous granules are observed in the neutrophil cytoplasm; granules are also seen in the lymphocyte and monocyte cytoplasm. The disease is inherited and rare. It has been treated with marrow transplantation.

May-Hegglin Anomaly.—These blue inclusion bodies are similar to the Döhle bodies present in neutrophils but are usually larger and have more sharply defined borders. Platelets may be decreased in number but some giant forms can be present. The disorder is inherited and most patients have no clinical symptoms.

Alder-Reilly Anomaly.—Heavy dark azurophilic granulation is observed in neutrophils, eosinophils, basophils, and sometimes lymphocytes and monocytes. This anomaly is inherited and is often associated with mucopolysaccharidoses.

Reactive or Atypical Lymphocytes.—Reactive or atypical lymphocytes (also called variant or transformed lymphocytes or virocytes) are particularly associated with infectious mononucleosis; however, many other viral infections also show such alterations. They generally show the different stages of immune responsiveness of B and T lymphocytes in the peripheral blood and immune system. In general, the cytoplasm increases in amount and appears to be reacting to a stimulus. Although the cells have been more specifically classified morphologically, they tend to have one or several of the following characteristics:

The cytoplasm tends to become more intensely blue in color (*cytoplasmic basophilia*). The basophilia tends to be localized, either peripherally, with an increased blue color around the outer edge of the cell, or radially, with areas of blueness radiating from the more central nucleus to the outer edges of the cell like spokes of a wheel. Radial and peripheral basophilia may be combined, in which case the cell is described as resembling a fried egg or a flared skirt. The reactive cell may also show increases or decreases in cytoplasmic volume. Cells with increased cytoplasmic volume, when observed on films prepared with Wright's stain, tend to show indentations by adjacent structures, especially RBCs. The cytoplasm appears to be flowing around and almost engulfing such structures. The cells also tend to have an increased number of nonspecific azurophilic granules in the cytoplasm.

Reactive or atypical lymphocytes also show nuclear changes. There is generally a sharper separation of chromatin and parachromatin. The nucleus may become loose and delicate, resembling an earlier developmental stage; this is referred to as a reticular appearance, hence the term *reticular lymphocyte*. In other cases, the nucleus becomes oval or kidney-shaped with heavy clumps of deeply stained chromatin; these are called plasmacytoid changes since the cells resemble plasma cells.

Such atypical lymphocytes have been classified as Downey type I, II, and III lymphocytes. However, in the laboratory it is sufficient to note the presence of reactive lymphocytes, as the three types have similar diagnostic significance. The reactive lymphocyte may resemble the lymphoblast, and it may be necessary to rule out a leukemic process in such cases of reactive lymphocytosis.

Türk Cells.—These are darkly staining cells having plasmacytoid characteristics. They are classified as atypical lymphocytes or plasma cells by different authors and are associated with viral infections.

Smudge or Basket Cells.—These are damaged white cells. They are cellular fragments consisting of battered or frayed nuclei with no cytoplasmic material. Basket cells are not counted as part of the white cell differential, and a few damaged cells are encountered in most peripheral blood films. They are not significant unless present in large numbers. They may be associated with CLL, and in some cases of CLL and acute leukemias the number of basket cells may be greater than the usual lymphocyte count.

COUNTING RETICULOCYTES

Reticulocytes are young red cells that have matured enough to have lost their nuclei but not their cytoplasmic RNA. They do not have the full amount of hemoglobin. The number of reticulocytes is a measure of the regeneration or production of RBCs. Reticulocytes appear in a blood film stained with Wright's stain as polychromatic RBCs because of the basophilic cytoplasmic remnant of the immature red cell RNA. Supravital stains may also reveal basophilic stippling and Howell-Jolly bodies. The inclusions seen as basophilic stippling represent precipitation of the RNA as pinpoint particles in the red cells; this precipitation is seen in toxic conditions such as lead or heavy metal poisoning. Basophilic stippling is also visible with Wright's stain. Howell-Jolly bodies are seen in pathologic conditions in which one or more larger spherical bodies consisting of nuclear material are found in the red cell (see also under Erythrocyte Alterations).

Normal Erythropoiesis and Reticulocytes

In the circulating blood 0.5% to 1.5% of the red cells are usually reticulocytes. This is based on a normal red cell life span of 120 ± 20 days and a normal red cell count necessitating replacement of approximately 1% of the adult circulating red cells each day. The range represents technical or counting errors in the method. A reticulocyte count above this level (reticulocytosis) is clinically significant, indicating that the body is attempting to meet an increased need for red cells. Such an increase in reticulocytes is observed when red cells are be-

ing hemolyzed within the body. The bone marrow sends out red cells at an increased rate until only the younger cells are available to be released, although increased red cell production is probably taking place at the same time. The demand may be so great in some instances that nucleated red cells are sent from the bone marrow.

Clinical Uses for Reticulocyte Counts

The reticulocyte count is used to follow therapeutic measures for anemias in which the patient is deficient in, or lacking, one of the substances essential for manufacturing red cells. When the deficiency has been diagnosed, therapy is begun. This consists of supplying the missing essential substances to the body and waiting for the body to react by increasing red cell production. New red cells will be released rapidly into the circulating blood, many before they are fully matured, in response to therapy. The corresponding increase in the reticulocyte count indicates a favorable response to therapy. The response to therapy in iron deficiency anemia (treated with iron) and pernicious anemia (treated with vitamin B_{12}) is followed by reticulocyte counts. As the total red cell count and the hemoglobin concentration reach normal levels, red cell regeneration slows to the normal rate, allowing more time for maturation of the red cells in the bone marrow. This is indicated by the presence of fewer reticulocytes in the circulating blood.

Specimen Requirements

Anticoagulated whole blood or capillary blood from the finger, toe, or heel may be used. Venous blood should be anticoagulated with EDTA. Heparinized blood should be avoided as the staining quality is poor. If anticoagulated whole blood is used, the test should be performed within 1 or 2 hours after the specimen is drawn.

Manual Methods for Counting Reticulocytes

RNA content can be detected in reticulocytes by exposing the living cells to a supravital stain. Manual methods for preparing reticulocyte slides for counts require supravital staining of the red cells, whether the end result is a dry film or not. In supravital staining the living blood cells are mixed with the stain, as opposed to making a film and staining it. One method consists of spreading the stain on the slide and drying it; the blood is then added to the dried stain and mixed, and the usual blood smear is prepared. Another method uses the same slide preparation, but the stain is mixed with a drop of blood and cover-slipped, and the mixture is sealed on the slide and viewed in the liquid form under the microscope. A third method is to mix blood and stain in a small test tube, allow time for the staining reaction to occur, and then prepare a blood film from the mixture; the prepared blood film is then viewed microscopically (Procedure 11–12). In some procedures the resulting film is counterstained with Wright's stain, using the method previously described. This is not an essential step and it may be omitted, as in the procedure to be described here. Such counterstaining with Wright's stain may be helpful in differentiating basophilic stippling and Howell-Jolly bodies from reticular RNA. The first two methods described

employ an alcoholic solution of the dye; the third method uses a saline solution.

Dyes Used to Stain Reticulocytes Using Manual Methods

Brilliant cresyl blue or new methylene blue is used for the staining of reticulocytes. New methylene blue dye gives consistent results and a sharp blue staining of the RNA reticulum. In addition to the dye, the stain should contain an ingredient to preserve the red cells (provide an isotonic condition). The method to be described in this section requires that its stain must prevent coagulation. Brilliant cresyl blue contains sodium citrate, which prevents coagulation, and sodium chloride, which provides

---

Procedure 11–12. Manual Reticulocyte Count

1. Two drops of blood (capillary or venous) are added to three drops of reticulocyte dye in a small test tube. If the hemoglobin is low, more blood should be used to ensure proper staining and good films.
2. The blood and dye are mixed thoroughly and allowed to stand for 15 minutes.
3. The cells are resuspended by mixing well, and at least three thin films are made on slides, using small drops of the blood-stain mixture. The usual procedure for making blood films is used. The films must be completely and *rapidly* dried.
4. When the films are dry, the reticulocytes are counted. A total of 1,000 erythrocytes (500 on each of two slides) is counted, using the oil-immersion ($\times 100$) objective.
5. The count is made in an area of the smear considered to be medium thin, where the erythrocytes are well distributed and not touching (about 100 cells per oil-immersion field).
6. The reticulocytes seen in the count are included in the total 1,000 cells counted; however, they are tallied and recorded separately. Separate counts should be recorded for the two slides in order to compare the distribution of reticulocytes.
7. The reticulocytes appear as greenish blue cells with the reticulum showing as a deep blue network of strands or granules within the cells (Fig 11–35).

8. If the two slides counted do not agree within 5 cells when the reticulocyte count is 3% or less (30 reticulocytes per 1,000 cells), another 500 cells must be counted on a third slide. If agreement within 5 cells cannot be met after counting all three slides, the procedure must be repeated from the beginning with new slides. If the reticulocyte count is greater than 3%, a reasonable difference between the counts on the two slides is allowable. This will be determined by the quality assurance system of the laboratory and is somewhat dependent on the experience of the person performing the procedure.
9. It is essential to focus the microscope carefully and continually when counting reticulocytes. The dye will stain platelet granules and leukocyte granules, and these or precipitated stain may be mistaken for reticulocytes. Inadequate drying will cause the red cells to contain highly refractile areas resembling remnants of RNA. Artifacts in red cells must not be confused with reticulocytes.
10. Reticulocytes are usually reported as a percentage of the total number of erythrocytes counted. However, more meaningful results are attained by correcting the reticulocyte count for the patient's hematocrit and for red cells prematurely released by the marrow, as indicated by the presence of "shift cells" (see under Reporting Reticulocyte Results).

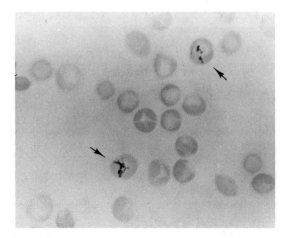

FIG 11–35.
Reticulocytes stained with new methylene blue (oil-immersion objective).

isotonicity. New methylene blue contains sodium oxalate, which prevents coagulation, and sodium chloride. These supravital dyes precipitate the RNA in the reticulocytes, coloring it blue.

Preparation of Stains

1. *Brilliant cresyl blue:* Dilute 1.0 g of brilliant cresyl blue and 0.4 g of sodium citrate to 100 mL with 0.85 g/dL NaCl. Filter before using.
2. *New methylene blue:* Dilute 0.50 g of new methylene blue N (color index 52030), 0.70 g of NaCl (CP grade), and 0.13 g of sodium oxalate (CP grade) to 100 mL with deionized water. Filter before using.

Calculations for Manual Reticulocyte Count

The reticulocyte count is reported as the percentage of reticulocytes in the total red cells counted. The following general formula can be used:

$$\frac{\text{Reticulocytes}}{\text{RBCs}} \times 100 = \%\ \text{reticulocytes}$$

This formula can be derived from a simple proportion relating the number of reticulocytes counted in a given number of red cells to the number of reticulocytes per 100 red cells, which is the percentage of reticulocytes. *Example:* On each of two slides 500 red cells are counted. The first slide shows 16 reticulocytes and the

second shows 20 reticulocytes. What is the percentage of reticulocytes in the blood?

$$500 + 500 = 1,000 \text{ cells counted}$$

$$20 + 16 = 36 \text{ reticulocytes per 1,000 cells counted}$$

$$\frac{36 \text{ reticulocytes}}{1,000 \text{ cells}} = \frac{x}{100 \text{ cells}}$$

$$x = \frac{36 \times 100}{1,000} = 3.6 \text{ reticulocytes per 100 cells}$$

$$= 3.6\% \text{ reticulocytes}$$

Reporting Reticulocyte Results

The classic reporting unit for the reticulocyte count is in percent reticulocytes counted while counting 1,000 erythrocytes, reticulocytes included. The reference values vary from 0.9% to 2.0% for adults with a 2% to 10% accuracy for manually counted cells.

Absolute Reticulocyte Count

There is a relation between the percentage of reticulocytes calculated and the total erythrocyte count. A meaningful reticulocyte count should indicate the total production of erythrocytes regardless of the concentration of erythrocytes in the blood. The reticulocyte count can also be reported as an absolute value by multiplying the reticulocyte count in percent by the total red cell count. This reporting method provides a comparable basis for following the progress or treatment of anemias and is the preferred way of reporting reticulocyte values.

Reticulocyte Count Corrected for a Low Hematocrit (Anemia)

Since a decreased hematocrit and an increased reticulocyte count ratio can exaggerate the red cell production response, the reticulocyte count can be corrected for the degree of anemia present by application of a factor involving hematocrit values. The patient's hematocrit is compared with a normal hematocrit (considered to be 42% for women and 45% for men) and then related to the patient's reticulocyte count as shown below:

Corrected reticulocyte count (%)
= patient's reticulocyte count (%)
$$\times \frac{\text{patient's Hct}}{\text{normal Hct}}$$

Reticulocyte Production Index

The use of this correction compensates for the amount of time it takes for reticulocytes to mature in the peripheral blood, especially for instances where the anemia is severe and the subsequent erythropoietic response involves early release of red cells from the bone marrow. A reticulocyte production index factor can be applied to correct the reticulocyte count for abnormally early release of red cells from the marrow into the peripheral blood. Premature release of cells from the marrow does not necessarily indicate increased marrow production. Abnormally early release of the red cells from the marrow into the peripheral blood is indicated by the presence of nucleated RBCs or polychromatic macrocytes ("shift" cells) on blood films prepared with Wright's stain. Reticulocytes normally spend approximately 2 days in the bone marrow before being released into the blood, and approximately 1% of the circulating red cells are replaced each day. When the hematocrit and rate of marrow release are normal, the apparent reticulocyte percentage may be considered an index of production, or maturation, and set equal to 1.

Normal reticulocyte production index = 1

However, if reticulocytes are being released directly into the blood before maturation in the marrow, as evidenced by the presence of nucleated forms or shift cells on the blood film, the count is corrected by dividing the apparent reticulocyte count by 2 (the usual number of days of maturation).

If the presence of polychromatic red cells is observed on a Wright's-stained blood film, a reticulocyte production index factor must be applied. The maturation time, in days, for the reticulocyte is as follows*:

Maturation factor (days)	Hematocrit (% units)
1	45
1.5	35
2	25
3	15

The corrected reticulocyte count is referred to as the reticulocyte production index. If no nucleated cells or shift cells are seen in the blood, the reticulocyte count is divided by 1 (i.e., left unchanged).

*Method for Reticulocyte Counting, Proposed Standard, Villanova, Pa, National Committee for Clinical Laboratory Standards, 1985; 5(June): H16-P, p 229.

When there is both an abnormally low hematocrit and shift cells on the blood film, both corrections should be applied to the apparent reticulocyte count. The following general formula can be used:

Reticulocyte production index

$$= \frac{1}{2}\left[\text{patient's reticulocyte count (\%)} \times \frac{\text{patient's Hct}}{\text{normal Hct}} \right]$$

The factor $\frac{1}{2}$ represents division by a maturation factor of 2. The maturation factor can vary, depending on the severity of the anemia. Marrow can respond to anemia by a two- to fivefold increase in red cell production.

Precautions and Technical Factors When Counting Reticulocytes Manually

Careful focusing of the microscope is essential when counting reticulocytes. Stained platelet granules and leukocyte granules must not be mistaken for reticulocytes. Precipitated stain might also be mistaken for reticulum within the erythrocytes. To minimize this possibility, the dye must be filtered immediately before use. Immediate drying of the film will prevent the formation of the crystalline-like artifacts that sometimes appear in the red cells and resemble remnants of RNA.

The proportions of dye and blood must be altered if the patient is anemic. More blood must be used. If the procedure is followed carefully, the distribution of reticulocytes on the blood films will be good. With experience, the problem of agreement will be primarily a result of the distribution of reticulocytes on the films and not misidentification of reticulocytes. Reticulocytes have a lower specific gravity than mature red cells and rise to the top of a blood-stain mixture. Therefore, the specimen must be well mixed before the incubation period and immediately before the three slides are made. The slides must be made in a uniform fashion to ensure random sampling.

Procedures employed for reticulocyte counts vary in different clinical laboratories, although the principles are the same. Variations include the manner in which the stain and cells are mixed, the total number of red cells counted and the number of slides observed, the use of a Miller disk in the eyepiece of the microscope to help define the field to be counted, counterstaining of the reticulocyte film with Wright's stain, and the use of corrections for the patient's hematocrit and the presence of shift cells.

Automated Reticulocyte Counts

With the use of an automated procedure, the process of counting reticulocytes is very much enhanced. The flow cytometry principle is employed, cells are stained with a fluorochrome dye that preferentially stains RNA, and the cells are counted by a fluorescent technique. The RNA-containing reticulocytes will fluoresce when exposed to ultraviolet light. The instrument can count thousands of reticulocytes in just a few seconds with an accuracy of about 0.1%.

Reference Values*

Reticulocytes: adult male: 1.1%–2.1%
             adult female: 0.9%–1.9%
Absolute reticulocyte count: 50×10^9/L

COUNTING EOSINOPHILS

Occasionally it will be necessary to count specific types of leukocytes, such as eosinophils. The eosinophil count is not a routine hematologic test. The relative number of eosinophils can be determined by doing differential studies on a stained blood film, but occasionally it is important to determine the total number of eosinophils in a particular volume of blood. For this purpose a direct method for counting eosinophils has been devised. It is similar in many respects to the counting methods for red and white blood cells.

Clinical Uses for Eosinophil Count

The reference value for the absolute eosinophil count is less than 0.4×10^9/L (400/µL) for a healthy, nonallergic subject. A low eosinophil count (eosinopenia) will be found in hyperadrenalism (Cushing's disease) and shock, and after the administration of adrenocorticotropic hormone (ACTH).

It has been shown that the administration of a single 25-mg dose of ACTH intramuscularly to subjects with

*Williams WJ, Beutler E, Erslev A, et al: *Hematology*, ed 4. New York, McGraw-Hill Book Co. 1990, p 1703.

normal adrenocortical function results in a reduction of the total number of circulating eosinophils. This effect has been used as a test of adrenocortical function, but it is not specific, and the value of the test is limited. An inverse relation exists between adrenocortical activity and the number of circulating eosinophils. A modification of the Randolph method is used for random eosinophil counts before and after the administration of ACTH.

An increase in the number of eosinophils (eosinophilia) may be seen in cases of trichinosis, widespread metastatic carcinoma, allergies (particularly asthma), skin disease (eczema), and infectious diseases (e.g., scarlet fever).

Direct Method for Eosinophil Count

One direct manual method is that devised by Randolph (Procedure 11–13).† Whole blood is diluted with staining solution. The specimen used can be venous blood preserved with EDTA or capillary blood from a finger puncture. Phloxine, which is present in the diluting fluid, serves to stain the eosinophils red; sodium carbonate and water help to lyse the white cells (except eosinophils), and the red cells are lysed by propylene glycol. If heparin is present in the diluting fluid, it will prevent clumping of the white cells. Sodium carbonate will also enhance the staining of the eosinophil granules. In the modification of the Randolph method described in this section, sodium carbonate is omitted.

Diluent for the Randolph Method (Modified)

One diluent used is a combination of phloxine B and methylene blue in propylene glycol. Another diluent that can be used is a hypotonic solution of eosin. A Unopette system containing phloxine B is also available for performing this test.

Preparation of Phloxine B and Methylene Blue Diluent

1. *Solution A.* Dissolve 0.5 g of phloxine B in 1,000 mL of 50 mL/dL propylene glycol in deionized water.

2. *Solution B.* Dissolve 0.5 g of methylene blue

†Randolph TG: Differentiation and enumeration of eosinophils in the counting chamber with a glycol stain, a valuable technique in appraising ACTH dosage. *J Lab Clin Med* 1949; 34:1696.

and 1000 mL of 50 ml/dL propylene glycol in deionized water.

3. Mix 1 part of solution B in 9 parts of solution A immediately before use.

Equipment for Eosinophil Count, Randolph Method (Modified)

The blood for the eosinophil count is diluted using an eosinophil Unopette system with phloxine B diluent. Alternately, a Thoma white cell diluting pipette along with the selected diluent can be used. A special counting chamber is used for this procedure—the Levy chamber with Fuchs-Rosenthal ruling. This chamber usually has a depth of 0.2 mm and has two ruled areas of 16 mm^2 each.

Procedure 11–13. Eosinophil Count: Modified Randolph Method

1. Blood (venous blood preserved with EDTA or heparin or capillary blood is satisfactory) is diluted with the propylene glycol-dye diluent. Using the Unopette system, this results in a 1:32 dilution. Duplicates should be prepared.
2. The pipettes are well mixed for 2 minutes and mounted on two sides of a counting chamber.
3. The cells are allowed to settle for 20 minutes, with the chambers covered to prevent evaporation during this waiting period. During this period, lysis of the red cells and staining of the eosinophils occur. Cells should be counted within 30 minutes after dilution.
4. Eosinophils are counted under low power in each of the four ruled areas (the total area counted is 64 mm^2). The eosinophils are identified in the counting chamber by their brightly red-stained granules. The remainder of the leukocytes do not stain, and the erythrocytes are destroyed by the diluent.

Calculation for Manual Eosinophil Count

In calculating the total eosinophil count, the following factors are taken into consideration: (1) the total number of eosinophils counted, (2) the dilution of the blood (1:32 with the Unopette system), and (3) the volume of the diluted blood, which is equal to the depth of

the chamber (0.2 mm) times the area in which the cells are counted (64 mm^2), or 12.8 μL. The number of eosinophils per liter of blood is given by the equation:

$$\frac{\text{Eosinophils counted} \times 32 \;(\text{in } 64 \text{ mm}^2)}{12.8 \; \mu L} = \text{eosinophils}/\mu L$$

$$= \text{eosinophils} \times 10^9/L$$

The mean reference value for the eosinophil count is about 0.12 × 10^9/L or 120/μL.*

Precautions and Technical Factors for Manual Direct Eosinophil Count

Venous or capillary blood may be used for this test. The type of blood used should be noted, as simultaneous counts with venous and capillary blood have shown capillary blood to give values 25% higher.

If the two solutions (A and B) are used for the diluting fluid, they are stable separately, but the final mixture of the two dyes must be used within 4 to 8 hours. After 8 hours, the dyes will precipitate (see above).

Technical errors should be minimized. The same technical factors apply that were described for other cell counts. To avoid undue rupture of the eosinophil membrane, gentle shaking of the pipettes is suggested.

The approximate error in the eosinophil count is ±20% when the Fuchs-Rosenthal counting chamber is used. Greater errors are seen when hemocytometers with Neubauer ruling are used.

Indirect Method for Eosinophil Count

The direct counting method can be double-checked by use of an indirect counting method. To do this, a WBC count is done on the specimen and two blood films are prepared and stained with Wright's stain. The indirect eosinophil count can be calculated as follows:

Eosinophils/μL
= eosinophils in differential (%) × WBC count

If the indirect and direct methods give counts that differ significantly, the procedures should be repeated.

---

*Williams WJ, Beutler E, Erslev A, et al: *Hematology,* ed 4. New York, McGraw-Hill Book Co, 1990, p 836.

In current laboratory practice, because of the widespread use of the automatic cell counter and its calculation capabilities for absolute cell count data, the direct counting methods for eosinophils have been rendered absolute.

Reference Values (for Nonallergic Population)

Absolute count: $<0.4 \times 10^9$/L
Mean: 0.12×10^9/L

RED BLOOD CELL OSMOTIC FRAGILITY TEST

The osmotic fragility test is a laboratory procedure that is helpful in the diagnosis of types of anemia in which the physical properties of the RBCs are altered. In simple terms, the osmotic fragility test reflects alterations in the shape of the RBC and whether or not it tends to be easily hemolyzed. The shape of the red cell is dependent on the volume, surface area, and functional state of the red cell membrane.

When red cells are introduced into a hypotonic solution of sodium chloride, they take up water and swell until a critical volume is reached, and then hemolysis, or rupture, occurs. When the critical volume is reached, the cells are spherical. In this shape the cell has the maximum volume for its surface area, and any further increase in volume would require an increase in the area of the cell membrane. As the cell takes up water it becomes increasingly fragile.

A red cell that is already spherical has an increased osmotic fragility in hypotonic solutions because it can swell only a little before it bursts. Conversely, one that is flat or has a large surface area compared to its volume has a decreased osmotic fragility in hypotonic solutions, because it can swell considerably before it reaches a spherical shape and bursts. The osmotic fragility is thus a measure of the rate of hemolysis of the red cell when exposed to hypotonic solutions of sodium chloride. When the rate of hemolysis of the red cell is increased, the osmotic fragility is increased, and when the rate of hemolysis is decreased, the osmotic fragility is decreased. An increase in the osmotic fragility of a red cell is sometimes referred to as a decrease in the resistance of the cell to rupture.

Clinical Significance

In certain diseases or conditions, the osmotic fragility of the red cell is characteristically increased or decreased. Since the resistance of the red cell membrane corresponds to its geometric configuration, red cell populations comprised of spherocytes demonstrate increased hemolysis, while those comprised of flattened red cells (such as sickle cells, target cells, or hypochromic cells) demonstrate decreased hemolysis. Hypochromic red cells are very thin, contain very little hemoglobin, and therefore swell to a large extent before reaching their critical volume. Diminished fragility is seen in the presence of obstructive jaundice, in iron deficiency anemias, in thalassemia, in sickle cell anemia, after splenectomy, and in a variety of anemias where target cells are seen. In conditions where the red cells are already spheroid, as in congenital hemolytic anemia, hereditary spherocytosis, and wherever spherocytes are found, increased fragility of the cell is demonstrated.

Specimens

A sample of freshly drawn venous blood, anticoagulated with heparin or defibrinated with glass beads, is preferred for the measurement of osmotic fragility. The blood should be drawn with as little physical trauma to the cells as possible. Heparin is the anticoagulant of choice because it causes less distortion of the red cells, but prolonged exposure to heparin will result in distortion of the red cells, so the test should be done as soon as possible after collection. Defibrination with glass beads is another means of preventing clotting. Freshly drawn venous blood is placed in a flask containing small glass beads. The flask is rotated, exposing the blood to the beads. On agitation, the fibrin coats the beads and is removed from the blood.

A normal or control specimen must be drawn at the same time as the sample of the patient's blood. The patient's results are interpreted by comparison with the results for the control specimen. Both specimens are treated in exactly the same way.

Methods for Determination of Osmotic Fragility

Manual and automated methods are available for estimating the osmotic fragility of the RBC. In the manual methods, the test blood and normal ("control") blood are

placed in a series of graded-strength sodium chloride solutions and any resultant hemolysis is compared with a
100% standard (blood and distilled water). In one manual method the results can be read after incubation for 20
minutes at room temperature (20° C); this is called an *immediate testing method*. In another, incubation for 24
hours at 37° C is required. Incubation at 37° C enhances
the changes in red cell fragility. Fragility curves that ap-

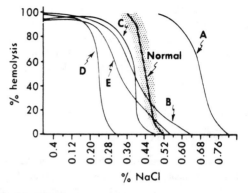

FIG 11–36.
Osmotic fragility curves. *(A)* Hereditary spherocytosis. *(B)*
Thalassemia major. *(C)* Thalassemia minor. *(D)* Hb E dis-
ease. *(E)* Iron deficiency anemia. (From Bauer JD: *Clinical
Laboratory Methods,* ed 9. St Louis, Mosby–Year Book,
Inc, 1982. Used by permission.)

Procedure 11–14. Osmotic Fragility Test Using the Unopette System (Manual Method)

1. Label ten conical centrifuge tubes for the control
   specimen and ten for the patient specimen: one
   tube for each of the sodium chloride solutions.
2. Using a 20-µL Unopette pipette measure well-
   mixed blood into each reservoir. Use a new pipette for each reservoir. This must be done very
   carefully and slowly, as any disturbance of the
   red cells may alter the results. Carefully rinse the
   pipette with the solution in the reservoir. Mix
   sample in reservoir.
3. Incubate the cell suspensions undisturbed at
   room temperature for 20 minutes.
4. Mix contents of reservoirs thoroughly and transfer carefully to labeled centrifuge tubes. Centrifuge at 2,000 rpm for 5 minutes.
5. Carefully decant the supernatant solutions into
   photometer cuvettes and read in a spectrophotometer at 540 nm (the same wavelength used to
   read hemoglobin). The percent transmittance
   should be set to read 100%*T* using water as a
   blank.
6. Record the percent transmission for each cuvette. Convert the readings to absorbance.
7. Calculate the percent hemolysis for each supernatant in the following way:

Percent hemolysis
$$= \frac{\text{absorbance of supernatant}}{\text{absorbance of 100\% hemolysis tube}} \times 100$$

Using linear graph paper, plot the percent hemolysis
on the vertical axis and the NaCl concentration on
the horizontal axis; include the control results (Fig
11–36).

---

pear normal in immediate testing methods may appear
abnormal when the test is done after incubation of the
blood. Thus, the incubation test is helpful in detecting
mild cases of spherocytosis and nonspherocytic hemolytic anemia. It is advisable to perform both tests (immediate and incubation) on each sample submitted for analysis.

The osmotic fragility test using the Unopette system
set up manually to be read immediately (after 20-minute
incubation period) is described in this section (Procedure
11–14).

Reagents

1. *Buffered NaCl stock solution (10 g/dL).* Weigh
180.0 g of NaCl (dry for 24 hours in a desiccator before weighing), 27.31 g of dibasic sodium phosphate
($Na_2\ HPO_4$), 4.86 g of monobasic sodium phosphate
($NaH_2PO_4 \cdot 2H_2O$). Dilute to 2 L with distilled water. This
solution is stable for several months at room temperature if
it is kept in a well-stoppered bottle. The pH is important; it
must be 7.4.

2. *Buffered NaCl (1 g/dL) prepared from the stock
solution.* Mix 20 mL of buffered 10 g/dL NaCl with 180
mL of distilled water.

3. *Working NaCl solutions.* Prepare from the 1 g/
dL solution, using distilled water as the diluent, in the
following concentrations: 0.85, 0.65, 0.60, 0.55, 0.50,

0.40, 0.35, 0.30, and 0.00 g/dL. Other concentrations can be included when necessary.

4. The Unopette System with the above concentrations in designated reservoirs is available for this procedure. The volume of buffered NaCl solutions in each reservoir is 1.98 mL.

Interpretation of Test Results

The control values should be plotted on the same graph as the patient values. The control results are fundamental for the correct interpretation of the test results. They must fall within the established normal range for the patient's results to be considered valid. A difference of more than one tube between the patient and the control is significant.

The osmotic fragility test is best reported as a curve on linear graph paper, always including the control results and indicating the saline solution concentrations at which (1) hemolysis begins, (2) hemolysis is complete, and (3) 50% hemolysis occurs. The patient's results are interpreted from the appearance of the completed graph line and not from one isolated point on the graph. The tube having the highest concentration of saline in which hemolysis is complete determines complete hemolysis. Nonincubated hemolysis begins at 0.45% to 0.50% NaCl and is complete at 0.20% to 0.30% for normal RBCs. The mean corpuscular fragility, which is the same as 50% hemolysis, is normally seen in the tubes having 0.40 to 0.45 g/dL NaCL. Since the 0.00% NaCl tube represents 100% hemolysis, it must be clear. If it is not clear for the control specimen, the test must be repeated. These results must be obtained at a pH of 7.4 and at 20° C.

Blood films are prepared from both the control and the patient's blood and stained with Wright's stain. The results of the osmotic fragility test should be verified by the red cell morphology observed on the stained film.

SICKLE CELL SCREENING TESTS

When blood from a patient with sickle cell anemia or sickle cell trait is deprived of oxygen, the red cells become sickle-shaped. This phenomenon is demonstrated in the laboratory when tests are done to screen for this sickling effect. Both sickle cell anemia and sickle cell trait are inherited. The disease and the trait are caused by the presence of an abnormal hemoglobin, Hb S, instead of the normal Hb A (see under Forms of Hemoglobin). The degree of sickling depends on the concentration of Hb S in the RBC.

Solubility Test

When normal red cells are added to a reagent solution of buffered sodium hydrosulfite (dithionite), the red cells immediately lyse owing to the saponin which is also present in the reagent. In contrast, red cells containing Hb S (and non-S sickling hemoglobins), in a reduced state after being added to the dithionite reducing agent, form liquid crystals and give a turbid appearance to the mixture. With the presence of Hb S, there is an increased turbidity of the red cell lysate when treated with sodium dithionite owing to the decreased solubility of deoxygenated Hb S. Preprepared dithionite reagent is available commercially for sickle cell screening tests. If a positive result is found using the dithionite test, a hemoglobin electrophoresis should be performed on the specimen. Because deterioration of reagents can cause false-negative or false-positive results, it is important to run positive and negative controls each time the procedure is performed.

REFERENCE VALUES FOR ROUTINE HEMATOLOGIC PROCEDURES

Reference values for any laboratory determination depend on many factors, and probably the most meaningful values are those peculiar to the particular institution and locale. The reference values for a normal population presented in this section are from several sources. Table 11–2 shows reference values for adult peripheral blood and Table 11–3 shows reference values for the leukocyte count, leukocyte differential, and hemoglobin concentration at various ages.

TABLE 11–2.

Adult Reference Values for Peripheral Blood (Mean ±2 SD)

Test*	Williams et al.†	Wintrobe‡	Coulter Counter§
White cell count ($\times 10^9$/L)	7.8(4.4–11.3)	7.0(4.3–10.0)	4.8–10.8
Red cell count ($\times 10^{12}$/L)			
Male	5.21(4.52–5.90)	5.4(4.5–6.3)	4.7–6.1
Female	4.60(4.10–5.10)	4.8(4.2–5.5)	4.2–5.4
Hemoglobin (g/dL)			
Male	15.7(14.0–17.5)	16(14.0–18.0)	14–18
Female	13.8(12.3–15.3)	14(12.0–16.0)	12–16
Hematocrit (L/L)			
Male	0.46(0.42–0.50)	0.46(0.41–0.51)	0.42–0.52
Female	0.40(0.36–0.45)	0.42(0.37–0.47)	0.37–0.47
Mean corpuscular volume (MCV) (fL)	88.0(80–96.1)	91(82–101)	80–94 81–99
Mean corpuscular hemoglobin (MCH) (pg)	30.4(27.5–33.2)	31(27–34)	27–31
Mean corpuscular hemoglobin concentration (MCHC) (g/dL)	34.4(33.4–35.5)	34(31.5–36)	33–37
Red cell distribution width (RDW) (%)	13.1(11.5–14.5)		11.5–14.5
Platelet count ($\times 10^9$/L)	311(172–450)	140–440	130–400

*SI units, as recommended by the International Committee for Standardization in Hematology. See Chapter 4.
†Data from Williams WJ, Beutler E, Erslev A, et al: *Hematology,* ed 4. New York, McGraw-Hill Book Co, 1990, pp 10, 18.
‡Data from Wintrobe MM: *Clinical Hematology,* ed 8. Philadelphia, Lea & Febiger, 1981, pp 1051, 1885.
§Data from Coulter Electronics, Inc., Hialeah, FL.

TABLE 11–3.

Leukocyte Count, Leukocyte Differential, and Hemoglobin Concentration for a Normal Population at Various Ages*†

		Leukocyte Differential Count ($\times 10^9$/L)							
	Total	Neutrophils							
Age	Leukocytes ($\times 10^9$/L)	Total	Band	Segmented	Eosinophils	Basophils	Lymphocytes	Monocytes	Hemoglobin (g/dL)
12 mo	11.46 (6.0–17.5)	3.5 (1.5–8.5) 31%	0.35 3.1%	3.2 (1.0–8.5) 28%	0.30 (0.05–0.70) 2.6%	0.05 (0.0–0.20) 0.4%	7.0 (4.0–10.5) 61%	0.55 (0.05–1.1) 4.8%	12.6 (11.1–14.1)
4 yr	9.1 (5.5–15.5)	3.8 (1.5–8.5) 42%	0.27 (0–1.0) 3.0%	3.5 (1.5–7.5) 39%	0.25 (0.02–0.65) 2.8%	0.05 (0–2.0) 0.6%	4.5 (2.0–8.0) 50%	0.45 (0–0.8) 5.0%	12.7 (11.2–14.3)
6 yr	8.5 (5.0–14.5)	4.3 (1.5–8.0) 51%	0.25 (0–10) 3.0%	4.0 (1.5–7.0) 48%	0.23 (0–6.5) 2.7%	0.05 (0–0.2) 0.6%	3.5 (1.5–7.0) 42%	0.40 (0–0.8) 4.7%	13.0 (11.4–14.5)
10 yr	8.1 (4.5–13.5)	4.4 (1.8–8.0) 54%	0.24 (0–1.0) 3.0%	4.2 (1.8–7.0) 51%	0.20 (0–0.60) 2.4%	0.04 (0–0.2) 0.5%	3.1 (1.5–6.5) 38%	0.35 (0–0.8) 4.3%	13.4 (11.8–15.0)
21 yr	7.4 (4.5–11.0)	4.4 (1.8–7.7) 59%	0.22 (0–0.7) 3.0%	4.2 (1.8–7.0) 56%	0.20 (0–0.45) 2.7%	0.04 (0–0.2) 0.5%	2.5 (1.0–4.8) 34%	0.30 (0–0.8) 4.0%	15.5 (13.5–17.5) 13.8 (12.0–15.6)

*Data from Williams WJ, Beutler E, Erslev A, et al: *Hematology,* ed 4. New York, McGraw-Hill Book Co, 1990, p 18.
†Means are shown, with ranges in parentheses.

BIBLIOGRAPHY

Bessman JD: *Automated Blood Counts and Differentials.* Baltimore, Johns Hopkins University Press, 1986.

Boggs DR: *White Cell Manual,* ed 4. Philadelphia, FA Davis Co, 1983.

Brown B: *Hematology: Principles and Procedures,* ed 5. Philadelphia, Lea & Febiger, 1988.

College of American Pathologists: *Surveys Manual, Section 2, Appendix 1: Glossary of Terms, Hematology—Coagulation/Clinical Microscopy.* Northfield, Ill, College of American Pathologists, 1990.

Diggs LW, Sturm D, Bell A: *The Morphology of Human Blood Cells,* ed 5. Abbott Park, Ill, Abbott Laboratories, 1985.

Henry JB: *Clinical Diagnosis and Management by Laboratory Methods,* ed. 18. Philadelphia, WB Saunders Co, 1991.

Hillman RS, Finch CA: *Red Cell Manual.* Philadelphia, FA Davis Co, 1985.

Method for Reticulocyte Counting, Proposed Standard, Villanova, Pa, National Committee for Clinical Laboratory Standards, 1985; 5(June):H16–P.

Pittiglio D, Sacher R: *Clinical Hematology and Fundamentals of Hemostasis.* Philadelphia, FA Davis Co, 1987.

Powers L: *Diagnostic Hematology.* St. Louis, Mosby–Year Book, Inc, 1989

Procedure for Determining Packed Cell Volume by the Microhematocrit Method, Approved Standard. Villanova, Pa, National Committee for Clinical Laboratory Standards, 1985; 5(May): H7-A.

Rapaport SI: *Introduction to Hematology,* ed 2. Philadelphia, JB Lippincott Co, 1987.

Reference Procedure for Human Erythrocyte Sedimentation Rate (ESR) Test, Approved Standard. Villanova, Pa, National Committee for Clinical Laboratory Standards, 1988; 8(August):H2-A2.

Reference Procedure for the Quantitative Determination of Hemoglobin in Blood, Approved Standard. Villanova, Pa, National Committee for Clinical Laboratory Standards, 1984; 4(February):H15-A.

Williams WJ, Beutler E, Erslev A, et al: *Hematology,* ed 4. New York, McGraw-Hill Book 6, 1990.

Wintrobe MM: *Clinical Hematology,* ed 8. Philadelphia, Lea & Febiger, 1981.

12 Coagulation and Hemostasis

Key Terms

Coagulation cascade	Intrinsic system of coagulation
Coagulation factors	Nomenclature of Blood Clotting Factors
Common pathway	Plasmin
Extrinsic system of coagulation	Platelet aggregation
Fibrin	Platelet plug
Fibrinogen	Prothrombin
Fibrinolysis	Thrombin
Hemophilia	Thromboplastin
Hemostasis	

HEMOSTASIS

Hemostasis is the cessation of blood flow from an injured blood vessel. It is one of the most important natural defense mechanisms of the body. The process of hemostasis involves numerous interdependent factors that are controlled carefully by the body for the purpose of preventing bleeding. When there is an injury to a blood vessel, the hemostatic process is designed to repair the break. Thus, hemostasis is the process whereby the body retains the blood within the vascular system, in spite of the many traumas that injure the blood vessel walls. Activation of both the hemostatic and inflammatory responses are simultaneous after injury to a blood vessel.

The most immediate response of the body to bleeding is *vasoconstriction*. In this process, the damaged blood vessel constricts, decreasing the blood flow through the injured area. A platelet plug can then form, which helps to further inhibit the bleeding. Finally, coagulation factors present in the blood interact, forming a fibrin network or clot, to stop the bleeding completely. Slow lysis of the clot begins, and final repair to the site of the injury thus takes place.

Coagulation and hemostasis are complicated mechanisms which are not completely understood. The discussion in this chapter is simplified, but certain basic concepts must be presented before coagulation or hemostasis procedures are carried out.

HEMOSTATIC MECHANISM

The hemostatic mechanism is the entire process by which bleeding from an injured blood vessel is controlled and finally stopped. It is a series of physical and biochemical changes that are normally initiated by an injury to the blood vessel and tissues and that culminate in the transformation of fluid blood into a thrombus or clot, which effectively seals the injured vessel. The entire hemostatic mechanism can be divided into three parts: extravascular effects, vascular effects, and intravascular effects.

A bleeding tendency can result from a defect in any of the phases of repair; that is, (1) the vascular system itself may be prone to injury; (2) the platelets may be inadequate in number to form the emergency platelet plug; (3) the **fibrin** clotting mechanism may be inadequate; or (4) the fibroblastic repair may be inadequate. Excessive abnormal bleeding is usually the result of a combination of defects.

Extravascular Effects

Extravascular effects consist of (1) the physical effect of the surrounding tissues, such as muscle, skin, and elastic tissue, which tend to close and seal the tear in the vessel that is injured, and (2) the biochemical effects of certain substances that are released from the injured tissues and react with plasma and platelet factors. The latter factors are called the **extrinsic system of coagulation.**

Vascular Effects

The inner monolayer of cells on the blood vessel, the vascular endothelium, is very important to the hemostatic process. If trauma or injury disrupts this cell layer, the underlying basement membrane of the vessel is exposed. Basement membrane contains collagenous material and when circulating platelets make contact with this collagenous material, biochemical and structural changes occur that result in the formation of platelet aggregates and fibrin clots. These platelet aggregates can plug the gaps in the endothelial lining and thus prevent more stimulation by the collagen layer—the **platelet plug** is formed.

Vascular effects are also concerned with the blood vessels themselves, which constrict almost instantaneously when injured. The vasoconstriction phenomenon tends to pass off within a relatively short time, but it may be enhanced and prolonged by local release of a vaso-constricting substance, serotonin. Serotonin is released from the platelets as they adhere to the margins of the injury in the wall of the blood vessel. It promotes local, direct, biochemically stimulated narrowing of the torn blood vessel and of locally intact blood vessels in the same vicinity as the injury.

Intravascular Effects

The intravascular factors take part in an extremely complicated sequence of physiochemical reactions that transform the liquid blood into a firm fibrin clot. This process requires the initiation of a platelet plug. This is followed by reinforcement with fibrin derived from the activation of the **intrinsic system of coagulation.** All the factors necessary for the intrinsic system are contained within the blood. Many natural inhibitors and accelerators are brought into action during this time.

The Function of Platetets

Platelets have three important functions: (1) to react to injury of vessels by forming an aggregate plug or platelet mass that can physically slow down or stop blood loss; (2) to help activate and be a participant in plasma coagulation to more effectively serve as a barrier to extensive blood loss; and (3) to maintain the endothelial lining of the blood vessels.

Hemostatic Platelet Plug

When endothelial cells are damaged, displaced, or become degenerate, the platelets in the bloodstream are exposed to the underlying collagen and subendothelial factor, von Willebrand's factor VIII:vWF. The contact with collagen results in changes taking place in platelet function which, in turn, result in adherence of the platelets to the damaged area of the blood vessel. During this process, fibronectin is secreted by the endothelial cells. Fibronectin has been shown to assist in bonding platelets to the collagen substrate. An additional protein factor VIII:vWF, is necessary for optimal platelet-collagen binding to occur. Adherence to the collagen initiates platelet activation. Upon activation, platelets take on a different shape, becoming more spherical, with long, irregular arms. This greatly increases the surface area of the platelet and facilitates interaction with other platelets and proteins in the coagulation cascade process. Platelets also aggregate with one another as a result of changes which take place on their outer coats. The mass of platelets grows and forms the primary hemostatic plug in vivo. This plug must be stabilized by fibrin strands produced during plasma protein coagulation in order for the plug to be anything other than temporary. A bleeding time test can assess platelet plug formation which is dependent on platelet concentration (the platelet count), platelet qualitative function, and vessel integrity.

Platelets in Coagulation

The role of platelets in the coagulation process is varied. They secrete proteins that serve as cofactors, their outer coat contains reacting surfaces for some coagulation steps, and they participate directly in initiated coagulation at the contact phase.

Platelet factor 3 (PF3) is a phospholipoprotein that is contained on or within the plasma membrane and is needed in activating certain of the coagulation factors. Platelets possess receptors to bind coagulation protein factors V, VIII, and Xa. Activation occurs on the surface of the platelets. These are specific receptor molecules on the platelet membrane or outer coat. These receptors are glycoproteins that bind to coagulation proteins and to substances that facilitate platelet-platelet and platelet-endothelium interactions.

The endothelia of blood vessels are repaired and maintained with help from products that are secreted by the platelets. One such product is platelet-derived growth factor (PDGF).

COAGULATION

Most of the clinical conditions requiring coagulation studies involve the intrinsic system of coagulation. The **coagulation factors,** their nomenclature, and procedures for analyzing some of the more important coagulation factors are discussed in this section.

The blood coagulation mechanism is complicated and involves many factors. Knowing which factor is not performing its proper function is of critical importance to the physician. This knowledge is gained through the use of several different laboratory tests. The proper formation of a blood clot after a scratch or cut depends on healthy functioning of all the factors. In an individual having a weakness or deficiency in one or several of the factors, severe trauma from a serious injury or from surgical treatment can result in collapse of the clotting mechanism. This in turn will result in a most drastic manifestation—severe hemorrhage. This has been dramatically demonstrated in persons whose clotting mechanism is adequate for everyday living but who, during such common surgical procedures as dental extractions or tonsillectomies, erupt into severe bleeding. It is of the utmost importance, therefore, that the laboratory tests in this area be accurately performed. Most of these tests employ macroscopic observations.

The topic of blood coagulation is not completely understood and much research is still in progress in this field. It is generally agreed that all the elements necessary for clot formation are normally present in the circulating blood. The fluidity of the blood, therefore, depends on a balance between the coagulant and anticoagulant factors.

The mechanism of coagulation takes place in three major steps: (1) the formation of **thromboplastin,** (2) the formation of **thrombin,** and (3) the formation of fibrin. Various clotting factors, or constituents, are involved in this mechanism.

Coagulation Factors

The coagulation factors are fundamentally protein, with the exception of calcium and the phospholipid of the platelets. Most of the factors are zymogens and become active enzymes after proteolytic or structural change. Most of the active enzymes are serine proteases.

The process of coagulation is a series of biochemical reactions in which inactive proenzymes are converted to active enzyme forms, which then, in turn, activate other proenzymes. The coagulation process is thus a true cascade of factor activities, all interrelated to other factors. It is a carefully controlled process which responds to injury while continuing the maintenance of blood circulation.

Nomenclature

To standardize the complex nomenclature that is used by those involved in coagulation studies, the International Committee on **Nomenclature of Blood Clotting Factors** was established in 1954 to standardize the terminology (Table 12–1). Twelve coagulation factors are described and designated by Roman numerals

Roman numerals have been assigned to the various coagulation factors in the order of their discovery and do not indicate anything about the sequence of the reactions. No factor has been assigned the Roman numeral VI. The numerals used denote the factors as they exist in the plasma, except for factor III, tissue thromboplastin, which is not normally present in plasma but is found in tissue. Factor III is not a single substance but a variety of substances. The lower-case *a* denotes activated forms and cofactors for the coagulation factors. All coagulation factors, except factor III, circulate in an inactive, or precursor, form. In addition to the factors denoted by Roman numerals, some other essential coagulation reactants are: phospholipid (or phospholipoprotein), the phospholipoprotein of platelets, PF3; prekallikrein, the active form of kallikrein; kininogen; and protein C, a vitamin K–dependent factor that is an inactivator of thrombin-activated factors V and VIII.

Factor I (Fibrinogen)

The term **fibrinogen** has been in use for many years. Fibrinogen is the soluble precursor of the clot-forming protein, fibrin. It is a plasma protein (globulin) with a molecular weight of 340,000 daltons. It is present in the plasma of normal persons at a concentration of 200 to 400 mg/dL. A minimum of 60 to 100 mg/dL is required for normal coagulation.

Fibrinogen is synthesized by the liver but does not require vitamin K for its production. In severe liver disease a moderate lowering of the plasma fibrinogen level may occur, although rarely to the degree where hemorrhage occurs.

By the action of thrombin, peptides are split from the fibrinogen molecule, leaving a fibrin monomer. Fibrin monomers aggregate to form polymers.

TABLE 12–1.

Nomenclature of the Coagulation Factors

Factor*	Name	Synonym(s)
I	Fibrinogen	
II	Prothrombin	Prethrombin
III	Tissue thromboplastin	Tissue factor
IV	Calcium	
V	Proaccelerin	Labile factor, accelerator globulin (AcG)
VII	Proconvertin	Stable factor, serum prothrombin conversion accelerator (SPCA), autoprothrombin I
VIII	Antihemophilic factor (AHF)	Antihemophilic globulin (AHG), antihemophilic factor A, platelet cofactor I
IX	Plasma thromboplastin component (PTC)	Antihemophilic factor B (AHB), Christmas factor, autoprothrombin II, platelet cofactor II
X	Stuart-Prower factor	Stuart factor, autoprothrombin III
XI	Plasma thromboplastin antecedent (PTA)	Antihemophilic factor C
XII	Hageman factor	Glass or contact factor
XIII	Fibrinase	Laki-Lorand factor, fibrin stabilizing factor (FSF)
	Prekallikrein (PK)	Fletcher factor
	High-molecular-weight kininogen (HMWK)	Fitzgerald factor

*When factors have been activated, they have the designation *a* after their Roman numeral.

Fibrinogen is relatively stable to heat and storage, but may be irreversibly precipitated at 56°C. It has a half-life of 3 to 4 days.

Factor II (Prothrombin)

Thrombin is generated from a precursor, **prothrombin.** *Prothrombin* is also a term that has been used for many years. Prothrombin is synthesized by the liver through the action of vitamin K. It is a protein (globulin) with a molecular weight of about 69,000 daltons, and is normally present in the plasma in a concentration of approximately 8 to 15 mg/dL. It is utilized in the clotting mechanism to such a degree that little remains in the serum. In normal plasma, there is an excess of prothrombin relative to the amount of thrombin needed to clot fibrinogen. Nature has provided a wide margin of safety for this important substance. About 20% of the normal concentration must be present to assure hemostasis. Pro-

thrombin is heat-stable and has a half-life of 70 to 110 hours.

Factor III (Tissue Thromboplastin)

Thromboplastin or tissue factor is the name given to any substance capable of converting prothrombin to thrombin. In coagulation, two separate mechanisms utilize thromboplastin: as intrinsic or blood thromboplastin and extrinsic or tissue thromboplastin. All injured tissues yield a complex mixture of as yet unclassified substances that possess potential thromboplastic activity. During clotting of whole blood, platelets appear to be the source of thromboplastin. The clot-accelerating activity of tissues has been assigned the name factor III by the International Committee on Nomenclature of Blood Clotting Factors.

Complete thromboplastins and partial thromboplastins are used in different laboratory diagnostic procedures. The term *partial thromboplastin* is used to designate thromboplastic reagents that are found to clot hemophilic plasma less rapidly than normal plasma. Complete thromboplastins are able to produce clotting as rapidly with hemophilic plasma as with normal plasma.

Tissue thromboplastin is a high-molecular weight lipoprotein that is found in almost all body tissues and is found in increased concentrations in the lungs and brain.

The molecular weight depends on the type of tissue from which the particular thromboplastin is derived—it can range from 45,000 to over 1 million daltons. Tissue thromboplastin is found in increased concentrations in red cell membranes, platelets, brain tissue, placenta, and lung.

Factor IV (Calcium)

It has been known for many years that calcium in the ionized state is essential for coagulation, and the term *factor IV* is used for calcium when it participates in this process. The exact mechanism by which calcium acts is not completely understood. The fact that it is essential for clotting makes possible the use of anticoagulants that bind calcium. By binding calcium, fibrin formation cannot take place and clotting does not occur.

Calcium appears to function mainly as a bridge between the phospholipid surface of platelets and several clotting factors. Binding sites or loops of prominent carboxyglutamic acid on several factors allow bridging with the calcium-phospholipid complex. The calcium ion concentration is very important in in vitro studies of coagulation.

Factor V (Proaccelerin)

Factor V is essential for the prompt conversion of prothrombin to thrombin in the clotting of whole blood as well as in the presence of tissue thromboplastins. It is synthesized in the liver, and acquired deficiencies have been observed in liver disease. When factor V levels decrease to 30% of normal, bleeding occurs. Factor V is a globulin with a molecular weight of about 330,000 daltons. It is labile, deteriorating rapidly in plasma, especially in oxalated plasma (not so quickly in citrated plasma). The activity of factor V in plasma deteriorates even when the plasma is frozen. It is the most unstable of the coagulation factors. Factor V is consumed in the clotting mechanism and is therefore not found in serum. Its activity decreases within a few hours when human blood or plasma is stored at or above room temperature. It has a half-life of about 12 to 36 hours in the plasma.

For this reason, the term *labile factor* has been used for factor V.

Factor VII (Proconvertin)

Factor VII is not destroyed or consumed in the clotting process, so it is present in both plasma and serum. It is a beta globulin with a molecular weight of 60,000 daltons. It is synthesized in the liver and requires vitamin K for its production. An acquired deficiency of factor VII results from any disorder that decreases its synthesis in the liver. It has a very short biological half-life, 4 to 6 hours, which results in a rapid disappearance from the blood when factor VII production is halted. This may occur during drug therapy with coumarin or in a congenitally deficient patient. It remains at a high level in stored blood as well as in serum. There is evidence to suggest that the activity of factor VII actually increases during the clotting process. Its presence can be monitored by the prothrombin test.

Factor VIII (Antihemophilic Factor)

The production site of factor VIII is not certain. It is a beta globulin with a high molecular weight of about 1.2 million daltons. Factor VIII is unaffected by vitamin K deficiency and coumarin-type drugs. It is lost rapidly from the bloodstream, having a half-life of 6 to 10 hours. This rapid clearance occurs in normal persons as well as in those with a congenital deficiency.

Factor VIII circulates as a complex made up of two functional subunits. One unit, designated *factor VIII:C* is a coagulation factor. Factor VIII:C represents the ability of the factor VIII molecule to correct coagulation abnormalities associated with hemophilia A. This unit is measured by the various factor VIII assays used routinely in the laboratory. The other subunit is called vonWillebrand's factor, designated factor *VIII:vWF*, which facilitates platelet adherence to subendothelial surfaces. Factor VIII:vWF is necessary for normal platelet adhesion. It is not necessary for the coagulation mechanism. It is present in plasma, platelets, megakaryocytes, and endothelial cells. The larger part of the complex is made up of VIII:vWF. It is strongly antigenic and a portion of the molecule participates in platelet aggregation induced by the antibiotic ristocetin. Laboratory tests utilizing immunoassay are used to measure antigenic activity while the basis of another test is the portion of the molecule which makes possible platelet aggregation in the presence of ristocetin.

Hemophilia refers to a sex-linked coagulation disorder. It has been demonstrated that the coagulation defect can be corrected by the use of normal plasma. The terms *antihemophilic factor (AHF)* and *antihemophilic globulin (AHG)* have been used to designate the procoagulant present in normal plasma but deficient in the plasma of patients with hemophilia. The term *hemophilia A,* the classic "bleeder's disease," is adopted to designate the hereditary disease with a deficiency in factor VIII:C subunit. These people generally have normal levels of the vonWillebrand factor VIII:vWF subunit.

Factor IX (Plasma Thromboplastin Component)

Factor IX is a stable protein factor, an alpha or beta globulin, with a molecular weight of 55,000 to 62,000 daltons. It has a half-life of about 20 hours, is not consumed during clotting, and is not destroyed by aging. It is present in both serum and plasma, and there is probably no significant loss of the factor in blood or plasma stored at 4°C for 2 weeks. Factor IX is an essential component of the intrinsic thromboplastin-generating system. It is synthesized in the liver and requires vitamin K for its production. The disease resulting from a deficiency of this factor is known as hemophilia B. Hemophilia B is also inherited as a sex-linked recessive disorder. Its clinical symptoms are identical to those of hemophilia A and the disorder can be divided into mild, moderate, or severe, paralleling the level of factor IX present.

Factor X (Stuart-Prower Factor)

This is a relatively stable factor that is not consumed during the clotting process and therefore is found in both serum and plasma. It is an alpha globulin weighing 59,000 daltons that requires vitamin K for its synthesis in the liver. Factor X works with other substances to form the thromboplastins that convert prothrombin to thrombin. It helps to form the final common pathway through which products of both the intrinsic and the extrinsic thromboplastin-generating system act. Factor X is stable for several weeks to 2 months when stored at 4°C. It has a half-life of from 24 to 65 hours.

Factor XI (Plasma Thromboplastin Antecedent)

Factor XI is a beta globulin weighing 160,000 to 200,000 daltons. Its synthesis takes place in the liver and vitamin K is not required. It circulates as a complex with another protein, high-molecular-weight kininogen (HMWK). Only part of Factor XI is consumed during the clotting process so it is present in the serum as well as the plasma. It is essential for the intrinsic thromboplastin-generating mechanism.

Factor XII (Hageman Factor)

Factor XII is a stable gamma globulin weighing 80,000 daltons. It is not consumed during the clotting process and is therefore found in both serum and plasma. It is synthesized in the liver and does not depend on vitamin K for its synthesis. Factor XII is converted to an active form when it comes in contact with glass. The natural counterpart of glass is not known, but platelets or damaged endothelium may be involved in this primary activation process. Factor XII is involved in the initial phase of the intrinsic coagulation pathway.

Factor XIII (Fibrinase)

Factor XIII is an alpha globulin with a high molecular weight. Its site of production is not fully known, but is believed to be in the liver for the plasma factor. Platelet XIII factor is synthesized by megakaryocytes. There is evidence that it is an enzyme (fibrinase) that catalyzes the polymerization of fibrin. This factor is inhibited by ethylenediaminetetraacetic acid (EDTA). Very little factor XIII is present in the serum, the major portion being used up in the polymerization of fibrin. It acts to stabilize the fibrin clot and also further acts to assist in linking the endothelial cell protein, fibronectin, to collagen and fibrin residues. This is extremely important in tissue growth and repair.

Prekallikrein (PK, Fletcher Factor)

Prekallikrein is a precursor for a serine protease, kallikrein, which also activates plasminogen. Kallikrein is a chemotactic factor used to recruit phagocytes and can stimulate the complement cascade. PK is found in the plasma in association with HMWK. It is produced in the liver but it is not dependent on vitamin K for its synthesis.

High-molecular-weight Kininogen (HMWK, Fitzgerald Factor)

High-molecular-weight kininogen can be acted upon to yield kinin. It serves as a cofactor for reactions involving factor XII and activation of factor VII. It is the precursor molecule of bradykinin, an important inflammatory mediator involving vascular permeability and dilation, pain production at sites of inflammation, and synthesis of prostaglandin. HMWK is produced in the liver and is not dependent on vitamin K for its synthesis.

Properties of Coagulation Factors

Coagulation factors can be divided into three groups based on their properties:

1. *The fibrinogen group* (thrombin-sensitive) consists of factors I, V, VIII, and XIII. Thrombin acts on all of these factors. Thrombin enhances factors V and VIII by converting them to active cofactors. It also activates factor XIII and converts fibrinogen (factor I) to fibrin. All of these factors are used up in the coagulation process so they are not found in serum. They are not absorbed by barium sulfate and therefore remain present in absorbed plasma. Factor V and VIII are relatively labile and are therefore not present in plasma that has been stored. In addition to the presence of these fibinogen factors in plasma, these factors are also found within platelets.

2. *The prothrombin group* (vitamin K–dependent) consists of factors II, VII, IX, and X. Vitamin K is essential for synthesis of all these factors. Coumarin-type drugs, which inhibit vitamin K, cause a decrease in these factors. Factors VII, IX, and X are not consumed in the coagulation process and are therefore present in serum as well in plasma. All four factors are absorbed by barium sulfate. They are stable and are therefore well preserved in plasma that has been stored.

3. *The contact group* consists of factors XI, XII, prekallikrein, and HMWK. These factors are not consumed in the coagulation process, are not dependent on vitamin K for their synthesis, and are not absorbed out of plasma by barium sulfate. They are relatively stable.

Mechanism of Coagulation

Stages of Coagulation

The complex mechanism of coagulation takes place in three major stages.

Stage 1: Generation of thromboplastic activity. The thromboplastic activity necessary to convert prothrombin to thrombin is produced in stage 1 through the interaction of platelets with factors XII, XI, IX, and VIII (the intrinsic pathway), or through the release of tissue thromboplastin from the injured tissues (the extrinsic pathway). Plasma factor VII activates the tissue thromboplastic substances. Various tests will detect stage 1 deficiencies but the one test of choice for screening purposes and for identification of stage 1 deficiencies is the activated partial thromboplastin time (APTT) test.

Stage 2: Generation of thrombin. The plasma or tissue thromboplastin plus factor VII produced in stage 1, in the presence of plasma factors V and X, converts prothrombin to the active enzyme thrombin. Laboratory tests are available to detect deficiencies in stage 2. The one-stage prothrombin time (PT) test detects deficiencies best in stages 2 and 3. Abnormal formation of a clot results from a deficiency of any of the coagulation factors or the presence of an inhibitor or anticoagulant. The anticoagulants EDTA, oxalate, and citrate remove calcium to prevent clotting in vitro. Heparin and coumarin drugs prevent the conversion of prothrombin to thrombin, also preventing the clotting mechanism from functioning in vivo.

Stage 3: Conversion of fibrinogen to fibrin. Thrombin converts fibrinogen to fibrin, and a fibrin clot is formed that is stabilized by the presence of factor XIII. The thrombin time test measures the concentration and activity of fibrinogen in stage 3.

The presence of calcium ions is necessary in all three stages of the clotting mechanism.

PATHWAYS FOR THE COAGULATION CASCADE

The final product in the clotting process is the production of a fibrin clot. A series of events must take place involving many reactions and feedback mechanisms before the clot is formed. By means of the intrinsic or extrinsic pathway, or both, leading to a **common pathway,** the various precursors, factors, and other reactants respond normally in an orderly, controlled process—the **coagulation cascade.**

The Intrinsic vs. Extrinsic Coagulation Pathway

All factors required for the intrinsic pathway are contained within the blood. The extrinsic pathway uses thromboplastin (factor III) which is released from the damaged cells and tissues outside the circulating blood.

Intrinsic Pathway (Activation of Factor X)

In the *intrinsic* pathway, all the necessary components are found within the circulating blood. It is thought that tissue injury, following exposure to foreign substances such as collagen, activates the intrinsic pathway. Injury to endothelial cells can begin this process. In this pathway, a complex involving factors VIII and IX, in association with calcium and phospholipid on the platelets, ultimately activates factor X. To accomplish this, factor IX is first activated by the action of factor XIa (in the presence of calcium ions) which has previously been activated by factor XII (Fig 12–1). Factors XI and XII are known as contact factors because their activation is initiated by contact with subendothelial basement membrane that is exposed at the time of a tissue or blood vessel injury.

Although the complex reactions which occur in the intrinsic pathway take place relatively slowly, they account for the majority of the coagulation activities in the body. A laboratory test that monitors the intrinsic pathway leading to fibrin clot formation is the partial thromboplastin time (PTT) test, The PTT measures factors XII, XI, X, IX, VIII, V, II, and I.

Extrinsic Pathway (Activation of Factor X)

Extrinsic is used to indicate the pathway taken when tissue thromboplastin, a substance not found in the blood, enters the vascular system. Factor VII is activated

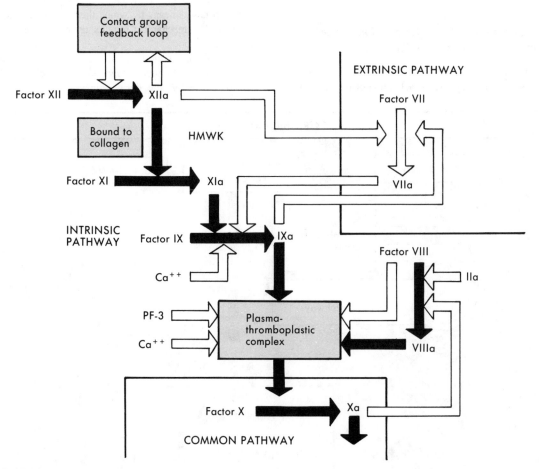

FIG 12–1.
Major reactions of the intrinsic pathway. Generation of factor IXa and the plasma thromboplastin complex. HMWK = high-molecular-weight kininogen. (From Powers LW: *Diagnostic Hematology.* St Louis. Mosby–Year Book, Inc, 1989, p 170. Used by permission.)

to its VIIa form in the presence of calcium (factor IV) and tissue thromboplastin (factor III) which, in turn, activates factor X to Xa. Thromboplastin is released from the injured wall of the blood vessel. Only activated factor VII is needed in the extrinsic pathway, bypassing factors XII, XI, IX, and VIII (used in the intrinsic pathway to activate factor X to its activated form, Xa) (Fig 12–2). In addition to quickly providing small amounts of thrombin which leads to fibrin formation, the thrombin generated in the extrinsic pathway can enhance the activity of factors V and VIII in the intrinsic pathway. To monitor the extrinsic pathway leading to fibrin clot formation in the laboratory, the PT test is performed. The PT measures factors VII, X, V, II, and I.

The Common Pathway (Formation of the Fibrin Clot From Factor X)

By means of either extrinsic, intrinsic, or a combination of both pathways, the activation of factor X to Xa

occurs. Once Xa is formed, another cofactor, V, in the presence of calcium and PF3, converts factor II, prothrombin, to the active enzyme, thrombin. The activation of thrombin is slow, but once it is generated, it further amplifies the coagulation process. Thrombin acts to convert fibrinogen to fibrin (Fig 12–3). Activation of factor XIII during this process results in the formation of a stronger, more durable clot.

FIBRINOLYSIS

Besides having a system for clot formation, the body also has a means by which the fibrin clot may be removed. The mechanism for clot removal is not completely understood.

As soon as the clotting process has begun, **fibrinolysis** is initiated to break down the fibrin clot that is formed. Normally, the fibrinolytic system functions to

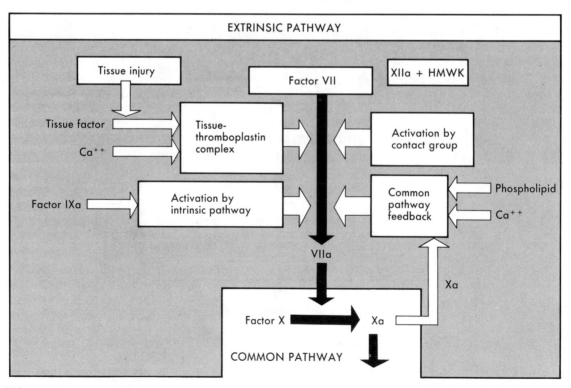

FIG 12–2.
Major reactions of the extrinsic pathway. Generation of factor VIIa following activation of tissue factors. (From Powers LW: *Diagnostic Hematology.* St Louis, Mosby–Year Book, Inc, 1989, p 168. Used by permission.)

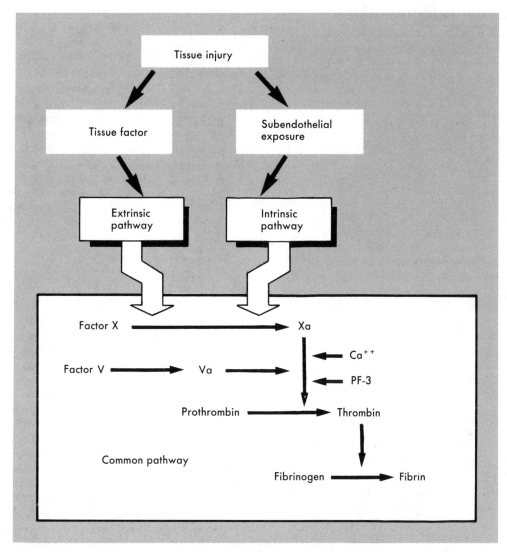

FIG 12–3.
Overview of coagulation. Relationship between the three pathways, common, extrinsic, and intrinsic, emphasizing the major events of the common pathway. *PF-3* = platelet factor 3. (From Powers LW: *Diagnostic Hematology.* St Louis, Mosby–Year Book, Inc, 1989, p 162. Used by permission.)

keep the vascular system free of fibrin clots or deposited fibrin. There is evidence that the fibrinolytic system and the coagulation system are in equilibrium in normal persons. As a general rule, fibrinolysis is increased whenever coagulation is increased.

The active enzyme that is responsible for digesting fibrin or fibrinogen is **plasmin.** Plasmin is not normally found in the circulating blood, but is present in an inac-

tive form, plasminogen. Plasminogen is converted to plasmin by certain proteolytic enzymes. These plasminogen activators are found in small amounts in most body tissues, in very low amounts in most body fluids, and in urine. The decomposition products of fibrin formed during fibrinolysis are removed from the blood by the reticuloendothelial system.

TESTS FOR HEMOSTASIS AND COAGULATION

The tests involved in the study of hemostasis may be divided into three main categories according to the three lines of defense against hemorrhage that were discussed earlier in this chapter: (1) tests for the vascular factor, (2) tests for the platelets, and (3) tests for the factors involved in coagulation. Tests for the vascular factor include the capillary fragility test (also known as the cuff test, tourniquet test, or capillary resistance test) and tests for bleeding time. Tests for the platelet factor include the platelet count, platelet aggregation assays, platelet adhesiveness studies, the bleeding time, and the clot retraction test. There are numerous tests for the plasma factors and whole blood factors involved in coagulation; these include the venous clotting time, the PT, and the PPT.

Tests for Vascular Factors

Capillary Fragility Test

This test measures the ability of the capillaries to withstand increased stress. In this test, a blood pressure cuff is placed above the patient's elbow and inflated to a maximum pressure of 100 mm Hg. A specified time interval and pressure is determined by the exact method used by the laboratory. The arm is examined before the pressure is applied to see if any petechiae are present. Petechiae are collections of red blood cells around minute vessels; when these are present, small reddish spots will be seen on the skin. Any petechiae are noted by making a circle around them with ink. The pressure is maintained for 5 minutes, the cuff is removed, and the number of petechiae are counted that have appeared in a circle 5 cm in diameter drawn below the bend of the elbow. A normal value is zero to ten petechiae of less than 1 mm diameter, appearing within 10 minutes, and a positive reaction is indicated by more than ten. A positive test result indicates capillary weakness, thrombocytopenia, or both.

Bleeding Time Tests

Bleeding time tests measure the time required for cessation of bleeding after a standardized capillary puncture to a capillary bed. The time required will depend on capillary integrity, the number of platelets, and the platelet function. There must be an adequate number of circu-lating platelets for a normal bleeding time. Below a platelet count of $50 \times 10^9/L$ the bleeding time is almost always prolonged.

A number of different bleeding time tests have been devised. Two that are used are the Ivy bleeding time test (Procedure 12–1)* and the Duke bleeding time test (Procedure 12–2). The Duke test is included in this discussion for historical purposes only.† The chief difficulty in performing these tests is in the production of an adequate and standardized skin puncture. An adequate test depends greatly on the skin wound, and therefore on the skill of the laboratorian. Capillary bleeding is tested, and wounds more than 3 mm deep are likely to involve vessels of greater than capillary size, whereas wounds that are shallow are not likely to adequately test the capillaries and the hemostatic factors involved.

A modification of the Ivy bleeding time test devised by Mielke et al. is considered to be the best bleeding time test (Procedure 12–3).‡ In this test, a plastic template is made with a slit or slits 1 mm wide and 1 cm long. With a calibrated gauge, a disposable blade is fitted on the holder so that it protrudes through the bottom of the template exactly 1 mm. The same procedure is employed as for the Ivy method, and a blood pressure cuff is used. Two incisions 9 mm long and 1 mm deep are made. The average of the two bleeding times is reported. A commercial, disposable product utilizing a modification of this method, called the Simplate, is available.

Under the conditions of the test, bleeding is believed to be controlled by capillary retraction and the formation of a platelet plug in the wounds. Tissue factors are also thought to play a role, especially tissue tonus (contraction). Defects in the clotting mechanism have little effect on the bleeding time. The bleeding time is prolonged when there is a combination of poor capillary retraction and platelet deficiency.

The bleeding test is positive (bleeding time is prolonged) in thrombocytopenic purpura and in constitutional capillary inferiority. Normal bleeding times are

---

*Ivy AC, Shapiro PF, Melnick P: The bleeding tendency in jaundice. *Surg Gynecol Obstet* 1935; 60:781.

†Duke WW: The relation of blood platelets to hemorrhagic disease: Description of a method for determining the bleeding time and coagulation time and report of three cases of hemorrhagic disease relieved by transfusion. *JAMA* 1910; 14:1185.

‡Mielke CH, Kaneshiro IA, Maher JM, et al: The standardized normal Ivy bleeding time and its prolongation by aspirin. *Blood* 1969; 34:204.

Procedure 12–1. Ivy Bleeding Time Test

1. A blood pressure cuff is placed on the upper arm, and the forearm is cleaned with medicated alcohol below the antecubital fossa area and allowed to dry. The area used should be relatively free of veins.
2. The cuff is inflated to 40 mm Hg, and this pressure is maintained throughout the test.
3. Two skin punctures 3 mm deep are made in the cleaned area. The punctures should be made in rapid succession, using a disposable capillary lancet.
4. Timing is started as soon as bleeding begins.
5. Blood is removed every 30 seconds as it accumulates over the wounds by blotting lightly with the flat side of a piece of blotting paper or other absorbent paper. Care should be taken not to apply any pressure or disturb the lips of the wounds (Fig 12–4).
6. The time at which bleeding ceases is reported to the nearest 30 seconds. Remove the blood pressure cuff and stop the timing.
7. Normal values are 2 to 6 minutes; values of 6 to 10 minutes are considered borderline and the test should be repeated.

Procedure 12–2. Duke Bleeding Time Test

1. An ear lobe (or heel, in an infant) is cleaned carefully with medicated alcohol. An earlobe on which the patient has been lying is not used.
2. A stab wound 3 mm deep is made in the margin of the ear lobe (or heel) using a disposable lancet.
3. Timing is started as soon as bleeding begins.
4. Drops of blood are blotted every 30 seconds without touching the wound with the blotting paper. The patient must remain quiet throughout the test.
5. The time at which bleeding ceases is reported to the nearest 30 seconds.
6. Normal values are 1 to 3 minutes; borderline values are 3 to 6 minutes.

Procedure 12–3. Template (Mielke Modification) Bleeding Time Test

1. A disposable blade is fitted onto a holder so that the blade protrudes through the bottom of the template exactly 1 mm.
2. A site on the forearm is selected away from obvious blood vessels.
3. A blood pressure cuff is placed on the arm and inflated to 40 mm Hg.
4. The skin is cleaned with alcohol and allowed to dry.
5. Two cuts are made. This device gives cuts exactly 9 mm long and 1 mm deep. With such shallow cuts, venules are virtually never cut.
6. After 5 to 15 seconds of no bleeding (venospasm occurs during the first 5 to 15 seconds after the cuts have been made), bleeding usually starts. Timing starts when the bleeding begins.
7. While the cuts are bleeding, the blood is blotted as necessary from the sides of the cuts to avoid disturbing the clot as it is formed (see Fig 12–4).
8. It should be noted that small scars may result from this test.
9. Normal values are 3 to 10 minutes

---

found in hemophilia and other defects of the clotting mechanism.

Simplate Bleeding Time Test: The procedure is similar to the Mielke template modification of the Ivy bleeding time test, except that a commercially available disposable apparatus is used to make the incisions. The Simplate II lancet device (Organon Teknika Corp., Durham, N.C.), contains dual spring-loaded blades within a plastic holder. When the trigger is depressed, the edge of the blades (each 5 mm in length) will spring forward 1 mm from the housing making parallel cuts 1 mm deep and 5 mm long. The incision made is therefore 5 mm long and 1 mm deep. With this very shallow cut being made, venules are rarely cut. The normal range for this procedure is from 2.3 to 9.5 minutes. The patient should be bandaged with a butterfly bandage over the puncture site and advised to keep it in place for 24 hours.

Precautions in Bleeding Time Tests.—Bleeding time tests are not always significant because normal

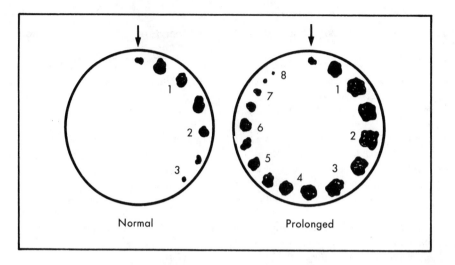

FIG 12–4.
Bleeding time determination. Appearance of blood spots on filter paper from a patient with a normal bleeding time *(left)* and from a patient with a platelet defect *(right)*. (From Powers LW: *Diagnostic Hematology.* St Louis, Mosby–Year Book, Inc, 1989, p 474. Used by permission.)

bleeding times are found in patients who have defects in the clotting mechanism. Bleeding time is prolonged in conditions where there is a combination of poor muscle contraction in the blood vessels and platelet deficiency. Obtaining an adequate bleeding time depends greatly on the depth of the skin puncture. In the Ivy method and its modifications, the blood pressure cuff must be maintained at 40 mm Hg throughout the test.

The template method is considered the best bleeding time test because the skin punctures are uniformly deep.

Tests for Platelet Factors

Tests for the platelet factors involved in hemostasis include the platelet count (see under Counting Platelets, Chapter 11), assays of platelet aggregation or adhesiveness, the bleeding time tests described above (template, and Ivy methods), the prothrombin consumption test, and the clot retraction test. The bleeding time tests are especially concerned with platelets—the number of platelets present and their ability to form a plug. Prolonged bleeding times will generally be found when the platelet count is below 50×10^9/L and where there is platelet dysfunction. A bleeding time test should not be done unless a platelet count has been done shortly before. It is not recommended that bleeding times not be done when the platelet count is $<50 \times 10^9$/L.

Platelet Aggregation Studies

The response of platelets during the hemostatic process includes a change in shape, increasing surface adhesiveness and the tendency to aggregate with other platelets to form a plug. Measurement of **platelet aggregation** is an essential part of the investigation of any patient with suspected platelet dysfunction. An aggregating agent is added to a suspension of platelets in plasma (plasma-rich plasma, PRP) and the response is measured turbidometrically as a change in the transmission of light. There are a variety of commercially available instruments devised to conduct this test. These instruments are called *aggregometers.*

When an aggregating reagent (including thrombin, adenosine diphosphate, epinephrine, serotonin, arachidonic acid, ristocetin, snake venoms, collagen) is added to PRP being stirred in a cuvette at a constant temperature, platelets start to aggregate and the transmission of light increases. The PRP appears turbid at the beginning of the test. With the addition of the aggregating reagent, larger platelet aggregates begin to form and because of this, the PRP begins to clear and there is a corresponding increase in the light being transmitted. The increased change in optical density or transmission of light is recorded as a function of time on a moving strip recording. The platelet response curve consists of distinct phases that will vary with the concentration and type of aggregating reagent used.

Platelet Retention or Adhesiveness Test

This test measures the ability of platelets to adhere to glass surfaces. When anticoagulated blood is passed through a plastic tube containing glass beads at a constant rate, some platelets will adhere to the glass beads. The percentage difference of the platelet count done prior to and after passage through the glass bead column is calculated. The normal range is 75% to 95% platelet retention. The platelet adhesiveness test is nonspecific. It is abnormal in several platelet functional disorders.

Clot Retraction Tests

Normal blood will clot completely and the clot will begin to retract within 1 hour. At the end of 18 to 24 hours, the clot should have retracted completely and serum should be expressed (Fig 12–5). The clot should be tough and elastic and not easily broken with an applicator stick. Retraction is primarily dependent on normal platelet function but hematocrit level and the fibrinogen level also can affect clot retraction. The extent of the retraction is influenced by the amount of fibrin formed, the presence of intact platelets within the fibrin network, and physical interference from trapped red blood cells. When the platelet count is less than 100×10^9/L, poor clot retractility is usually seen.

If the tube of blood is incubated in a water bath at 37°C and observed periodically, clot retraction is complete in 4 hours for a normal subject, but may be poor or absent 24 hours later in a patient with inadequate thrombosthenin (a protein component of platelets, important in

a clot reaction), or a low platelet count. This test is not considered to be a very sensitive measure of platelet dysfunction.

Prothrombin Consumption Test (PCT)

This test is done to determine the amount of prothrombin remaining in the serum after clotting has occurred. Normally, prothrombin is used up as it is converted to thrombin. If blood is allowed to clot for 1 hour while being incubated at 37°C, normally 95% or more of the prothrombin that was present in the plasma is consumed in this clotting process. The PCT is done by performing a prothrombin assay on serum after the blood has clotted (using the 1-hour incubation specimen) and calculating the amount of prothrombin consumed. Reference values will vary with the reagent system used by the laboratory, but normal PCT times are usually greater than 18 to 20 seconds. Increased serum prothrombin results from a quantitative or qualitative platelet deficiency.

Tests for Plasma Coagulation Factors

To assess potential defects in the coagulation cascade, screening tests are first performed. Common screening tests of the plasma coagulation system are the one-stage PT, the APTT, and the thrombin time. Other related tests for coagulation are bleeding time, platelet counts, and clot retraction tests. Once it has been determined by the coagulation screening tests that the patient

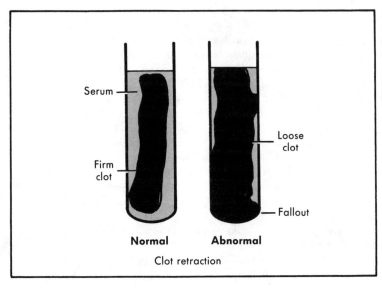

FIG 12–5.
Clot retraction. Normal and abnormal appearance of a clot after 24 hours' incubation. (From Powers LW: *Diagnostic Hematology.* St Louis, Mosby–Year Book, Inc, 1989, p 476. Used by permission.)

Serum

Firm clot

Loose clot

Fallout

Normal   **Abnormal**

Clot retraction

has a coagulation disorder, the exact factor, deficiency, or abnormality should be identified.

In monitoring anticoagulant therapy, the PT is most generally employed when the patient is receiving coumarin drugs. Heparin therapy is usually followed by determining the APTT and thrombin time, although the whole blood coagulation time is occasionally used.

The manual methods for doing coagulation tests have been replaced in most laboratories by automated and semiautomated equipment. Several instruments are available that can do coagulation tests such as PTs and PTTs. Some of these instruments can detect the formation of the clot photoelectrically, thus eliminating the error associated with visual timing of clot formation.

Two nonautomated techniques for performing plasma clotting tests are discussed in this section: the PT and the APTT.

Specimens for Coagulation Tests

Improper specimen collection and handling is a major problem for coagulation assays. Screening coagulation assays are performed on plasma that has been processed from blood anticoagulated with a citrate solution. The citrate reversibly binds calcium ions and prevents the various steps in the coagulation process that begin with the activation of factor IX and VII from taking place. Binding the calcium does not inhibit the contact phase of coagulation so it is critical that no activation of this process be made while collecting the blood or processing it.

By a long-established convention for coagulation tests, nine volumes of carefully drawn blood is mixed with one volume of citrate anticoagulant. Blood must be collected into containers made from nonreactive materials which will not interact or activate the coagulation mechanism. Either a syringe or evacuated tube system can be used to collect the specimen. A clean entry into the vein must be made. The blood should flow quickly and smoothly into the container. The method of collection to ensure the highest quality of specimen for coagulation tests is to use a "two-syringe" method. This is the best way to prevent contamination of the blood specimen with traces of tissue juices that would activate the coagulation process. Two plastic syringes should be used to prevent activation of the contact phase of coagulation. The first syringe is used to withdraw a few milliliters of blood, then a new syringe is attached and the specimen collected for coagulation testing. The tourniquet should not be left in place for a prolonged time as extended stasis can result in endothelial injury and the release of plas-

minogen activators. As soon as the blood is drawn into the syringe, the needle is removed and the blood allowed to flow down the inside of the specimen tube. The tube of blood and anticoagulant should be covered and gently mixed several times without shaking or foaming. Shaking the tube will result in activation of platelets and the contact system.

The ratio of blood to anticoagulant is important. For specimens with high hematocrits where there is a reduced plasma volume, the use of special tubes with reduced anticoagulant volume is often employed. For hematocrit values of about 0.55 mL/dL, the National Committee for Clinical Laboratory Standards (NCCLS) recommends that adjustment be made from the anticoagulant to blood ratio usually used.

Evacuated collection tubes are available with 3.2% buffered citrate anticoagulant in them. There is less direct contact with the actual blood specimen when these tubes are used which allows easier adherence to the universal precautionary regulations being so strongly applied in health care facilities. If the evacuated tube system is used, blood should be collected into the citrated tubes for coagulation studies after blood has been drawn for other tests. The coagulation testing specimen should be the second or third tube obtained. If only a single coagulation tube is needed, an extra tube of blood is drawn prior to the blood being drawn into the citrate tube. This is done so the coagulation specimen is not part of the first flow of blood out of the vein. The same precautions in venipuncture technique and handling procedures for the specimen should be used as described for the syringe method to ensure that the specimen is collected in the best possible way, eliminating false coagulation assay results. It is important that the correct ratio of blood to anticoagulant be maintained, so the vacuum citrate tube must be allowed to fill completely.

The carefully collected blood specimen is transported to the laboratory as quickly as possible and centrifuged. The cell-free plasma-anticoagulant mixture is separated from the cellular elements. It is important to check the sample for microclot formation by using a wooden applicator stick. The plasma to be tested should be kept refrigerated in a tightly covered clean tube until it is tested. The screening coagulation tests are performed on plasma.

General Information About Coagulation Tests

Most coagulation assays are performed on plasma and require the addition of calcium in order to perform the test (see above). The only acceptable anticoagulant is citrate, usually a buffered sodium citrate (3.2% or 3.8%). Other anticoagulants, such as EDTA, oxalate, or heparin, are not acceptable. Most of the coagulation assays are done at 37°C. Reagents and aliquots of plasma should be prewarmed to 37°C before tests are performed. Coagulation tests must be performed in duplicate with the mean of the two tests being the reported result. It is recommended that the duplicate results agree within 10% of the shorter result.* (see also under Reporting of Results). The end point of the reaction can be determined by a number of methods, including visual or automatic end-point determinations.

The manufacturer's instructions for reagents and instruments must be followed carefully. For coagulation assays, an ongoing program of quality control should be in place and followed.

Quality Control.—Control specimens are reconstituted daily from a lyophilized aliquot or frozen controls are used. At least one control specimen should be abnormal with prolonged coagulation times. Once a control is thawed or reconstituted, it should not be refrozen or reused. Control specimens should be run at the beginning of work each day or at the beginning of each shift and when large numbers of tests are performed, an abnormal control should be run at least once every 20 samples. Control samples should be handled and tested under conditions similar or identical to the patient samples for that laboratory. Values for controls are reported along with the values for the patient.

Reference Ranges.—Laboratories must develop their own reference ranges for control specimens representing a normal population for their particular facility. When new reagents are implemented, with major changes in collection techniques, or when new instruments are introduced into the laboratory, reference values should be reestablished.

Reporting of Results.—Patient PT and APTT tests should be reported in seconds to the nearest tenth of a second, along with the control specimen reference values

Collection, Transport, and Preparation of Blood Specimens for Coagulation Testing and Performance of Coagulation Assays, Approved Guideline. Villanova, Pa, National Committee for Clinical Laboratory Standards, 1986; 6(December):H21-A, p 599.

established for the laboratory. Results must be reported clearly marked for "patient" or "control."

Prothrombin Time (Quick's One-stage Method)†

This test was devised on the assumption that when an optimal amount of calcium and an excess of thromboplastin are added to decalcified plasma, the rate of coagulation depends on the concentration of prothrombin in the plasma. The PT is therefore the time required for the plasma to clot after an excess of thromboplastin and an optimal concentration of calcium have been added. It measures the functional activity of the extrinsic (and common) coagulation pathways. It is a test of generation of thrombin (stage 2) and conversion of fibrinogen to fibrin (stage 3) of the clotting mechanism (Procedure 12–4).

Specimens for the PT test must be anticoagulated with sodium citrate. A ratio of one part of citrate to nine parts of blood must be maintained. The blood must be free of clots when visually examined before the test. If more than 4 hours elapse before the PT is measured, there will be progressive inactivation of some of the factors. (See also Specimens for Coagulation Tests.)

The normal values for the PT range from 10 to 13 seconds. A normal PT shows that the elements of stages 2 and 3 of the coagulation mechanism are probably not disturbed. This finding, coupled with a prolonged venous clotting time, places the abnormality within stage 1. The PT is used to follow the progress of patients treated with coumarin-type oral anticoagulant drugs used to inhibit clotting, (especially for preventing postoperative thrombosis and pulmonary embolism) and to screen for factor deficiencies in hemorrhagic diseases. Antithrombotic drugs are commonly used and they can present some very real hazards to the patient. If the degree of anticoagulation is insufficient, rethrombosis or embolism can occur. If there is too much anticoagulation, fatal hemorrhage can take place. The laboratory tests for coagulation can provide information whereby therapeutic balance is maintained. The laboratory is responsible for advising the physician about the level of anticoagulation achieved. Two categories of antithrombotic drugs are the coumarins, which act as vitamin K antagonists, and heparin. Coumarin drugs, are monitored by use of the one-stage PT test.

The reagents necessary for the PT test are primarily

†Quick AJ: *Bleeding Problems in Clinical Medicine.* Philadelphia, WB Saunders Co, 1970, p 43.

calcium chloride and thromboplastin. These reagents must be prepared in specific concentrations or purchased commercially. A commercial control is tested with each batch of prothrombins. Each prothrombin control must be prepared before use according to the manufacturer's directions. Control values and limits will vary with the brand of control used. The laboratory will establish its own reference range for the control specimens. Proper use of the control can detect deterioration of the thromboplastin, use of a calcium solution of the wrong concentration, or use of the wrong incubation temperature.

Use of automatic pipetting devices is recommended when performing the PT test manually. Many of the automated instruments used in laboratories incorporate automatic pipetting as a part of the testing process. All plasma samples are tested at least in duplicate and usually in triplicate. Determinations must agree within certain limits; the allowable difference between the results of duplicate or triplicate tests varies with the PT. Normal duplicate results should agree within ±0.5 second of each other; therapeutic results within ± seconds. The mean clotting time is calculated and the result reported to the nearest 0.1 second. Depending on the reagents used and on the type of method or instruments employed, the normal reference value for PT is between 10 to 13 seconds. A control plasma is tested in the same manner as the patient plasma is tested and the control value is reported along with the patient result. Laboratories will establish acceptable reference ranges for the control specimens they use. The test must be repeated if the allowable error is exceeded.

Precautions and Technical Factors.—The PT test should be done within 4 hours of blood collection. The plasma may be frozen and stored up to 1 week without appreciably affecting the result of the test.

When using the thromboplastin-calcium reagent, it is important to mix the suspension very well. The blood for this test must be free of clots; if any clots are present, a new specimen must be drawn. The ratio of anticoagulant to blood specimen must be 1:10 (0.5 mL of anticoagulant and 4.5 mL of whole blood). The PT test must be done within 4 hours after the blood is drawn, because of progressive inactivation of certain factors. If a PT of more than 1 minute is obtained, the test should be repeated on a new sample. All plasma samples are tested at least in duplicate (often in triplicate). A control specimen must be used to detect deterioration of the thromboplastin, inaccurately prepared reagents, or an incorrect incu-

---

Procedure 12–4. Prothrombin Time

1. As soon as possible after collection, centrifuge the blood specimen at 3000 rpm for at least 10 minutes. Separate the plasma from the cells as soon as possible after centrifugation.
2. Pipette 0.2-mL portions of the thromboplastin–calcium chloride reagent into small test tubes or cups.
3. Incubate the tubes containing the thromboplastin–calcium chloride mixture and the tubes containing portions of the plasma for patient and control at 37°C. Allow a minimum of 1 minute for the thromboplastin and plasma to reach 37°C.
4. Add 0.1-mL samples of plasma to the tubes containing the thromboplastin–calcium chloride reagent. Start the stopwatch simultaneously. At this point, automated instruments use mechanical agitation or an optical beam to measure formation of the clot. Automated methods will start the timing process simultaneously as the test plasma is added using automatic pipettes and will stop when the fibrin web or clot is formed.
5. Mix the tubes and leave them in the water bath (37°C) for a minimum of 7 to 8 seconds. Then remove them and tip them gently back and forth until a clot is formed. The clot is best seen by tilting against a bright light.
6. Stop the stopwatch immediately when a clot is observed, and record the time.

---

bation temperature, all of which could result in inaccurate test values.

Automated Prothrombin Time Testing.—Automated or semiautomated methods using fibrometers or fully automated methods using optical density readings are used for screening coagulation tests (PT and APTT tests) by many laboratories. These instruments automatically pipette all necessary reagents for the testing process. The principle of the test is the same as for the nonautomated methods described, but the end point of the reaction—the formation of the fibrin clot—is detected photoelectrically. A sudden change in optical density occurs as the clot is formed, timing automatically is stopped, and the clotting time recorded. The clotting time is recorded to the nearest 0.1 second. In some instruments, the result is printed out on tape.

Activated Partial Thromboplastin Time and Partial Thromboplastin Time

The APTT test is the single most useful procedure available for routine screening of coagulation disorders (Procedure 12–5). The APTT adds an activator of factor XII which increases activation, shortens the clotting times, and improves reproducibility. Both APTT and PTT are major screening tests of the intrinsic pathway function. The nonactivated PTT test uses the glass walls of the test tube used for the test to activate factor XII, resulting in poor reproducibility. The nonactivated PTT is seldom done.

The APTT measures deficiencies mainly in factors VIII, IX, XI, and XII, but can detect deficiencies of all factors except VII and XIII. The tests are based on the observation that when whole thromboplastin is used, as for the PT test, the times obtained for hemophilic plasma are about the same as those for normal plasma. With a partial thromboplastin solution or platelet substitute, the times obtained for hemophilic plasma are much longer than those for normal plasma. One important use of the APTT test is in the control of patients on heparin therapy. The sensitivity of the thromboplastin reagent must be evaluated before this test is used as a heparin control.

A phospholipid substitute for platelets acts as a partial thromboplastin. It is more sensitive to the absence of factors involved in intrinsic thromboplastin formation than are the more complete tissue thromboplastins used in the PT tests.

An unsensitized test may be used (PTT) or sensitization (that is, activation) may be obtained by separate addition of a kaolin suspension (APTT).* Kaolin ensures maximal activation of the coagulation factors. The major difference between the PTT and APTT tests is that the APTT is activated by kaolin. By addition of kaolin, the slow contact phase of the coagulation cascade is speeded up. By activation of the contact factors, more consistent and reproducible results are achieved.

Generally, a normal APTT is less than 35 seconds with a range from 25 to 40 seconds. Control plasmas must be run and their values carefully monitored. Deviations in control results can be due to temperature

---

*Proctor RR, Rapaport SL: The partial thromboplastin time with kaolin. *Am J Clin Pathol.,* 1961; 36:212.

changes, different reagent lots, the technique being used, or instrument malfunction, if automation or semiautomation is being employed. Patient results are always reported along with control values. All test results must be repeated if the control results do not fall within the established reference range for the control specimens. Since thromboplastin reagents are manufactured by several different commercial companies, and laboratories do not all use the same reagent product, APTT test (and PT test) results cannot be directly compared from one laboratory to those from another laboratory. Each laboratory must therefore determine its own reference range for normal and abnormal controls used for these tests.

The APTT test result will be prolonged in contact factor and intrinsic factor deficiencies. The presence of an inhibitor, such as the lupus anticoagulant, in the patient's plasma may also be the cause of a prolonged APTT. The APTT is used to monitor heparin concentration during intravenous administration. The APTT is not sensitive to minor abnormalities in some common pathway factors, but is is useful to screen mild to moderate deficiencies of factors VIII and IX and the contact factors. Deficiencies of these factors represent the most common and potentially serious disorders.

If an abnormal PTT or APTT is determined, differential studies should be done for specific factor deficiencies.

Specimens for the PTT and APTT tests are collected by using sodium citrate as the anticoagulant, with nine parts of whole blood to one part of anticoagulant. The specimen should be collected carefully and preserved on ice until it reaches the laboratory.

The principle of this test relies on the assumption that during anticoagulation, the calcium present in the blood is bound to the anticoagulant. After centrifugation, the plasma contains all the intrinsic coagulation factors except calcium (removed during anticoagulation) and platelets (removed during centrifugation). Under carefully controlled conditions and with properly prepared reagents, calcium, a phospholipid platelet substitute (the partial thromboplastin), and kaolin are added to the plasma to be tested using the APTT test. (For the PTT test, kaolin is not added.) The time required for the plasma to clot is the APTT. The normal times proposed by the reagent manufacturer should be followed.

Control specimens are always run along with the patient's specimen. Normal control results must always fall within the normal control range; if they do not, something is wrong with the reagents, equipment, or tech-

---

Procedure 12–5. Activated Partial Thromboplastin Time (APTT) With Kaolin Added

1. As soon as possible after the blood has been collected, centrifuge the anticoagulated specimen at 3,000 rpm for at least 10 minutes.
2. Remove the plasma from the cells immediately and place on ice.
3. Warm the calcium reagents at 37°C.
4. Pipette 0.1 mL of activated platelet substitute suspension (kaolin plus partial thromboplastin) into the desired number of tubes (duplicates for patient and control samples) and incubate at 37°C for a minimum of 1 minute.
5. Add 0.1 mL of plasma (patient or control) to the activated thromboplastin mixture already incubating in the tubes. Mix well and allow to incubate for at least 2 minutes. The minimum incubation time for this mixture is 2 minutes. Incubation times over 5 minutes may cause loss of certain factors in the plasma coagulation system being measured.
6. Add 0.1 mL of the calcium chloride reagent to the plasma-thromboplastin reagent mixture and start the stopwatch immediately.
7. Mix the tube once, immediately after adding the calcium reagent. Allow the tube to remain in the water bath for about 25 seconds.
8. After 25 seconds, remove the tube from the water bath. Wipe off the outside of the tube so that the contents can be clearly seen. Gently tilt the tube back and forth. The clot is best seen by tilting against a bright light. The end point is the appearance of fibrin strands.
9. At the appearance of fibrin strands, stop the stopwatch and note the time.
10. Control and patient plasmas must always be tested in duplicate and the two results averaged to obtain the final result. The duplicate results should agree within 1.5 seconds when the APTT is less than 45 seconds. If they do not, another test should be done. When the clotting time is longer, duplication of results is more difficult and the allowable range of variation is wider. If formation of the clot has not started by the end of 2 minutes, the test may be stopped and the results reported as greater than 2 minutes.

---

nique being used. When the control is out of range, the entire test must be repeated.

Precautions and Technical Factors.—The PTT test may be done without the addition of kaolin. In this case the normal results range from 40 to 100 seconds, with 120 seconds or longer being considered abnormal. Use of kaolin gives maximal activation of the coagulation factors and therefore more consistent and reproducible results.

If there are enough stopwatches, more than one test can be done at a time by starting the separate incubations at intervals to allow time for the manipulations and observations of the clots.

Citrated blood should be centrifuged within 30 minutes of collection and may be stored on ice for up to $1\frac{1}{2}$ hours. Plasma allowed to sit longer than the recommended time will give abnormal results.

When kaolin suspensions are used, it is necessary to mix the solutions vigorously before any pipetting is done, as kaolin in suspension settles out very quickly.

Tests for Whole Blood Clotting Time (Lee-White Method)

This test is not very reliable for the detection of mild or moderate procoagulant defects. In gross defects it gives an abnormal result. It is not recommended as a single screening test of procoagulant function, but it is sometimes used to monitor heparin therapy, although it has been largely replaced by the APTT time and thrombin time tests.

The Lee-White method for determining venous blood coagulation time is still in general use in some laboratories (Procedure 12–6).* Capillary blood clotting tests are unreliable because the sample is contaminated with thromboplastin from the tissue juice. The Lee-White test measures the time required for freely flowing blood to clot after it has been removed from the body. The results are influenced by the nature of the surface of the test tube used and by the diameter of the tube. Tem-

---

*Lee RI, White PD: A clinical study of the coagulation time of blood. *Am J Med Sci* 1913; 145:495.

perature and agitation of the blood sample also influence the test results; vigorous agitation of the tubes shortens the clotting time. Only when these factors are carefully controlled and there is no mixture of tissue fluid with the blood sample can the venous clotting time be regarded as representing the *intrinsic coagulative power* of the blood. Contamination with tissue thromboplastin because of a poor venipuncture will shorten the clotting time. This test in no way differentiates between deficiencies in the clotting factors and the presence of anticoagulants, both of which can prolong the clotting time.

Procedure 12–6. Lee-White Venous Clotting Time Test

1. Make a clean venipuncture. It is important that the vein be penetrated without excessive probing. Start a stopwatch as soon as the blood enters the syringe, and draw 5 mL of blood.
2. Place 1 mL of blood carefully into each of three small serologic tubes (inner diameter, 8 mm).
3. Allow the tubes to stand undisturbed at room temperature for 10 minutes.
4. After the 10-minute waiting period, tip the first tube gently at 1-minute intervals until the blood is completely clotted.
5. After the blood in the first tube has clotted, tip the second tube in a similar fashion at 1-minute intervals until clotting is observed.
6. After the blood in the second tube has clotted, tip the third tube every 30 seconds until clotting is observed.
7. Report the clotting time of the third tube to the nearest 30 seconds. The normal range is 15 to 25 minutes.

Precautions and Technical Factors.—In doing the venipuncture to obtain the blood specimen, the vein should be penetrated cleanly with as little probing as possible. Any excessive probing could introduce tissue juices into the specimen, which would contaminate it with thromboplastin and thus shorten the clotting time.

If the tubes containing the blood are clotted at the end of the initial 10-minute waiting period, the test is unsatisfactory and must be repeated. One cause of such early clotting could be contamination with tissue thromboplastin.

Vigorous agitation of the tubes can also shorten the clotting time. Some procedures for this test require that the three tubes used for the blood specimen be rinsed out with saline solution before their use. The surface of the tubes and their inner diameter influence the clotting time.

The venous clotting time test, when properly performed, may be considered a screening test for abnormalities of the clotting mechanism. When there is a deficiency of any of the factors required for clotting, the venous clotting time will be abnormal. This is also true when an abnormal inhibitor is present in the blood. This test cannot differentiate between an inhibitor or a plasma factor deficiency; other more specific tests must be performed.

Other Tests for Coagulation

Several other tests for specific coagulation factors are done in a coagulation laboratory. These include the prothrombin consumption test, thromboplastin generation test, plasma recalcification time (plasma clotting time), thrombin time, fibrinogen titer, quantitative tests for fibrinogen, Russell viper venom time, reptilase time, and various coagulation factor assays. Specific tests for von Willebrand's factor such as that employing ristocetin reagent are also commonly performed.

BIBLIOGRAPHY

Brown B: *Hematology: Principles and Procedures,* ed 5. Philadelphia, Lea & Febiger, 1988.

Collection, Transport, and Preparation of Blood Specimens for Coagulation Testing and Performance of Coagulation Assays, Approved Guideline. Villanova, Pa, National Committee for Clinical Laboratory Standards, 1986; 6 (December): H21-A.

Pittiglio D, Sacher R: *Clinical Hematology and Fundamentals of Hemostasis.* Philadelphia, FA Davis Co, 1987.

Powers L: *Diagnostic Hematology.* St Louis, Mosby–Year Book, Inc, 1989.

Rapaport SI: *Introduction to Hematology,* ed 2. Philadelphia, JB Lippincott Co, 1987.

Williams WJ, Beutler E, Erslev A, et al: *Hematology,* ed 4. New York, McGraw-Hill Book Co, 1990.

13 Urinalysis

Key Terms

Albuminuria	Nonglucose reducing substances
Amorphous material	(NGRS)
Bilirubin	Oval fat bodies
Casts	Peroxidase
Crystals, normal and abnormal	pH
Cytocentrifugation	Phase-contrast microscopy
Diazo reaction	Physical properties
Ehrlich's aldehyde reaction	Porphobilinogen
Epithelial cells; renal, transitional	Protein error of pH indicators
(urothelial), and squamous	Proteinuria
Glomerular filtrate	Pyuria
Glycosuria	Refractometer
Hematuria	Sediment, organized and unorganized
Hemosiderin	Specific gravity
Jaundice	Tamm-Horsfall mucoprotein
Ketosis	Urinary system
Leukocyte esterase	Urine
Lithiasis	Urobilinogen
Nephron	

Of all the diagnostic procedures performed in the laboratory, the analysis of the **urine** is perhaps the oldest. Urine samples are readily available, and many of the routine tests are relatively simple to perform. The simplicity of the tests in no way means that they are unimportant or should be performed sloppily or in haste. It cannot be overemphasized that it is extremely important in the urinalysis department, as well as in the other departments of the laboratory, to do careful, accurate work at all times.

In general, urine can be considered a fluid composed of the waste materials of the blood. It is formed in the kidney and excreted from the body by way of the urinary system.

The **urinary system** consists of two kidneys and ureters, the bladder, and the urethra. The urine is formed in the **nephron** (working unit of the kidney), passed on to the bladder for temporary storage by way of the ureters, and then eliminated from the body by way of the urethra (Fig 13–1).

KIDNEY AND URINE

Kidney Function

The kidney functions as a means of eliminating waste materials from the body. Another definition of this important organ is that it is a regulator of the extracellular fluid. The extracellular fluid is a water solution containing numerous dissolved substances; it consists of all the liquid in the body, outside the individual tissue cells. It includes the liquid part of the blood plasma, the lymph, and the interstitial fluid, which is the fluid in the space between the cells of the body. The kidney regulates the extracellular fluid in such a way as to keep its composition constant. Since the extracellular fluid is the environment of the individual body cells, even slight changes in its composition may result in death.

The kidney acts to eliminate excess water from the body and thus to maintain the volume of the extracellular fluid. This is clear from the relationship between the amount of water or fluid that is ingested daily and the amount of urine that is eliminated from the body. Waste products of metabolism such as urea and creatinine are

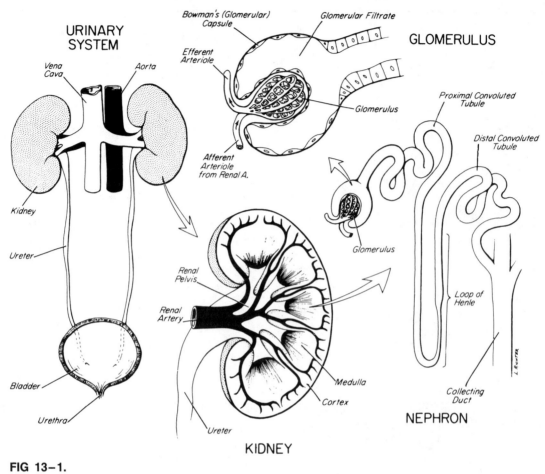

FIG 13–1.
The urinary system.

eliminated from the body through the urine, maintaining the composition of the extracellular fluid. Foreign substances such as drugs or excess substances from the diet are also eliminated in the urine. Composition is also maintained by the retention of substances necessary for normal body function such as proteins, amino acids, and glucose. Larger particles are retained in the blood because they are unable to be filtered or cross into Bowman's capsule (a function of particle size), and certain substances such as glucose are actively reabsorbed from the renal tubules back into the blood. Acidity and osmotic pressure of the extracellular fluid are maintained by various mechanisms, such as filtration, reabsorption, and secretion, which have the net effect of regulating the electrolyte balance and osmotic pressure of body fluids.

Formation of Urine

Urine is formed in the nephron, which is the working unit of the kidney (see Fig 13–1). Each kidney contains about 1.2 million nephrons. Each nephron consists of two main parts: the glomerulus, or renal corpuscle, and the renal tubules. The formation of urine involves three processes, namely filtration, reabsorption, and secretion.

The glomerulus is the portion of the nephron made up of blood vessels. All of the blood in the body circulates through the kidney (one-fourth of the heart's output at a time), eventually going to a glomerulus. The glomerulus is a small structure, consisting of a knot or tuft of blood capillaries. Blood enters the glomerulus from the renal circulation through the afferent arteriole and leaves through the efferent arteriole. Urine formation begins with the glomerulus, the structure that delivers the blood, with its waste products and essential constituents, to the working portion of the kidney.

The renal tubular portion of the nephron begins with *Bowman's capsule,* also called the glomerular capsule. Bowman's capsule is a cup-shaped structure or sac that encircles the glomerulus (see Fig 13–1). As blood circulates through the glomerulus, it is filtered into Bowman's capsule. The function of the glomerulus is filtration. The glomerular capillaries are covered by the inner layer of Bowman's capsule, forming a semipermeable membrane. This membrane passes all substances with molecular weights less than about 70,000 daltons. This is basically the blood plasma without proteins and fats, as these molecules are too large to pass through the glomerular membrane. The filtrate is an ultrafiltrate of blood and is referred to as the **glomerular filtrate.** This is the first step in urine formation. However, the glomerular filtrate is significantly altered by reabsorption of some materials and secretion of others before it becomes urine.

The remainder of the nephron after the glomerulus consists of a series of renal tubules, which have certain functions. Beginning with Bowman's capsule, the tubules (which are only one cell layer thick) are as follows: the proximal convoluted tubule, the loop of Henle, and the distal convoluted tubule. The total length of these tubules in each nephron is 30 to 40 mm. The nephron ends with the distal convoluted tubule (see Fig 13–1).

All of the nephrons of each kidney eventually come together into progressively larger and larger tubules. These are the collecting tubules, and they combine to form the ureter, which delivers the urine to the bladder for temporary storage and then elimination from the body through the urethra. The fluid in the collecting tubule is urine.

Anatomically, the kidney is arranged in two portions: an outer, highly vascular area called the cortex, and a central area called the medulla (see Fig 13–1).

Blood enters the kidney through the renal artery, which branches into smaller and smaller units, finally forming the afferent arterioles going to the glomeruli. The efferent arterioles, which leave the glomerulus, run close to the corresponding renal tubules of the nephron, facilitating reabsorption and secretion between the blood and glomerular filtrate. The efferent arterioles eventually join to form the renal vein.

An extremely large amount of blood is filtered through the kidney each day. In fact, about 180 L of glomerular filtrate is produced daily, while only 1 or 2 L of urine is eliminated from the body. Clearly, much of the glomerular filtrate must be reabsorbed into the body. The majority of the water in the glomerular filtrate (87.5%) is reabsorbed into the body in the proximal convoluted tubule, the first portion of the nephron after the glomerular capsule. The water is actually passively reabsorbed along with sodium ions (Na^+), 87.5% of which are actively reabsorbed by the sodium pump mechanism. Along with the water, chloride, and bicarbonate ions (Cl^- and HCO_3^-) and 40% to 50% of the urea in the filtrate are also passively reabsorbed at this point.

All threshold substances such as glucose, amino acids, creatine, pyruvate, lactate, and ascorbic acid, which normally are present in the blood and not in the urine, are actively transported across the cell membrane of the proximal tubule and reabsorbed into the blood. Phosphate is reabsorbed in the proximal convoluted tubule under hormonal control and depending on the body's tissue and fluid electrolyte balance. In addition, 90% of the uric acid and most of the protein passing through the glomerulus are reabsorbed in the proximal tubule. Creatine is not reabsorbed and may be excreted in the proximal tubule, as are sulfates, glycuronides, and hippurates.

As the modified glomerular filtrate passes through the loop of Henle, it loses both water and sodium in the descending portion and then sodium without water in the ascending portion.

In the distal tubule the remainder of the sodium is reabsorbed. This is influenced by the hormone aldosterone. The pH of the urine is determined in the distal tubule, especially through excretion of hydrogen and ammonium ions (H^+ and NH_4^+) in exchange for Na^+. Potassium is also excreted and exchanged for sodium in the distal tubules. The remainder of water is reabsorbed in the distal tubules under the influence of antidiuretic hormone (ADH).

The body's electrolyte balance is controlled by the kidney, with the result that the urinary pH differs from the blood pH. Urine is generally more acid than blood, because acid substances are produced as end products of metabolism. These substances are buffered in blood by a bicarbonate–carbonic acid buffer system. They pass into the glomerular filtrate as salts, but sodium must be returned to the blood to conserve its concentration of base and maintain its pH within narrow limits. This is done by exchanging Na^+ for H^+, resulting in elimination of acid from the blood and in acidification of the urine. Urine has a normal pH of 5 or 6, while blood is slightly basic at about pH 7.4. Potassium ions (K^+) are also exchanged for Na^+ in competition with H^+. When it is necessary to retain more Na^+, ammonia (NH_3) is formed from glutamine and combines with H^+ to form NH_4^+, allowing for greater exchange of H^+ for Na^+. The osmotic pressure is controlled in the distal tubules through the secretion of antidiuretic hormone (ADH), which is controlled by the osmotic pressure of blood. Urea, the major waste product of nitrogen (protein) metabolism, is eliminated from the body through the urine. Urea is not actively reabsorbed or secreted by the kidney; instead, it moves passively into and out of the nephron with water. With average rates of urine flow, about 60% of the urea is reabsorbed and 40% is excreted in the urine.

In summary, in the adult more than 1 L of blood flows through the kidney each minute. The blood is filtered through the glomerulus into Bowman's capsule, producing the glomerular filtrate, which is an ultrafiltrate of plasma. The glomerular filtrate has a pH of 7.4 and an osmolality (measure of the concentration of solutes) similar to that of plasma, about 285 mOsm/kg of water, with a specific gravity of about 1.008. The filtrate is modified by reabsorption and some secretion in the proximal tubules. In the distal tubules more water is absorbed and the urine is acidified. The rate of flow of the filtrate is reduced as it passes through the tubules and water is reabsorbed into the blood. The rate of flow is 130 mL/min in the proximal tubules; 16 mL/min in the loop of Henle, and 1 mL/min as the urine enters the collecting tubules. The filtrate is concentrated and acidified as it passes through the tubules; by the time it reaches the collecting tubules the resulting substance, urine, has a pH of approximately 6 and an osmolality of about 800 to 1,200 mOsm/kg.

Composition of Urine

The composition of urine varies a great deal, depending on such factors as diet and nutritional status, metabolic rate, the general state of the body, and the state of the kidney or its ability to function normally. Urine is a complex aqueous mixture consisting of 96% water and 4% dissolved substances, most of which either are derived from the food eaten or are waste products of metabolism. The dissolved substances consist primarily of urea (the principal end product of protein metabolism) and sodium chloride (NaCl). The substances present in

normal urine may be divided into organic and inorganic compounds. The major ones are:

Normal organic substances
   Urea
   Uric acid
   Creatinine

Normal inorganic substances
   As cations:
      Sodium (Na^+)
      Potassium (K^+)
      Ammonium (NH_4^+)

   As anions:
      Chloride (Cl^-)
      Phosphate (PO_4^{3-})
      Sulfate (SO_4^{2-})

Many other substances are normally present in urine in lesser amounts. Other products of nitrogen metabolism include amino acids, ammonia, traces of proteins, glycoproteins, enzymes, and purines. Excretion of urea and these substances is related to protein intake.

The amount of creatinine excreted is not related to dietary factors, but to the amount or mass of muscle in the body. Each individual excretes a uniform amount of creatinine every day, and this may be used to determine the completeness of timed urine collections. Since creatinine is normally filtered through the glomerulus and none is reabsorbed into the blood, increased concentrations of blood creatinine imply impaired glomerular filtration, and therefore blood creatinine may be used as an indicator of renal function.

Other constituents found in small amounts in normal urine include calcium, intermediary metabolic products such as oxalate, hormonal metabolites, biogenic amines (catecholamines), enzymes, and small or trace amounts of sugars, proteins, cholesterol, fatty acids, vitamins, and metals.

Normal but concentrated urine will commonly crystallize certain chemicals out of solution at room or refrigerator temperature. Therefore, a routine urinalysis will commonly show crystals of uric acid or its salts, the urates, at an acid pH, while phosphates will commonly crystallize out of solution in concentrated urine of an alkaline pH. Such crystallization will show grossly as cloudiness or turbidity of the urine, and the crystals are identified morphologically by microscopic examination.

Although they are the primary constituents of urine, urea and sodium chloride do not crystallize out of urine specimens.

Normal urine specimens also contain certain formed elements, which are observable in the microscopic examination of the urinary sediment. These include red blood cells, white blood cells, renal tubular epithelial cells, transitional epithelial cells, squamous epithelial cells, histiocytes, and a few hyaline casts. All of these formed elements are found in very small numbers in normal urine, and increased numbers represent an abnormal (pathologic) situation.

Many abnormal substances occur in urine in various conditions. It is important to know the relative amounts of these substances, because some of them are present in small amounts in normal urine. These abnormal substances may exist as dissolved substances or as solids, which are seen in the microscopic examination of the urinary sediment. Some of the more important substances that are considered abnormal in the urine are:

Acetone and acetoacetic acid
Bile (or bilirubin)
Blood (red blood cells)
Casts
Cystine
Epithelial cells (renal type)
Fat
Glucose
Hemoglobin
Protein
Spermatozoa
Sulfonamides
Urobilinogen
White blood cells (or pus)

ROUTINE URINALYSIS

Definition

The physical, chemical, and microscopic analysis of the urine is known as *urinalysis*. The routine urinalysis is an important part of the initial examination of patients in all branches of medicine. It is made up of a number of different tests and observations. Some of these tests are chemical and others are not. When the urinalysis is performed in an orderly fashion and the results are recorded accurately, the combination of observations and test re-

sults will provide a valuable picture of the patient's general health pattern.

In general the urinalysis will provide information concerning (1) the state of the kidney and urinary tract, and (2) information about metabolic or systemic (nonrenal) disorders. Tests for the presence of protein, blood, nitrite, and leukocyte esterase together with the physical properties and the finding of casts, cells, and certain crystals are most helpful in assessing and treating renal and urinary tract disease. On the other hand, tests for glucose, ketone bodies, bilirubin, and urobilinogen are useful indicators in metabolic and systemic disorders such as diabetes and jaundice.

Components of the Routine Urinalysis

The routine urinalysis generally consists of three parts as shown in Table 13–1.

Physical Properties

These include an assessment of color, transparency, odor, foam, and specific gravity. Abnormalities in any of these must be accounted for in subsequent parts of the urinalysis.

Chemical Tests

These are generally done as screening or semiquantitative tests using multiple reagent strips. Tests for protein and glucose are basic to any urinalysis. Other chemical tests have become routine as they have been added to the readily available multiple reagent strips. Different combinations are available for use in different clinical situations. For example, in an obstetric clinic, tests for glucose, protein, blood, and leukocyte esterase are especially desirable. In certain instances, positive findings in the chemical screen may require confirmation with other chemical tests or indicate the likelihood of certain findings in the microscopic examination of the urinary sediment.

Microscopic Examination of the Urinary Sediment

This is especially helpful in assessing the presence of kidney and urinary tract disease. The presence of certain findings in the microscopic examination will explain abnormal physical and chemical tests. Certain tests have long been part of the routine urinalysis. As early as 1821, William Prout's set of routine urine tests included

TABLE 13–1.

Possible Routine Urinalysis Protocol

Physical properties	Color
	Transparency
	Odor
	Foam
	Specific gravity (urinometer or refractometer)
Chemical screening tests (reagent strips)	pH
	Specific gravity (reagent strip)
	Protein
	Blood
	Nitrite
	Leukocyte esterase
	Glucose
	Ketones
	Bilirubin
	Urobilinogen
Microscopic examination of urinary sediment	Red blood cells
	White blood cells
	Epithelial cells
	Casts
	Bacteria and other microorganisms
	Crystals
	Other components

observations of the daily urinary volume, color, specific gravity, and pH (estimated by the reaction of litmus paper to urine). The presence of protein and sugar were also determined—protein by heat, and sugar by taste or high specific gravity (over 1.030). Analysis of the urinary sediment has also been traditional since the development of medical microscopy, with the pioneering course taught by Alfred Donne in Paris in 1837. Early microscopists differentiated pus cells from crystals and amorphous deposits in cloudy urine, while casts of coagulated albumin were found to be associated with Bright's disease.

Considerations in Performing the Urinalysis

Certain factors must be kept in mind and understood when performing the routine urinalysis. These include:

1. The basic principle on which the test is based, including the specificity of the test for the substance being measured and common interfering substances.

2. The sensitivity of the test, which is the lowest concentration of substance than can be detected by the method.

3. The range of concentrations of the substance over which changes in the concentration can be detected.

4. A general idea of the clinical application of the substance being tested for and its correlation to other findings in the urinalysis.

5. The need for additional or confirmatory tests. These include such tests as quantitative tests for urinary sugar and protein and further procedures such as thin-layer chromatography to identify reducing sugars other than glucose, such as galactose, that may be present in the urine.

For example, the finding of protein in the urine is an especially helpful indicator of renal or urinary tract disease. Both the amount of protein and the presence or absence of other findings in the sediment will help indicate the site and nature of the disease. Chemical tests for blood, nitrite, and leukocyte esterase are also helpful in assessing the cause of proteinuria.

Urinary glucose may indicate the metabolic disorder diabetes mellitus. This is further indicated when ketone bodies, a reduced pH, increased urine output of a pale urine specimen with a high specific gravity when measured with a urinometer or refractometer are found.

Collection and Preservation of Urine Specimens

The collection and preservation of urine specimens and the relative advantages of random vs. 24-hour collections are discussed in the section on urine specimen collections in Chapter 2. Important considerations in the proper collection and handling of urine for routine examination include the container used, the collection procedure, and the conditions of storage and preservation from the time of collection until the specimen is tested. Some aspects of the collection procedure may be out of the hands of the laboratory. A good working relationship and good avenues of communication are necessary between all members of the medical team to ensure that a suitable specimen is collected and delivered to the laboratory for examination.

For routine urinalysis, a freely voided specimen, rather than one obtained by catheterization, is usually suitable. If the specimen is likely to be contaminated by vaginal discharge or hemorrhage, a clean-voided midstream specimen as required for bacteriologic examination (described in Chapter 2) may be necessary. It may be necessary to pack the vagina or use a tampon to avoid vaginal contamination. Although any random urine specimen voided during the day may be used for routine urinalysis, a fairly concentrated specimen is preferable to a dilute one. The first specimen voided in the morning is usually the most concentrated one, as fluids are not taken while the patient is asleep but dissolved substances are still excreted by the kidneys. A concentrated specimen is especially desirable when examining for protein and the contents of the urinary sediment. When testing for the presence of glucose, the best specimen to use is one voided 2 or 3 hours after a meal (postprandial). This is the major exception to the recommended use of the first morning specimen for routine tests.

It is of primary importance that the containers used to collect the urine specimen be clean and dry. Although several types of container are suitable for this purpose, disposable inert plastic containers are usual.

Probably the most important consideration is that the urine specimen be fresh or suitably preserved, usually by refrigeration. Ideally, the urine should be examined within 30 minutes of collection, as decomposition begins within this time, urine being an excellent culture medium for bacterial growth. If this is impossible, the urine must be preserved in some way. The most common and simple method of preservation is to refrigerate the specimen. It can be kept in this way for 6 to 8 hours with no gross alterations, and such a refrigerated specimen should be examined within this time period. Chemical preservatives are usually reserved for 24-hour urine collections, as they may interfere with parts of the routine urinalysis.

Decomposition of urine primarily involves the growth of bacteria. At room temperature, bacteria reproduce rapidly. This bacterial growth results in a cloudy-looking specimen. Changes in pH also occur as a result of bacterial growth. These changes interfere markedly with other tests. Other substances, namely phosphates and urates, may precipitate out of solution, adding to the turbidity of the urine specimen.

Some of the other changes that occur on prolonged standing at room temperature are the following: the pH becomes alkaline because of the breakdown of urea by the bacteria to form ammonia; red blood cells, white blood cells, and casts disintegrate; sugar decomposes, acetone evaporates, acetoacetic acid is converted to acetone; bilirubin is oxidized to biliverdin; and urobilinogen is oxidized to urobilin. It can be seen from these many changes that it is most important that only fresh urine specimens be used in performing a urinalysis.

In summary, for routine urinalysis the urine specimen must be collected in a suitable clean, dry container. In most cases the first specimen freely voided in the morning is preferred, although a specimen collected 2 to 3 hours after eating is preferable when testing for glucose. The specimen must be examined when fresh, ideally within 30 minutes, or suitably preserved, such as by refrigeration for up to 6 to 8 hours.

Classification of Urinalysis Tests

There are certain general categories of urinalysis tests grouped according to their degree of accuracy: *screening* tests, *qualitative* (or *semiquantitative* tests), and *quantitative* tests. Most of the tests performed in the urinalysis laboratory are either screening or qualitative (semiquantitative) tests.

Screening Tests

Screening tests tell only whether a substance is present or absent, and the results are reported as *positive* or *negative*. For most screening tests any random sample of urine can be used, but the first morning specimen is recommended. A specimen obtained 2 to 3 hours after a meal is preferred for the urine glucose test.

Qualitative or Semiquantitative Tests

Qualitative tests give a rough estimate of the amount of substance present. They are also classified as *semiquantitative* tests. Results of qualitative tests were traditionally graded in a plus system as negative, trace, 1+, 2+, 3+, or 4+, or in some cases as small, moderate, or large. With the development of dry reagent strip tests commonly used in routine urinalysis together with the computerization of laboratory reports, many of these tests are semiquantitated as a concentration of substance and reported in units such as grams or milligrams per deciliter or liter. The method used will depend both on the test being performed and the institution. The most important consideration being continuity within a given institution. For most of these tests an early-morning specimen is preferred, the exception again being tests for glucose.

Quantitative Tests

These tests determine accurately the amount of the substance that they detect. They are much more time-consuming than screening, qualitative, or semiquantitative tests, and for this reason they are not done routinely in the urinalysis laboratory. The two most common quantitative tests performed in urinalysis are those for sugar and for protein. The results of a quantitative test are usually reported in milligrams per deciliter, grams per deciliter, milliequivalents per liter, milligrams per 24 hours, grams per 24 hours, or milliequivalents per 24 hours. For quantitative tests a complete 24-hour timed urine specimen is needed. An appropriate preservative should be added to the container, and the specimen should be stored in the refrigerator until the test is done. The total volume of the 24-hour specimen is measured and recorded; the urine is thoroughly mixed before a measured aliquot is withdrawn for analysis (see Chapter 2).

Confirmatory Tests

In many cases it is necessary to confirm the presence of a substance in urine that is indicated on the basis of initial screening tests. The confirmatory test is used to establish the accuracy or correctness of another procedure. It is used both to decide if an analyte is actually present in low-level (trace) reactions, and to further estimate the quantity of analyte present. The confirmatory test is not just a repeat test using the same methodology. Rather, it is an alternative method with at least the same or better specificity, is based on a different principle, or has equal or better sensitivity than the original test. Examples of common confirmatory tests in urinalysis when positive results are seen on the chemical screen by reagent strips include: a protein precipitation test for protein; use of another reagent strip for glucose with greater differentiation of values; testing high specific gravity values with a refractometer; testing with a tablet test for bilirubin; looking for red cells, leukocytes, and casts in the microscopic analysis of the urine sediment. Other confirmatory tests which might be requested by the physician based on routine urinalysis include: quantitative protein or protein electrophoresis; bacterial culture; and cytology using a cytocentrifuged and stained preparation.

PHYSICAL PROPERTIES OF URINE

The first part of a routine urinalysis usually involves an assessment of **physical properties,** such as volume, color, transparency, odor, and foam. Another physical property, specific gravity, is discussed in a separate sec-

tion. Observation of physical properties is probably the easiest part of a urinalysis. However, these simple observations are extremely useful both for the eventual diagnosis of the patient and for the laboratory personnel who perform the complete urinalysis. Such tests often give clues leading to findings in subsequent portions of the urinalysis. For example, if a urine specimen is cloudy and red, the presence of red blood cells will probably be revealed by microscopic analysis of the urinary sediment. If red cells are not found, all parts of the urinalysis must be carefully rechecked for accuracy. Chemical tests for blood (hemoglobin) might be falsely-negative when ascorbic acid is present in urine; however, the presence of blood might be indicated by an abnormal red color and confirmed by the presence of red cells in the urinary sediment. If hemoglobin is present without red cells, the only indication of ascorbic acid interference might be the abnormal color of the urine.

Certain tests are performed when abnormal physical properties are observed. For example, a chemical test for the pigment bilirubin is necessary when it is suspected on the basis of abnormal color of the urine. These are only two examples of several situations in which the complete urinalysis may be evaluated by the laboratory for reliability before results are reported to the physician, or abnormal constituents are found in subsequent tests because abnormal physical properties were noted.

The final evaluation of urinalysis results will be described more completely after all parts of the routine urinalysis have been discussed. Physical properties are summarized in Table 13–2.

Volume

Normal Volume

Although it is a physical property, the volume of the urine is not measured as part of a routine urinalysis. However, in certain conditions the volume of urine excreted in 24 hours is a valuable aid to clinical diagnosis. In normal adults with normal fluid intake, the average 24-hour urine volume is 1,200 to 1,500 mL. It can, however, normally range from 600 to 2,000 mL. The total volume of urine excreted in 24 hours must be measured when quantitative tests are performed, since it enters into the calculation of results in these tests.

Under normal conditions, there is a direct relation between urine volume and water intake. That is, if water intake is increased, the kidney will protect the body from excessive retention of water by eliminating a larger vol-

TABLE 13-2.

Physical Properties of Urine

Physical Property	Description	Possible Cause
Normal color	Yellow (straw) Amber	Urochrome, the chief pigment in normal urine with uroerythrin and urobilin
Abnormal color	Pale	Dilute urine
	Dark yellow or brown-red (amber)	Concentrated urine
	Yellow-brown or green-brown	Bilirubin or biliverdin
	Orange-red or orange-brown	Urobilin (excreted colorless as urobilinogen)
	Bright orange	Phenazopyridine (aminopyrine drugs)
	Clear red	Hemoglobin
	Cloudy red	Red blood cells
	Dark red or red-purple	Porphyrins
	Clear dark red-brown	Myoglobin
	Dark brown and black	Melanin, homogentisic acid, phenol poisoning
	Green, blue, orange	Drugs, medications, foodstuffs
Transparency	Clear	
	Hazy	Mucus, phosphates,
	Cloudy	bacteria, urates, pus,
	Turbid	blood, fat, casts, crystals
Odor	Aromatic	Normal, volatile acids
	Ammoniacal	Breakdown of urea by bacteria on standing
	Putrid or foul	Urinary tract infection
	Sweet or "fruity"	Ketone bodies
Foam	White, small amount	Normal
	Yellow, large amount	Bilirubin or bile pigments

ume of urine than normal. Conversely, if water intake is decreased, the kidney will protect the body against dehydration by eliminating a smaller amount of urine.

Abnormal Volume

There are various situations that result in abnormal urine volumes.

Polyuria.—The term *polyuria* refers to the consistent elimination of an abnormally large volume of urine, over 2,000 mL/24 hr.

Diuresis.—*Diuresis* refers to any increase in urine volume, even if the increase is only temporary.

Oliguria.—*Oliguria* refers to the excretion of an abnormally small amount of urine, less than 500 mL/24 hr.

Anuria.—The complete absence of urine formation is *anuria*.

Nocturia.—The excretion of urine at night is called *nocturia*.

These terms merely describe abnormalities in urine volume. Each abnormality has several possible causes, reflecting various abnormal conditions. It is the responsibility of the physician, with the aid of the routine urinalysis and other clinical or laboratory findings, to determine the actual cause and significance of volume changes.

Color

Normal Color

The color of normal urine varies considerably, even in one person in a single day. Numerous words have been used to describe the range of normal color (few institutions agree on exact terms). In general, it can be said that normal urine is some shade of yellow. The exact name that is attached is not as important as the recognition that the color is normal. It is advisable for each institution to use precise terms to define normal color. The terms *yellow, straw,* and *amber* are often used. Straw is generally used to describe a lighter-colored urine with normal yellow pigment. The term yellow is preferable to straw as it is less ambiguous. Amber refers to a darker color with red or orange pigments in addition to yellow. Another system commonly used is to make a notation only if the color is abnormal.

Urine that is more highly colored has a greater concentration of normal waste products because its volume is diminished. Color, however, is not an adequate measure of concentration. Specific gravity or osmolality values are preferred.

The color of normal urine seems to result from the presence of three pigments: urochrome, uroerythrin, and urobilin. Urochrome is a yellow pigment and is present in larger concentrations than the other two. Uroerythrin is a red pigment, and urobilin is an orange-yellow pigment.

Abnormal Color

The ability to recognize normal color is, of course, necessary to ensure the recognition of abnormal color. Several abnormal colors are of pathologic significance and require special attention.

Pale.—Pale urine suggests that the urine is dilute. The paleness results from a large volume with correspondingly low concentrations of normal constituents, as in polyuria. Pale urine is often associated with diabetes mellitus or diabetes insipidus. In cases of diabetes mellitus, a pale-greenish urine is characteristic. However, the large sugar content in diabetes mellitus results in a high specific gravity when measured with the urinometer or refractometer, whereas dilute urine is characterized by low specific gravity. Pale, foamy urine specimens are seen, along with large amounts of protein, in the nephrotic syndrome.

Dark Yellow or Brown-red (Amber).—Highly colored dark yellow or brown-red urine is indicative of very concentrated constituents and a correspondingly low volume. It is often seen in conditions associated with fever, where water is eliminated through sweat rather than the kidney. When such concentrated and acid urine is excreted, a pink or red precipitate of urates or uric acid, also referred to as brick dust, is often seen.

Yellow-brown or Green-brown.—This is a very characteristic and alarming color to the experienced observer which has also been referred to as "beer-brown." It indicates the presence of **bilirubin,** a highly colored bile pigment, which is related to the clinical condition **jaundice** if it is also present in the blood. Urine specimens containing bilirubin will foam considerably when shaken, and the foam will have a vivid yellow color. This is not true of other highly colored urine specimens. Whenever bilirubin is suspected, it is the responsibility of the laboratory worker to perform a chemical test to detect it. This is extremely important, for bilirubin may appear in the urine before clinical jaundice develops and detection will lead to early treatment of the condition, whatever its cause. On standing, urine containing bilirubin may become green as a result of the oxidation of bilirubin to biliverdin, a green pigment. Unfortunately, this might result in a negative or reduced chemical test for bilirubin.

Orange-red or Orange-brown.—This color is very similar to that of urine containing bilirubin and results from a related pigment, urobilin. In fact, urines that are tested for bilirubin on the basis of color should also be tested for **urobilinogen.** The cause of clinical jaundice may be discovered by observing the presence or absence of either or both of these pigments in the urine. When freshly voided, the pigment urobilin is present in a colorless form, urobilinogen. The urine slowly takes on color on standing because of oxidation of urobilinogen to urobilin. If shaken, urine containing urobilin will not produce a colored foam, and chemical tests will be negative or reduced when oxidation to urobilin has taken place.

Bright Orange (Orange-red, Orange-brown, or Red).

—This is very similar to the color of urine containing bilirubin or urobilinogen, although it is somewhat more vivid. In this case the color is caused by the presence of phenazopyridine (Pyridium) or other aminopyrine drugs, which have been given to the patient as a urinary analgesic. The presence of this substance presents a problem because it interferes with or masks several tests such as tests for bilirubin, urobilinogen, protein, and ketone bodies on reagent strips.

Clear Red.

—Urine that is clear and red characteristically contains hemoglobin, the color pigment of red blood cells. The hemoglobin results from increased red cell destruction in the body (intravascular hemolysis), which has several causes such as an incompatible blood transfusion reaction, autoimmune hemolytic anemia, paroxysmal nocturnal hemoglobinuria, march hemoglobinuria, glucose-6-phosphate dehydrogenase deficiency, and certain infections and drugs. The urine may be bright red, red-brown, or even black as a result of the conversion of hemoglobin to methemoglobin. Urine with this color should be tested chemically for the presence of hemoglobin.

Cloudy Red.

—This is similar to the clear red color. However, it is caused by the presence of red blood cells, rather than merely hemoglobin; hence the cloudy appearance. It is important to differentiate **hematuria** (red cells in urine) from hemoglobinuria (hemoglobin in urine). This may be most easily done by observation under the microscope. However, if the urine is very dilute, red blood cells will lyse, resulting in hemoglobinuria. For this reason the specific gravity is important to the physician in determining whether the cause of red urine is hematuria or hemoglobinuria. The intensity of the red will depend on the number of red cells present; the urine ranges from smoky red or reddish-brown to a highly colored cloudy specimen.

Dark Red or Red-purple.

—Described as the color of port wine, this is characteristic of the presence of porphyrins in the urine.

Dark Red-brown.

—Also referred to as cola-colored, this is characteristic of myoglobin, the form of hemoglobin contained in muscles. It is especially associated with cases of extensive muscle injury, from trauma or extreme exercise. Reagent strip tests for blood (hemoglobin) also detect myoglobin. Detection is an important finding as it is thought to be nephrotoxic.

Dark Brown or Black.

—This color may result from melanin or homogentisic acid. In both cases the urine is colorless when voided and becomes black on standing. Both are the result of serious conditions, and the color must not be overlooked. Melanin is associated with melanoma, a type of tumor. Homogentisic acid is associated with alkaptonuria, a result of an inborn error in the metabolism of tyrosine. Phenol poisoning may also result in an olive-green to black urine. Specific chemical tests for all these possible causes of black urine must be performed, since immediate diagnosis and treatment is imperative in each case. These conditions are rarely encountered. Some patients taking levodopa for parkinsonism may excrete urine which is dark brown or cola-colored.

Miscellaneous Colors.

—Various bizarre urine colors such as yellow, orange, red, pink, blue, green, and brown may result from such causes as vitamins, vegetables, fruits, certain chemicals, and dyes. These have very little clinical significance. However, they are important to the laboratory from a technical standpoint. Certain drugs interfere with other chemical tests that are performed as part of a routine urinalysis, and such interference may be suspected when the urine shows an unusual color. Each laboratory should have on hand reference materials to help determine the cause of possible interference. Some useful references include the following:

1. Hansten PD: *Drug Interactions,* ed 6. Philadelphia, Lea & Febiger, 1989.
2. Young DS, Pestaner LC, Gibberman V: Effects of drugs on clinical laboratory tests. *Clin Chem* 1975; 21:386D.
3. *Factors Affecting Urine Chemistry Tests*. Elkhart, Ind, Ames Division, Miles Laboratories, Inc, 1982.

4. *Urinalysis Today*. Indianapolis, Boehringer Mannheim Diagnostics, Boehringer Mannheim Corp, 1987.

Transparency

When voided, urine is normally clear; most urines, however, will become cloudy when allowed to stand. Cloudiness of a specimen when voided is usually of clinical significance and should not be disregarded.

The degree of cloudiness is observed in a well-mixed urine specimen at the time of urinalysis. When cloudiness is noted, it must be accounted for in the microscopic analysis of the urinary sediment, since it is caused by solid materials that will be visible under the microscope.

As with color, numerous words have been used in attempts to describe the degree of transparency of a urine specimen. Again, it is advisable that a particular institution use only one system of nomenclature. For example, the transparency may be said to vary from clear to hazy, cloudy, very cloudy, and turbid.

Schweitzer et al. advocate the use of a limited number of descriptors which are clearly defined as follows.*

Clear   No visible particulate matter present.
Hazy   Some visible particulate matter present; newsprint is not distorted or obscured when viewed through the urine.
Cloudy Newsprint can be seen through the urine but letters are distorted or blurry.
Turbid Newsprint cannot be seen through the urine.

Common constituents that cause cloudiness in urine, both generally normal and possibly significant or pathologic, are summarized in Table 13–3. A description of many of these constituents follows.

Normal Constituents Causing Cloudiness

Mucus.—The cloudiness that develops in most urine specimens on standing may result from the presence of *mucus* in the urine. Mucus is especially likely to solidify in urine stored under refrigeration and is of little clinical significance, although it is increased in inflammatory states of the lower urinary or genital tract.

*From Schweitzer SS, Schumann JL, Schumann GB: *J Med Technol* 1986; 3:11.

TABLE 13–3.

Common Constituents Causing Cloudiness in Urine

Generally Normal	Possibly Pathologic
Mucus	
Amorphous phosphates	Amorphous urates (also normal)
Normal crystals	Abnormal crystals
	Red blood cells
	White blood cells (pus)
Bacteria (old urine)	Bacteria (fresh urine)
	Other microorganisms (yeast, fungus, parasites)
Squamous epithelial cells	Epithelial cells (renal)
	Casts
Sperm, prostatic fluid	Fat
Powders, antiseptics	

Amorphous Phosphates, Carbonates, and Other Crystals.—Other substances commonly responsible for the development of cloudiness in urine are *amorphous phosphates* and occasionally *carbonates*. These are especially likely to form in alkaline urine on standing and are of no diagnostic significance.

Bacteria.—*Bacteria* are another common cause of cloudiness in urine specimens that have been allowed to stand. In this case, bacteria are not clinically significant. However, if the specimen is fresh or was collected under conditions suitable for bacteriologic examination, bacteria indicate a urinary tract infection.

Spermatozoa, Prostatic Fluid, Powders, Antiseptics.—*Spermatozoa* or *prostatic fluid* may also cause clouding of the urine, as may contamination with *powders* or certain *antiseptics*.

Possible Pathologic Constituents Causing Cloudiness

There are other causes of cloudiness in urine specimens that may have pathologic significance.

Amorphous Urates.—*Amorphous urates*, like amorphous phosphates, are often responsible for normal cloudiness in urine specimens. They appear as a white or pink cloud of material, which settles out as the urine stands, especially if it is refrigerated. Unlike amorphous phosphates, the urates are characteristic of acid urines. The characteristic appearance is often referred to as brick dust, seen as a pink to red precipitate usually in highly colored, concentrated urine. This precipitate is visible under the microscope. Amorphous urates may have pathologic significance when present in large numbers in various febrile conditions associated with highly concentrated urine, and also in some cases of gout and leukemia.

White Blood Cells or Pus.—The occurrence of *white blood cells,* or *pus,* in urine is another abnormal cause of cloudiness. The white blood cells will be seen as white cloudiness in the urine and, when present in large numbers, will give the urine a milky appearance. Along with the white cells, bacteria will often be present, giving the urine a particularly foul odor. Both bacteria and white blood cells should be confirmed in the microscopic analysis of the urinary sediments.

Red Blood Cells.—Another cause of cloudiness, already mentioned under Color, is the presence of *red blood cells.* These are especially pathologic, unless they are the result of vaginal contamination, and give the urine a characteristic smoky-red or reddish-brown appearance. They should be confirmed in the microscopic analysis of the sediment. If present in very small numbers they will be observed only on examination under the microscope.

Epithelial Cells.—These cells may be either normal or pathologic when present in the urine depending on the type of cell and source. Increased numbers of renal epithelial cells, which resemble leukocytes, are abnormal. However, large numbers of squamous epithelial cells from a female patient may only represent vaginal contamination of the specimen.

Fat.—Although only rarely present, *fat* may be a pathologic cause of cloudiness in the urine specimen. In this case the urine has an opalescent appearance. Fat may even be found floating on top of the urine specimen in cases of fat embolism or phosphorus poisoning.

Casts.—These are another constituent of the urinary sediment which are indicated by increased cloudiness in the urine. Casts may be formed from precipitated protein which forms a cast of the renal tubule. They resemble mucus. They may also be formed of or contain any of the elements previously mentioned. The presence of casts is an extremely significant finding in the urine.

Again, it is stressed that most urine specimens show some cloudiness, and the cause of the cloudiness should be accounted for in the microscopic analysis of the urinary sediment.

Odor

Normal Odor

Normal urine has a characteristic, faintly aromatic odor because of the presence of certain volatile acids.

Abnormal Odor

Bacterial Action.—If allowed to stand, urine acquires a strong *ammoniacal* odor. This is caused by the breakdown of urea by bacteria (which are invariably present in the urine specimen), resulting in the formation of ammonia. This odor is important as an indication that the urine specimen is probably too old for the urinalysis to have clinical significance. Along with the breakdown of urea, various other decomposition reactions will have occurred, altering or destroying other components that were present at the time the urine was voided. Urine heavily infected with bacteria may have a particularly unpleasant odor, which may be described as *foul* or *putrid*. This is also caused by the action of bacteria on urea, forming ammonia, plus the decay of proteins that are also present in infection. Practically, it cannot be distinguished from the smell of old urine. Therefore, foul-smelling urine will indicate urinary infection only if the specimen is known to be fresh.

Ketones.—Another characteristic odor that is significant clinically is a so-called *fruity,* or *sweet,* odor. This results from the presence of acetone and acetoacetic acid, especially in cases of diabetic **ketosis.**

Amino Acid Metabolism Errors.—In certain extremely rare disorders of amino acid metabolism, a characteristic odor has helped in the diagnosis of the condition. These odors are generally observed by the mother or caretaker of a baby who has particularly unusual-smelling diapers. It is not expected that this will be noticed by laboratory personnel. The odors have been described as being like sweaty feet, maple syrup, cabbage or hops, mousy, rotting fish, and rancid. Each has a specific amino acid disorder associated with it.

Foodstuffs.—Finally, the ingestion of certain foodstuffs will result in a characteristic urine odor. Probably the most obvious is the odor of asparagus. This is of no clinical significance.

Foam

Normal Foam

Normal urine will foam slightly when stoppered and shaken, and the foam will be white.

Abnormal Foam

High Protein Concentration.—When high concentrations of protein are present in the urine, a large amount of white foam may be seen if the urine container is securely closed and shaken. This is especially true of conditions like the nephrotic syndrome as large amounts of protein (albumin) are lost from the body into the urine. The foam that is formed looks like beaten egg white; the substance responsible for the foam in both cases is albumin. This observation should be confirmed by the chemical test for protein and the specimen will probably contain significant numbers of casts and other microscopic findings such as **oval fat bodies.**

Bile Pigments, Bilirubin.—When certain bile pigments are present, especially bilirubin, the urine will foam significantly and show a vivid yellow color. This is a simple test for the detection of bilirubin, which should be performed on abnormally dark urine specimens. However, it is not a confirmatory test, and all urine specimens suspected of containing bilirubin should be tested chemically whether the foam test is positive or negative.

SPECIFIC GRAVITY

Urine is a mixture of substances dissolved and suspended in water. In normal urine, these dissolved substances are primarily urea and sodium chloride. **Specific gravity** is a measure of the amount of dissolved substances in a solution. The specific gravity of urine is used as a measure of the ability of the kidney to regulate the composition and osmotic pressure of the extracellular fluid by concentrating or diluting the urine.

Clinical Aspects

Clinically, the specific gravity of urine may be used to obtain information about two general functions: the state of the kidney, and the state of hydration of the patient. If the kidney is performing adequately, it is capable of producing urine with a specific gravity ranging from about 1.003 to 1.035. However, if the renal epithelium is not functioning adequately, it will gradually lose the ability to concentrate and dilute the urine. The ability to concentrate urine is one of the first functions lost when the kidney is impaired. Deficiency or failure to respond to ADH will also result in failure to concentrate urine.

The specific gravity of the protein-free glomerular filtrate is about 1.007. Without any active work on the part of the kidney, this will increase to 1.010 as a result of simple diffusion as the filtrate passes through the kidney tubules. Thus, if the kidney has completely lost its ability to concentrate and dilute the urine, the specific gravity will remain at 1.010. If it is known that the kidney is functioning adequately, the state of hydration may be reflected by the specific gravity. For example, if the urine is consistently very concentrated, dehydration is implied.

Although normal specific gravity may range from 1.003 to 1.035, it is usually between 1.010 and 1.025. Since the specific gravity is a reflection of the amount of dissolved substances present in solution, it varies inversely with the volume of urine (this is because a fairly constant amount of waste is produced each day). Therefore, if the urinary volume increases because of increased water intake, and the amount of waste produced remains constant, the specific gravity of the urine decreases. In other words, if the urinary volume is high the specific gravity is low, and vice versa, assuming the kidney is functioning normally. With an individual on a restricted fluid diet for 12 hours, the normal kidney is capable of concentrating urine to a specific gravity of about 1.022 or more. If the individual is placed on a very high fluid diet, the normal kidney is capable of diluting the urine to a specific gravity of about 1.003. The concentrated first urine specimen passed in the morning should have a specific gravity greater than 1.020 if the kidney is functioning normally.

Two frequently observed cases where specific gravity does not vary inversely with urinary volume are diabetes mellitus and certain types of renal disease. With diabetes mellitus an abnormally large urinary volume associated with an abnormally high specific gravity is observed. This is caused by the presence of large amounts of dissolved glucose, which raises the specific gravity of the urine. In certain types of renal disease such as glomerulonephritis, pyelonephritis, and various anomalies, there is a combination of low specific gravity and low urinary volume. This results from the inability of the renal tubular epithelium either to excrete normal amounts of water or to concentrate the waste products. The specific gravity in these cases may eventually be fixed at about 1.010.

The loss of concentrating ability is seen in the disease diabetes insipidus, an impairment of ADH. This rare condition results in extremely large volumes of urine with very low specific gravity, ranging from 1.001 to 1.003.

Abnormally high specific gravity values, usually greater than 1.035 and up to 1.050 or more, may also be encountered after certain diagnostic x-ray procedures in which a radiographic dye is injected intravenously to obtain a pyelogram of the kidney. Such high specific gravity readings will be accompanied by delayed false-positive reactions for protein with the sulfosalicylic acid procedure, and the dye may crystallize out of the urine as an abnormal colorless crystal resembling plates of cholesterol.

Measures of Urine Solute Concentration

Although specific gravity is a convenient measure of the urine solute concentration, it is not the only one available. Other measures are osmolality, refractive index, and ionic concentration.

Specific Gravity

This is a measure of the amount of dissolved substances present in a solution. Specific gravity is the weight of a solution compared to the weight of an equal volume of water. More specifically, it is the ratio of the density (weight per unit volume) of a solution compared to the density (weight per unit volume) of an equal volume of water at a constant temperature. From this definition, it is clear that the specific gravity of water is always

1.000. Since it is a ratio, specific gravity has no units. Specific gravity in urine is measured with a urinometer, a specialized hydrometer which is calibrated to measure specific gravity in urine at a given temperature. It is always reported to the third decimal place. Specific gravity is dependent both on the weight (density) and the number of particles in the solution.

Osmolality

This is another method of determining solute concentration. It is a measure of the number of solute particles per unit amount of solvent. Thus it is dependent only on the number of particles in solution. It is determined with an osmometer by measuring the freezing point of a solution, since the freezing point is depressed in proportion to the amount of dissolved substances present. In normal persons with a normal diet and fluid intake, the urine will contain about 500 to 850 mOsm/kg of water.

Refractive Index

Another measure of solute concentration, reported in the urinalysis laboratory as specific gravity, is refractive index. The refractive index of a solution is the ratio of the velocity of light in air to the velocity of light in solution. This ratio varies directly with the number of dissolved particles in solution. Although not identical to specific gravity, refractive index varies and corresponds with specific gravity. Measurement is made with a **refractometer** which is calibrated to give results in terms of specific gravity. Results agree well with urinometer readings.

Ionic Concentration

Finally, reagent strips have been developed to give specific gravity values of urine. These strips actually measure ionic concentration which relates to specific gravity. Values are reported as specific gravity. However, substances which are dissolved in urine must ionize in order to be measured by this method. Certain substances which may be present in urine, such as glucose or certain radiopaque dyes, do not ionize, therefore, specific gravity results obtained with the urinometer or refractometer will be significantly higher than with the reagent strip if the urine contains significant quantities of nonionizable, dissolved substance.

The Urinometer

The specific gravity of urine was traditionally measured with a urinometer. The urinometer is a glass float weighted with mercury, with an air bulb above the weight and a graduated stem on the top (Fig 13–2). It is weighted to float at the 1.000 graduation in deionized water when placed in a glass urinometer cylinder or appropriate sized test tube. It is important that the cylinder, or test tube, be of the correct size so that the urinometer can float freely. The specific gravity of the urine is read directly from the graduated scale in the urinometer stem. The procedure for measuring specific gravity with the urinometer is described in Procedure 13–1. It has generally been replaced by the refractometer or reagent strip method. It has the disadvantage of being time-consuming and requires a relatively large volume (at least 15 mL) of urine.

Calibration

To obtain correct specific gravity readings in urine, the urinometer must be weighted to read exactly 1.000 in

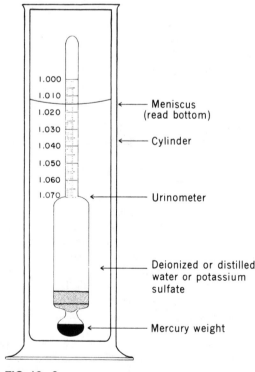

1.000
1.010
1.020 ←——— Meniscus (read bottom)
1.030
1.040 ←——— Cylinder
1.050
1.060
1.070 ←——— Urinometer

←——— Deionized or distilled water or potassium sulfate

←——— Mercury weight

FIG 13–2.
Urinometer and urinometer cylinder.

deionized water. Two methods may be used to test the urinometer calibration: the specific gravity value may be read from the scale in deionized or distilled water, or it may be read in a solution of known specific gravity.

1. *Calibration in deionized or distilled water.* Exactly the same procedure is followed as for urine. The reading on the urinometer scale should be exactly 1.000. If it is not, a correction must be applied to all values obtained for urine specimens with the urinometer. For example, suppose the urinometer reads 1.002 in deionized water. The specific gravity of water is 1.000. Therefore the urinometer correction is 0.002. In this case, the apparent reading is greater than it should be, and 0.002 must be subtracted from subsequent specific gravity readings. If a urine specimen has an apparent specific gravity of 1.037, this value minus 0.002 results in the corrected specific gravity of 1.035 for the urine specimen.

2. *Calibration in potassium sulfate (K_2SO_4) of specific gravity 1.015.* Any solution of a known specific gravity can be used to check the urinometer. A solution of K_2SO_4 with a specific gravity of 1.015 may be prepared by diluting 20.29 g of K_2SO_4 to 1 L in deionized water. A reading is obtained in the known solution following exactly the same procedure as in urine or water. The reading on the urinometer scale should be exactly 1.015. If it is not, a correction must be applied to all urine specimen readings obtained with that urinometer. For example, if the urinometer reads 1.012 in the K_2SO_4 solution, the correction is 1.015 minus 1.012, or 0.003. In this case, the reading is less than it should be. Therefore, 0.003 must be added to all specific gravity readings. For the urine specimen in the preceding example, the apparent reading in this case would be 1.032. The corrected specific gravity is 1.035.

Few urinometers read exactly 1.000 or 1.015 in water or potassium sulfate, respectively. Therefore, it is necessary to calibrate each urinometer before it can be used with accuracy. In addition, the correction can change from day to day, so it is necessary to calibrate the urinometer each day before urine specific gravity readings are determined.

Temperature Correction

By definition, the specific gravity of a solution is dependent on temperature. Urinometers are calibrated to read 1.000 in water at a particular temperature. If the urine specimen is either warmer or cooler than the urinometer calibration temperature, the result will be inaccurate. For precise work 0.001 should be added to the urinometer reading for each 3° C that the urine specimen is above the calibration temperature, and 0.001 should be subtracted from the urinometer reading for each 3° C below the calibration temperature.

Most urinometers are calibrated at 60° F, which is 16° C. The calibration temperature is stated on each urinometer. Since room temperature is approximately 18 to 22° C, it is acceptable to report the specific gravity reading directly from the scale if the reading is made when the urine specimen is at room temperature. However, a significant error will result if the reading is taken on a urine specimen that has been refrigerated. The temperature of a refrigerated urine specimen is 4° C, which is 12° less than 16° C. The temperature correction in this case is $(12°/3°) \times 0.001 = 0.004$. Assuming that the specimen reads 1.015 at 4° C, its actual specific gravity is $0.015 - 0.004 = 0.011$. Instead of applying this correction, the urine specimen should be allowed to warm up to room temperature before its specific gravity is determined.

Correction for Abnormal Dissolved Substances

The specific gravity represents the amount of dissolved substances present in urine. In determining the specific gravity of a urine specimen, the clinician is interested in assessing the kidneys' ability to concentrate and dilute normal waste products. In certain instances the specific gravity of a urine specimen is elevated because of the presence of abnormal constituents such as glucose, which may give the impression that the kidney is adequately concentrating the urine when in reality it is not. For this reason it is important to know how to correct for the presence of abnormal substances such as glucose.

Each gram of glucose present per 100 mL of urine will raise the specific gravity 0.004. Urine specimens of persons with diabetes mellitus often contain as much as 3 or 4 g of glucose per 100 mL of urine. This would represent a considerable error in the apparent specific gravity, as seen in the following example.

Assume that the apparent specific gravity of a urine specimen is 1.020. However, it is determined that this urine contains 4 g of glucose per 100 mL of urine. Therefore, the specific gravity is elevated 4×0.004, or 0.016, because of the presence of glucose. The actual specific gravity of this specimen in terms of normal urine constituents is $1.020 - 0.016$, or 1.004.

In this example the urinary specific gravity was

Procedure 13–1. Specific Gravity With Urinometer

1. Check the cleanliness of the urinometer cylinder. Clean the urinometer cylinder at the end of each day following the standard procedure for chemically clean glassware. A dirty cylinder will result in a thin, hard-to-read meniscus.
2. Calibrate the urinometer in deionized or distilled water before use each day. Follow the same procedure as with urine.
3. Fill the test tube to about 1 in. from the top with well-mixed urine. (Be sure the test tube is the correct size for the urinometer—that is, that the urinometer is able to float freely. All tubes should be of the same size and filled to the same level with urine.)
4. Grasp the urinometer stem at the top and insert slowly. Avoid wetting the stem above the water line, as excessive wetting of the stem will cause the urinometer to be depressed, and this will result in an inaccurate reading. Twirl the urinometer slightly as it is inserted, and note the reading as soon as it comes to rest. Be sure the urinometer floats freely away from the sides of the container while reading results.
5. See that the following requirements are met when reading the specific gravity:
   a. Use a clean urinometer.
   b. Make sure there are no bubbles around the urinometer.
   c. Avoid wetting the stem above the water line.
   d. Have the urinometer float freely about 1 in. off the bottom of the container.
   e. Read on a flat level surface.
   f. Read at the bottom of the thick meniscus.
   g. Keep the eye at the same level in relation to the urinometer for each reading.
   h. Recalibrate the urinometer each day.
6. Apply the appropriate correction to the results when necessary, and report the corrected specific gravity.
7. Rinse the urinometer in fresh water and dry the stem before proceeding to the next specimen.
8. When all determinations are complete, clean the urinometer and cylinder. Store the clean urinometer floating in fresh deionized water in the cylinder.

lower than normal. However, in diabetes, urinary function is often normal in spite of the large sugar content. For this reason, it is common to find diabetic urine specimens with specific gravity values well above 1.030. When values above 1.030 are discovered, diabetes is often suspected, and the laboratorian should expect to find indications of large amounts of sugar in the urine. This is not to say, however, that all specimens with abnormally high specific gravity readings contain sugar.

It is not usual for the laboratory to correct specific gravity readings for the presence of sugar when laboratory results are reported. Instead, the clinician will be aware that the specific gravity is elevated because of the presence of sugar and take this into account in the assessment of kidney function. If the results are corrected by the laboratory, this must be noted on the report form and the values both before and after correction must be reported.

Another abnormal substance that raises the specific gravity of a urine specimen is protein. Protein raises the specific gravity 0.003 for every gram per 100 mL of urine. However, unlike glucose, 1 g/100 mL represents an extremely large amount of protein and is seldom seen. Therefore, it is generally unnecessary to correct the urinary specific gravity when protein is present unless the amounts of protein present are extremely large.

The Refractometer

The refractive index of urine is closely correlated with the specific gravity. Since the development of the Goldberg refractometer, a temperature-compensated small hand-held instrument, measurements of the refractive index have become common in routine urinalysis (Fig 13–3). They have the advantage that they require only a drop of urine, while the urinometer requires at least 15 mL of specimen. In addition, the refractometer is simple to operate and rapidly gives reliable results. Its

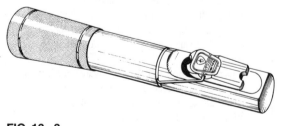

FIG 13–3.
Refractometer.

major disadvantage is its cost. The procedure for measuring specific gravity with a refractometer is given in Procedure 13–2.

Although the refractometer actually measures the refractive index, the scales of the instrument are calibrated in terms of total solids (g/100 g) for plasma or serum, or in terms of specific gravity for urine. Up to a value of 1.035, the urinary refractive index and specific gravity agree. Few normal urines have values greater than 1.035; higher values suggest the presence of unusual solutes in the specimen such as glucose, protein, or radiopaque compounds. Beyond a value of 1.035, the refractive index is poorly correlated with the specific gravity and should be reported only as greater than 1.035, rather than extrapolated to a higher value.

Calibration

The refractometer should be calibrated each day with deionized water and two standard solutions, such as sodium chloride (NaCl) solutions of known refractive index. The distilled water should read 1.000. The NaCl solutions may be the same standards that are used in the determination of osmolality. These may be purchased standards. Various concentrations should read as follows:

mOsm/kg H_2O	Specific Gravity (Refractometer) ±0.001
500	1.008
750	1.011
1,100	1.017
1,600	1.024

Corrections

Refractive index changes with temperature, but the Goldberg refractometer compensates for temperature changes in the solution being measured. Therefore, it is not necessary to correct for changes in temperature of the urine.

Since refractive index is a measure of dissolved particles in solution, the presence of substances such as glucose, protein, or radiopaque dyes will act to raise the specific gravity when measured with the refractometer. The effect is similar to that when measured with the urinometer and the same corrections should be applied. With values greater than 1.035, unusual substances such as radiopaque dye should be suspected when not explained by other findings, such as high glucose concentration. The presence of unusual crystals of these dyes in the microscopic analysis of the urine sediment is often associated with very high specific gravity readings with the refractometer. These substances will not be measured by the reagent strip method. Thus the presence of unusual crystals might be correlated with specific gravity readings greater than 1.035 by refractometer.

Procedure 13–2. Specific Gravity With Refractometer

1. Clean surface of instrument prism and cover by rinsing with water. Wipe dry.
2. Close the coverplate of the instrument.
3. Apply a drop of urine to the exposed portion of the measuring prism, at the notched bottom of the cover, using a disposable pipette. The liquid will be drawn into the space between the prisms by capillary action.
4. Hold the instrument up to a light source or position in the refractometer stand so that light passes over the chamber.
5. Looking through the eyepiece, make the reading on the specific gravity scale at the point where the dividing line between the bright- and darkfields crosses the scale.
6. Rinse the chamber and cover with water and wipe dry.

Reagent Strips

The reagent strips for specific gravity actually measure ionic concentration. Both Multistix (Ames Division, Miles Laboratories, Inc., Elkhart, IN) and Chemstrip (Boehringer Mannheim Diagnostics Division of Boehringer Mannheim Corp., Indianapolis, IN) have multiple reagent strips with test areas for specific gravity. The test is based on a pK_a change of certain pretreated polyelectrolytes in relation to the ionic concentration of the urine. The polyelectrolytes in the reagent strip contain acid groups which dissociate in proportion to the number of ions in solution. This produces hydrogen ions which reduce the pH. The pH change is indicated by the color change of an acid-base indicator. The system is buffered so that any change in color is related to pK_a change, and not pH of the urine itself. Readings are made at 0.005-intervals from 1.000 to 1.030 by comparison with a color

chart. The procedure for measuring urine specific gravity with reagent strips is the same as that used for all reagent strips as described in Procedure 13–3.

Corrections and Limitations

Dissolved substances must ionize in order to be detected by the reagent strips for specific gravity. Therefore, substances like glucose or radiopaque dyes which do not ionize will not affect the reagent strips, giving different values than those obtained by urinometer or refractometer. Although this may give a better picture of the concentrating ability of the kidney, it is important that the clinician understand which methodology is used by the laboratory for specific gravity, and if the results are "corrected" or not, to adequately interpret the specific gravity results.

Highly buffered alkaline urine may cause low readings, and 0.005 may be added to readings from urines with pH equal to or greater than 6.5. Unlike readings with the urinometer or refractometer, elevated specific gravity readings may be obtained in the presence of only moderate (100–750 mg/dL) amounts of protein. Finally, urine specimens containing urea at concentrations over 1 g/dL will cause low readings relative to more traditional methods.

CHEMICAL TESTS IN ROUTINE URINALYSIS

Most of the chemical tests that are done as part of the routine urinalysis use dry reagent strips. Reagent strips are available both as single tests for a specific chemical substance and combinations of single test referred to as *multiple reagent strips*. Two products are described in this section: the Chemstrip products and the Multistix and other Ames reagent strip and tablet tests are used to make important decisions in diagnosis, treatment, and monitoring of disease.

Reagent strips are plastic strips that contain one or more chemically impregnated test sites on an absorbent pad. When the chemicals on the test site come into contact with urine or a control solution, a chemical reaction occurs. The reaction is indicated by a color change which is compared with a special color chart which is provided with the reagent strip, usually printed on the bottle. The intensity of the color formed is generally proportional to the amount of substance present in the specimen or control when observed at a specific time. Some areas are used as screening tests which tell if a substance is present or absent, others are semiquantitated, giving a rough estimate of the amount of substance present. Results can be read visually, or in special instruments which automatically read specific reagent strips.

There are several advantages to dry reagent strip tests over the more traditional chemical tests on which they are based. They are more convenient, giving rapid results with a minimum of time and personnel. They are generally cost-effective and stable. Their use is relatively easy to learn; however, the basic principles must be understood and the proper technique followed. This reduces chances for error. They are completely disposable and require only small samples, sufficient to wet the test area. Finally, they are space-saving, in terms of storage, use, and cleanup.

Because they are so apparently easy to use, reagent strip tests are candidates for abuse. Reliable, reproducible results depend on correct technique. Manufacturer's directions must be followed. These will differ for the same substance tested with different products. It is essential that the laboratorian understand the principle and specificity of each chemical test area; to be aware of precautions or limitations and interferences that occur; and to know the sensitivity and significance of positive or negative results.

In certain instances, additional confirmatory tests are necessary when positive results are obtained with the reagent strip tests. These may be in the form of tablet tests, or more traditional chemical tests. These are described as necessary below and in Procedure 13–3.

Reagent Strip Tests: General Procedure and Precautions

Manufacturer's Directions

General directions that apply to all reagent strip tests are included in this section. However, it is imperative that the specific directions of the manufacturer be followed for all reagent strip tests. Tests are continually changed and reformulated in this highly competitive market. Each container of reagent strips is supplied with a product insert. This contains the most up-to-date information for the successful performance of the test in question. Inserts include directions for use, warnings, procedure limitations, specimen handling information, storage, and expected values. Information on interfering substances that may produce false-negative or false-positive reactions are included. For each new lot number of reagent strips, the laboratorian should study the product insert, compare it to the previous insert, noting any changes, and file it with the laboratory procedure manual.

The Urine Specimen

The specimen to be tested must be fresh, or adequately preserved, well mixed, not centrifuged, and at room temperature.

Sampling or Wetting

The first step in using the reagent strip is adequately sampling the specimen or wetting the reagent strip. Although this sounds easy, it is a common source of error. The strip must be adequately moistened so that all test areas of the strip are brought into contact with the sample. However, care must be taken not to leave the strip in contact with the sample too long, or chemicals will be leached out of the strip and be unavailable for the chemical reaction to occur. Therefore, the strip is inserted into the specimen only briefly, for 1 second or less. Another problem is runover between chemicals on adjacent pads. This is avoided by drawing the edge of the strip along the edge of the urine container as it is removed, touching the edge of the strip to absorbent paper, and holding the strip horizontally while waiting for and reading results.

Storage

Reagent strips must be kept in tightly capped or stoppered containers. They will deteriorate rapidly when exposed to moisture, direct sunlight, heat, or volatile substances. Each container contains a dessicant or drying agent to protect it from moisture. It should not be removed. The dessicant is contained within the original stopper in the Chemstrip products. Store containers at recommended temperatures, generally under 30° C but not refrigerated or frozen. Keep strips in their original container. Do not mix strips from different containers. Remove only the number of strips needed at a time, and close the container tightly. Do not touch the test areas. Keep the test areas away from detergents or other contaminating substances such as bleach (hypochlorite) that may be present in the work area.

Expiration and Discoloration

Each container of reagent strips is marked with a lot number and expiration date. Do not use strips after the expiration date. Write the date opened on each container. Once opened, use strips within 6 months. Watch test areas for possible deterioration by comparing the color of the dry reagent to a negative test block on the color chart. If deterioration is suspected, test the strip with a known control solution.

Timing

Read the results at the time stated by the manufacturer for each chemical test. This is absolutely necessary if results are to be semiquantitated. Very different results will be seen for the same specimen at different times. In general, the Ames products are read during the kinetic phase of reactions, and timing is absolutely critical. The Chemstrip products are generally read at an end point or stable phase allowing all results to be read at 1 minute with results stable for 2 minutes. An advantage of using an automated or semiautomated instrument to read reagent strips is that it controls the exact time at which all of the chemical reactions are read.

Reading Results: Color Comparison

Whenever results depend on color comparison, individual interpretation is a possible source of error. Adequate light is essential in visual interpretation. Hold the strip next to the most closely matched color block for each chemical test. Be sure to correctly orient the reagent strip to the color chart when reading results, a problem with new personnel or students. The use of automated or semiautomated instruments will eliminate individual differences in color interpretation and improve the reproducibility of results. Report results in a consistent manner as established for your institution.

Control Solutions

Several commercial control products are readily available. A control product should be used to test every parameter of the reagent strip in use and limitations of the control product should be known. Each opened bottle of reagent strips should be tested by every shift during which it is used. Test reagent strips when bottles are newly opened.

AUTOMATION IN URINALYSIS

Although multiple reagent strips were developed to be read visually, instruments have been developed to measure electronically the intensity of the color reactions produced on the reagent strips. The instruments are reflectance photometers. They measure the intensity of light that is produced by the chemical reaction between the analyte in question and the chemicals impregnated on each test portion of the reagent strip. The intensity of light produced is proportional to the amount of analyte in the specimen being tested. The instruments contain a microprocessor which controls and coordinates reflectance measurements at each test area. It mechanically moves the reagent strip through the photometer to ensure accurate and consistent timing, and displays or prints out the results for each test area. In addition, it displays error codes when the strips are inserted improperly or otherwise mishandled. Actual instruments vary in the way the strips are inserted into the instrument, the degree of automation, and the manner in which patient specimens are identified and results are displayed or printed.

There are many advantages to instrumentation. The readings are more reproducible and unbiased. Visual readings may vary from person to person, especially with respect to color interpretation and timing. The instruments are programmed to read each test area at a specific

---

Procedure 13–3. General Procedure for Urine Reagent Strips

1. Test fresh, well-mixed, uncentrifuged urine.
2. Completely immerse all chemical areas of the reagent strip briefly—not over 1 second.
3. Remove excess urine from the reagent strip by drawing the strip along the lip or rim of the urine container as it is removed.
4. Avoid possible mixing of chemicals from adjacent reagent areas.
5. Read each chemical reaction at the time stated. Timing is critical for semiquantitation of results.
6. Use adequate light. Hold the strip close to the color block on the chart supplied by the manufacturer and match carefully for each chemical test. Be sure the strip is properly oriented to the color chart: horizontal for Multistix, vertical for Chemstrip products.
7. Record the results in consistent units as established for your laboratory.

time, which, although very important, is sometimes difficult to do manually. It is also possible to analyze a greater number of specimens in less time than is possible manually. Printed results decrease the incidence of transcription (clerical) errors. Results can also be interfaced with the laboratory computer system to further minimize clerical errors and save time in reporting results. It should be remembered that the instrument does not alter the chemical methodology of the reagent strip but it does increase reproducibility.

Before the instrument is used, it must be calibrated. This is done with a reference standard strip provided by the manufacturer. After this calibration is done, the reflectance readings are compared to calibration curves which are stored in the microprocessor. These are used to estimate the concentration of each analyte.

Although these instruments are fairly simple and relatively easy to use, several important factors must be kept in mind. The person using the instrument must read the operating manual carefully and follow the directions exactly. Short cuts cannot be tolerated. The instrument must be maintained on an established, regular schedule. The instrument must be kept clean and free from contamination. One person should be responsible for maintenance.

The microscopic analysis of urine has also been automated by the Yellow IRIS (International Remote Imaging Systems, Chatsworth, CA). This is an integrated system which uses multiple reagent strips and instrumentation for the chemical analysis of the urine specimen. An aliquot of the urine is presented to a video microscope in a single layer of particles which are analyzed by computer according to size and number. A laboratorian views low-power and high-power digitized images on a color monitor and makes final identification by selecting an appropriate category on the monitor screen.

The use of instrumentation for the chemical analysis of urine should provide time for other parts of the urinalysis, leaving valuable time for careful microscopic analysis of the urinary sediment. Care must be taken with standardization and controls, and the instrument must not be misused. The laboratorian must still be aware of the principles and limitations of the tests. A gross examination of the urine specimen must not be omitted, and the instrumental results must be checked against the gross appearance and correlated with findings in the urinary sediment before final results are reported.

pH

One function of the kidney is to regulate the acidity of the extracellular fluid. Some information about this function, and other information as well, may be obtained by testing the urinary **pH.**

The pH is the unit that describes the acidity or alkalinity of a solution. In ordinary terms, acidity refers to the sourness of a solution, while alkalinity refers to its bitterness. Lemon juice is an example of a sour, or acidic, solution; baking soda (sodium bicarbonate) is a bitter, or alkaline, substance in solution. In chemical terms, acidity refers to the hydronium ion (H_3O^+) concentration of a solution and alkalinity refers to its hydroxyl ion (OH^-) concentration. These concentrations are usually expressed in terms of pH.

All solutions can be placed somewhere on a scale of pH values from 0 to 14. There are some solutions that are neither acidic nor basic. These solutions are neutral and are placed at 7 on the pH scale. Water is an example of a neutral solution; its pH is 7. Water is neutral because the concentration of hydronium ions is equal to the concentration of hydroxyl ions.

A solution with more hydronium ions than hydroxyl ions is an acidic solution. On the pH scale an acidic solution has a value ranging from 0 to 7. The farther it is from 7, the greater the acidity. For instance, solutions of pH 2 and pH 5 are both acidic; however, a solution of pH 2 is more acidic than a solution of pH 5. In simpler terms, a solution of pH 2 is more sour than a solution with a higher pH value. For example, lemon juice has a pH of about 2.3, while orange juice has a pH of about 3.5.

An alkaline solution has a pH value greater than 7. It can be anything from 7 to 14; the farther it is from 7, the greater the alkalinity, or the more bitter the solution.

Clinical Aspects

Regulation of the pH of the extracellular fluid is an extremely important function of the kidney. Normally, the pH of blood is about 7.4 and varies no more than ±0.05 pH unit. If the blood pH is 6.8 to 7.3, marked acidosis will be seen clinically; if it is 7.5 to 7.8, marked alkalosis will be observed. A pH less than 6.8 or greater than 7.8 will result in death. The carbon dioxide produced in normal metabolism results in a tremendous amount of acid, which must be eliminated from the blood and extracellular fluid, or death will result. This acid is normally eliminated from the body by the lungs and the kidneys.

Because the kidney is generally working to eliminate excess acid, the pH of urine is normally between 5 and 7, with a mean of 6. The kidney is capable of producing urine ranging in pH from 4.5 to 8.0. The urine is normally acidified through an exchange of hydrogen ions for sodium ions in the distal convoluted tubules. In renal tubular acidosis this exchange and the ability to form ammonia are impaired, resulting in a relatively alkaline urine. Certain metabolic acid-base disturbances may also be reflected in measurements of urinary pH as the kidney attempts to compensate for changes in blood pH. Such acid-base disturbances are classified as metabolic or respiratory acidosis and alkalosis, and measurements of titratable acidity, ammonium ion, and bicarbonate concentration are used in these distinctions.

Although the kidney is essential in controlling the pH of blood and extracellular fluid, measurements of urinary pH are not necessarily used to obtain information about this role. The routine urinalysis includes a measurement of urinary pH for the following reasons:

1. Freshly voided urine usually has a pH of 5 or 6. However, on standing at room temperature, urea is converted to ammonia by bacterial action. The production of ammonia raises the hydroxyl ion concentration, resulting in an alkaline urine specimen. Therefore, unless it is known that a urine specimen is fresh, an alkaline pH probably indicates an old urine specimen.

2. Alkalinity of freshly voided urine, especially if persistent throughout the day, may indicate a urinary tract infection. Other urinalysis findings in infection include positive reagent strip tests for nitrite and leukocyte esterase and large numbers of bacteria and possibly white cells (neutrophils) in the urine sediment.

3. The urinary pH helps in the identification of crystals of certain chemical compounds that are often seen in the urine sediment. Certain crystals are associated with acid urine, pH under 7, and others with alkaline urine, pH 7 and over. Knowledge of the urine pH is of great importance in the identification of crystals and may be the major reason for testing the pH of a urine specimen.

4. If the urine specimen is dilute and alkaline, various formed elements, such as casts and red blood cells, will rapidly dissolve.

5. Persistently acidic urine may be seen in a variety of metabolic disorders, especially diabetic acidosis resulting from an accumulation of ketone bodies in the blood.

6. Persistently alkaline urine may be seen in some infections, in metabolic disorders, and with the administration of certain drugs.

7. It is sometimes necessary to control the urinary pH in the management of kidney infections, in cases of renal calculi (stones), and during the administration of certain drugs. This is done by regulating the diet; meat diets generally result in acidic urine and vegetable diets in alkaline urine.

Methods of Measuring Urinary pH

In most instances a precise measure of the urinary pH is not necessary. A rough estimate obtained with an indicator is sufficient. Such indicators include nitrazine paper and a methyl red and bromthymol blue double indicator system. Multiple reagent strip tests make use of a methyl red and bromthymol blue indicator system. If a more precise measurement of urinary pH is clinically necessary, a pH meter may be employed.

Reagent Strip Tests

Principle and Specificity.—Both the Chemstrip and Multistix products utilize a methyl red and bromthymol blue double indicator system that measures urine pH in a range from 5 to 9. They are available as multiple reagent strips in combination with other tests for urinary constituents. The methyl red is used to indicate a pH change from 4.4 to 6.2 with a color change from red to yellow. Bromthymol blue indicates a pH change from 6.0 to 7.6 as seen by a color change from yellow to blue. Follow the reagent strip test procedure as described in Procedure 13–3.

Sensitivity and Results.—Multistix products: report values in 0.5-pH units from 4.0 to 8.5. Chemstrip products: report values in 1-pH units from 5 to 9.

Precautions, Interferences, Limitations

1. No interferences are known.
2. The pH value is not affected by the buffer concentration of the urine.
3. The specimen must be tested when fresh, since

bacterial growth may result in a significant shift to an alkaline pH, giving falsely alkaline values.

4. Be careful not to wet the reagent strip excessively so that the acid buffer from the protein area runs into the pH area causing an orange discoloration.

Nitrazine Paper

Nitrazine paper such as pHdrion paper (Micro Essentials Laboratory, Brooklyn, N.Y.) makes use of a universal pH indicator, sodium dinitrophenolazo-naphthol disulfonate, which has a pH range from 4.5 to 7.5. There is a color change from yellow to blue as the pH value increases. The color is easily matched against reference color charts.

Limitations.—Most nitrazine paper is manufactured with color charts ranging from pH 3 or 4 to pH 9. However, nitrazine paper has an accurate range of only 4.5 to 7.5. For this reason, only results that compare with colors 5, 6, and 7 are accurate. If the moistened paper compares with a color below 5, the result should be reported as acidic. If the moistened paper compares with a color greater than 7, the result should be reported as alkaline.

pH Meter

Principle.—The most accurate measurement of pH is made with a pH meter. Such accuracy is only rarely necessary in urinalysis; however, the principles of use of the pH meter will be discussed at this time. The pH meter is more commonly used in the clinical laboratory to measure the pH of blood and to check the pH of certain reagents such as buffers that are prepared for use in the laboratory.

The pH meter consists of three basic parts: (1) a glass-bulb electrode; (2) a reference electrode, which is usually a calomel electrode; and (3) a sensitive meter or measuring device. The glass-bulb electrode contains a solution of a certain fixed pH or hydrogen ion concentration. When the electrodes are placed in a solution of unknown pH, an electrical potential is produced between them that depends on the hydrogen ion concentration of the solution compared to the fixed concentration of the solution in the glass bulb. This potential, which is proportional to the hydrogen ion concentration of the test solution, is measured with the aid of the reference electrode. The potential of the reference electrode is compared to the potential of the pH electrode (the glass-bulb electrode) and is measured by means of the meter. The

meter is an electronic voltmeter (potentiometer) that measures millivolts (mV). Results are read from an arbitrary pH scale of 0 to 14 pH units or from a millivolt scale. A reading of 0 mV is equivalent to a pH of 7.0.

The procedure will vary with different pH meters and the manufacturer's instructions should be followed. However, certain considerations and precautions, such as standardization, apply to all instruments. (See Procedure 13–4).

Procedure 13–4. Use of pH Meter

1. Before the pH meter can be used to test the pH of unknown solutions, it must be standardized or calibrated. This is done by immersing the electrodes in a buffer solution of known pH at a particular temperature and then adjusting the instrument with the calibration knob to the correct value. The buffer that is chosen for standardization should be close to the expected pH of the test sample, and a second buffer with a different known pH should be tested, and the instrument adjusted accordingly, to ensure that the pH meter is accurate over a range of values. For example, the buffers used for calibration might have pH values of 7 and 4. Standard buffer solutions are commercially available. The pH meter should be standardized each time it is used.
2. The pH electrodes are fragile and should be treated accordingly. The manufacturer's directions about storage and activation should be followed carefully. In some cases the electrodes are stored in water, in other cases in saline or buffer.
3. The electrodes are immersed in the unknown solution, and a reading is taken from the pH scale.
4. Before and after use the electrodes should be sprayed clean with deionized or distilled water and carefully dried with an appropriate tissue.
5. Since the pH varies with temperature, the buffer used and the urine sample to be tested must be within 5° C of each other.

PROTEIN

Clinical Aspects

As stated earlier, the routine urinalysis will provide information about possible renal disease or information about metabolic or systemic disorders. In the detection and diagnosis of renal disease, probably the most significant single finding is that of urinary protein. The presence of protein when correlated with certain chemical tests, especially tests for blood, nitrite, and leukocyte esterase, and findings in the microscopic analysis of the urinary sediment, are part of the eventual diagnosis.

The occurrence of protein in the urine is termed **proteinuria.** Proteinuria is an abnormal condition, probably the most important pathologic condition found in a routine urinalysis. In general it may be the result of glomerular damage, tubular damage, or overflow from the excessive production of low-molecular-weight proteins such as hemoglobin, myoglobin, or immunoglobulins.

Normally, the glomerular filtrate, the initial stage in the formation of urine, is an ultrafiltrate of blood plasma without cells, larger protein molecules, and certain fatty substances. There is a very small amount of protein present in normal urine. However, this is less than 10 mg/dL of urine and is not detectable by normal tests for urinary protein. The normal glomerular membrane allows the passage of proteins with molecular weights of 50,000 to 60,000 or less. These are normally reabsorbed in the proximal convoluted tubules. Albumin has a molecular weight of about 67,000. This is a fairly small molecule, and some albumin is normally filtered through the glomerulus. However, this is normally reabsorbed in the convoluted tubules.

Glomerular Damage.—Proteinuria (generally **albuminuria**) is a consistent finding in glomerular disease. If the glomerular membrane is damaged, larger protein molecules find their way into the glomerular filtrate and are detected in the urine. This increased glomerular permeability usually begins with the passage of the smaller albumin molecules, and the larger globulin molecules remain in the blood plasma. The reagent strip tests for protein are actually most sensitive to the presence of albumin and may miss other protein molecules. This is not a problem in the great majority of renal diseases, where the major urinary protein is albumin. It is a problem when certain abnormal proteins such as the low-molecular-weight globulins associated with diseases such as multiple myeloma are present, as they might be missed with the reagent strip tests.

Tubular Damage.—A very small amount of protein (albumin) does find its way into the glomerular filtrate. In normal situations, all of this protein is reabsorbed back into the blood through the renal convoluted tubules. Although the concentration of protein that normally filters into the glomerular filtrate is extremely small and only 1 in 180 parts of the glomerular filtrate is eliminated from the body as urine (the rest is reabsorbed), failure to reabsorb any protein from this large volume of glomerular filtrate will result in fairly large amounts of protein in the urine. In other words, another cause of proteinuria is decreased reabsorption of protein by the renal tubular cells.

It is usually impossible to say which mechanism is responsible for the occurrence of proteinuria; it is most likely a combination of the two. The important consideration is that it indicates renal disease.

Although proteinuria is indicative of renal disease, additional tests are needed for the final diagnosis. These include observations of the urinary sediment, especially for the presence and types of casts; a determination of the amount of protein excreted per day by quantitative tests, and the type of protein by electrophoresis; and the patient's clinical history.

Proteinuria in Normal Persons.—There are situations in which small amounts of urinary protein may occur transiently in normal persons. In particular, they may be found in young adults after excessive exercise or exposure to cold, or in so-called orthostatic proteinuria, which occurs in persons engaged in normal activity but disappears when they lie down. In general, the proteinuria associated with renal disease is consistent, while that found in normal persons is transient. To determine the cause of the proteinuria, it is often necessary to quantitatively determine the amount of protein in a 24-hour urine collection. Tests for orthostatic proteinuria are made on urine collections obtained both when the patient is at rest and after the patient has been walking and standing, but not sitting.

Consistent Microalbuminuria.—Although screening tests for proteinuria should not be so sensitive that they detect the very small amount of protein that may be normally present in urine, it is sometimes desirable to detect the consistent passage of very small amounts of protein (microproteinuria). This is especially true of patients with diabetes mellitus. In these patients, it is thought that the early development of renal complications can be predicted by the early detection of consistent microalbuminuria. This early detection is desirable as it is felt that better control of blood glucose levels will delay the progression of renal disease. The methodology for the detection of microalbuminuria includes nephelometry, radial immunodiffusion, and radioimmunoassay. More recently, a relatively simple tablet test, Micro-Bumintest (Ames Division, Miles Laboratories, Inc., Elkhart, IN) has been developed to detect very small amounts of albumin. The principle of this test is analogous to the reagent strip tests; however, the sensitivity of Micro-Bumintest is 4 to 8 mg albumin per deciliter of urine, compared with a sensitivity of 15 to 30 mg/dL for the Ames reagent strip tests.

Proteinuria and Casts.—There is a correlation between the presence of casts and protein in the urinary sediment since casts are made of precipitated protein. **Tamm-Horsfall mucoprotein** is a type of protein which is normally secreted by the renal tubules. It is a product of the kidney and not present in the blood plasma. This is the protein that forms the matrix of most urinary casts. Thus, the occurrence of casts with proteinuria distinguishes an upper urinary tract (kidney) disorder from a disorder of the lower urinary tract. Bacterial infections of the kidney are often indicated by the presence of white blood cells and bacteria in the urinary sediment in addition to protein in the urine. In these cases the amount of protein excreted is usually fairly small. White blood cells and bacteria in the urinary sediment in the absence of urinary protein probably indicate a lower urinary tract infection without renal involvement.

The implications of protein in the urine are extremely serious. Extensive renal destruction is incompatible with life, and any renal destruction is permanent. Therefore, prompt diagnosis and treatment are vitally important. In addition, the loss of protein from the blood plasma will result in severe water balance problems, since the osmotic pressure of the blood is largely dependent on the concentration of plasma proteins. This is readily seen in the edema that is often associated with kidney disorders.

Methods of Measurement

Tests for urinary protein are of two major types:

1. Tests which are based on the use of the **protein error of pH indicators.** This is the methodology employed in the various reagent strip tests commonly used to screen urine for protein.

2. Tests which are based on the precipitation of protein by a chemical or coagulation by heat. These are generally tube tests which are used both as screening tests for urine protein and as confirmatory tests which are used when the reagent strip shows a positive result.

Many equally acceptable tests fit into these two categories, and the test that is used will depend on the individual laboratory situation, patient population, and volume of work. It is important to learn the general principle, which can then be applied to the particular test that is used in practice.

Reagent Strip Tests

Principle

Reagent strip tests for urinary protein involve the use of pH indicators—substances that have characteristic colors at specific pH values. At a fixed pH, certain pH indicators will show one color in the presence of protein and another color in its absence. This phenomenon is referred to as the **protein error of indicators** because it is often a problem in the laboratory, but it is put to use in testing for urinary protein. In this case the pH of the urine is held constant by means of a buffer, so that any change of color of the indicator will indicate the presence of protein.

The reagent strip tests for urine protein are available either individually, or in various combinations with other tests as multiple reagent strips. They differ in the buffer and pH indicator system impregnated on the strip; otherwise they are analogous. The general procedure for using reagent strips as discussed in Procedure 13–3 should be followed.

Specificity

The reagent strip tests for urinary protein are more sensitive to the presence of albumin than they are to other proteins such as globulin, hemoglobin, Bence Jones protein, and mucoprotein. If these proteins are present in the urine without albumin, false-negative results may be obtained. In other words, a negative reagent strip does not rule out the presence of protein. Therefore, depending on the patient population, it may be necessary for a given laboratory to test all urine specimens with both a reagent strip and precipitation method for urinary protein so as not to miss certain abnormal proteins such as those seen in new, undiagnosed cases of multiple myeloma.

Contents of Reagent Strips

Multistix, Albustix (Ames).—The Ames products protein test areas are impregnated with a citrate buffer and tetrabromphenol blue. The buffer provides a pH of approximately 3. At this pH tetrabromphenol is yellow in the absence of protein, and yellow-green, green, or blue in its presence. The shade of the color is dependent on the amount of protein present.

Chemstrip.—The Chemstrip products use tetrachlorophenol and tetrabromsulfophthalein as the indicator with a buffer. This gives essentially the same color change in the presence of protein as the Ames products.

Results

Reagent strips may be reported in a plus system or semiquantitated in milligrams per deciliter to give a rough estimate of the amount of protein present. Laboratories with automated reagent strip readers and computerized reports are more likely to employ a numerical system of specific units. When reading results, color must be matched closely with the color chart, which may be technically difficult. The protein portion of the reagent strip is one of the most difficult to interpret. This is particularly true of trace readings. Automated instruments that read reagent strips are helpful, but not foolproof. The tablet test, Micro-Bumintest, is useful in interpreting trace readings. Although developed for the detection of microalbuminuria in diabetic patients, the use of this test will help differentiate the negative and trace readings on reagent strips when this distinction is clinically desirable. Micro-Bumintest is based on the same principle as the reagent strip tests for protein. Reagents are provided in a tablet form. Results are easier to interpret and the test is more sensitive than the reagent strip tests.

Because of the difficulty in interpreting protein readings, along with the fact that the reagent strips are much more sensitive to albumin than to any other protein, which could be missed altogether, many laboratories confirm all questionable or positive reagent strip results with precipitation methods.

Sensitivity

Multistix and Albustix detect 15 to 30 mg/dL albumin, Micro-Bumintest detects 4 to 8 mg/dL albumin, and Chemstrip detects 6 mg/dL albumin.

Precautions, Interferences, Limitations

1. If the urine is exposed to the reagent strip for too long, the buffer may be washed out of the strip, resulting in the formation of a blue color whether protein is present or not (false-positive result).

2. If a urine specimen is exceptionally alkaline or highly buffered, the reagent strip tests may give a positive result in the absence of protein (false-positive result).

3. Contamination of the urine container with residues of disinfectants containing quaternary ammonium compounds or chlorhexidine may cause false-positive results due to alterations of pH (increased alkalinity).

4. Chemstrip products may give false-positive results during therapy with phenazopyridine and when infusions of polyvinylpyrrolidone (blood substitutes) are administered according to product inserts.

5. The test areas are more sensitive to albumin than to globulin, hemoglobin, Bence Jones protein, or mucoprotein. Therefore, the presence of these proteins may give negative reactions for specimens that test positive with precipitation methods (false-negative result).

6. The presence of large amounts of bilirubin or other strong colors or pigments may interfere with color interpretation, making the results impossible to read.

7. The reagent strip tests for protein are not affected by turbidity, radiographic contrast media, most drugs and their metabolites, and urine preservatives, which occasionally affect other protein tests.

Precipitation Tests

Principle

In the precipitation tests for urinary protein, the protein is either precipitated out of the urine specimen by means of a chemical, which is usually a strong acid, or it is coagulated out of solution with heat. The results are read in terms of the amount of precipitate or turbidity that is formed. The amount of turbidity or precipitation is roughly proportional to the amount of protein present in the urine specimen, and these results are generally graded in a plus system as negative, trace, 1+, 2+, 3+, or 4+. Coagulation tests depend on the fact that protein is more insoluble at the isoelectric point (a particular pH) of the protein molecule. At the isoelectric point, protein will readily precipitate out when heat is applied. For the proteins found in urine, the isoelectric point is approximately pH 5; therefore, in these tests the pH of the test solution and urine is adjusted in some way to 5.

Since the results in precipitation tests are determined by the presence of either turbidity or a precipitate, it is important that the urine be free from particles before the test is performed. For this reason, the procedure includes a step to clear the urine specimen. This is usually done by centrifuging the specimen and testing the clear supernatant for the presence of protein. When the urine is centrifuged, the solid material left after collecting the supernatant is the urinary sediment, which is observed under the microscope.

Precipitation tests for urinary protein include Roberts' test and Heller's test, which are ring or contact tests; Exton's sulfosalicylic acid test and various modifications; and many tests that make use of acetic acid, salt, and heat, which are variously called the heat and acetic acid test, the salt and acetic acid test, and Purdy's test.

Specificity

Precipitation tests will detect all proteins, albumins and globulins, unlike the reagent strip tests, which are more sensitive to albumin. To identify the actual type of protein present, further tests such as electrophoresis, immunoelectrophoresis, immunodiffusion, or ultracentrifugation may be necessary.

Sources of Error

1. Turbidity in the urine specimen itself poses a problem in the precipitation tests for protein. Some urines are turbid when they are voided and many become turbid as they are cooled. Such urines must be clarified before they are tested. This is usually done by centrifugation. Turbidity does not interfere with the reagent strip tests for protein.

2. Mucin is a normal constituent of urine that may give false-positive results in certain precipitation tests for urinary protein. Interference by mucin may be avoided by acidifying the urine with acetic acid to precipitate the mucin, then filtering to remove the precipitated mucin, and finally testing the clear filtrate. However, interference may be avoided simply by adding sufficient sodium chloride or other salt to raise the specific gravity to a level that will keep the mucin in solution.

3. The presence of organic iodides in radiographic contrast media will precipitate in the acid test solution, giving a delayed positive reaction in the sulfosalicylic acid tests for protein. This interference is suspected when very high specific gravity values, greater than 1.035 by urinometer or refractometer, are obtained and the reagent

strip test for protein is negative. Unusual crystals of the radiographic media may be found in the urinary sediment in such cases.

4. Metabolites of drugs such as tolbutamide (an oral drug used to treat diabetes), which are excreted in urine, are insoluble in acid and give false-positive results in the protein precipitation methods. Other drugs which may give false-positive reactions are massive doses of penicillins, sulfisoxazole and sulfonamide metabolites, and the anti-inflammatory drug tolmetin (Tolectin). These substances do not affect the reagent strip tests for protein.

5. The occurrence of a highly buffered alkaline urine might result in a reduced or false-negative reaction if the buffer is sufficient to neutralize the acid in the acid precipitation procedure.

6. The presence of Bence Jones protein will produce varying results depending on methodology. In the precipitation tests that depend on the coagulation of protein by heat, positive reactions will be observed only at certain temperatures. Bence Jones protein is an unusual gamma globulin (an immunoglobulin) which precipitates when heated to 40 to 60° C. It will not be seen at temperatures less than 40° C or greater than 60° C. However, it will be detected by cold precipitation methods such as the sulfosalicylic acid method. It may be missed altogether by reagent strip methods which are more sensitive to albumin.

Sulfosalicylic Acid Test

Principle.—This test is based on the cold precipitation of protein with a strong acid, namely sulfosalicylic acid. Various concentrations of sulfosalicylic acid have been described for use in tests for urinary protein. In the procedure used at the University of Minnesota Hospital and Clinic, a 7-g/dL solution is employed so that 11 mL of cleared urine, resulting from the routine 1:12 concentration of the urinary sediment, can be used. The free sulfosalicylic acid in the working reagent serves to precipitate any protein in the specimen. It will detect albumin, globulins, glycoproteins, and Bence Jones protein. Since the test does not rely on heat for precipitation, Bence Jones protein will precipitate like any other protein.

Sulfosalicylic acid procedures may give false-positive results with compounds used for diagnostic radiographic procedures. The reaction in this case is delayed somewhat and the precipitate is rather fluffy and crystalline in appearance, unlike the normal protein precipitate. Such interference is suggested by specific gravity values greater than 1.035 by urinometer or refractometer and may be confirmed by checking the patient's history for the use of diagnostic radiographic procedures. When this interference occurs, the reagent strip results for protein should be used.

The sulfosalicylic acid test is described in Procedure 13–5. A positive reaction is the presence of turbidity. The amount of turbidity that is formed is roughly proportional to the amount of protein in the specimen. The results are graded as negative, trace, 1+, 2+, 3+, or 4+. Since the results depend on the degree of turbidity, it is important to begin with a urine specimen that is free of turbidity. A filtered or centrifuged specimen should be used.

Sulfosalicylic Acid Reagent (7 g/dL).—Weigh 70 g of 5-sulfosalicylic acid ($C_7H_6O_6S \cdot 2H_2O$) and dilute to exactly 1,000 mL with deionized water in a volumetric flask.

Sensitivity.—Sulfosalicylic acid tests for urine protein detect 5 to 10 mg of protein in 100 mL of urine.

BLOOD (HEMOGLOBIN AND MYOGLOBIN)

Clinical Significance

Together with tests for protein, and the microscopic analysis of the urinary sediment, tests for blood in urine are used as indicators of the state of the kidney and urinary tract. Chemical tests for blood in urine also react with hemoglobin and myoglobin (which is muscle hemoglobin). Although the chemical tests are more sensitive to the presence of hemoglobin and myoglobin than to intact red cells, most positive reactions are actually caused by the presence of red cells (erythrocytes). Blood in the urine may represent bleeding at any point from the glomerulus to the urethra and the actual location is important to the diagnosis and treatment of the patient. A distinction between red cells, hemoglobin, and myoglobin is also of clinical significance. Therefore, tests for blood are included in the routine urinalysis, and test areas for blood appear on most multiple reagent strips. Before reagent strip tests were available, the detection of blood in the urine was based on gross observation of blood through a change in the appearance (color) of the urine

---

> ### Procedure 13–5. Sulfosalicylic Acid Test for Protein
>
> 1. Centrifuge a 12-mL aliquot of urine. Note the clarity of the centrifuged urine.
> 2. Decant 11 mL of the supernatant urine into a test tube.
> 3. Add 3 mL of 7-g/dL sulfosalicylic acid reagent.
> 4. Stopper the tube.
> 5. Mix by inverting the tube twice.
> 6. Let stand exactly 10 minutes.
> 7. Invert *twice*.
> 8. Observe the degree of precipitation and grade the results according to the following descriptions. To avoid making the test too sensitive, examine negative and trace reactions in ordinary room light, avoiding a Tyndall effect (scattering of light by colloidal particles), which might result from examination in too bright a light. If an agglutination viewer is available, use it to grade results higher than trace.
>
> *Negative:* no turbidity or no increase in turbidity (0.005 g/dL or less)
> *Trace:* barely perceptible turbidity in ordinary room light (0.010 g/dL)
> *1+:* distinct turbidity but no granulation (0.050 g/dL)
> *2+:* turbidity with granulation but no flocculation (0.20 g/dL)
> *3+:* turbidity with granulation and flocculation (0.50 g/dL)
> *4+:* clumps of precipitate or tube of solid precipitate (1.0 g/dL or more)

---

and the presence of red cells in the microscopic examination of the urinary sediment. Without a chemical test for hemoglobin, its presence would be missed.

It is clinically significant to differentiate between red cells and hemoglobin in the urine. Since tests for hemoglobin are positive in the presence of both free hemoglobin and red cells, it would seem that this differentiation is made mainly by the finding of red cells in the microscopic analysis of the urinary sediment. However, the presence of hemoglobin and the absence of red cells in the urine does not necessarily mean that the hemoglobin was originally free urinary hemoglobin. Red cells rapidly lyse in urine, especially when it has a specific gravity of

1.006 or less or is alkaline. For this reason urine should be absolutely fresh when examined for the presence of red cells. In addition, the specific gravity and pH of the urine will be useful in differentiating between red cells and free hemoglobin in the urine.

Hematuria

Hematuria is the presence of red blood cells in the urine. It results from a great variety of renal diseases, including both lesions of the kidney itself and bleeding at any other point in the urinary tract. Hematuria is a sensitive, early indicator of renal disease, and usually is accompanied by the presence of hemoglobin. Although blood will not be present in every voided specimen in every case of renal disease, occult blood (i.e., blood that is not grossly visible but is found by laboratory tests) may be present in almost every renal disorder. There may be little correlation between the amount of blood and the severity of the disorder, but its presence may be the only indication of renal disease. Other laboratory findings besides the presence of occult blood indicate the presence of renal disease. Protein is usually present along with blood, and findings in the microscopic analysis of the urinary sediment, such as the presence of casts, especially red cell casts and dysmorphic red cells, are particularly useful in detecting renal disorders.

Hemoglobinuria

Hemoglobinuria, or the presence of free hemoglobin in the urine, results from a variety of conditions and disease states. It may be the result of hemolysis in the bloodstream, (intravascular hemolysis), in a particular organ, in the kidney or lower urinary tract, or in the urine sample itself. The detection of intravascular hemolysis is important because the passage of free hemoglobin through the glomerulus and subsequent uptake by renal proximal convoluted epithelial cells is damaging to the nephron. When hemoglobin is released into the bloodstream it is normally bound to haptoglobin, which is a protein. This hemoglobin-haptoglobin complex is a large molecule which is not filtered through the glomerulus. However, there is a limited amount of haptoglobin in the blood and once it is saturated, the excess hemoglobin is filtered through the glomerulus into the renal tubules. Hematologic disease states resulting in hemoglobinuria include hemolytic anemias, hemolytic transfusion reactions, paroxysmal nocturnal hemoglobinuria, paroxysmal cold hemoglobinuria, and favism. Severe infectious diseases such as yellow fever, smallpox, and malaria also

result in hemoglobinuria, as do poisonings with strong acids or mushrooms, severe burns, and renal infarction. Finally, significant amounts of free hemoglobin occur whenever excessive numbers of red cells are present as a result of various renal disorders, infectious or neoplastic diseases, or trauma in any part of the urinary tract.

Myoglobinuria

Myoglobinuria is the presence of myoglobin in the urine. It is a rare finding. Chemical tests for occult blood are equally sensitive to the presence of hemoglobin and myoglobin. Myoglobinuria may result from traumatic muscle injury (such as from traffic accidents), excessive unaccustomed exercise, and beating or other crush injury. It is also seen in certain infections, after exposure to toxic substances and drugs, and in rare hereditary disorders.

The detection of myoglobinuria is important, as myoglobin is rapidly cleared from the blood and excreted into the urine as a red-brown pigment. Large amounts of myoglobin are damaging to the kidney and may result in anuria. It seems that myoglobin is more damaging than hemoglobin to the kidney.

Differentiation (Hematuria, Hemoglobinuria, Myoglobinuria)

This may be difficult. It is done with a combination of gross observations of urine and serum (or plasma) and certain chemical tests. The occurrence of blood in urine will result in a coloration ranging from frankly bloody, to slightly smoky, pink, amber, red-brown, or brown. In general, with hemoglobin and myoglobin the urine specimen is brown or red-brown in color. Although the presence of red blood cells would result in cloudiness, and hemoglobin or myoglobin by themselves would leave a clear specimen, other constituents often accompany all three entities, leading to cloudiness of the specimen. A gross observation of the serum or plasma accompanying these specimens is useful. If the urine contains only red blood cells, the serum would be normally colored. If intravascular hemolysis has occurred, the serum would appear to be hemolyzed (red). If rhabdomyolysis, which is the acute destruction of muscle fibers, occurs, myoglobin is released into the blood and is rapidly cleared into the urine, so that the serum appears normal in color.

In all cases, the reagent strip test for blood is positive. If red cells are present, they should be detectable in the microscopic examination of the urine sediment. With both hemoglobin and myoglobin, red cells would be absent, or very few would be present. In the case of rhabdomyolysis resulting in myoglobinemia and myoglobinuria, markedly elevated serum creatinine kinase (CK) is typical owing to the destruction of muscle. CK levels are not affected as markedly by hemolysis.

Unfortunately, myoglobin-induced renal failure may not be seen clinically until a week or more after the clinical event, and by then myoglobin is no longer present in the urine. In some cases, it may be helpful to use serum lactate dehydrogenase (LD) isoenzymes values to differentiate hemolysis from rhabdomyolysis. The total LD is elevated in both cases, but the LD_1 and LD_2 isoenzymes predominate in hemolysis, and the LD_4 and LD_5 isoenzymes with rhabdomyolysis.

Reagent Strip Tests

Principle and Specificity

The reagent strip tests for blood (hemoglobin, myoglobin) in urine make use of the **peroxidase** activity of the heme portion of the hemoglobin molecule. The reagent strips are impregnated with an organic peroxide, together with the reduced form of a chromogen. A positive reaction is seen when the peroxidase activity of the heme portion of the hemoglobin molecule catalyzes the release of oxygen from peroxide on the reagent strip. The released oxygen reacts with the reduced form of a chromogen, forming an oxidized chromogen which is indicated by a color change. This reaction is summarized as:

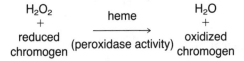

The reagent strips are equally sensitive to hemoglobin and myoglobin. Intact red blood cells are hemolyzed when they come into contact with the reagent strip, and the released hemoglobin reacts as described. It is essential that well-mixed urine be tested for the presence of blood. This is especially important when only a few intact red blood cells are present in the urine specimen. If intact red cells are allowed to settle and the supernatant urine is tested, false-negative results will be obtained.

Since the reaction is based on the peroxidase activ-

ity, other substances with peroxidase activity also give positive reactions. In urine specimens this peroxidase activity may be present in white blood cells and bacteria.

As in any of the reagent strip tests which depend on the release of oxygen and subsequent oxidation of a chromogen, the presence of ascorbic acid (or vitamin C) in the specimen will cause false-negative or delayed results. When present in sufficient quantity, the ascorbic acid acting as a strong reducing agent will react with the released hydrogen peroxide rather than the chromogen. This is seen as an inhibited or delayed color reaction. This interference is suspected when the reagent strip test for blood is negative, yet red blood cells are observed in the microscopic analysis of the urine sediment. The presence of ascorbic acid may be confirmed by testing the urine with a reagent strip test for ascorbic acid.

Contents of Reagent Strips and Results

Multistix, Hemastix (Ames).—The Ames reagent strips for blood contain cumene hydroperoxide (an organic peroxide) with the chromogen tetramethylbenzidine. A positive reaction is seen as a color change from yellow to shades of green, then blue. The presence of intact red cells is seen as the presence of green spots on the reacted test area. Results are compared to the color chart and reported as negative, trace, small (+), moderate (++), or large (+++).

Chemstrip.—The Chemstrip reagent strips for blood contain dimethyl dihydroperoxyhexane (organic hydroperoxide) and tetramethylbenzidine as the chromogen. The manufacturer claims to have eliminated interference due to ascorbic acid concentrations as high as 500 mg/dL by sealing the test area with an iodate-impregnated mesh layer. The iodate reacts with ascorbic acid present in the urine, thus removing it as an interfering substance. A positive reaction is seen as a color change from yellow to shades of green and blue, analogous to those seen with the Ames strips. Intact red cells are seen as green spots on a yellow background.

Sensitivity

Multistix and Hemastix detect 0.015 to 0.062 mg/dL hemoglobin (approximately equivalent to 5–10 intact red blood cells per microliter). Chemstrip detects 5 red cells per microliter, or hemoglobin from 10 red cells per microliter.

Precautions, Interferences, Limitations

1. The presence of strong oxidizing cleaning agents, such as hypochlorite bleach, may cause false-positive reactions due to oxidation of the chromogen in the absence of peroxidase.

2. False-positive reactions may be seen from microbial peroxidase activity associated with urinary tract infection.

3. False-negative or delayed reactions may be seen in urine specimens containing ascorbic acid. This is seen after ingestion of large doses of vitamin C or when included as a reducing agent in certain parenteral antibiotics, such as tetracycline. The Ames strips may show false-negatives at the trace level with ascorbic acid concentrations of 5 mg/dL or greater, according to the manufacturer. Chemstrip products claim to be unaffected by the ingestion of "reasonable quantities of ascorbic acid."

4. Elevated specific gravity or elevated protein may reduce the color reaction.

5. False-negative results occur when formalin is used as a urinary preservative.

6. Extremely high nitrite levels (over 10 mg/dL), seen rarely in severe urinary tract infections, may delay the color reaction.

NITRITE

Clinical Significance

Tests for the presence of nitrite in the urine have been included in the routine urinalysis as a rapid method of detecting asymptomatic urinary tract infection. Screening tests for nitrite are most useful when combined with tests for **leukocyte esterase,** another indicator of urinary tract infection. Therefore, combination leukocyte esterase and nitrite reagent strips are available, in addition to the multiple reagent strips.

The presence of urinary nitrite indicates the existence of a urinary tract infection. It is especially useful in detecting asymptomatic infections, where a positive nitrite test will alert the physician to the need for urine culture. When certain, but not all, bacteria are present in the urinary tract, they will convert nitrate, a normal constituent of urine, to nitrite, an abnormal constituent. However, urine must be retained (incubated) in the bladder for a sufficient period (generally 4 hours) for this reaction to take place. Thus, a first morning urine collection

is the specimen of choice when testing for nitrite. A specimen collected at least 4 hours after previous voiding is also acceptable. Unfortunately, a common complaint with urinary tract infection is frequent urination, making collection of an adequate specimen difficult.

The early detection of urinary tract infection is important for the prevention of kidney damage. It is felt that most urinary tract infections begin in the lower urinary tract, as a result of fecal contamination. Most infections are due to organisms that are normally present in the feces, such as *Escherichia coli*. The infection is introduced into the normally sterile urinary tract via the urethra, and ascends to the bladder, ureters, and finally the kidney. The early detection and subsequent treatment of infection is important in preventing infection of the kidney and subsequent renal failure. From this discussion it should be apparent that due to anatomical differences, urinary tract infection is much more common in women than men. In fact, other than just after birth or in old age, urinary tract infection is typically a disease of women.

Traditionally, urinary tract infections are diagnosed through quantitative urine culture, in which the organism that causes the infection is cultured and identified (see Chapter 16). Nitrite tests are merely screening tests that aid, but in no way replace, quantitative urine cultures. The existence of urinary tract infections is suggested by other findings in the routine urinalysis. These include the presence of white blood cells and bacteria with lower urinary tract infections in addition to the presence of casts, especially white cell or pus casts with upper urinary tract infection (pyelonephritis). Chemical tests suggestive of urinary tract infection include the presence of leukocyte esterase, protein, and a more alkaline urinary pH.

Reagent Strip Tests

Principle and Specificity

Chemical tests for nitrite are based on the Griess test. This involves a **diazo reaction.** Nitrite will react with an aromatic amine (*p*-arsanilic or sulfanilic acid) in an acid medium to produce a diazonium salt. The diazonium salt is then coupled with another aromatic ring (quinolin) to give an azo dye which is seen as a pink or red color. The test is specific for nitrite. However, many false-negative reactions occur. Thus a negative reaction does not rule out a significant urinary tract infection. In addition, it is possible for a false-positive reaction to occur due to bacterial contamination of the specimen by in vitro conversion of nitrate to nitrite. This is prevented by testing fresh urine specimens. The intensity of color formation is related to the amount of nitrite in the urine and does not necessarily indicate the degree of bacterial infection.

Contents of Reagent Strips

Multistix.—The Ames reagent strips for nitrite contain *p*-arsanilic acid and 1,2,3,4-tetrahydrobenzo-(h)-quinolin-3-ol.

Chemstrip.—The Chemstrip reagent strips for nitrite contain sulfanilamide and 3-hydroxy-1,2,3,4-tetrahydro-7,8-benzoquinoline.

Results

Report as positive or negative. Report any overall pink coloration as positive. Pink spots or pink edges are a negative reaction.

Sensitivity

Multistix detects 0.06 to 0.1 mg/dL nitrite ion. Chemstrip detects 0.05 mg/dL nitrite in 90% of urines tested.

Precautions, Interferences, Limitations

1. The test is primarily useful if positive. If the nitrite test area shows a negative reaction, urinary infection cannot be ruled out and there are many causes of false-negative reactions.

2. The urine must be retained in the bladder for 4 hours or more for adequate conversion of nitrate to detectable nitrite. Therefore, a first morning specimen is preferred or a specimen that has been retained in the bladder for at least 4 hours since the last voiding. This may be difficult because frequent urination is common in urinary tract infections.

3. Organisms must contain the reductase enzyme necessary to reduce nitrate to nitrite. This is true of most of the gram-negative enteric pathogens that cause urinary tract infections. The gram-positive enterococci and yeast, however, do not.

4. There must be sufficient dietary nitrate present for bacteria to reduce nitrate to nitrite or false-negative reactions may occur with significant bacterial infection.

Examples include starvation, fasting, or intravenous feeding. Vegetables are an important source of nitrates.

5. False-negative reactions may occur due to further degradation of nitrite to nitrogen.

6. Sensitivity may be reduced in urine with high specific gravity, although this is not typical of bacterial infection.

7. The presence of ascorbic acid in concentrations of 25 mg/dL or greater may cause false-negative results owing to reduction of the diazonium salt by ascorbic acid. This interference by ascorbic acid is true of any diazo reaction.

8. The urine specimen should be as fresh as possible to prevent false-positive reactions due to in vitro conversion of nitrate to nitrite by bacterial contamination.

9. Medications such as phenazopyridine that color urine red or that turn red in an acidic medium may cause false-positive results.

LEUKOCYTE ESTERASE

Clinical Significance

Chemical tests for leukocyte esterase have been included on the urine reagent strip tests as another means of detecting urinary tract infection. These tests are based on the measurement of leukocyte esterase which is present in azurophilic or primary granules of granulocytic leukocytes. These granulocytes include polymorphonuclear neutrophils (PMNs or neutrophils), monocytes (histiocytes), eosinophils, and basophils. In practice, positive reactions occur with increased neutrophils. Conditions associated with sufficient quantities of other granulocytes to give positive reactions are extremely rare, if they ever occur. Lymphocytes and the various epithelial cells which make up the kidney and urinary tract do not contain leukocyte esterase and are not measured in this test.

The detection of leukocyte esterase as an indicator of infection is useful, since neutrophils are generally increased in response to bacterial infection. When bacteria infect the urinary tract, at any point from the urethra to the kidney, the presence of increased numbers of white cells, particularly neutrophils, is typical. Neutrophils are also seen in the urinary sediment. However, a frequent problem is the rapid lysis of neutrophils in urine, a result of their phagocytic activity. Once lysed they are not detectable in the microscopic analysis of the sediment. However, the test for leukocyte esterase depends on its release from the azurophilic or primary granules of granulocytes. Thus the leukocyte esterase test is positive whether lysed or intact cells are present in the urine.

Urine normally contains 0 to 2 white cells per high-power field in the microscopic analysis of the urinary sediment. This normal occurrence of white cells is not sufficient to cause a positive reaction with the leukocyte esterase test. In fact, the reaction requires 5 to 15 leukocytes per HPF to give a positive reaction. Therefore, the absence of leukocyte esterase does not rule out a urinary tract infection. However, the presence of leukocyte esterase is helpful, especially when combined with an elevated (alkaline) urine pH and the chemical detection of nitrite in the urine together with the presence of bacteria and white cells in the urine sediment.

Increased leukocyte esterase may be seen in conditions where bacteria are not seen in the urine sediment or cultured. These include inflammatory conditions which may occur without bacterial infection, bacterial infection after treatment with antibiotics, and infections by organisms such as trichomonads and chlamydia which are not seen on standard culture media.

Reagent Strip Tests

Principle and Specificity

Tests for leukocyte esterase utilize a diazo reaction, much like the reagent strip tests for nitrite. In this case, the test area contains an ester which is hydrolyzed by leukocyte esterase to form its alcohol (which contains an aromatic ring) and acid. The aromatic ring is then coupled with a diazonium salt, present in the test area, to form an azo dye which is seen as the formation of a purple color. Chemstrip uses an indoxyl ester and Multistix uses a pyrrole amino acid ester. The reaction is specific for esterase which is present in granulocytic leukocytes, thought to be the only source of esterase in urine. The presence of red blood cells and bacteria does not affect the reaction.

Contents of Reagent Strips

Multistix.—The Ames reagent strips for leukocyte esterase contain a derivative of a pyrrole amino acid ester and a diazonium salt.

Chemstrip.—The Chemstrip reagent strips for leukocyte esterase contain indoxylcarbonic acid ester and a diazonium salt.

A positive reaction is seen as the formation of a purple color. The intensity is roughly proportional to the amount of leukocyte esterase present. Trace readings are generally interpreted as negative.

Sensitivity

Multistix requires 5 to 15 cells per HPF for a positive reaction. Chemstrip requires 10 cells per microliter.

Precautions, Interferences, Limitations

1. The presence of repeated trace and positive values are clinically significant and indicate the need for further testing to determine the cause of the presence of neutrophils (granulocytes) in the urine (pyuria). They may include microscopic analysis of the urinary sediment, Gram's stain, and quantitative urine culture.

2. False-positive reactions may be seen with strong oxidizing agents, as, for example, contaminants in urine containers.

3. The presence of leukocytes from vaginal contamination can cause false-positive results.

4. The test is not affected by the presence of blood, bacteria, or epithelial cells.

5. There are several causes of reduced or false-negative results. These include several drugs (antibiotics) such as cephalexin, cephalothin, tetracycline, and gentamicin.

6. Urine preservatives, especially formalin, may cause false-positive results and should not be used.

7. Decreased test results may be seen with elevated glucose (over 3 g/dL), high specific gravity, oxalic acid, and high levels of albumin (over 500 mg/dL).

8. As with any diazo reaction, the presence of very large amounts of ascorbic acid may inhibit the reaction owing to reduction of the diazonium salt.

9. The presence of substances which color urine, such as nitrofurantoin or bilirubin, may make color interpretation difficult.

10. Results are especially useful clinically when combined with the reagent strip test for nitrite. Therefore, strips which combine nitrite and leukocyte esterase are available, in addition to the multiple reagent strips with up to ten different test areas.

GLUCOSE (SUGAR)

Chemical screening tests for glucose are generally included in every routine urinalysis. However, these are not necessarily included to obtain information about the state of the kidney or urinary tract. Rather, the occurrence of glucose (also called *dextrose*) in the urine indicates the metabolic disorder diabetes mellitus should be suspected. Tests for urinary glucose are commonly used for the diagnosis and management of this disease, together with tests for blood glucose.

Any condition in which glucose is found in the urine is termed **glycosuria** (or glucosuria), which comes from the Latin words for glucose and urine. Tests for glucosuria were among the earliest laboratory tests. The "taste test" was used by the Babylonians and the Egyptians to detect diabetes by tasting for the presence of sugar in what would normally be a salty solution, while Hindu physicians noticed that "honey urine" attracted ants.

Clinical Aspects

The occurrence of glucose in the urine is not normal. The blood glucose concentration normally varies between 60 and 110 mg/dL depending on the method of analysis. After a meal it may increase to 120 to 160 mg/dL. Normally all the glucose in the blood is filtered by the glomerulus and reabsorbed into the blood. However, if the blood glucose concentration becomes too high (usually greater than 180–200 mg/dL) the excess glucose will not be reabsorbed into the blood and will be eliminated from the body in the urine. Other factors which might result in glucosuria are reduced glomerular blood flow, reduced tubular reabsorption, and reduced urine flow.

The lowest blood glucose concentration that will result in glycosuria is termed the *renal threshold,* and it varies somewhat from person to person. The most common condition in which the renal threshold for glucose is exceeded is diabetes mellitus. In simplified terms, diabetes mellitus is a deficiency in the production of, or an inhibition in the action of the hormone insulin. Insulin has the effect of lowering the blood glucose concentration. As a result of the deficiency of insulin, the blood glucose concentration exceeds the renal threshold, and glucose is spilled over into the urine. Tests for diabetes mellitus include tests for blood glucose in addition to tests for urinary glucose. Additional tests, such as those for glycated hemoglobin may also be used to monitor diabetes mellitus.

Although diabetes mellitus is suspected in cases of glycosuria, the occurrence of glycosuria is not diagnostic of the condition, since there are many other causes. For example, glycosuria may be observed after large amounts of sugar or foods containing sugar are eaten, in cases of acute emotional strain where glucose is liberated by the liver for energy, and after exercise. It may also be associated with pregnancy, certain types of meningitis, hypothyroidism, certain tumors of the adrenal medulla, and some brain injuries.

In addition, certain abnormal conditions are characterized by the presence in the urine of sugars other than glucose. These are generally reducing substances or sugars which require detection by methods other than those employed in the reagent strip tests which are specific for glucose. *Galactosuria* is the presence of the sugar *galactose* in the urine. It results from a metabolic error where the enzyme galactose-1-phosphate uridyltransferase is lacking so that galactose is not metabolized, resulting in increased galactose in the blood (galactosemia) and urine. This condition results in permanent physical and mental deterioration which may be controlled by early detection and dietary restriction of galactose. Therefore, urine from young pediatric patients should be screened with a nonspecific copper reduction test for reducing substances which will detect galactose and other reducing sugars in addition to glucose.

Methods of Measurement

Virtually all tests for urinary glucose may be classified as one of two types:

1. *Specific tests for glucose* are based on the use of the enzyme *glucose oxidase*. The reagent strip tests for urine glucose are of this type.

2. *Nonspecific tests* for sugar in general are based on the ability of glucose to act as a *reducing substance*. The Clinitest tablet test (Ames Division, Miles Laboratories, Inc., Elkhart, IN) is an example of a copper reduction test for reducing substances.

Reagent Strip (Glucose Oxidase) Tests

Principle and Specificity

The reagent strip tests for urinary sugar are specific for glucose because they are based on the use of the enzyme glucose oxidase. An enzyme is often described as a biological catalyst, a substance that must be present before a chemical reaction will occur. Glucose oxidase, like most enzymes, is absolutely specific. It will react only in the presence of glucose and it will not react with any other substance.

Glucose oxidase will oxidize glucose to gluconic acid and at the same time reduce atmospheric oxygen to hydrogen peroxide. The hydrogen peroxide formed will, in the presence of the enzyme peroxidase, oxidize the reduced form of a dye to the oxidized form which is indicated by the color change of an oxidation-reduction indicator. This reaction is diagrammed below:

Step 1:

Glucose (in urine)

$$+ O_2 \text{ (from air)} \xrightarrow[\text{oxidase}]{\text{glucose}} \text{gluconic acid} + H_2O_2$$

Step 2:

$$H_2O_2 + \text{reduced form of dye} \xrightarrow{\text{peroxidase}}$$
$$\text{oxidized form of dye} + H_2O$$

The glucose oxidase, peroxidase, and reduced form of the oxidation-reduction indicator are all impregnated on a dry reagent strip or paper strip. The products that are commercially available differ in the chromogen used as the oxidation-reduction indicator and the substance that is impregnated with the reactants.

It must be remembered that **nonglucose reducing substances (NGRS)** will not be detected by tests that are specific for glucose; therefore, specimens from infants and young pediatric patients and specimens in which NGRS are suspected should always be subjected to nonspecific (usually copper reduction) tests for reducing substances in addition to the specific tests for glucose.

Contents of Reagent Strips and Results

Multistix, Diastix (Ames).—The Ames multiple reagent strips and Diastix test for urine glucose contain glucose oxidase, peroxidase, buffer, a blue background dye, and potassium iodide as the chromogen. In a positive reaction oxidation of potassium iodide results in the formation of free iodine, which blends with the background dye to give shades of green through brown. Results can be semiquantitated by comparison to color blocks to 2 g/dL at exactly 30 seconds.

Chemstrip.—The Chemstrip products for urine glucose contain glucose oxidase, peroxidase, buffer, and tetramethylbenzidine as the indicator. A positive reaction is seen as a color change from yellow to shades of green, then blue. The multiple reagent strips can be semiquantitated by comparison to color blocks to 1 g/dL at 60 seconds. The glucose areas on the Chemstrip, uG and uGK, are impregnated differently than on the multiple reagent strips, which allows for semiquantitation over a range to 5 g/dL. The timing is also extended to 2 minutes.

Clinistix (Ames Division, Miles Laboratories, Inc., Elkhart, IN).—This is the original test for urine glucose. It utilizes *o*-toluidine as the color indicator, with glucose oxidase and peroxidase. Positive results are seen as a color change from red to purple. Results are read at 10 seconds, and should be reported as positive or negative only.

Tes-Tape (Eli Lilly & Co., Indianapolis, IN).—This is another example of a very early test for urine glucose. It also utilizes glucose oxidase, peroxidase, and an indicator. The reagents are impregnated on a tear strip of special paper, and the indicator is yellow in its reduced form and green to blue in its oxidized form. Results are read as the appearance of a green color at 30 seconds and reported as positive or negative.

Sensitivity

Reagent strip tests will generally detect glucose in amounts ranging from 40 to 125 mg/dL (see product inserts for exact amounts). Since the reagent strip tests for glucose are generally more sensitive to the presence of glucose than the copper reduction tests, they may give a positive reaction in the presence of very small amounts of glucose, while tests for reducing substances will give a negative reaction.

Interferences and Limitations

Since reagent strip tests are all specific for glucose, most interferences result in reduced or false-negative results. The exception is the possible contamination by bleach or other strong oxidizing agents which would react with the reduced form of the dye present on the reagent strip resulting in false-positive results in the absence of glucose. This shows the importance of utilizing contamination-free urine containers and work surfaces.

1. Large urinary concentrations of ascorbic acid, from therapeutic doses of vitamin C or from drugs such as tetracyclines in which ascorbic acid is used as a reducing agent, may inhibit or delay color development. This is true of any test that depends on the release of hydrogen peroxide, which acts as an oxidizing agent in the oxidation of the color indicator (chromogen) from a reduced to an oxidized form. In these cases, the ascorbic acid will act as a reducing agent, reacting with the released hydrogen peroxide (rather than the chromogen in the reagent strip) resulting in a false-negative or delayed positive reaction. This was especially troublesome in the earlier tests for glucose in urine. According to product inserts, Multistix products are inhibited by ascorbic acid concentrations of 50 mg/dL or greater in specimens containing small amounts of glucose (75–125 mg/dL). With Chemstrip, the manufacturer claims that by adding iodate to the test area, interference by ascorbic acid has been eliminated at glucose concentrations of 100 mg/dL or above. However, owing to possible false-negative results, Chemstrip recommends that tests be repeated on urine voided at least 10 hours after the last administration of vitamin C.

2. Ketone bodies will reduce sensitivity of the Multistix tests for glucose giving falsely low results. With small amounts of glucose (75–125 mg/dL) moderately high ketones (40 mg/dL) may cause false-negative reactions. However, according to product inserts, a ketone level this high is unlikely in a diabetic with such a low glucose level.

3. Sodium fluoride is an enzyme inhibitor and will therefore cause false-negative results in tests which utilize glucose oxidase. It should not be used as a preservative.

4. Both Chemstrip and Multistix are buffered so that pH does not affect results. Clinistix is influenced by the pH of the urine.

5. Urine must be at room temperature when tested.

Refrigerated specimens will give falsely low results due to decreased enzyme activity.

6. The reactivity of the glucose oxidase tests decrease as the urine specific gravity increases, so that sensitivity is greater in very dilute urine specimens.

7. Hypochlorite or chlorine bleach or strong oxidizing agents and cleaners such as hydrogen peroxide, which may be introduced as contaminants in the urine container, cause false-positive results due to oxidation of the dye resulting in a color change.

Copper Reduction Tests for Reducing Sugars

General Principle and Specificity

Tests that are based on the reducing ability of glucose are not specific for glucose. In these tests, the glucose is merely acting as a reducing agent, and any compound with a free aldehyde or ketone group will give the same reaction. Glucose is not the only reducing substance that may be found in urine. The NGRS include uric acid, creatine, galactose, fructose, lactose, pentose, homogentisic acid, ascorbic acid, chloroform, and formaldehyde. All these substances and glucose have the ability to reduce a heavy metal from a higher to a lower oxidation state. Usually copper(II) ions are reduced to copper(I) ions. Since this is an oxidation-reduction reaction, the reducing substance is oxidized to a higher oxidation state. When glucose is the reducing agent, it is oxidized to gluconic acid. A positive reaction is indicated by a color change, which varies in intensity in proportion to the amount of reducing substance present in the urine specimen. A commonly used copper reduction test for urinary sugar that will be discussed in detail is the Clinitest tablet test which is based on Benedict's qualitative test for reducing substances. Although often thought of a test for glucose, it must be remembered that Clinitest will give the same reaction with any reducing substance that may be present in the urine, either naturally or as a contaminant. In cases where the presence of a reducing sugar other than glucose—for instance, galactose—is suspected in the urine, a nonspecific test must be performed. Although specific reagent strip tests for glucose are commonly used as screening tests for the presence of glucose, all specimens obtained from young pediatric patients should be tested by a nonspecific method as well.

If the presence of an NGRS is indicated by a negative test specific for glucose coupled with a positive nonspecific test for reducing substances, the NGRS must eventually be identified. The method that is used to identify the NGRS is usually thin-layer chromatography or the resorcinol test for fructose. Remember that common table sugar is sucrose. This is a nonreducing sugar and will not react with copper reduction or glucose oxidase tests.

Clinitest Tablet Test (Ames)

Principle.—The Clinitest tablet test is a nonspecific test for urinary sugar which, as mentioned, is based on Benedict's qualitative test which utilizes the ability of glucose (or any reducing substance) to reduce copper(II), or cupric ions, to copper(I), or cuprous ions, in the presence of heat and alkali.

A positive reaction is semiquantitated as a change in color ranging from blue to green, yellow, and orange depending on the amount of sugar present. The overall reaction is:

$$CuSO_4 + 2NaOH \rightarrow Cu(OH)_2 + Na_2SO_4$$
(bluish)

Rapid reaction (occurs as if one step)

$$\downarrow \text{heat}$$

CuO
(Black)

$$\downarrow \text{reducing substance (e.g., glucose)}$$

Cu_2O + oxidized form of reducing
(yellow to red) substance (e.g., gluconic acid)

This reaction may be shortened to:

$$2Cu^{2+} + \text{reducing sugar (e.g., glucose)} \xrightarrow[\text{heat}]{\text{alkali}}$$

Cu_2O + oxidized sugar (e.g., gluconic acid)

The Clinitest tablet may be thought of as a solid form of Benedict's qualitative reagent. The tablet combines copper sulfate, anhydrous sodium hydroxide, citric acid, and sodium carbonate in an effervescent tablet. The interaction of sodium hydroxide with citric acid and water results in moderate boiling making an external boiling water bath unnecessary.

Results are semiquantitated at 15 seconds after boiling stops by comparison with a permanent color chart supplied with the tablets. Results must be read at this time since the reaction continues and will result in falsely high values if observed at a later time.

Both a five-drop and a two-drop Clinitest method have been described by the manufacturer and color charts are available for both (see Procedure 13–6). The two-drop method was developed in response to a "pass-through" phenomenon which may occur if more than 2 g/dL of sugar is present in the urine. Such concentrations of urinary glucose are possible in patients with diabetes mellitus. In the pass-through phenomenon, after the addition of the Clinitest tablet, the solution goes through the entire range of colors and back to a dark greenish brown because of carameiization of the large amount of sugar in the urine by heat. The final color does not compare with any section of the color chart; however, it corresponds most closely to a color indicating a significantly lower result. Thus it is extremely important to observe the entire Clinitest reaction from the addition of the tablet to the end so that this pass-through to a lower color is not missed and a falsely low result is not reported.

Contents of the Clinitest Tablet.—The Clinitest tablet contains copper sulfate, citric acid, sodium carbonate, and anhydrous sodium hydroxide.

Sensitivity.—Clinitest reagent tablets will detect as little as 250 mg/dL sugar (0.25 g/dL). This is less sensitive than the reagent strip tests for glucose. Thus it is possible to see a positive reagent strip reaction for glucose with a negative Clinitest if only a small amount of glucose is present in the urine.

Precautions and Interferences.—Observe the precautions in the information supplied by the manufacturer.

1. The bottle must be kept tightly closed at all times to prevent absorption of moisture and must be kept in a cool, dry place, away from direct heat and sunlight. The tablets normally have a spotted bluish-white color. If not stored properly they absorb moisture or deteriorate from heat, turning dark blue or blackish. In this condition they will not give reliable results. They are also available individually packaged in aluminum foil to help prevent absorption of moisture. Although they are more

---

Procedure 13–6. Clinitest Tablet Test for Reducing Sugars (Five-drop Method)

Follow the directions supplied with the Clinitest tablets.

1. Place five drops of urine in a test tube and add ten drops of water.
2. Add one Clinitest tablet.
3. Watch while boiling takes place, but do not shake.
4. Wait 15 seconds after boiling stops, then shake the tube gently, and compare the color of the solution with the color scale.
5. Report results with the same units as used for reagent strip glucose results, such as trace, 0.25, 0.5, 0.75, 1.0 or 2.0 g/dL.
6. Watch the solution carefully while it is boiling. If it passes through orange to a dark shade of greenish brown, the sugar concentration is more than 2.0 g/dL and the result should be recorded as greater than 2.0 g/dL without reference to the color scale. Urines showing this pass-through phenomenon should be retested with the two-drop method.

Clinitest Tablet Test for Reducing Sugars (Two-drop Method)

Follow the directions supplied with the Clinitest tablets.

1. Place two drops of urine in a test tube and add ten drops of water.
2. Add one Clinitest tablet.
3. Watch while boiling takes place, but do not shake.
4. Wait 15 seconds after boiling stops, then shake the tube gently, and compare the color of the solution with the color scale supplied for the two-drop method.
5. Watch the test throughout the entire reaction and waiting period, as the pass-through phenomenon may also occur with the two-drop test with concentrations of sugar over 10 g/dL.
6. Report the results as negative, trace, 0.5, 1.0, 2.0, 3.0, 5.0, and over 10 g/dL.

---

expensive in this form it is useful when a limited number of tests are performed.

2. The bottom of the test tube becomes very hot during the Clinitest reaction. Hold the test tube at the lip (not bottom) or place in a test tube rack to avoid burns.

3. Do not mix the test tube before the 15-second wait after boiling stops. Mixing before this time may cause falsely low values due to reoxidation of the cuprous ions to cupric ions by atmospheric oxygen.

4. Clinitest tablets will react with sufficient quantities of any reducing substance in the urine, including other reducing sugars such as lactose, fructose, galactose, maltose, and pentoses. Use reagent strips that are specific for glucose to confirm the presence or absence of glucose.

5. Since it is a reducing substance, large amounts of ascorbic acid (over 250 mg/dL) may cause false-positive results.

6. It has been reported that urine specimens that have a low specific gravity and contain glucose may give a slightly elevated result with Clinitest.

7. Nalidixic acid, cephalosporins, and probenecid may result in false-positive reactions if present in large quantities.

8. The presence of radiographic contrast media may result in reduced or false-negative reactions.

Quantitative Tests for Urine Sugar or Glucose

Occasionally it is necessary to determine exactly how much sugar is present in a urine specimen. In this case, the qualitative result is not sufficient, and a quantitative result is required. Results of quantitative urinary sugar determinations are typically reported in terms of grams per 24 hours of urine excretion. For these tests a complete 24-hour urine collection is required. The total volume of the specimen must be measured and the specimen preserved with a suitable chemical preservative that will not interfere with the reaction employed to test the specimen. Two methods that are often used are Benedict's quantitative method and the Somogyi method for quantitative urinary sugar. The exact procedure may be found in one of the many textbooks of clinical laboratory procedures. Both these methods are based on the reducing ability of glucose and make use of the reduction of copper(II) to copper(I).

KETONE BODIES

Clinical Aspects

Ketone bodies are a group of three related substances: acetone, acetoacetic (or diacetic) acid, and β-hydroxybutyric acid. Their structural similarity is illustrated in Figure 13–4. They are normal products of fat metabolism and are not normally detectable in the blood or urine.

In fat catabolism (the phase of metabolism in which fats are broken down for energy), acetoacetic acid is produced first. It is converted to either β-hydroxybutyric acid or acetone. All three ketone bodies are utilized as a source of energy and are eventually converted to carbon dioxide and water. When normal amounts of fat are utilized by the body, the tissues are able to use the entire ketone production as an energy source. However, if more fat than normal is metabolized, the body is unable to utilize all the ketone bodies. The clinical result is an increased concentration of ketones in the blood *(ketonemia)* and in the urine *(ketonuria)*. **Ketosis** is the combination of increased ketones in both the blood and urine.

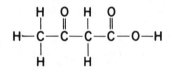

Acetoacetic Acid

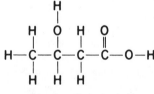

β-hydroxybutyric Acid

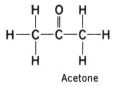

Acetone

FIG 13–4.
The ketone bodies.

Whenever fat (rather than carbohydrate) is used as the major source of energy, ketosis and ketonuria may result. The two outstanding causes of ketone accumulation are diabetes mellitus and starvation. In diabetes mellitus, the body is unable to use carbohydrate as an energy source and attempts to compensate by resorting to fat catabolism, which results in accumulation of the ketones. In starvation, the body is depleted of stored carbohydrate and must resort to fat as an energy source. In like manner, ketosis is seen in cases of dehydration, and conditions associated with fever, vomiting, and diarrhea. The same situation may occur in cases of severe liver damage. Most carbohydrate is stored as liver glycogen. In liver damage, there is not stored glycogen; hence the body must again resort to fat for energy. Finally, a ketogenic diet will result in ketone accumulation. A ketogenic diet is one that is high in fat and low in carbohydrates—specifically, a diet containing more than 1.5 g of fat per 1.0 g of carbohydrate. Low carbohydrate diets used for weight reduction may be ketogenic diets.

Since the presence of ketone bodies in urine is an early indication of lack of insulin, reagent strips which combine tests for glucose and ketones are often used by diabetics for home monitoring of their disease. Also, reagent strip tests for ketones have been advocated for home testing in persons on weight reduction diets. The physiologic effect of ketone accumulation in the blood and urine (ketosis) is serious. Acetoacetic acid and β-hydroxybutyric acid contribute excess hydrogen ions to the blood, resulting in acidosis. As mentioned under pH, acidosis is an extremely serious condition and results in death if allowed to continue. Therefore, the body attempts to compensate for excess acid in the blood by eliminating acid through the urine. The kidney is capable of producing urine with a pH as low as 4.5. Thus, the occurrence of ketones in the urine is associated with a low urinary pH. Before insulin was used in the treatment of diabetes mellitus, acidosis was the cause of death in two-thirds of all cases. In the treatment of diabetes mellitus, it is important to control the amount of insulin so that ketosis and acidosis do not occur. A typical urine specimen from an uncontrolled diabetic is pale and greenish, contains a large amount of sugar, has a high specific gravity by refractometer or urinometer, a low pH, and contains ketone bodies.

Another physiologic effect of ketosis concerns the substances acetone and acetoacetic acid. Both have been found to be toxic to brain tissue when present in increased concentrations in the blood. Of the two, aceto-acetic acid is the more toxic.

Methods of Measurement

When ketones accumulate in the blood and urine, they do not occur in equal concentrations. Of the ketones, 78% are present as β-hydroxybutyric acid, 20% as acetoacetic acid, and only 2% as acetone. However, most of the tests for ketones are sensitive to the presence of acetoacetic acid. There are no simple laboratory tests for β-hydroxybutyric acid.

The commonly used tests for ketone bodies are based on the sodium nitroprusside (nitroferricyanide) reaction and are available as dry reagent strips or tablet tests. They are all more sensitive to the presence of acetoacetic acid than to acetone, or sensitive only to acetoacetic acid. Before the development of the dry reagent strip or tablet tests, the nitroprusside reaction was employed as a ring test—Rothera's test (also known as Legal's test). Specimens which tested positive with Rothera's test were further tested with a ferric chloride reaction called Gerhardt's test which, although specific for acetoacetic acid, detected only large amounts, indicating severe ketosis. This test is now more commonly used as a quick test for the presence of salicylates in urine.

Specimen Requirements

It was mentioned above that in the normal formation of ketone bodies, acetoacetic acid is produced first and β-hydroxybutyric acid and acetone are produced from it. Similarly, if a urine specimen containing all three ketone bodies is allowed to stand after it is voided, the β-hydroxybutyric acid and acetoacetic acid will be converted to acetone. Since it is volatile, acetone will eventually disappear from the urine specimen. This means that urine should be tested for ketone bodies when fresh, or a false-negative result may be obtained. Heat accelerates this conversion; therefore, refrigeration should be used to preserve the urine if it cannot be tested immediately.

Reagent Strip Tests for Ketone Bodies

Principle and Specificity

The reagent strip tests for ketone bodies are based on a color reaction with sodium nitroprusside (nitroferri-cyanide). Acetoacetic acid will react with sodium nitroprusside in an alkaline medium to form a purple color. If glycine is added, the test is slightly sensitive to acetone. The Ames products Multistix and Ketostix have been formulated to react only with acetoacetic acid. They do not react with acetone. The Chemstrip products include glycine and detect both acetoacetic acid and larger amounts of acetone. None of the reagent strips detect β-hydroxybutyric acid (see Procedure 13–3).

Contents of the Reagent Strips and Results

Multistix, Ketostix (Ames).—The Ames reagent strips for ketone contain sodium nitroprusside in an alkaline buffer. They are specific for acetoacetic acid and change color from buff pink to maroon when acetoacetic acid reacts with nitroprusside. Results are read from the color chart as negative or as varying degrees of positive which indicate the relative amount of acetoacetic acid present. Color blocks represent negative, trace (5 mg/dL), small (15 mg/dL), moderate (40 mg/dL), and large (80–160 mg/dL).

Chemstrip.—The Chemstrip reagent strips for ketone contain sodium nitroferricyanide, glycine, and an alkaline buffer. They react with acetoacetic acid and acetone to form a violet dye complex. A positive result is indicated by a color change from beige to violet. Results are read from the color chart as negative, small, moderate, or large.

Sensitivity

Multistix and Diastix detect 5 to 10 mg/dL aceto-acetic acid. Chemstrip detects 9 mg/dL acetoacetic acid and 70 mg/dL acetone in 90% of urines tested.

Dilution for Large Amounts of Ketones

When a patient is monitored with repeated determinations of acetone and acetoacetic acid in plasma or urine, the concentrations of these compounds may start at very high levels and fall, but still give results that correspond to large on the color chart. Repeated reports of large do not reflect the changes as they occur. In such instances, semiquantitative results can be obtained by doing the analyses on several dilutions of each specimen until a large result is no longer seen. The report on this analysis should show that such dilutions have been done and state when a reading of large is no longer obtained. An example of such a report would be: undiluted, large;

1:2 dilution, large; 1:4 dilution, moderate. This applies to both tablet and reagent strip tests.

Acetest Tablet Test

Acetest (Ames Division, Miles Laboratories, Inc., Elkhart, IN) is a test for acetone and acetoacetic acid based on a color reaction with sodium nitroprusside. The principle is virtually identical to that of the reagent strip tests. In addition to urine, Acetest can be used to test whole blood, plasma, or serum, as described in Procedure 13–7.

Contents of the Tablet

The Acetest tablet contains sodium nitroprusside (nitroferricyanide), glycine, and a strongly alkaline buffer.

Precautions

Observe the precautions in the literature supplied with the product. Do not use black or discolored tablets.

Procedure 13–7. Acetest Tablet Test for Ketones

Follow the manufacturer's directions.
1. Place the tablet on a clean surface, preferably a piece of white paper.
2. Place one drop of urine, serum, plasma, or whole blood on the tablet.
3. For testing urine, compare the color of the tablet with the color chart 30 seconds after application of the specimen.

   For testing serum or plasma, compare the color of the tablet with the color chart 2 minutes after application of the specimen.

   For testing whole blood, 10 minutes after the application of the specimen remove the clotted blood from the tablet and compare the color of the tablet with the color chart.

   If acetone and acetoacetic acid are present, the tablet will show a color varying from lavender to deep purple. Report the results as negative, small, moderate, or large, as the manufacturer directs.

Sensitivity

Acetest detects 5 to 10 mg/dL of acetoacetic acid and 20 to 25 mg/dL of acetone.

Precautions, Interferences, Limitations

1. Tests based on a reaction with nitroprusside may give color reactions similar to those produced by acetoacetic acid and acetone in urine specimens containing phthaleins (Bromsulphalein, phenolsulfonphthalein), very large amounts of phenylketones, or the preservative 8-hydroxyquinoline.

2. The presence of various pigments, drugs, or substances causing abnormal highly colored urine specimens presents problems when reading ketone results. False-positive reactions may occur due to the formation of a color which may be interpreted as positive, or true-positive reactions may be masked in these urine specimens.

3. Low-level false-positive reactions may be seen in highly pigmented urine specimens or in specimens containing large amounts of levodopa metabolites.

4. False-positive reactions may be seen with 2-mercaptoethanesulfonic acid (mesna) or other compounds containing sulfhydryl groups. In this case, a positive reaction is seen initially, but the color fades to normal by the time specified for reading the color reaction. This interference is especially problematic when automatic reagent strip readers are employed as these instruments are programmed to read the various chemical reactions in a shorter time frame than is done with visual readings. If such interference is suspected, reagent strips should be checked visually, and the visual result reported. If the color persists and interference is still suspected, a drop of glacial acetic acid may be added to the test area on the reagent strip or the Acetest tablet. If the color is due to a sulfhydryl group, it will fade, whereas color due to diacetic acid will remain.

5. False-negative or reduced reactions might be seen in improperly stored specimens if acetoacetic acid is converted to acetone by bacterial action.

Gerhardt's Test for Acetoacetic Acid and Salicylates

Of the ketone bodies, Gerhardt's test is specific for diacetic acid; however, it is capable of detecting only large amounts of acetoacetic acid. Therefore any specimen giving a positive result in Gerhardt's test must also give a positive result in the various nitroprusside tests.

Gerhardt's test has been used as a means of determining the severity of ketosis. A positive result indicates severe ketosis, and treatment must be started immediately. For this reason, Gerhardt's test was performed whenever a positive reaction occurred with Rothera's test.

Rather than performing Gerhardt's test, a measure of the severity of ketosis may be obtained with reagent strip or tablet tests by diluting the original, concentrated specimen until a moderate result is obtained, as described above. For example, if the specimen required a 1:3 dilution for a moderate reaction, the result would be reported as: undiluted, large; 1:3 dilution, moderate. This method has virtually eliminated the need for Gerhardt's test in routine urinalysis. Gerhardt's test is included in this section because it is a simple test for salicylates in the urine and therefore can be used as an emergency test in case of aspirin overdose or poisoning. For this purpose, however, it is also being replaced by a commercial test, the Phenistix (Ames Division, Miles Laboratories, Inc., Elkhardt, IN) reagent strip test for phenylketones, which also reacts with metabolites of aspirin or other salicylates.

Procedure 13–8. Gerhardt's Test for Acetoacetic Acid and Salicylates

1. Place 5 mL of urine in a test tube. Add ferric chloride reagent dropwise until any precipitate of ferric phosphate dissolves. This generally takes only five to ten drops of ferric chloride, and ferric phosphate does not always precipitate.
2. Observe the color of the solution. If acetoacetic acid or salicylates are present, a red-brown to Bordeaux red color will develop.
3. To confirm the presence of acetoacetic acid, divide the test solution in half and boil one portion for 5 minutes. If the color disappears or becomes lighter after boiling, acetoacetic acid was present. If the color remains unchanged after boiling, salicylates are present.
4. Report the results as positive or negative for acetoacetic acid or salicylates.

Principle

Both acetoacetic acid and salicylates react with a 10-g/dL solution of ferric chloride ($FeCl_3$), forming a Bordeaux red color, as described in Procedure 13–8. Whenever a Bordeaux red color develops when ferric chloride is added to urine, the presence of acetoacetic acid or salicylates must be confirmed. As mentioned previously, acetoacetic acid is converted to acetone in the presence of heat. Gerhardt's test is specific for acetoacetic acid and does not detect acetone. Therefore, to confirm the presence of acetoacetic acid, the test solution is heated by boiling. After boiling, the Bordeaux color will not be present if acetoacetic acid was present in the urine. Since salicylates are unaffected by heat, the color will remain after boiling if the original specimen contained salicylates.

Reagent

The reagent is a 10-g/dL ferric chloride solution.

BILIRUBIN AND UROBILINOGEN

As mentioned earlier, the routine urinalysis is used to provide information concerning the state of the kidney and urinary tract, or other metabolic or systemic disorders. Tests for urine bilirubin and urobilinogen are used as indicators of the latter, in particular as indicators of liver function. In order to better understand this, the following information on normal liver function and the formation and excretion of bilirubin and urobilinogen is included.

Normal Liver Function

The liver is a large and complex organ, absolutely necessary for numerous body functions. The liver is responsible for many metabolic, storage, excretory, and detoxifying functions. More specifically, the liver is a major factor in the metabolism of carbohydrates, lipids, and proteins, in terms of both intermediary metabolism and the synthesis of many essential compounds. Many necessary enzymes and coenzymes for carbohydrate, lipid, and protein metabolism are present only in cells of the liver. Glycogen is formed, stored, and converted back to glucose in the liver. Energy derived from food is made available to the cells of the body through the process of glycolysis of the high energy bonds in adenosine triphosphate (ATP), which were formed by oxidative phosphorylation in the cells of the liver.

The liver is the site of detoxification of various substances. These toxic substances may be formed in normal body metabolism and converted or detoxified by the liver; an example is the formation of urea from the ammonia produced in protein metabolism. Toxic substances introduced into the blood from the intestine (such as dyes, heavy metals, and drugs) are excreted by the liver. The liver is essential in the formation and secretion of bile, bile pigments, and bile salts, which are necessary for digestion. These substances are derived from bilirubin, a major byproduct of the destruction of red blood cells. In addition, the liver is the site of formation and synthesis of many of the factors involved in the clotting of blood.

These important functions of the liver may be altered when the liver is diseased or damaged. Numerous laboratory tests are available to determine both the existence of liver disease and the extent, location, and type of damage so that appropriate treatment can be initiated. There is no one test that will give a complete clinical view of liver function; instead, a carefully selected group of tests may be requested by the physician depending on the process in question. These include tests for the presence and concentration of bilirubin in the blood and the urine.

Normal Formation and Excretion of Bilirubin and Urobilinogen

Bilirubin is a normal product resulting from the breakdown of red blood cells. Individual red blood cells do not exist indefinitely in the body; they are degraded after approximately 120 days. As part of red blood cell degradation, the heme portion of the hemoglobin molecule is converted to the bile pigment bilirubin by the *reticuloendothelial system (RES),* primarily by RES cells in the liver, spleen, and bone marrow. A total of approximately 6 g of hemoglobin is released each day as red blood cells are eliminated from the body. The cells of the RES first phagocytose the red cells, then convert the released hemoglobin through a complex series of reactions in which the heme portion of the molecule is finally converted to bilirubin. Bilirubin is a vivid yellow pigment.

An increase in the concentration of bilirubin in the blood indicates the presence of jaundice. Although it is useful in the bile, bilirubin is a waste product that must eventually be eliminated from the body. When it is formed by the RES cells, bilirubin is not soluble in water. Therefore it is transported from the RES cells through the blood to the liver cells as a bilirubin-albumin complex. This water-insoluble form of bilirubin is often referred to as *free* bilirubin or *unconjugated* bilirubin.

Bilirubin is normally excreted from the body by the liver by way of the intestine. It is excreted by the liver rather than the kidney because free bilirubin linked to albumin cannot pass through the glomerular capsule of the kidney. When free bilirubin reaches the liver, it is converted to a water-soluble product by the Kupffer cells of the liver. It is made soluble by conjugation with glucuronic acid and other hydrophilic substances to form bilirubin glucuronide.

Water-soluble bilirubin, often referred to as *conjugated* bilirubin, can be eliminated from the body by way of the kidney or the intestine. Normally, conjugated bilirubin is excreted by the liver into the bile, transported to the common bile duct and then to the gallbladder, where it is concentrated and emptied into the small intestine.

In the intestine, most of the bilirubin is converted to urobilinogen. Bilirubin is reduced to urobilinogen by the action of certain bacteria that make up the intestinal flora. Urobilinogen is actually a group of colorless chromogens, all of which are referred to as urobilinogen. Approximately half of the urobilinogen formed in the intestine is absorbed into the portal blood circulation and returned to the liver. In the liver, most of the urobilinogen is excreted into the bile once again and returned to the intestine.

A very small amount of urobilinogen escapes this liver clearance and is therefore excreted from the body by way of the urine. This represents only about 1% of the urobilinogen produced in 1 day. Urobilinogen in the intestine is either eliminated from the body unchanged or oxidized to the colored compound urobilin. Incidentally, urobilin is the substance that gives the feces their normal color. The net effect is that, in normal circumstances, 99% of the urobilinogen formed from bilirubin is eliminated by way of the feces.

It is therefore apparent that the urine normally contains only a very small amount of urobilinogen and no bilirubin. As mentioned, unconjugated bilirubin cannot be excreted by the kidney and is absent in urine. However, conjugated bilirubin can pass through the renal glomerulus, and if it is present in abnormal concentration in the blood, it will be excreted by the kidney.

Clinical Importance

Tests for urinary bilirubin and urobilinogen were formerly performed only when indicated by abnormal color of the urine or when liver disease or a hemolytic condition was suspected from the patient's history. Because they are part of most multiple reagent strips they are now included in the routine urinalysis. The presence of bilirubin in the urine is an early sign of liver cell disease (hepatocellular disease) and obstruction of the bile flow from the liver. It is especially useful in the early detection and monitoring of hepatitis, a highly infectious disease of particular importance to laboratory workers.

The presence of urobilinogen in the urine is increased in any condition that causes an increase in the production of bilirubin and any disease that prevents the liver from its normal function of returning urobilinogen to the intestine via the bile. The physician usually needs information about urinary bilirubin and urobilinogen in addition to serum bilirubin levels to determine the liver disorder or cause of jaundice. The clinical significance of these substances and laboratory tests for them are described in the following paragraphs.

Bilirubin

Clinical Significance

Tests for urinary bilirubin (along with urobilinogen) are important in the detection of liver disease and the determination of the cause of the clinical condition known as jaundice. Normally, there is no detectable bilirubin in the urine with even the most sensitive methods. However, finding even very small amounts of bilirubin in urine is important as it may be present in the earliest phases of liver disease. *Jaundice* is a condition that occurs when the serum bilirubin concentration becomes greater than normal and there is an abnormal accumulation of bilirubin in the body tissues. Since bilirubin is a vivid yellow pigment, its accumulation in the tissues results in yellow pigmentation of the skin, the sclera or white of the eyes, and the mucous membranes. The causes of jaundice are numerous and must be discovered as soon as possible so that treatment may be started.

There are several classifications of the various types of jaundice; one of them describes three types: prehepatic (hemolytic), hepatic (hepatocellular), and posthepatic (obstructive).

Hemolytic (Prehepatic) Jaundice.—*Prehepatic* jaundice is also known as *hemolytic* jaundice. It occurs in conditions where there is increased destruction of red cells—for instance, in infants with blood group incompatibilities, in neonatal physiologic jaundice, and in hemolytic anemias. The liver is basically normal, so there is an increased formation of conjugated bilirubin and subsequently of urobilinogen. While there is an increased concentration of urobilinogen in the stool, the liver cannot pick up or reexcrete the large amount of urobilinogen returned to it via the portal circulation. Therefore, more urobilinogen goes into the general blood circulation and is eliminated in the urine. In summary, prehepatic, or hemolytic, jaundice is characterized by increased free bilirubin in the blood and increased urobilinogen in the feces and urine. However, all the bilirubin that is conjugated by the liver goes into the intestine, where it is converted to urobilinogen, and no bilirubin is found in the urine.

Hepatocellular (Hepatic) Jaundice.—*Hepatic* jaundice is also known as *hepatocellular* jaundice. This type of jaundice is probably the most varied and difficult to understand. It results from conditions that involve the liver cells directly and prevent normal excretion. Such a condition might be specific damage such as conjugation failure in neonatal physiologic jaundice, where there is an enzyme deficiency. Diseases of conjugation failure result in an increased concentration of unconjugated bilirubin in the blood. Disturbances of the transport mechanisms by which conjugated bilirubin is passed into the bile canaliculi are characteristic of hepatocellular jaundice. Diffuse or overall hepatic cell involvement occurs in conditions such as viral hepatitis, toxic hepatitis caused by heavy metal or drug poisoning, and cirrhosis. In these cases the ability of the liver cells to remove and conjugate free bilirubin is decreased, resulting in increased amounts of free bilirubin in the blood. Bilirubin that is conjugated by the liver is not excreted into the bile, resulting in increased amounts of conjugated bilirubin in the blood, which can now be eliminated by the kidney.

Of the conjugated bilirubin that reaches the gut, urobilinogen is formed, half of which is absorbed into the portal circulation and returned to the liver for excretion. However, the diseased liver cells are unable to remove the urobilinogen which is then excreted in the urine. Thus urobilinogen in the urine is useful for the detection of early hepatitis; however, as the disease progresses to later stages, the liver is unable to form and pass conjugated bilirubin into the bile, so that the formation, reabsorption, and amount of urobilinogen in the urine are also decreased.

Obstructive (Posthepatic) Jaundice.—*Posthepatic* jaundice is also known as *obstructive* jaundice. This occurs when the common bile duct is obstructed by stones, tumors, spasms, or stricture. As a result, the conjugated bilirubin is regurgitated back into the liver sinusoids and the blood. If the blockage is sufficiently extensive, liver cell function may be impaired so that both free and conjugated bilirubin are found in the blood. The conjugated bilirubin will be excreted by the kidney and therefore found in the urine. Since conjugated bilirubin is unable to reach the intestine, no urobilinogen is formed and it is absent in the blood and urine. Since urobilinogen is not formed, urobilin is absent and the stools have a characteristic chalky white to light brown color.

Requirements for Testing

A chemical test for bilirubin should be included in the urinalysis when indicated on the basis of urine color or when requested by the physician. Urine containing bilirubin will typically have a yellow-brown color and produce a yellow foam when shaken. If only small amounts of bilirubin are present these signs may be lacking, or the urine may appear only slightly darker than normal. In addition, bilirubin is not stable in solution but will be oxidized to biliverdin, which is a green pigment. Thus, urine containing bilirubin will typically be yellow-brown when voided and will turn green or green-brown on standing, especially if exposed to light. Tests for bilirubin will not be positive when converted to biliverdin, so the urine must be examined when fresh.

Methods of Measurement

Several methods have been used to test for bilirubin in urine. One of the oldest laboratory methods is the foam test for bilirubin. It was used by the early Greeks to help determine the cause of jaundice. However, this method of simply shaking the urine and looking for the presence of a yellow foam is not sufficient today. Several chemical tests for bilirubin are available. Smith's test involves the use of tincture of iodine diluted with nine times its volume of alcohol. This reagent is overlaid on the urine, and the interface is observed for the presence of an emerald green ring. Gmelin's test makes use of fuming nitric acid, which may be combined with the urine in a number of ways. The results involve a play of colors; green and violet are associated with the presence of bilirubin. Harrison's test depends on precipitation of bilirubin with barium chloride and subsequent oxidation of the bilirubin to biliverdin with Fouchet's reagent. The formation of biliverdin gives the barium chloride a green color, which constitutes a positive reaction. The reagent strip and tablet tests which are routinely used to test for bilirubin are based on diazotization. A detailed description follows.

Reagent Strip Tests

Principle and Specificity.—The reagent strip tests for bilirubin are based on a diazo reaction. Bilirubin is coupled with a diazonium salt in an acid medium to form azobilirubin. A positive reaction is seen as the formation of a colored compound. The tests differ in the diazonium salt used, and thus the color produced. Although specific for bilirubin, false-positive reactions are seen in situations where there are other highly colored pigments in the urine. This is especially true when metabolites of drugs such as phenazopyridine are present which give the gross urine specimen a characteristic vivid red-orange color which might be mistaken for bilirubin and mask or give atypical color reactions on the reagent strip.

Contents of Reagent Strips and Results

Multistix.—The Ames reagent strips for bilirubin use a 2,4-dichloroanilinediazonium salt buffered to an acid pH. The formation of azobilirubin is seen as a brownish to purplish color. Results are read as small (+), moderate (++), or large (+++) by careful comparison with the color chart provided.

Chemstrip.—The Chemstrip reagent strips for bilirubin use 2,6-dichlorobenzene-diazonium-tetra fluoroborate which is buffered to an acid pH. This reacts with bilirubin to form a red-violet azo dye which is seen as a color change from white to beige-pink or light red-violet. Results are also read as small (+), moderate (++), or large (+++) by careful comparison with the color chart provided. According to the manufacturer, even the slightest pink color represents a positive (significant) result.

Sensitivity.—Multistix will detect 0.4 to 0.8 mg/dL bilirubin. Chemstrip will detect 0.5 mg/dL bilirubin.

Precautions, Interferences, Limitations.—As for all reagent strips, observe the precautions and follow the instructions supplied by the manufacturer and as described in Procedure 13–3. Report results as established for your laboratory.

1. The reagent strip tests for bilirubin are difficult to read and the color formed after reaction with urine must be carefully compared with the color chart supplied by the manufacturer. Proficiency in reading these results comes with experience and is essential for reliable results. Many negative urine specimens as well as specimens containing varying amounts of bilirubin should be tested to gain experience and proficiency. In addition, control specimens that are positive for bilirubin should be tested daily to maintain proficiency.

2. Since the reagent strip tests are significantly less sensitive for bilirubin than the Ictotest tablet test or oxidation methods such as Harrison's test, it may be necessary to routinely test all urine specimens suspected of containing bilirubin, but which are negative with the reagent strip tests, with a more sensitive method.

3. Since colors are difficult to interpret, it has been recommended that all positive reactions with reagent strips be confirmed with another method, such as the Ictotest tablet test.

4. Atypical colors, which are unlike any of the color blocks, may indicate that other bile pigments derived from bilirubin are present in the urine and may be masking the bilirubin reaction. This may indicate bile pigment abnormalities and the urine specimen should be tested with a more sensitive test, such as the Ictotest. Large amounts of urobilinogen may affect the color reaction but not enough to give a positive result.

5. False-positive tests for bilirubin may occur in any situation where substances are present which color the urine red or which turn red in an acid medium. These include urine specimens from patients who have received large doses of phenothiazine or chlorpromazine or from metabolites of phenazopyridine (Pyridium) or ethoxazene (Serenium). Unfortunately, the presence of these highly pigmented compounds may be mistaken for bilirubin in the gross urine specimen, and may mask the reaction of small amounts of bilirubin.

6. A yellow-orange to red color may be seen with indican (indoxyl sulfate). This can result in false-negative or false-positive readings.

7. Urine specimens must be tested when absolutely fresh as bilirubin is rapidly oxidized to biliverdin, especially when exposed to ultraviolet light. Since the test is specific for bilirubin, this oxidation will result in low or false-negative results.

8. As with all diazo reactions, the presence of an ascorbic acid concentration of 25 mg/dL or greater may cause false-negative reactions.

9. Elevated nitrite concentration as seen in urinary tract infection may decrease sensitivity.

Ictotest Tablet Test

Principle and Specificity.—The Ictotest tablet test (Ames Division, Miles Laboratories, Inc., Elkhart, IN), is used as a confirmatory test for bilirubin when positive results are seen on the reagent strip, or in any condition in which bilirubin is suspected (see Procedure 13–9). It is more sensitive to bilirubin than either of the reagent strip tests. Ictotest is typical of various tests that use diazo compounds to demonstrate the presence of bilirubin as azobilirubin. The tablets are supplied with a special mat. Urine is placed on the mat, the liquid portion is absorbed, and the bilirubin remains on the outer surface of the mat. The tablet contains the reactive ingredients. When bilirubin is present, it reacts with a solid diazonium salt, resulting in a blue or purple color. Other ingredients in the tablet provide the proper pH and ensure solution of the tablet when water is added, so that the reaction can take place.

Contents of the Ictotest Tablet.—The Ictotest tablet contains 2,4-dichlorobenzenediazonium tetrachlorozincate and sulfosalicylic acid.

Sensitivity.—Ictotest will detect as little as 0.05 to 0.1 mg/dL bilirubin. This is more sensitive than either reagent strip test.

Precautions, Interferences, Limitations

1. Precautions and interferences are generally the same as for the reagent strips, as the principle of all products is the same. Large amounts of ascorbic acid may suppress results and the presence of vivid pigments may mask or cause false-positive results.

Procedure 13–9. Ictotest Tablet Test for Bilirubin

Observe the precautions and follow the instructions supplied by the manufacturer.

1. Place ten drops of urine on the center of either side of the special test mat supplied with the reagent tablets.
2. Place the Ictotest tablet in the center of the moistened area. Do not touch the tablet with your hands.
3. Place one drop of water onto the tablet. Wait 5 seconds, then place a second drop of water onto the tablet so that the water runs off the tablet onto the mat.
4. Observe the mat around the tablet for the appearance of a blue to purple color at 60 seconds.
5. Report the result as positive or negative according to the following criteria:
   Negative: The mat shows no blue or purple within 60 seconds. Ignore any color that forms after 60 seconds, or a slight pink or red that may appear.
   Positive: The mat around the tablet turns blue or purple within 60 seconds. Ignore any color change on the tablet itself.

---

2. Be sure to use the special mat provided. Either side may be used.

3. Observe the reaction at the time stated (60 seconds) since a confusing pink color may appear after this time.

4. The tablet must begin to dissolve, and water flow from the tablet to the mat for the reaction to occur.

5. It may be necessary to move or remove the tablet from the mat when reading results.

6. Tablets must be protected from exposure to light, heat, and ambient moisture. Deterioration is seen by a tan to brown discoloration of the tablet.

Urobilinogen

Clinical Significance

Urobilinogen is a byproduct of red blood cell degradation and results from intestinal reduction of bilirubin. Increased destruction of red cells may be accompanied by large amounts of urobilinogen in the urine. Therefore,

urobilinogen will be seen in conditions such as various hemolytic anemias, pernicious anemia, and malaria. In the absence of increased red cell destruction, the tests may be considered liver function tests. One of the first effects of liver damage is impairment of the mechanism for removing urobilinogen from the blood circulation and excreting it through the intestine. This results in removal of urobilinogen by the kidney and its presence in the urine. Tests for urinary urobilinogen are thus useful for the early detection of liver damage. Urobilinogen is found in the urine in conditions such as infectious hepatitis, toxic hepatitis, portal cirrhosis, congestive heart failure, and infectious mononucleosis.

Normally, 1% of all the urobilinogen produced is excreted in the urine and 99% is excreted in the feces. However, under certain conditions urobilinogen is completely absent from the urine and the feces. When the normal intestinal bacterial flora are destroyed, as by antibiotic therapy, urobilinogen cannot be produced. Urobilinogen is also absent if the liver does not conjugate bilirubin, or if there is biliary tract obstruction, such as from gallstones, resulting in failure of conjugated bilirubin to reach the intestinal tract.

Requirements for Testing

Tests for urobilinogen have become routine since their inclusion in multiple reagent strips. Urine should certainly be tested for urobilinogen when requested by the physician or whenever its presence is suspected on the basis of abnormal urine color. Urine containing urobilinogen will often show a characteristic orange-red or orange-brown color because of the presence of urobilin. Whenever a test for bilirubin is performed, a test for urobilinogen should also be done.

It is particularly necessary to use a fresh urine specimen when testing for urobilinogen, since it is unusually unstable and is rapidly oxidized to urobilin. This oxidation takes place so readily that most urine specimens that contain urobilinogen will show an abnormal color caused by partial oxidation to urobilin. The presence of urobilinogen and that of urobilin have the same clinical significance; however, they take part in different chemical reactions, and urine is more frequently tested for urobilinogen. Normally, 1 to 4 mg of urobilinogen is excreted in the urine each day. This is less than 1 Ehrlich unit* in each 2-hour urine collection period.

*The Ehrlich unit is a traditional measure of urobilinogen activity; 1 Ehrlich unit is equivalent to 1 mg/dL of urobilinogen.

Porphobilinogen

Another substance that is related to urobilinogen is **porphobilinogen.** The porphyrins are a group of compounds that are utilized in the synthesis of hemoglobin. The heme portion of hemoglobin is a type of porphyrin, namely ferroprotoporphyrin 9. In normal persons, porphyrins are eliminated from the body in the urine and feces, mainly as coproporphyrin I with a small amount of coproporphyrin III. However, certain errors of porphyrin metabolism lead to increased excretion of other porphyrins in the urine. These conditions are collectively called porphyrias, and in some of them porphobilinogen is present in the urine. The Watson-Schwartz test, which is described here as a test for urobilinogen, will also detect porphobilinogen.

Methods of Measurement

Tests for urobilinogen have traditionally employed **Ehrlich's aldehyde reaction** which is based on the formation of a characteristic cherry-red color when urobilinogen reacts with Ehrlich's reagent. In the reaction, urobilinogen, together with porphobilinogen and other Ehrlich-reactive compounds, reacts with *p*-dimethylaminobenzaldehyde in concentrated hydrochloric acid to form a colored aldehyde. This reaction is the basis of the test for urobilinogen on the Ames reagent strips and the Watson-Schwartz test which will be described in detail. An inverse Ehrlich's aldehyde reaction is the basis of the Hoesch test which is used for the detection of porphobilinogen in urine.

The Chemstrip reagent strips employ a different principle for the measurement of urobilinogen. They use a diazo reaction that results in the formation of a red azo dye. This reaction is specific for urobilinogen. Intermediate Ehrlich-reactive compounds and porphobilinogen are not detectable.

Reagent Strip Tests

Principle and Specificity.—As discussed above, the reagent strip tests for urobilinogen differ in basic principle and specificity.

The reagent strips manufactured by Ames have test areas for urobilinogen based on the Ehrlich reaction in which *p*-dimethylaminobenzaldehyde reacts with urobilinogen in a strongly acidic medium to form a colored aldehyde. However, the test is not specific for urobilinogen and reacts with substances known to react with Ehrlich's reagent. These substances include porphobilinogen, and various intermediate Ehrlich-reactive substances

such as sulfonamides, *p*-aminosalicylic acid, procaine, and 5-hydroxyindoleacetic acid. Therefore, urine specimens that give a positive reaction with these reagent strips should be confirmed with tests such as the Watson-Schwartz test, the Hoesch test, or with reagent strips such as Chemstrip, which are specific for urobilinogen.

The Chemstrip reagent strips for urobilinogen utilize a diazonium salt which reacts with urobilinogen in an acidic medium to form a red azo dye. The strips react with both urobilinogen and stercobilinogen. However, differentiation between these two substances is not diagnostically important as stercobilinogen is found in feces, not urine. Porphobilinogen and other Ehrlich-reactive substances are not detected with this procedure. This is helpful, as many interfering Ehrlich-reactive substances are commonly encountered in routine urinalysis. However, the existence of unsuspected or undiagnosed porphyria would be missed completely with this test.

Contents of Reagent Strips and Results

Multistix, Urobilistix (Ames).—The Multistix reagent strips utilize *p*-dimethylaminobenzaldehyde in an acidic medium. Results are seen as the formation of a red or reddish-brown color which varies with the amount of urobilinogen present. After a timed interval, the color is compared with a graded color chart. Results are reported in Ehrlich units (EU): 1 mg/dL urine is approximately 1 EU. Results that compare with 0.2 or 1.0 EU are reported as normal rather than negative, as the presence of up to 1 EU is found in normal urine specimens. The absence of urobilinogen is not detectable with this method. The Multistix and Urobilistix are formulated slightly differently and the appropriate color chart must be used.

Chemstrip.—The Chemstrip reagent strips are impregnated with the diazonium salt 4-methoxybenzene-diazonium-tetrafluoroborate in an acid medium. Results are seen as the formation of a red azo dye which is compared with a color chart which gives values in milligrams per deciliter. These are equivalent to Ehrlich units. As with the Ames strips, results are reported as normal rather than negative. Values up to 1 mg/dL are considered normal. The absence of urobilinogen is not detectable.

Sensitivity.—Multistix and Urobilistix will detect 0.2 mg/dL urobilinogen (approximately 0.2 EU/dL) in urine. The absence of urobilinogen cannot be determined. Chemstrip will detect 0.4 mg/dL urobilinogen. The absence of urobilinogen cannot be determined.

Precautions, Interferences, Limitations.—Observe the precautions and follow the instructions supplied by the manufacturer and as described in Procedure 13–3.

1. It is extremely important that fresh urine specimens be tested because urobilinogen is very unstable when exposed to room temperature or daylight. If it is not tested within an hour of voiding, the specimen should be refrigerated. Urine preservatives should not be used, as they may interfere. For example, formalin may be the cause of false-negative results with both tests. Urobilinogen, a colorless compound, is rapidly oxidized to urobilin, an orange-red pigment, which is not detected with either reagent strip test.

2. Interferences with the Ames reagent strips are generally those for the Watson-Schwartz test, e.g., sulfonamides, *p*-aminosalicylic acid, procaine, and 5-hydroxyindolacetic acid.

3. Both strips are affected by highly colored pigments or their metabolites in the urine specimen. These include ethoxazene, drugs containing azo dyes, nitrofurantoin, and riboflavin. Atypical color reactions may also be seen with high concentrations of *p*-aminobenzoic acid.

4. Interferences with the Chemstrip reagent strips are generally those for the reagent strip tests for bilirubin, namely substances which interfere with the diazo reaction such as ascorbic acid, nitrite, or highly colored pigments.

5. With both tests, the absence of urobilinogen is not detectable.

6. The normal urobilinogen concentration in urine is approximately 0.2 to 1.0 mg/dL. A result of 2 mg/dL may or may not be abnormal and requires further evaluation.

7. Although porphobilinogen may be detected with the Ames reagent strips, it is not a reliable method for the detection of porphobilinogen.

8. Porphobilinogen is not detectable with the Chemstrip reagent strips.

9. The presence of intermediate Ehrlich-reactive substances is a problem in any test based on the Ehrlich reaction. Thus, a combination of reagent strips with confirmation by the Hoesch test and Watson-Schwartz test is helpful in establishing the presence of abnormal concentrations of urobilinogen.

Ehrlich's Qualitative Aldehyde Reaction for Urobilinogen and Porphobilinogen (Watson-Schwartz Test)

Principle and Specificity.—The Watson-Schwartz test is used as a confirmatory test for the detection and differentiation of urobilinogen, porphobilinogen, and intermediate Ehrlich-reactive compounds, as described in Procedure 13–10. Ehrlich's aldehyde reaction occurs with urobilinogen but not with urobilin. Therefore, absolutely fresh urine is necessary for this test. In the presence of Ehrlich's reagent, urobilinogen gives a characteristic cherry-red color. This color is the result of the reaction of *p*-dimethylaminobenzaldehyde in concentrated hydrochloric acid with urobilinogen and porphobilinogen to form a colored aldehyde. The color is enhanced in the presence of saturated sodium acetate, which also inhibits color formation by skatoles and indoles, which might be present in the urine. However, porphobilinogen and certain intermediate Ehrlich-reactive compounds give the same cherry-red color with Ehrlich's reagent and sodium acetate and must be distinguished from urobilinogen. To do this, the test solution is extracted with the organic solvents chloroform and butanol. Urobilinogen is soluble in both solvents, porphobilinogen is not soluble in either,

TABLE 13–4.

Results of Watson-Schwartz Test

Result	Ehrlich's Reagent Plus Sodium Acetate	Chloroform Extract	Butanol Extract
Negative	No pink color		
Urobilinogen	Pink	Pink	Pink
Porphobilinogen	Pink	Colorless	Colorless
Intermediate Ehrlich-reactive compounds	Pink	Colorless	Pink

Procedure 13–10. Watson-Schwartz Test for Urobilinogen and Porphobilinogen

1. Place 1 volume (approximately 3 mL) of urine in a test tube. Add an equal volume of Ehrlich's reagent. Mix well by inversion.
2. Add 2 volumes of saturated sodium acetate and mix. A red or deep pink (cherry-red) color is a positive result and indicates the presence of urobilinogen, porphobilinogen, or other Ehrlich-reactive compounds. If the test is positive at this stage, split the colored solution into two parts, and continue with step 3.
3. Add a few milliliters of chloroform to one portion of the colored solution and shake vigorously. Observe whether the color is completely extracted into the lower chloroform layer. Extract the colored solution with chloroform as many times as is necessary. If the color is caused by urobilinogen, it will be extracted into the chloroform layer. Color caused by porphobilinogen or an intermediate Ehrlich-reactive compound will not be extracted by chloroform.
4. If the color is not extracted by chloroform, extract the other portion of the colored solution with a few milliliters of butanol to distinguish porphobilinogen from intermediate Ehrlich-reactive compounds. Color caused by urobilinogen or intermediate Ehrlich-reactive compounds will be extracted into the upper butanol layer.
5. Report the results as positive or negative for urobilinogen, positive for porphobilinogen, or positive for both urobilinogen and porphobilinogen (very rare). Do not report the finding of intermediate Ehrlich-reactive compounds.

---

and intermediate Ehrlich-reactive compounds are soluble in butanol but not in chloroform (Table 13–4).

Reagents

1. Ehrlich's reagent. Combine 0.7 g of *p*-dimethylaminobenzaldehyde, 150 mL of concentrated hydrochloric acid, and 100 mL of deionized water.
2. Saturated sodium acetate in deionized water.

3. Chloroform.
4. Butanol.

Precautions, Interferences, Limitations

1. Fresh urine should be cooled to room temperature before the test is carried out to prevent the "warm aldehyde" reaction. This is a weak Ehrlich reaction that takes place at body temperature with a chromogen (probably indoxyl) that is present in normal urine.
2. The sodium acetate solution must be saturated for complete color enhancement. To ensure saturation, there should be a layer of undissolved crystals on the bottom of stock and working reagent bottles.
3. Sulfonamides, procaine, 5-hydroxyindoleacetic acid, and other compounds are intermediate compounds which may make interpretation of the test difficult.
4. In patients receiving methyldopa (Aldomet), a strong color reaction is often observed. However, unlike the situation with porphobilinogen, there is an approximately equal distribution of the pink or red color between the aqueous and butanol layers.

Hoesch Test for Porphobilinogen

Principle.—This is a confirmatory test for porphobilinogen. It may be used to confirm results with the Watson-Schwartz test, or to confirm results when a positive Ames reagent strip test is seen together with a negative reaction on Chemstrip which is specific for urobilinogen.

The test is based on an inverse Ehrlich's aldehyde reaction in which an acid solution is maintained by adding a small volume of urine to a relatively large volume of Ehrlich's reagent (see Procedure 13–11).

Reagents

1. Hydrochloric acid 6 mol/L. Make a 1:2 dilution of concentrated hydrochloric acid in deionized or distilled water.
2. Hoesch reagent. Dissolve 2.0 g *p*-dimethylaminobenzaldehyde in 6 mol/L HCl and dilute to 100 mL.

Sensitivity.—The Hoesch test will detect about 2.0 to 10 mg/dL of porphobilinogen. This is similar to the Watson-Schwartz test. It is, however, specific for porphobilinogen.

Procedure 13–11. Hoesch Test for Porphobilinogen

1. Pour approximately 2 mL of Hoesch reagent into a test tube.
2. Add two drops of well-mixed urine.
3. Observe for the appearance of an instantaneous cherry-red or bright-red color which appears on top of the solution. Agitate briefly, and look for a light to bright pink throughout the test tube.
4. Report results as positive or negative for porphobilinogen.

Precautions, Interferences, Limitations

1. A quantitative porphobilinogen test is necessary when either the Watson-Schwartz or Hoesch test is questionable.

2. Although the sensitivity is similar to the Watson-Schwartz test, it has been reported that the Watson-Schwartz test is more sensitive than the Hoesch test for porphobilinogen.

3. False-positive reactions have been reported with large doses of methyldopa, with indoles in some patients with intestinal ileus, and in the presence of phenazopyridine.

4. Very large quantities of urobilinogen (over 20 mg/dL) are needed to give a positive reaction; therefore, urobilinogen does not pose a practical problem.

5. Urosein, a pigment related to indoleacetic acid, may produce a rose color in response to strong HCl which may be confused with a positive porphobilinogen result. Such interference may be ruled out by separately testing the specimen in question with 6 mol/L HCl, along with the Hoesch reagent.

Schlesinger's Test for Urinary Urobilin

Principle.—Urobilin is an oxidation product of urobilinogen. Urobilin is colored and urobilinogen is colorless. Both compounds have the same clinical significance when present in urine; however, they undergo different chemical reactions (see Procedure 13–12).

Reagent.—The reagent used in this test is a saturated alcohol solution of zinc acetate.

Procedure 13–12. Schlesinger's Test for Urobilin

1. Mix equal parts of urine and alcohol–zinc acetate in a test tube. Filter the mixture.
2. Examine the filtrate for green fluorescence by viewing the tube from above as it is passed through the direct rays of a fairly strong light (e.g., Wood's light).
3. Report as positive or negative.

Quantitative Determination of Urinary Urobilinogen

Quantitative determinations of urinary urobilinogen are very similar to Ehrlich's qualitative aldehyde reaction. In the quantitative determination the reagents are measured volumetrically and the degree of color formation is measured with a photometer. One difference between this and other quantitative tests is related to the freshness of the specimen. Because urobilinogen is so rapidly oxidized to urobilin, it is impossible to employ a complete 24-hour urine collection. Instead, a complete 2-hour collection is used. A specimen collected between 1 and 3 P.M. is preferred, since excretion of urobilinogen is highest during this period. The test must be performed within 30 minutes of collection because of the instability of urobilinogen. In addition, specimens must be protected from sunlight and other sources of intense heat. Therefore, they are collected in brown bottles and stored under refrigeration.

ASCORBIC ACID

Clinical Significance

Although ascorbic acid is not a normal constituent of urine, it is sometimes present. It is different from the constituents that are commonly tested for and have been described up to now. Most of the substances tested for in urine are either abnormal constituents or constituents that are present in abnormal concentrations and are the result of metabolic processes within the body. These substances must be detected because their presence in the urine reflects pathologic conditions. Ascorbic acid is not such a substance (although its presence in urine may result in a tendency to kidney stone formation in some persons). Its presence in the urine is important because of the interfering effect it has on other chemical tests, especially the reagent strip tests for glucose and blood that depend on the release of hydrogen peroxide by peroxidase. Although the manufacturers of these products continue to make modifications to reduce the inhibitory effect of ascorbic acid, it remains a problem.

Inhibiting quantities of ascorbic acid are found in the urine of patients who have ingested large quantities of vitamin C or who are receiving medications, such as intravenous antibiotics, which contain vitamin C. Quantities of vitamin C in excess of those required by the body for normal function are quickly eliminated through the urine.

The interfering effect of ascorbic acid results from its action as a strong reducing agent. In reagent strip tests for glucose and blood, hydrogen peroxide is used to oxidize a chromogen from a reduced form to a colored oxidized form. Ascorbic acid interferes by reducing the released hydrogen peroxide to water, preventing or delaying the desired oxidation of the chromogen indicator. These reactions are summarized below:

Desired reaction with peroxidase:

$$H_2O_2 + \text{reduced chromogen} \longrightarrow$$
(Released through peroxidase activity

$$\text{oxidized chromogen} + H_2O$$
(colored)

Effect of ascorbic acid:

$$H_2O_2 + \text{ascorbic acid} \longrightarrow$$
(reduced form)

$$\text{dehydroascorbic acid} + H_2O$$
(oxidized form)

As discussed previously, ascorbic acid will also interfere with the various reagent strip tests which are based on the diazo reaction. In these tests, the ascorbic acid may react with the diazonium salt which is formed, causing a reduced or false-negative reaction.

The presence of ascorbic acid in the urine may be suspected when a reagent strip test for blood is negative although the urinary sediment shows the presence of red cells. It may also be suspected when reagent strip tests for glucose on urine specimens from diabetic patients give inconsistent results, showing negative or reduced reactions even though the tests for ketones and the copper reduction tests for sugar are positive. In such cases ascorbic acid may be confirmed by a reagent strip test specific for ascorbic acid. If this is not available, a clinical history of ingestion of large doses of ascorbic acid, or retesting a urine specimen which is voided at least 10 hours after the last administration of vitamin C, may suffice.

Reagent Strip Test for Ascorbic Acid (Merckoquant) Principle and Specificity

No Ames or Chemstrip reagent strips are available which test for ascorbic acid. Ames previously produced an ascorbic acid strip, but it has been discontinued. Both companies maintain that they have minimized interference from ascorbic acid and thus test strips are not necessary. However, some institutions still find the presence of ascorbic acid troublesome. Therefore, we will describe one strip which is available, namely, the Merckoquant ascorbic acid test (available from E. Merck, Darmstadt, Federal Republic of Germany).

The Merckoquant strips are intended for the semiquantitative determination of ascorbic acid in foodstuffs, such as fruit and vegetable juices and in wine. However, they may be used to test urine for ascorbic acid by default, without reagent strips intended for urine. The reaction is based on the reduction by ascorbic acid of phosphomolybdate, a yellow complex, to molybdenum blue. The reaction is not specific for ascorbic acid but will react with other reducing substances.

Results are read by comparison with a color chart in milligrams per liter. This may require conversion to other units (i.e., mg/dL).

URINARY SEDIMENT

Urinary sediment refers to all solid materials suspended in the urine specimen. Very few urine specimens are absolutely clear, and even those that appear clear to the naked eye have some solid material suspended in them. In addition, many urine specimens obviously contain solid material, as evidenced by their cloudiness. Any amount of cloudiness that is visible to the naked eye must be accounted for in a microscopic analysis of the urinary sediment. The solid material present in urine specimens may be identified only under the microscope, and a microscopic examination of the urinary sediment is essential in any routine urinalysis. It may be the most important part of the urinalysis.

However, the examination of the urinary sediment is not a simple procedure, nor is it inexpensive. It requires well-trained, skilled, knowledgeable personnel, and it is time-consuming. Personnel need to be skilled in the use of the microscope, and aware of the various microscopic techniques and other aids that are helpful in identifying the various components of the urinary sediment that may be encountered. This includes an understanding of the clinical correlation or significance of the various elements of the urinary sediment. For all of these reasons, together with the need for cost containment in health care, it has been suggested that the microscopic analysis of the urinary sediment is not necessarily a part of every routine urinalysis. Rather, various protocols have been devised which call for the microscopic analysis only when abnormal findings are seen in the physical and chemical analysis of the urine, or when indicated by the patient's condition or clinical history. In this discussion, however, we assume that the microscopic analysis of the urine sediment is part of every routine urinalysis.

When the urinary sediment is to be examined, a concentrated portion of the urine is used rather than a well-mixed specimen. The sediment is concentrated before examination to ensure detection of less abundant constituents. To concentrate the sediment, a well-mixed, measured portion of urine is centrifuged. The clear supernatant is decanted and the solid material, which settles to the bottom during centrifugation, is examined under the microscope (the supernatant may be further tested for chemical constituents, such as urinary protein). The various parts of the sediment are identified and counted to give semiquantitative results. For these results to have any meaning, a constant amount of urine must be centrifuged and a constant volume of supernatant removed. Urine is therefore centrifuged in a graduated centrifuge tube. Results in this section are based on centrifuging exactly 12 mL of urine and removing exactly 11 mL of supernatant, leaving 1 mL of sediment for examination under the microscope. The actual volume used may be

different, but it must be consistent within each laboratory.

Various aids to the standardization of the preparation and examination of the urinary sediment are available. These include specially designed graduated centrifuge tubes with special devices or pipettes which allow for the easy decanting of the supernatent urine and retention of an exact volume of undisturbed concentrated urinary sediment. The sediment may be examined with a traditional glass microscope slide and coverglass, or specially designed slides of plastic or Plexiglas with wells or applied coverglasses may be used. Systems vary in the volume of urine to be concentrated, volume of sediment examined, number of tests per slide, slide chamber volume, depth of the test chamber, and type of coverglass material. These systems include the KOVA system (ICL Scientific, Fountain Valley, CA), the UriSystem (Fisher Scientific, Pittsburgh, PA), and the Count-10 system (V-Tech, Inc., Palm Desert, CA)

The urinary sediment consists of a great variety of material. Some of the constituents are normal, while others are abnormal and represent serious conditions. It is important to learn to identify both the normal and abnormal constituents. In general, the normal constituents are more easily seen under the microscope, and must be recognized so that they do not obscure the presence of the less obvious but more serious abnormal constituents. Recognition of the abnormal constituents is extremely important in the diagnosis and treatment of various renal diseases. They often give information about the state of the kidney and the urinary tract. In addition, the microscopic analysis of the sediment will help to confirm and account for findings in the chemical examination of the urine. For example, protein in the urine is often associated with the presence of **casts** and cellular elements in the sediment.

Urine Specimen Requirements

Type of Specimen

Although any freely voided collection is acceptable, the ideal specimen for microscopic analysis of the urinary sediment is a fresh, voided, first morning specimen. A first morning specimen is preferable since it is the most concentrated, and therefore small amounts of abnormal constituents are more likely to be detected. In addition, the formed elements are less likely to disintegrate in more concentrated urine.

Preservation

A fresh urine specimen is particularly important for reliable results. If the urine cannot be examined shortly after it is voided, it should be refrigerated. If it must be kept in the refrigerator for more than a few hours, a chemical preservative should be added. Formalin may be used as a preservative that will fix the various formed elements. However, it interferes with chemical tests. Other preservatives, such as toluene, may be used to prevent bacterial contamination. None of the preservatives are completely satisfactory, and fresh collections are definitely preferred. If preservatives that may interfere with various chemical tests are added, it is advisable to split the well-mixed specimen so that the sediment constituents are preserved, yet the chemical constituents are not affected.

Changes After Voiding

Changes that may occur as the urine stands include the following: Red blood cells become distorted because of the lack of an isotonic solution. They either swell or become crenated which makes them difficult to recognize, and they finally disintegrate. White blood cells also disintegrate in hypotonic solutions. Casts disintegrate, especially as the urine becomes alkaline, since they must have sufficient acidity and solute concentration to exist. Other components that are found only in acidic urine will disappear as the urine becomes alkaline. The increase in alkalinity results from the growth of bacteria and production of ammonia. Finally, bacteria multiply rapidly, obscuring various components.

Protection From Contamination

In addition to being a fresh first morning collection, the urine specimen should be clean and free of external contamination. This is sometimes a problem, especially with female patients, since vaginal contamination will result in the presence of epithelial cells, red cells, and white cells. In such cases it may be necessary to use a clean voided midstream specimen, which is also required for quantitative urine culture. It may also be necessary to pack the vagina or use a tampon in some cases to avoid vaginal contamination.

Urine Sediment Examination Techniques

Traditionally, the urinary sediment has been examined microscopically by placing a drop of urine on a microscope slide, applying a coverglass, and observing the preparation under the low-power ($\times 10$) and high-power ($\times 40$) objective of a brightfield microscope. Since the preparation is a wet mount, oil immersion cannot be used in this examination. When the sediment is examined with brightfield illumination, correct light adjustment is essential. The light must be sufficiently reduced, by correct positioning of the condenser and use of the iris diaphragm, to give contrast between the unstained structures and the background liquid. As described in Chapter 3 the condenser should be left in a generally uppermost position, at most only 1 or 2 mm below the specimen, and the desired contrast achieved by opening or closing the iris diaphragm. The condenser should not be "racked down." The correct light adjustment requires care and experience. Because of the difficulty of this traditional examination, various techniques have been developed and are described.

Microscopic Techniques

Brightfield Microscopy.—As mentioned above, this is the traditional method of observation of the urinary sediment. It is also the most difficult. Correct light adjustment is essential, and various translucent elements that may occur in the urine sediment are easily overlooked with this technique. Of particular difficulty are hyaline casts, mucous threads, and various cells. If only a brightfield microscope is available, the use of a suitable stain is encouraged. It should also be mentioned that certain constituents, such as crystals and pigmented casts, are best visualized with brightfield illumination.

Phase-contrast Microscopy.—Phase-contrast microscopy is useful in the examination of unstained urinary sediment, particularly for delineating translucent elements such as hyaline casts and mucous threads, which have a refractive index similar to that of the urine in which they are suspended. Some laboratories use a phase-contrast microscope for the routine examination of the urinary sediment. However, some elements are better visualized with brightfield, and the microscopist must be able to change from phase to brightfield with ease. For example, pigmented blood and red cell casts are better identified with brightfield microscopy where their characteristic color is easily recognized and aids in identification.

Interference Contrast Microscopy.—This is also useful in the examination of unstained urinary sediment, but it is expensive and therefore not used routinely. Since it gives an apparently three-dimensional view of the object being observed, inclusions such as granules or vacuoles within a cell or cast can be better visualized. Besides increasing contrast, the geometric shape is observable.

Polarizing Microscopy.—Polarized light, with or without a full-wave retardation plate (first-order red filter), may be used to study substances that polarize (bend or rotate) light when viewed with polarizing filters. Such birefringent bodies include various crystals and fat globules. Polarizing filters show the typical Maltese cross appearance (a light cross against a dark background) of anisotropic, doubly refractive fat globules (cholesterol), whether as free-floating fat in the urine, within oval fat bodies, or in fatty casts. Starch granules also polarize as a Maltese cross, but are easily identified with brightfield illumination and should not be confused with fat. Polarizing microscopy may also be useful in telling amorphous urates or phosphates from certain cocci (bacteria), and an unusual ovoid form of calcium oxalate from red blood cells. It may also help distinguish certain fibers from waxy casts.

Filters.—Filters can also aid in the examination of the urinary sediment. A colored filter placed over the microscope light source can help bring out details in various structures in the unstained sediment. The filter used should be of a color complementary to the detail being studied. A green filter is especially useful for the observation of cells and casts.

Staining Techniques

Various staining techniques may be used to increase contrast and therefore visualize various components in the urinary sediment. They are especially useful in enhancing cellular detail, either free or within casts. They are also useful in accentuating many, although not all, casts. Several stains are described, although the stain most often used for routine urinary sediment examination is a crystal violet and safranin stain, as described by Sternheimer and Malbin.

Acetic Acid.—Although not really a stain, acetic acid may be useful in differentiating white blood cells from red blood cells. A 2% solution of acetic acid may be added to a few drops of sediment in a test tube, or

flowed under the coverglass of a mounted urine sediment. The acetic acid will accentuate the nucleus of leukocytes and epithelial cells and lyse red cells. Also, certain crystals that are sometimes present in urine will be dissolved or converted to other forms by acetic acid.

Methylene Blue.—Also known as Löffler's solution, this is used to visualize the cellular structures of bacteria.

Crystal Violet and Safranin (Sternheimer-Malbin Stain).—This stain is useful in the identification of cellular elements. It is an all-purpose stain which is quick and easy to use. It is available as Sedistain (Clay Adams, division of Becton-Dickinson & Co., Parsippany, NJ) and KOVA stain (ICL Scientific, Fountain Valley, CA). The staining reactions of the various cellular elements that may be encountered are supplied by the manufacturer and available on package inserts. It is recommended that both stained and unstained sediment be mounted and observed, as the stain may cause precipitation of some constituents. This is especially a problem with alkaline urine specimens. In these cases the precipitated background material may obscure important pathologic constituents, while in other cases, as when crystals are to be identified, a stain is not useful.

Fat Stains.—Fat stains such as Sudan dyes (Sudan III) or oil red O may be used to stain neutral fat or triglycerides which do not polarize as a Maltese cross as does cholesterol. Fat stains are useful for the detection of free fat globules, fat in renal cells or macrophages (oval fat bodies), and fat within casts (free or in oval fat bodies). They may be used along with a general-purpose stain and with polarizing and phase microscopy.

Gram's Stain.—This routine microbiological stain is used to differentiate gram-negative (red) and gram-positive (purple) bacteria. A dry preparation (smear, film, or cytocentrifuged) is necessary, which is heat-fixed and then stained.

Cytocentrifugation

Although by no means a routine technique in urinalysis, the use of cytocentrifugation is being increasingly recognized as a very useful adjunct in the examination of the urinary sediment. Preparations may be stained with a

TABLE 13–5.

Grading Scale and Reporting System for Urinary Sediment

	No. per Low-power Field (av)—× 100 magnification						
Casts	Negative	0–2	2–5	5–10	10–25	25–50	>50
Abnormal crystals	Negative	0–2	2–5	5–10	10–25	25–50	>50
Squamous epithelial cells		Few		Moderate		Many	
Mucous threads		Present					
	No. per High-Power Field (av)—× 400 magnification						
Red blood cells	0–2	2–5	5–10	10–25	25–50	50–99	>100
White blood cells	0–2	2–5	5–10	10–25	25–50	50–99	>100
Normal crystals		Few		Moderate		Many	
Epithelial cells (renal tubular, oval fat bodies, transitional)		Few		Moderate		Many	
Miscellaneous (bacteria, yeast, *Trichomonas,* fat globules)		Few		Moderate		Many	
Sperm (males only)		Present					

Papanicolaou stain, the usual stain for cytologic studies in tumor detection. Since this stain is time-consuming, and requires several solutions which are difficult to maintain when not in use routinely, a Wright's stain, either the traditional procedure or a quick stain, may be sufficient.

Cytocentrifugation is useful in differentiating white blood cells from epithelial cells in addition to identifying the type of white blood cell present. As such, it is useful in the early detection of renal allograft rejection by the recognition of lymphocytes in the sediment. It is also useful in the detection of viral inclusion bodies as with cytomegalovirus, fungi, and certain casts. Traditionally, it is used for cytologic studies of precancerous or malignant cells.

Laboratory Procedure

Procedure 13–13 is based on the procedure used by the University of Minnesota Hospital and Clinic, Minneapolis. It uses a 12:1 concentration of the urine specimen and employs parts of the KOVA system. This includes a special graduated centrifuge tube (KOVA tube) and a special disposable pipette (KOVA petter) with a built-in plastic disk which, when inserted into the KOVA tube, retains exactly 1 mL of undisturbed concentrated urinary sediment. This procedure uses a traditional microscope slide and an 18- × 18-mm coverglass. Alternatively, standardized disposable slides such as those available with the KOVA system, or others, can be used, in which case, the grading system (Table 13–5) may require modification. Reference values are shown in Table 13–6.

TABLE 13–6.

Reference Values for Urinary Sediment*

Red blood cells	0–2/HPF
White blood cells	0–5/HPF
Casts	0–2 hyaline casts/LPF
Squamous epithelial cells	Few/LPF
Renal tubular epithelial cells	Few/HPF
Transitional epithelial cells	Few/HPF
Bacteria	Negative
Yeast	Negative
Abnormal crystals	Negative

*These values may be considered normal for constituents in the urinary sediment. They are based on a 12:1 concentration viewed with a low-power (×10) and high-power (×40) objective with a ×10 ocular.

Procedure 13–13. Microscopic Examination of the Urinary Sediment

1. Pour exactly 12 mL of well-mixed urine into a labeled, graduated centrifuge (KOVA) tube. If less than 12 mL is available, use 3 mL. If less than 3 mL is available, examine the sediment without concentration. This information must be included on the report form.
2. Centrifuge at a relative centrifugal force of 450 for 5 minutes. Let the centrifuge come to a stop without using the brake. Use of the brake will cause resuspension of the sediment and falsely low results.
3. Decant 11 mL of clear supernatant urine, leaving 1 mL to ensure consistency in grading results. This is easily accomplished with the KOVA system. Insert the KOVA Petter into the centrifuge tube. Push it to the bottom of the tube until it is firmly seated. Holding the Petter in place with an index finger, decant the supernatant urine. This will leave exactly 1 mL of sediment in the bottom of the tube.
    a. If a 3-mL specimen was used, do not use a KOVA Petter. Decant all liquid quickly, retaining a small drop in which to resuspend the sediment. This is approximately equivalent to a 12:1 concentration.
    b. If the KOVA Petter is not available, pour off 11 mL of supernatant urine in one even motion so as not to resuspend the sediment. Use a disposable pipette to bring the volume of sediment to exactly 1 mL with the clear supernatant urine. Removal of more than 11 mL and readjustment to 1 mL is preferable to removal of less than 11 mL.
4. Resuspend the sediment for examination by mixing thoroughly by squeezing the KOVA Petter.
5. Place a standardized drop of resuspended sediment on a microscope slide and cover with an 18- × 18-mm coverglass. (Alternatively, place the resuspended sediment in a standardized microscope slide following the manufacturer's directions.)
    a. The size of the drop is important. The fluid should completely fill the area under the coverglass but without overflowing the area or causing the coverglass to float.
    b. Take care that no bubbles appear when placing the coverglass over the sediment. If bubbles appear, a new preparation must be made on a clean slide. Bubbles are confusing and make enumeration impossible, since they prevent random distribution of the substances to be counted.
6. Examine two preparations for each urinary sediment. After removing a sufficient portion of the unstained sediment (usually enough for only one preparation) add a drop or two of stain (e.g., Sedistain) to the remaining portion of sediment and mix thoroughly. Alternatively, the sediment may be stained directly on the microscope slide before covering by adding a small portion of stain with the tip of a disposable glass pipette or wooden applicator to the drop of sediment on the slide. This method leaves an adequate amount of unstained sediment for further examination.
7. Place the preparation, either stained or unstained, on the microscope stage, and focus and adjust the light, using the low-power objective. Adjust the light by careful positioning of the condenser and iris diaphragm. The tendency is to have too much light, but the light must not be overly reduced. Be sure the sediment itself is brought into focus, rather than the coverglass. It is easier to achieve focus with specimens that are stained. Finally, vary the fine adjustment continuously to maintain focus.
8. Be systematic in the examination. Begin by looking around the four sides of the coverglass. Do not examine the preparation for more than 3 minutes, or drying will occur and the identifications will be inaccurate. First, look for the substances that are identified and graded under low power. Then change to high power, refocus and readjust the light, and search for the substances that are graded and identified under high power. All gradings are based on the average number of structures seen in a minimum of ten microscopic fields. To ensure accurate results, prepare two separate portions of sediment, and count the structures seen in five microscopic fields in each preparation (the first portion should be prepared and observed before the second is prepared). To obtain a meaningful average, observe and count structures in the four quadrants and center of each preparation. Describe separately the structures searched for under low and high power. Casts and

---

Procedure 13–13 (cont.)

---

cells are most important; look for these most carefully, observing the less important crystals and miscellaneous structures almost in retrospect.

9. Examine sediment preparations with the low- and high-power objectives as outlined below. Report results as indicated in this discussion and in Table 13–5. All entities encountered must be reported using the appropriate objective and within the grading scale established for the individual laboratory. For example, if a urinary sediment was examined and the microscopist found an average of 15 white blood cells, 3 hyaline casts, no red blood cells, and 2 squamous epithelial cells, the results would be reported as:

Concentration 12:1

Hyaline casts 2–5/LPF

Red cells 0–2/HPF

White blood cells 10–25/HPF

Few squamous epithelial cells

Low-power examination

With the low power (×10) objective, search for the following:

a. *Casts*. Since they tend to roll to the edges of the coverglass, look for casts around all four edges of the preparation, and then in the center. When a cast is discovered, change to high power to identify it. Grade and report casts on the basis of the average number seen in a minimum of ten low-power fields as shown in Table 13–5. If more than one type of cast is found in a single specimen, identify and grade each type separately.

b. *Mucous threads*. These are reported as present when significant numbers are viewed under low power. They are most apparent with phase-contrast microscopy.

c. *Crystals and amorphous material*. Look for these structures in the same way as for casts.
   (1) *Normal crystals* are reported as few, moderate, or many per high-power field, but may be more apparent under low power.
   (2) Grade *abnormal crystals* as the average number seen in a minimum of ten low-power fields (see Table 13–5). Remember, abnormal crystals must be confirmed before they are reported.
   (3) Since crystals are generally identified by shape rather than size, a combination of low- and high-power observation is necessary in the detection and identification of these structures.

d. *Squamous epithelial cells*. Report as few, moderate, or many per low-power field.

High-power examination

With the high power (×40) objective, search for the following:

a. *Red blood cells*. Grade and report on the basis of the average number seen in a minimum of ten high-power fields (see Table 13–5). Report the presence of unusual forms, such as dysmorphic red cells if encountered.

b. *White blood cells*. Grade and report on the basis of the average number seen in a minimum of ten high-power fields (Table 13–5). These are usually neutrophils (PMNs). If unusual cell types, such as lymphocytes or eosinophils, are morphologically identifiable, report this finding.

c. *Normal crystals*. Identify and report as few, moderate, or many per high-power field for each type of crystal encountered.

d. *Identify casts* which are graded under low power.

e. *Epithelial cells:* renal tubular, oval fat bodies (renal tubular cells with fat), and transitional. Estimate and report as few, moderate, or many per high-power field.

f. *Miscellaneous*. This category includes various cells forms and other structures which may be encountered in the urine sediment: yeast, bacteria, trichomonads, fat globules. Identify the cell or structure and report as few, moderate, or many per high power field. Report the presence of sperm as present in males only. It is considered a contaminant in routine urinalysis specimens from females and is not reported.

CONSTITUENTS OF URINARY SEDIMENT*

In general, the constituents of the urinary sediment are of a biological or chemical nature. The biological part (also called the **organized sediment**) includes the red blood cells, white blood cells, epithelial cells, fat of biological origin, casts, bacteria, yeast, fungi, parasites, and spermatozoa. (Casts are long cylindrical structures that result from the solidification of material within the lumen of the kidney tubules.) The biological portion is the more important part of the sediment, the cells and casts being of primary importance (unfortunately, they are also the most difficult to detect).

The chemical portion (also called the **unorganized sediment**) consists of crystals of chemicals and **amorphous material.** In general, it is less important than the biological portion. However, some abnormal crystals have pathologic significance. In addition, the crystalline or chemical portion is sometimes so large that it tends to obscure the more important parts, which must be searched for with great care.

Constituents of the urinary sediment that may be encountered on microscopic examination will now be described. Unless otherwise specified, the staining reactions are those of the Sternheimer-Malbin crystal violet safranin stain (Sedistain).

Cellular Constituents Derived From Blood

Red Blood Cells

Clinical Aspects.—Red blood cells are abnormal urinary constituents, and the presence of more than one to two per high-power field is always of pathologic significance. The condition in which red cells are found in the urine is termed *hematuria.* Often, the clinician will want to distinguish between hematuria and hemoglobinuria (free hemoglobin in the urine). This may be done by observing red cells under the microscope. However, red cells lyse so easily in urine that the specimen must be absolutely fresh when this distinction is attempted. In addition, lysis may occur within the urinary tract, yet not be intravascular.

*Photomicrographs in this section (Figs 13–5 to 13–16) courtesy of Dr. G. Mary Bradley and Karen M. Ringsrud, Department of Laboratory Medicine and Pathology, University of Minnesota, Minneapolis, and Dr. Patrick Ward, Department of Pathology, School of Medicine, University of Minnesota at Duluth, with permission from the University of Minnesota Medical School.

The degree of hematuria may vary from a frankly bloody specimen on gross examination to a specimen that shows no change in color. Blood may be seen as merely a tiny red button in the bottom of the centrifuge tube after centrifuging. The amount of blood detected in the chemical reagent strip test for hemoglobin should be quantitated in the microscopic analysis of the sediment. Hematuria may be the result of bleeding at any point along the urogenital tract and may be seen with almost any disease of the urinary tract. It is a sensitive early indicator of renal disease.

To determine the cause of hematuria, it is necessary to determine the site of bleeding. This involves various types of information, both laboratory and clinical. Part of this information will depend on other findings in the microscopic examination and other portions of the routine urinalysis. For example, bleeding through the glomerulus will often be accompanied by red cell casts, as seen in acute glomerulonephritis or disease of the glomerulus. This is an extremely serious situation, and red cell casts must be looked for carefully when red cells are found. There may be little correlation between the amount of blood and the severity of the disorder, yet the hematuria may be the only indication of renal disease. The occurrence of hematuria without accompanying protein and casts usually indicates that the bleeding is in the lower urogenital tract.

Microscopic Appearance.—Red cells are not easy to find under the microscope. Their detection requires careful examination. The high-power objective is used, and the light must be reduced by proper adjustment of the condenser and iris diaphragm or they will be missed. Their detection also requires continual refocusing with the fine adjustment of the microscope. The phase-contrast microscope is very useful in detecting red blood cells. Even after hemolysis has occurred, the red cell membrane is clearly visible with this technique.

In absolutely fresh urine, red cells will be unaltered or intact and appear much as they do in diluted whole blood. They have a characteristic bluish-green sheen, are intact biconcave disks that are especially apparent as they roll over, have a generally smooth appearance as opposed to the granular appearance of white cells, and are about 7 μm in diameter (Fig 13–5). However, they rapidly undergo morphologic changes in urine specimens and are rarely observed as described. This is because urine is rarely an isotonic solution with red cells (the solute concentration within the red cell is rarely the same as the solute concentration of urine). The urine may be

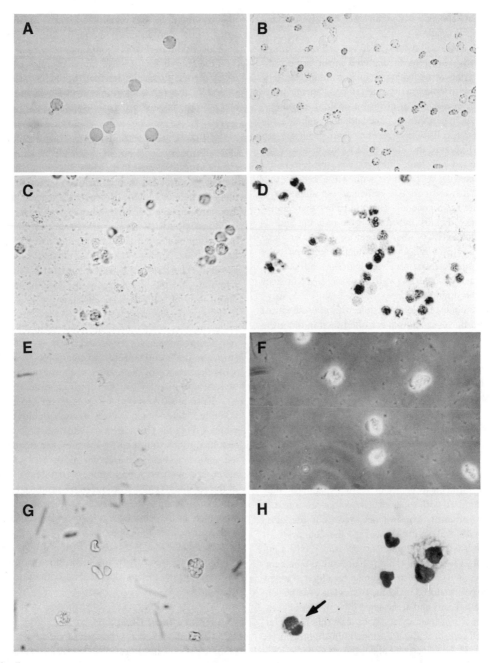

FIG 13-5.
Red cells and white cells in the urinary sediment. **A,** intact red cells (six), unstained, ×400. **B,** variety of red cell types: intact, crenated, and shadow, unstained, ×400. **C,** white cells and many bacteria, unstained, ×400. **D,** white cells and bacteria, stained with Sedistain, ×400. **E,** white cells and bacteria, unstained, ×400. **F,** white cells and bacteria, same field as **E** with phase-contrast illumination. **G,** dysmorphic red cells (four), white cells (two), unstained, ×400. **H,** eosinophil *(arrow),* neutrophils, possible renal tubular cell. Cytospin preparation, quick Wright's stain, ×1,000.

more or less concentrated than the blood, and the changes described below result.

Several changes may be seen in red cell morphology in the red cells which are encountered in the urine sediment. When the urine is hypotonic or dilute, as evidenced by low specific gravity, the red cells appear *swollen* and *rounded* because of diffusion of fluid into them. If the urine is hypertonic or concentrated (high specific gravity), the red cells appear *crenated* and *shrunken* (see Fig 13–5,B) because they lose fluid to the urine. When crenated, the red cells have little spicules, or projections, that cause them to be confused with white cells. However, a crenated red cell is significantly smaller than a white cell and has a generally smooth, rather than granular, appearance. Finally, when the urine is dilute and alkaline, the red cells will often appear as *shadow* or *ghost cells* (see Fig 13–5,B). In this situation the red cells have burst and released their hemoglobin; all that remains is the faint colorless cell membrane, a ghost or shadow of the original cell.

This membrane is clearly visible with phase-contrast illumination, however. Ghosts are often seen in old urine specimens. Eventually, even the ghosts will disappear as the cell completely disintegrates. Distorted or *dysmorphic* red cells may also be seen (see Fig 13–5,G). These misshapen red cells may indicate the presence of glomerular disease. The distortion is best seen with phase-contrast illumination. It is also possible to see nucleated red cells or sickle cells (in sickle cell disease) in urine. This is, however, extremely rare.

Structures Confused With Red Cells.—Red cells are not only difficult to detect in a urine specimen, they are often confused with other structures that are found in the urinary sediment. For instance, red cells are often confused with leukocytes; however, the leukocyte is larger and has a generally granular appearance plus a nucleus (see Fig 13–5). If morphologic differentiation is impossible, a drop of 2% acetic acid may be added to a new preparation or introduced under the coverglass. Acetic acid will lyse the red cells and at the same time stain (or accentuate) the nuclei of leukocytes. With a Sternheimer-Malbin stain, red cells in acidic urine may stain slightly purple or not at all. If the urine is alkaline, the alkaline hematin that is formed stains dark purple. The reagent strip tests for blood and leukocyte esterase are also helpful.

Yeast may also be confused with red cells in urine. However, yeast cells are generally smaller than red cells, are spherical rather than flattened, and vary considerably in size within one specimen (see Fig 13–7). In addition, since yeast reproduces by budding, the occurrence of buds or little outgrowths should identify yeast.

Bubbles or *oil droplets* are also confused with red cells, especially by the inexperienced. These vary considerably in size, are extremely refractive or reflective, and are obvious under the microscope.

Other Considerations.—The identification of red cells in urinary sediment may be aided by the use of a chemical test for blood. Red blood cells in the sediment should be correlated with a positive reagent strip test for blood and hemoglobin. However, since chemical tests are more sensitive to hemoglobin than to intact red cells, it is possible to have a negative reagent strip test when only a few intact red cells are present and no hemolysis has occurred. Such a situation is quite rare, although it is possible. The tests are sensitive to 5 to 10 red cells per microliter but the sensitivity of the reagent strips is reduced in urine with high specific gravity. False-negative or delayed reagent strip tests for blood are possible when large amounts of vitamin C are present. In this case, the sediment result can be confirmed by the use of a reagent strip test for ascorbic acid. Another clue would be the gross appearance of the urinary sediment, or a red button of cells in the bottom of the centrifuge tube.

False-positive reagent strip tests for blood are also possible. Unless hemoglobin or myoglobin is present without red cells (both are rare situations), the chemical test should be confirmed by the presence of red cells in the sediment. False-positive chemical tests (positive reagent strip with no hemoglobin, myoglobin, or red cells in the sediment) can be produced by residues of strongly oxidizing cleaning agents such as bleach in the urine container, or by peroxidase in microorganisms associated with urinary tract infections.

Red cells that are present in the urinary sediment should be reported by grading the average number of red cells seen in ten microscope fields according to the scale in Table 13–5.

White Blood Cells

Clinical Aspects.—The presence of a few white blood cells or leukocytes in the concentrated urine sediment is normal. More than an occasional white cell (1–5/HPF) is considered abnormal. The term *white blood cell* or *leukocyte* in urine usually refers to the presence of a neutrophilic leukocyte (polymorphonuclear neutrophil, or PMN). Unless otherwise specified, it is assumed that this is what is meant. However, any white cell type present in blood can also be found in the urinary sediment. The presence of lymphocytes and eosinophils are of particular diagnostic significance and are described later.

The presence of large numbers of white blood cells in the sediment indicates inflammation at some point along the urogenital tract. The inflammation may result from a bacterial infection or other causes. The presence of white blood cells is thus often associated with bacteria, but both bacteria and white cells can be present alone without the other. In bacterial infections, ingested bacteria are often seen within the cell. If the leukocytes originate in the kidney, rather than lower in the urinary tract (such as in the bladder), they may form cellular casts. Therefore, the presence of casts (usually cellular or granular) along with white blood cells and bacteria would help distinguish an upper (kidney) from a lower (bladder) urinary tract infection. Protein is usually present along with casts, and may or may not be present in a lower urinary tract infection.

The condition in which increased numbers of leukocytes are found in urine is termed **pyuria.** Pyuria may cause clouding of the urine, and when this is severe enough the urine will have a characteristic milk-white appearance. Under the microscope the white cells may appear singly or in clumps. The presence of clumps indicates infection and should be reported.

Microscopic Appearance.—Leukocytes must be searched for under the high-power objective, reduced light, and continual refocusing with fine adjustment. Typically, they are about 10 to 12 μm in diameter (about twice the size of red cells); however, this size difference may not be obvious. Leukocytes have thin cytoplasmic granulation and a nucleus. Even if the nucleus is not distinct, the center of the cell appears granular (see Fig 13–5). White cells are fragile and will disintegrate in old alkaline urine specimens. Various stages of disintegration may be observed in a single urine specimen. Neutrophil leukocytes are especially vulnerable in dilute alkaline urine specimens, and about 50% can be lost within 2 to 3 hours if the urine is kept at room temperature. In addition, the lobed nucleus tends to consolidate and the neutrophil appears as a mononuclear cell as the cell begins to degenerate. If the urine is dilute, the cell cytoplasm may expand out in petals, without granules, before the neutrophil disintegrates.

Phase-contrast microscopy is especially useful in the detection and identification of white blood cells in the urinary sediment, as is the use of a stain, such as the Sternheimer-Malbin stain. However, precipitation of the stain in the highly alkaline urines associated with white cells and bacteria may pose a problem. When stained, neutrophilic leukocytes show a red-purple nucleus and violet or blue cytoplasm, although the same urine specimen may have a variety of staining reactions, and extremely fresh cells may fail to stain.

Structures Confused With White Cells.—Other structures may be mistaken for leukocytes. Most often this occurs with red cells and epithelial cells. White cells are generally larger than red cells, appear granular, and have a nucleus. A 2% acetic acid solution may aid in their identification. There are several very different morphologic types of epithelial cells, but in general they are larger than white cells and have smaller nuclei. The nuclei are generally more distinct and are surrounded by more cytoplasm (Fig 13–6).

White cells should be reported by grading the average number of cells seen in ten microscope fields according to the scale in Table 13–5.

Other white blood cell types that may be seen in the urinary sediment include the following:

Glitter Cells.—These are larger, swollen neutrophilic leukocytes that appear in hypotonic urine with a specific gravity of about 1.010 or less. Their cytoplasmic granules are in constant random (brownian) movement giving a glittering appearance. These cells are especially striking under phase-contrast illumination. When stained, glitter cells have a light-blue or almost colorless cytoplasm and the brownian motion of the granules may or may not be observed. Once thought to indicate chronic pyelonephritis, glitter cells are also seen in dilute urine specimens from patients with lower urinary tract infections.

Eosinophils.—Eosinophils may be present in the urine sediment. They are morphologically very similar to neutrophils and difficult to distinguish, especially with a wet preparation under both brightfield and phase-contrast illumination. They are typically larger than neutrophils and oval or elongated. The cytoplasmic granules may not be prominent, but the presence of two or three distinct lobes of the nucleus with fresh specimens is helpful. **Cytocentrifugation** is useful in confirming the presence of

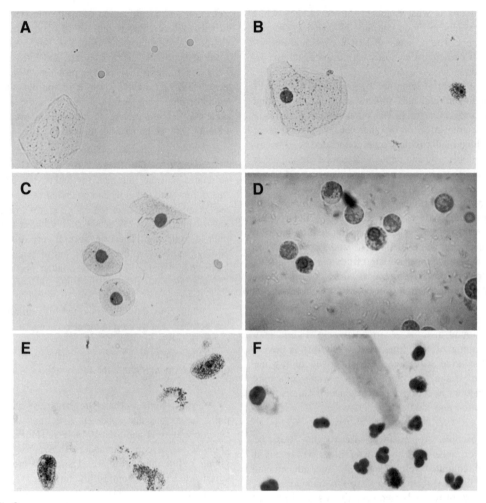

FIG 13–6.
Epithelial cells in the urinary sediment. **A,** squamous epithelial cell and three red cells, unstained, ×400. **B,** squamous epithelial cell and eosinophil. Cytospin preparation, quick Wright's stain, ×400. **C,** squamous epithelial cell *(folded),* two transitional epithelial cells, and red cell (dysmorphic). Cytospin preparation, quick Wright's stain, ×400. **D,** renal epithelial cells (two), white cells, red cells, and bacteria, stained with Sedistain, ×450. **E,** renal tubular epithelial cells (two, probably proximal) looking like granular casts, and amorphous material stained with Sedistain, ×400. **F,** renal tubular epithelial cell (one), several neutrophils, two eosinophils, hyaline cast. Cytospin preparation, quick Wright's stain, ×1,000.

eosinophils (Fig 13–5,H). They do not, however, stain as well on Wright's stain as they do in blood smears. Special eosinophil stains, such as Hansel's stain, is helpful. Increased eosinophils are associated with drug-induced interstitial nephritis, as seen with treatment with penicillins. Detection is important because the treatment is fast and effective: namely, discontinue the drug.

Lymphocytes and Other Mononuclear Cells.—
A few small lymphocytes are normally present in urine, even though they are rarely recognized. They are very difficult to distinguish from red blood cells, especially with the normal wet preparation of the urinary sediment, both under brightfield and phase-contrast illumination. They are only slightly larger than red cells, with a single

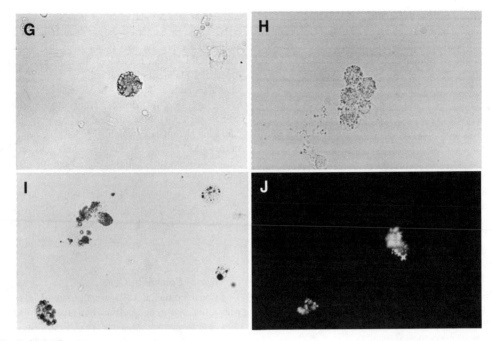

FIG 13–6 (cont.).
G, oval fat body, unstained, ×400. **H,** Clump of oval fat bodies, unstained, ×400. **I,** several oval fat bodies and free fat, stained with Sudan III, ×400. **J,** oval fat bodies showing the typical Maltese cross of cholesterol when viewed with polarized light, ×400.

round nucleus and scant cytoplasm. The presence of many small lymphocytes are seen in the first few weeks after renal transplant rejection and are a useful early indicator of this rejection process. If their presence is suspected, identification is most easily confirmed by cytocentrifugation and stain with Wright's stain. Since they are not granulocytes, lymphocytes will not react with the reagent strips for leukocyte esterase.

Monocytes, histiocytes, and macrophages may also be present in the urinary sediment. They are difficult to recognize on the standard wet preparation, but are generally larger than, and resemble, aging neutrophils. The cytoplasm is usually abundant, vacuolated, and granulated. These cells are granulocytes and capable of reacting with the reagent strips for leukocyte esterase. However, the sensitivity of the strips may not be sufficient to detect these cells which, even when present, are seen in relatively small numbers. Monocytes and histiocytes are associated with chronic inflammation and radiation therapy.

Macrophages may be present with various inclusions within the cytoplasm. These include ingested fat, **hemosiderin,** red cells, or crystals. As with lymphocytes, identification of other mononuclear cells is most easily confirmed by cytocentrifugation and staining with Wright's stain.

Epithelial Cells

The structures that make up the urinary system consist of several layers of epithelial cells, except for the single-layered tubules of the nephron. The epithelial cells of organs such as the urethra and bladder (besides contaminating cells of the male and female genital tracts) are continually sloughed off into the urine and replaced by cells originating from deeper layers. Therefore, urine always contains some epithelial cells.

The identification of the various epithelial cell types may be difficult yet clinically significant. They include **squamous, transitional (urothelial),** and **renal epithelial cells.**

Squamous Epithelial Cells

Squamous epithelial cells line the female urethra and the distal portion of the male urethra. They are the most commonly encountered type of epithelial cell in urine specimens. However, many of the squamous epithelial cells found in urine are the result of perineal or vaginal contamination. Squamous epithelial cells can be divided into intermediate and superficial squamous cells. They form the most superficial layer of cells which line the mucosa and are continually sloughed off and replaced by newer, deeper cells.

Squamous epithelial cells are very large, flat cells made up of a thin layer of cytoplasm and a single distinct nucleus (see Fig 13–6). The nucleus is about the size of a red blood cell, and the cell is about five to seven times the size of a red cell. A thin cell, it may be rectangular or round. Epithelial cells are large enough to be seen easily under low power and sometimes roll into cigar shapes, which are mistaken for casts. When stained, these cells show a purple nucleus and an abundant pink or violet cytoplasm. They are easily recognized until they begin to degenerate when they may eventually appear as an amorphous mass.

The presence of squamous epithelial cells is of little clinical significance unless present in large numbers. When the urine is contaminated by vaginal secretions or exudates, sheets of squamous epithelial cells accompanied by many rod-shaped bacteria or yeasts, or both, may be seen.

Clue Cell.—Another type of squamous epithelial cell that might be encountered in the urine is of vaginal origin and is referred to as a *clue cell*. These cells are covered with bacteria, *Gardnerella vaginalis*. They are coccobacilli and give the cytoplasm a characteristic refractile, stippled appearance. Clue cells indicate *G. vaginalis* vaginitis or bacterial vaginosis.

Transitional Epithelial (Urothelial) Cells

Transitional epithelial cells occur in multiple layers. They line the urinary tract from the kidney pelvis to the base of the bladder in the female, and the proximal part of the urethra in the male. As the cell layers become deeper, the cells become thicker and rounded, looking more and more like renal epithelial cells or white blood cells. Their size varies with the depth and place of origin in the transitional epithelium. However, in general they are about four to six times the size of a red blood cell,

and appear smaller and plumper than squamous epithelial cells. They are generally larger than renal tubular cells and have a round nucleus (sometimes two nuclei) as opposed to the lobular nucleus of the leukocytes. The more superficial bladder epithelial cells are large flat cells of a squamous nature. The cells become smaller and rounder as the layers become deeper. Transitional epithelial cells stain with a dark blue nucleus and varying amounts of pale blue cytoplasm, which may have occasional inclusions. Some of these cells have tails and are indistinguishable from the *caudate* cells of the renal pelvis (see Fig 13–6).

A few transitional epithelial cells are present in the urine of normal persons. Increased numbers are seen in the presence of infection. Clusters or sheets of these cells are seen after urethral or ureteral catheterization and with urinary tract lesions.

Renal Epithelial Cells

Renal epithelial cells are the single layer of cells which line the nephron from the proximal to the distal convoluted tubules, plus the cells lining the collecting ducts to the pelvis of the kidney. Their occurrence in urine is important, for it implies a serious pathologic condition and destruction of renal tubules, as does the presence of epithelial casts. Identification is difficult in wet preparations with both brightfield and phase-contrast illumination. Intact renal epithelial cells are from three to five times the size of red cells, i.e., slightly larger to twice as large as a neutrophil. Cells from the proximal and distal convoluted tubules are relatively large and elongated or oval with a granular cytoplasm. The granularity makes the proximal tubular cells, in particular, appear as small or fragmented granular casts (see Fig 13–6,E). The nucleus is extremely difficult to see in these renal epithelial cells in wet preparations. The use of cytocentrifugation and staining with Wright's stain will help visualize the nucleus and show these structures to be cells rather than casts. However, the traditional cytologic examination with the Papanicolaou stain is recommended.

Renal epithelial cells are very difficult to identify in wet preparations. They resemble both white blood cells and smaller transitional epithelial cells. Morphologically, renal epithelial cells closely resemble leukocytes, especially degenerating ones, but they are typically larger and have a single distinct nucleus (see Fig 13–6,D–F). Renal cells of the collecting tubules tend to be cuboid, and one side tends to be flat as opposed to the rounded cell more typical of transitional epithelial cells. As is the case with all epithelial cells, renal epithelial cells will not react with the leukocyte esterase reagent strips. This may be helpful in distinguishing them from neutrophils. However, they are associated with the presence of protein in the urine.

When stained, renal epithelial cells have a dark-purple nucleus and a small rim of orange-purple cytoplasm. Renal cells are often found in association with casts. The presence of epithelial or granular casts will help confirm their identification, and when renal cells are suspected, casts should be searched for with great care. The phase-contrast microscope is particularly useful in such situations.

Oval Fat Bodies.—These are a special type of renal epithelial cell that are filled with fat (lipid) droplets. Oval fat bodies are sometimes referred to as *renal tubular fat* or *renal tubular fat bodies*. They indicate a serious pathologic condition and must not be overlooked when present in the urinary sediment. The fat droplets are generally contained within degenerating or necrotic renal epithelial cells, although some oval fat bodies may be macrophages that have filled with fat. The fat droplets contained within these cells are highly refractive, coarse droplets that vary greatly in size (see Fig 13–6,G–I). Although they are considered cells filled with fat, the cell nucleus is generally not visible. Certain aids to the identification of oval fat bodies are available. When stained with Sternheimer-Malbin stain, fat globules do not become colored but appear highly refractive in a blue-purple background. When stained with fat stains such as Sudan III or oil red O, globules of triglyceride or neutral fat appear orange or red. Polarized light is useful for indicating the presence of cholesterol esters in the fat. Cholesterol esters are anisotropic or doubly refractive and show a typical Maltese cross pattern when viewed with polarizing filters (see Fig 13–6,J). However, triglycerides or neutral fat do not show this pattern with polarized light. The appearance of a Maltese cross pattern alone cannot be used to determine whether fat is present in urine, as many crystals, and urine contaminated with starch, give the same pattern. Fat should be confirmed by careful microscopic examination or specific staining.

Oval fat bodies are often seen along with fat droplets and fatty casts in the urinary sediment, and the other two components should be searched for carefully when one is present. Oval fat bodies resulting from tubular epithelial degeneration of the nephron are associated with large amounts of protein in the urine, as in the nephrotic syndrome. The fatty material in the tubular cells may be the lipoprotein that passes through the damaged glomerulus in this syndrome. The lipoprotein may be ingested by the renal tubular cell, which metabolizes it into cholesterol.

Fat Globules.—Although not a cellular constituent, the presence of fat globules is discussed now because of the relationship of fat globules to oval fat bodies. Fat globules may be found in the urinary sediment as highly refractive droplets of various sizes (see Figs 13–6,G–J and 13–12). When their source is biological (rather than contamination), a serious pathologic condition implying severe renal dysfunction exists. Such *lipuria* is also associated with the nephrotic syndrome and its various causes, diabetes mellitus, and conditions that result in severe damage of renal tubular epithelial cells such as ethylene glycol or mercury poisoning. Fat globules are found in association with oval fat bodies and fatty casts. Fat stains orange or red with Sudan III stains. The identification may be aided by the use of polarized light, as cholesterol will show a Maltese cross pattern when so viewed. Fat in urine may also come from extraneous sources such as unclean collection utensils or oiled catheters (see Fig 13–16,C). This is less common with the use of disposable urine collection containers.

Hemosiderin.—Occasionally, renal epithelial cells with granules of hemosiderin in the cytoplasm are seen in the urinary sediment. This occurs several days after a hemolytic episode, when free hemoglobin has passed through the glomerulus into the nephron. The hemosiderin granules appear as yellow or colorless granules which are morphologically similar to amorphous urates. Unlike urates, they will stain blue with a Prussian blue stain for iron. Besides their presence in desquamated renal epithelial cells, granules of hemosiderin may be seen as free granules in the sediment, in macrophages, and in casts.

Viral Inclusion Bodies.—Renal tubular epithelial cells may also be seen with viral inclusion bodies. This is especially characteristic of infection with cytomegalovirus. They are difficult to recognize on wet preparations. Cytocentrifugation and staining with the Papanicolaou stain is helpful in recognizing this condition.

Other Cellular Constituents

Bacteria

Under normal conditions the urinary tract is free of bacteria. However, most urine specimens contain at least a few bacteria because of contamination when the urine is voided. Bacteria multiply rapidly when urine stands at room temperature. In specimens that are obtained in a manner suitable for urine culture and kept under sterile conditions, the presence of bacteria may indicate a urinary tract infection. In this case, they are likely to be associated with the presence of white blood cells, although this is not always true. Bacterial infection should be confirmed by quantitative urine culture.

Bacteria are easily recognized morphologically. They are extremely small, only a few micrometers long. They may be either rods or cocci and may occur singly or in chains (Figs 13–5,C–F and 13–7,A,B). They are often motile, which helps in their identification. Bacteria are most often seen in alkaline urine and may be confused with amorphous material at first, but this will not be a problem as experience in observation is gained. Phase-contrast microscopy is very useful in the visualization of bacteria, which are difficult to see with brightfield illumination.

In lower urinary tract (bladder) infections, bacteria are generally, but not always, associated with the presence of leukocytes (PMNs). Mild proteinuria and a positive reagent strip test for nitrites or leukocyte esterase may also be seen. With upper urinary tract (kidney) infections, bacteria may be seen along with leukocytes and leukocyte, cellular, or granular casts. There may be moderate proteinuria and a positive reagent strip test for nitrites or leukocyte esterase.

Yeast

Yeast cells are occasionally seen in urine, especially from females and diabetic patients. They are often present as the result of contamination of the urine from a vaginal yeast infection. They are associated with the presence of sugar in the urine. Sugar is the energy source for yeast cells, which grow and multiply rapidly when it is present. For this reason yeast cells are often discovered in the urine of diabetics, along with a high sugar content, low pH, and ketones. However, yeast cells are also common contaminants from skin and air.

Yeast cells are often mistaken for red blood cells. They are generally smaller than red cells and show considerable size variation, even within a specimen. They have a typically ovoid shape, lack color, and have a smooth and refractive appearance. The most distinguishing characteristic is the presence of little buds, or projections, because of their manner of reproduction (see Fig 13–7,C–F). Pseudomycelial forms of *Candida* sp. (the type of yeast usually present) may also be seen as hyphae (filaments). These should not be mistaken for casts.

Trichomonas Vaginalis

Trichomonas vaginalis is the parasite most frequently seen in urine specimens. It may be present as the result of vaginal contamination. The organism is motile, which is an aid to its identification. When a urethral or bladder infection is suspected, the organism must be searched for immediately after the urine is voided. *Trichomonas* is a unicellular organism—a protozoan. It has a characteristic appearance with anterior flagella and an undulating membrane, the motility of which is helpful in identification as it appears to swim through the urinary sediment. The organisms are larger than typical leukocytes and may resemble transitional epithelial cells, especially when no longer motile. Phase-contrast microscopy is particularly useful in visualization, especially of the flagella (see Fig 13–7,G).

Other Parasites

Various other parasites may be seen in urine as the result of fecal or vaginal contamination and may be common to particular geographic areas. Examples are *Schistosoma haematobium* and amebas such as *Entamoeba histolytica,* and *Enterobius vermicularis,* or pinworm.

Spermatozoa

Spermatozoa may also be present as urinary contaminants. They are easily recognized, having oval bodies with long delicate tails, and they may be motile or stationary (see Fig 13–7,H).

Tumor Cells

Tumor cells and other cell forms with altered cytologic features may be found in the urinary sediment. However, these cell forms cannot be diagnosed from the usual urinary sediment preparation but require special collection, cytocentrifugation, and stains and examination by qualified personnel. If their presence is suspected from the examination of the sediment, the specimen should be referred accordingly.

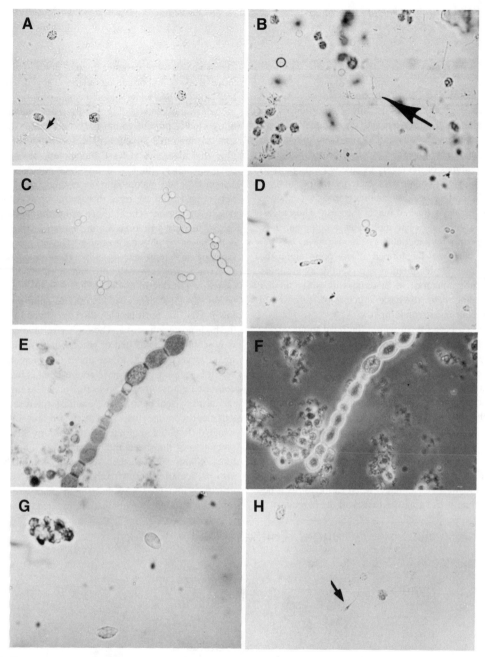

FIG 13–7.
Other cell forms in the urinary sediment. **A,** many bacteria with protoplast *(arrow),* four white cells, unstained, high power. **B,** many bacteria including protoplast *(arrow),* many white cells, and red cells, stained with Sedistain, ×440. **C,** yeast cells, unstained, high power. **D,** Several yeast cells with a few red cells, unstained, ×400. **E,** yeast cells with pseudohyphae, not to be confused with casts. Stained with Sedistain, ×400. **F,** yeast cells with pseudohyphae (same as **E**), phase-contrast microscopy, ×400. **G,** *Trichomonas vaginalis* unstained, ×400. **H,** sperm *(arrow);* white cells are also present. Stained with Sedistain, ×400.

Casts

Formation and Significance

Casts are at once the most difficult portion of the urinary sediment to discover and the most important. Their importance and their name derive from the manner in which they are produced. Casts are formed in the lumen of the tubules of the nephrons (the working units of the kidney) by solidification of material in the tubules. They are important because anything that is contained within the tubule is flushed out in the cast. Thus a cast represents a biopsy of an individual tubule and is a means of examining the contents of the nephron. It is believed that casts may be formed at any point along the nephron, either by precipitation of protein or by grouping together (conglutination) of material within the tubular lumen. In either case, the basic structure of the cast is a Tamm-Horsfall mucoprotein matrix.

Before casts can form within the renal tubules, certain conditions must exist. Since the cast is made of protein, there must be a sufficient concentration of protein within the tubule. In addition, the pH must be low enough to favor precipitation and there must be a sufficient concentration of solutes. Since these conditions most likely exist in the distal tubules, it is felt that cast formation is more likely in the distal than in the proximal convoluted tubules. For the same reasons, casts are not likely to be found in dilute alkaline urine, since these conditions do not favor their formation. This also means that the urine must be examined when fresh, for as it becomes alkaline with aging the casts will disintegrate.

Since casts represent a biopsy of the kidney, they are extremely important clinically. They often contain red blood cells, white blood cells, epithelial cells, fat globules, and bacteria (Fig 13–8). These inclusions are not normally present within the renal tubule; they represent an abnormal situation. The formation of casts implies that there was at least a temporary blocking of the renal tubules. Although a few hyaline casts made of Tamm-Horsfall mucoprotein are normal, increased numbers of casts indicate renal disease rather than lower urinary tract disease. The number of hyaline casts may increase in mild irritations of the kidney associated with dehydration or physical exercise. The presence of other types of casts represents a serious (pathologic) situation.

Casts are extremely difficult to see and must be searched for carefully with reduced light and the low-power objective. They are found and enumerated under low power, but must be identified as to type by means of the high-power objective. The refractive index of the cast is nearly the same as that of glass, which means that the image is very difficult to see under the microscope. It is for this reason that phase-contrast and interference-contrast microscopy are so useful in the examination of the urinary sediment. Phase-contrast microscopy gives sufficient contrast that structures are not overlooked, while differential interference microscopy gives an appreciation of the shape and inclusions within these structures. Stains such as the Sternheimer-Malbin stain are also particularly useful for the discovery of casts in the urinary sediment. Casts that might otherwise be overlooked in brightfield examination, especially by the inex-

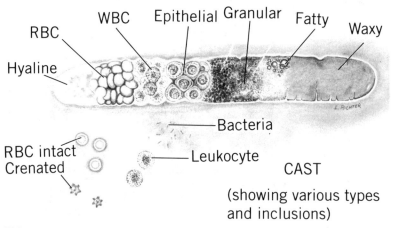

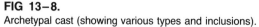

FIG 13–8.
Archetypal cast (showing various types and inclusions).

perienced observer, become obvious when so stained, although the presence of mucous strands in the sediment might be confusing, especially when searching for hyaline casts.

As might be imagined from the shape of the tubular lumen, casts are cylindrical bodies and have rounded ends. To be identified as a cast, a structure should have an even and definite outline, parallel sides, and two rounded ends. Although they vary somewhat in size, casts should have a uniform diameter (about seven or eight times the diameter of a red cell) and be several times longer than wide (see Fig 13–8).

Although casts ideally have parallel sides and two rounded ends, this is not always the case. Casts take on the shape of the tubule in which they are formed. They may be serpentine or convoluted and are often folded. One end may taper off to a tail or point (Fig 13–9). Such structures have been referred to as *cylindroids,* but they should be considered to be, and enumerated along with, hyaline casts. Cylindroids are often confused with strands of mucus, and care must be taken to avoid this mistake. In addition, casts may be fragmented or broken, and waxy casts typically show blunt, rather than rounded ends. Judgment is necessary in the enumeration of such structures. The whole urinary sediment picture must be considered so that important pathologic findings are reported. Conversely, the occurrence of only one questionable cast, with no other pathologic indicators, should not be reported.

Classification of casts is not always simple. In the laboratory it is done mainly on the basis of morphologic groupings: hyaline, finely granular, coarsely granular, waxy, cellular, or fatty. However, a urine specimen may contain more than one morphologic type, and a particular cast may be of mixed morphology—for instance, one end may be hyaline and the other cellular. This is shown in the extreme in Figure 13–8. A classification on the basis of composition and origin has been described by Lippman. This system recognizes only three main types of casts: hyaline, epithelial, and blood. The system is especially useful for understanding cast formation, but it is not completely practical for use in the laboratory, where only morphologic classification is possible.

Casts are felt to arise either by precipitation of protein within the renal tubule or by conglutination of material within the tubular lumen. Both types of casts may contain inclusions. Casts formed by protein precipitation may trap any other substance, such as leukocytes, fat, bacteria, red cells, desquamated renal tubular epithelium, or crystals that may be present. Casts formed by either mechanism may appear coarsely or finely granular or waxy, as cells disintegrate when the cast is retained in the tubule before being flushed out of the kidney. Structures will also disintegrate if the urine specimen stands.

In any case, casts have a protein matrix, and the presence of casts in the urine is virtually always accompanied by proteinuria. Tamm-Horsfall protein is a specific mucoprotein that has been identified immunologically and found to be present in all casts. Other immunoproteins have been identified in certain casts, although they are not found exclusively in any particular type of cast or disease state.

The following morphologic classification is based on appearance, physical properties, and existence of cellular components. The appearance of a cast when it is seen in the urine may not be the same as when it was originally formed in the renal tubule. If the cast is retained in the kidney (as happens in oliguric patients), cells present in it change in appearance. As the cells degenerate in the cast, their cytoplasm becomes granular. This is followed by loss of cell membranes, resulting in large or coarse granules. As these granules degenerate further, the cast shows smaller or fine granules. The final step in this degeneration is complete lack of structure, with the protein changed or coagulated into a thick, very refractive, opaque substance with a waxlike appearance. These are the most serious casts pathologically, as the formation of the waxy material implies a greatly lengthened transit time, or shutdown of the portion of the kidney where the structure evolved.

The width or diameter of a cast is important clinically. Since casts are generally formed within the distal convoluted tubules of the nephron, which have a fairly constant diameter, there is normally little variation in cast diameter, although casts from small children are narrower than those from adults. *Narrow* casts probably result from swelling of the tubular epithelium, as in an inflammatory process, with narrowing of the tubular lumen. They are not particularly important and tend to be of a hyaline type. *Broad* casts are much more serious. Their diameter is several times greater than normal. This is felt to result from their formation in dilated renal tubules or in collecting tubules (several nephrons empty into a common collecting tubule, which has a greater diameter than the renal tubule). Severe chronic renal disease or obstruction (stasis) will often result in dilation and destruction of renal tubules. Cast formation in the collecting tubules must result from urinary stasis in the

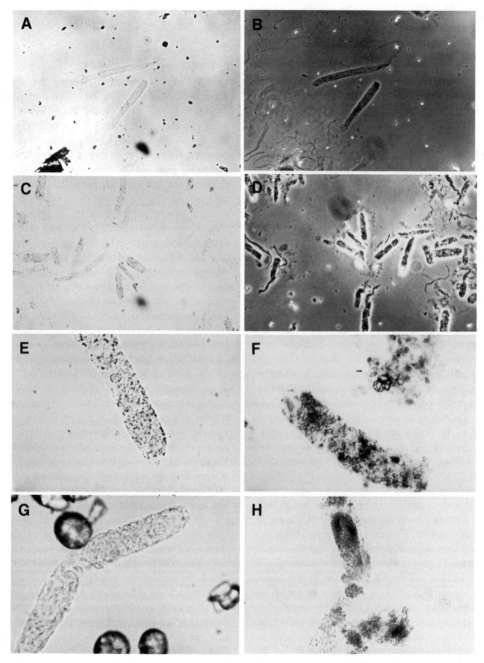

FIG 13–9.

Hyaline and granular casts in the urinary sediment. **A,** two hyaline casts, unstained, ×100. **B,** two hyaline casts, same field as **A,** also showing mucous threads, phase-contrast microscopy, ×100. **C,** several hyaline casts with fine granulation, unstained, ×100. **D,** several hyaline casts with fine granulation, same field as **C.** Mucous threads and other cells are also present. Phase-contrast microscopy, ×100. **E,** granular cast with one cell, unstained, ×640. **F,** granular cast, stained, ×400. **G,** granular cast and uric acid crystals, unstained, ×400. **H,** granular cast and possibly renal tubular epithelial cells (degenerating), stained with Sedistain, ×400.

TABLE 13–7.

Casts, a Morphologic Classification

Hyaline casts
Cellular casts
   White blood cell (leukocyte, neutrophil, or pus) casts
   Epithelial cell casts
   Red blood cell (blood and blood pigment) casts
Granular casts
   Coarsely granular casts
   Finely granular casts
Waxy casts
Fatty casts (oval fat body casts)
Pigmented casts
   Hemoglobin (blood) casts
   Myoglobin casts
   Bilirubin casts
Inclusion casts
   Hemosiderin casts
   Crystal casts
   Bacterial casts

group of nephrons feeding a single collecting tubule. If not, the fluid pressure would be far too great for cast formation to occur. This represents serious stasis, and the presence of a significant number of broad casts in the urine sediment is considered to be a bad sign. Broad casts can be of almost any type, but because of the degree of stasis necessary for their formation, most tend to be waxy.

The types of casts that are encountered in the microscopic analysis of the urinary sediment will now be described in a morphologic classification. These are summarized in Table 13–7. Staining reactions that are described pertain to the Sternheimer-Malbin crystal violet safranin stain (Sedistain).

Hyaline Casts

Hyaline casts are colorless, homogeneous, nonrefractive, semitransparent structures (Fig 13–9,A–D). They are the most difficult casts to discover under the microscope. They require careful adjustment of light with the brightfield microscope; the light is adjusted to give contrast by lowering the condenser slightly and closing the iris diaphragm. Phase-contrast and interference microscopy are especially valuable tools in the search for hyaline casts. Stain is also useful; hyaline casts stain a uniform pale pink or pale blue. However, they may take up a minimum of stain and remain difficult to visualize. Hyaline casts may be difficult to distinguish from mucous threads when they are present in the urine, both when stained and when observed by phase-contrast microscopy.

Hyaline casts result from precipitation of Tamm-Horsfall protein within the lumen of kidney tubules. Since the casts are believed to result from gel formation, they include any material that may be present, such as cells or cellular debris.

Although they are generally of the classic shape for identification as a cast (i.e., parallel sides, uniform diameter, definite borders, and rounded ends), very interesting modifications, representing molds of the tubular lumen where they are formed, may be observed. Some hyaline casts are broad, while others are thin and elongated; serpentine and folded forms are not unusual. Cylindroids are hyaline casts with one end that has not rounded off. They should be enumerated and reported as hyaline casts.

Hyaline casts are soluble in water and even more soluble in slightly alkaline solution. They are therefore more likely to be found in concentrated, acidic urine and may not form in advanced renal failure because of the inability to concentrate the urine or maintain the normal acid pH. In addition, hyaline casts dissolve if the urine stands and becomes alkaline. Hyaline casts may be further classified according to their inclusions as hyaline cellular (name type of cell present), hyaline granular, and hyaline fatty casts.

Simple hyaline casts are the least important clinically, and a few (less than two per low-power field) may be seen in urine from normal persons. They may be seen in large numbers (20 or 30 per low-power field) in moderate or severe renal disease.

Cellular Casts

These casts contain intact white cells, red cells, or epithelial cells (Fig 13–10). They are called white cell (or pus) casts, red blood cell (or blood) casts, and epithelial casts. A truly cellular cast appears to result from clumping, or conglutination, of cells rather than simply precipitation of protein, although they are still incorporated in a protein matrix. Alternatively, smaller numbers of the same cell types may be embedded in a hyaline cast.

Cellular casts indicate the presence of cells in the renal tubules. Whenever this occurs, although there are a variety of causes and different degrees of severity, a serious situation exists.

Cellular casts are more easily detected under the mi-

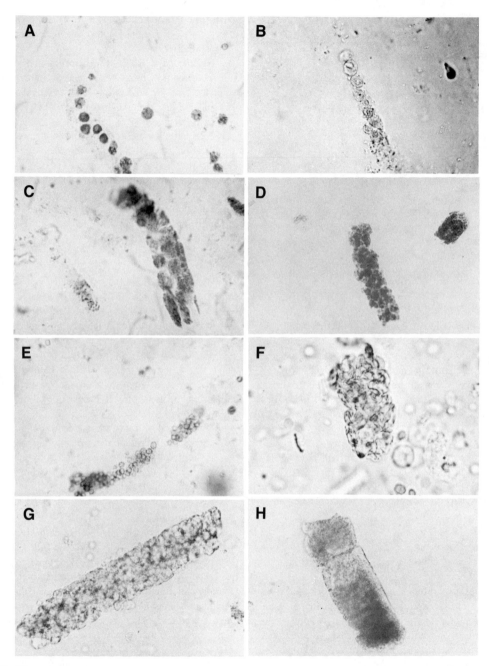

FIG 13–10.
Cellular casts in the urinary sediment. **A,** white blood cell cast, stained with Sedistain, ×450. **B,** epithelial cell cast, un-stained, ×400. **C,** cellular (probably epithelial cell) cast, stained with Sedistain, ×450. **D,** cellular (possibly red cell) cast, stained with Sedistain, ×400. **E,** red blood cell cast, stained with Sedistain, ×450. **F,** red blood cell cast, unstained, oil immersion. **G,** red blood cell (or blood) cast, unstained, ×400. **H,** blood pigment cast, unstained, ×400.

croscope than hyaline casts, since the cells give them a definite structure compared with homogeneous solidified protein. They must still be searched for with care, however, and proper illumination of the brightfield microscope is essential. Phase-contrast or interference microscopy and stains and cytocentrifugation are useful tools in the examination of the urinary sediment for cellular casts. The various types of cellular casts are described in the following paragraphs.

White Blood Cell Casts

These casts are also referred to as leukocyte casts, or pus casts when neutrophilic leukocytes are present. When leukocytes are present in a cast, it is obvious that the cells originated in the kidney. The leukocytes may enter the nephron from the blood by passing through the glomerulus into the glomerular capsule in glomerular diseases. More commonly, they probably enter the nephron from the blood by squeezing through the cells making up the renal tubules, often in response to a bacterial infection within the tubular interstitium. Such phagocytic neutrophils are typically seen in pyelonephritis, a renal infection. In such cases leukocytes and bacteria are also present in the urinary sediment. The presence of casts (particularly white cell casts) along with white cells and bacteria is used to distinguish an upper from a lower urinary tract infection.

White cell casts are seen fairly easily in the urinary sediment with the brightfield microscope (see Fig 13–10,A). The cells are fairly prominent, and the characteristic multilobular nucleus can usually be seen. Small leukocytes stain purple to violet, while large ones may be pale blue, in a pink matrix. As the cells disintegrate within the cast, their cytoplasm becomes granular, cell borders merge, and nuclei become indistinct, resulting in a granular cast when the cells are no longer distinguishable. The number of cells in a cast varies—some casts are packed with cells while others show only a few cells in a hyaline matrix. White cell casts packed with cells still have a protein matrix, and should have parallel sides and rounded ends. It is sometimes difficult to distinguish such a white cell cast from a clump of leukocytes (pseudoleukocyte cast), which may originate lower in the urinary tract. The presence of strands of mucus to which the white cells adhere is another complication. Yet it is important not to report such pseudocasts as casts, which imply renal involvement or disease.

It may also be difficult, if not impossible, to distinguish a leukocyte cast from an epithelial cast, especially when cells begin to deteriorate. Here, the best indicator is probably the nature of other constituents in the urinary sediment. Leukocytes and bacteria in the sediment would be associated with leukocyte casts, while epithelial casts are more likely to be accompanied by cells appearing to be renal epithelium. Glitter cells are often seen when phagocytic neutrophils are present. When a morphologic distinction is impossible, the cast should be reported merely as a cellular cast, rather than misidentifying it. The physician will use information about other constituents in the sediment, the results of other urinalysis and laboratory tests, and the patient's case history in arriving at a diagnosis.

Epithelial Cell Casts

Epithelial casts represent a most serious situation, although they are very infrequently seen in the urine, as renal tubular disease (nephrosis) is relatively rare. They may be seen in cases of exposure to nephrotoxic substances such as mercury or ethylene glycol (antifreeze), or in infections with viruses such as cytomegalovirus or hepatitis virus. They result from destruction or desquamation of the cells that line the renal tubules. These cells are responsible for the work done by the kidney. The damage may be irreversible, depending on the severity of the disease process. The time needed to replace renal epithelial cells, if the basement membrane is left intact, is unknown; however, cells do not show maximum concentrating ability for several months after severe loss of tubular epithelium.

The epithelial cast often appears to consist of two rows of renal epithelial cells, implying tubular desquamation (see Fig 13–10,B,C). However, the cells may also vary in size, shape, and distribution, showing a varying amount of protein matrix. When the cells are haphazardly arranged in the cast in varying stages of degeneration, cellular damage and desquamation from different and separate portions of the renal tubule is implied. The epithelial cast does not remain constant once formed, but undergoes a series of changes. These changes result from cellular disintegration as the cast remains within the kidney, as a result of decreased urine flow (stasis). Therefore, a range of epithelial casts from cellular to coarsely granular, finely granular, and finally waxy may be seen. The waxy type represents the most serious situation, as prolonged blockage of renal flow is required for them to form. All of these types of casts are often seen in the same specimen; such specimens are re-

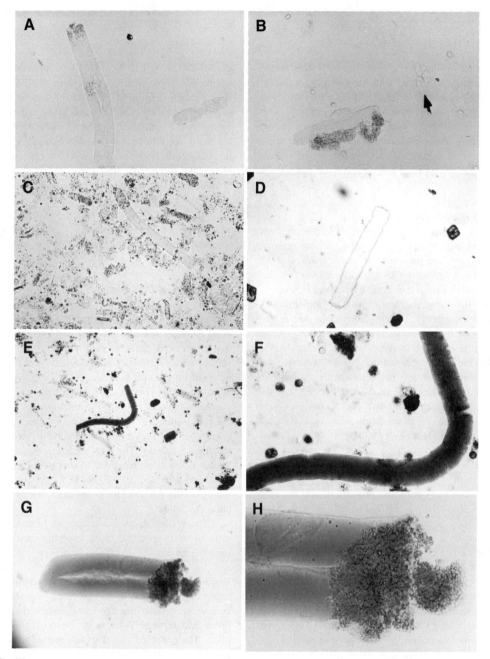

FIG 13–11.

Waxy and other casts in the urinary sediment. **A,** waxy cast *(left),* granular to waxy cast *(right),* unstained, ×160. **B,** waxy cast and two granular casts. A clump of renal tubular epithelial cells is also present *(arrow).* Unstained, ×160. **C,** mixture of casts including, waxy, granular, hyaline, unstained, ×100. **D,** broad waxy cast. Note broken ends and compare with diaper fibers (see Fig 13–16,F). Unstained, ×100. **E,** mixture of casts including waxy, granular, and hyaline, from same patient as **C.** Stained with Sedistain, ×100. **F,** enlarged view of the cast in **E,** showing a broad cast in transition from granular to waxy. Stained with Sedistain, ×400. **G,** broad waxy cast with central fissure and granular end. Stained with Sedistain, ×160. **H,** high-power view of the granular end of the broad waxy cast in **G,** also showing the presence of fat globules, ×400.

ferred to as "telescoped" urinary sediments (see Fig 13–11,C,E,F).

Epithelial casts may be difficult to distinguish from white cell casts, as previously discussed. When stained, the cells have a blue-purple nucleus and lighter blue-purple cytoplasm in a pink matrix. Phase-contrast and interference microscopy are also helpful in this examination, as is cytocentrifugation.

Red Blood Cell, and Blood and Blood Pigment Casts

The observation of red blood cell casts in the urinary sediment is a significant diagnostic finding and indicates a serious renal condition. Their presence must not be missed. The red cells enter the nephron by leakage through the glomerular capsule. It is possible that they bleed into the renal tubules at a point beyond the glomerular capsule; however, this would be a far less common path, as red cell casts are almost always associated with diseases that affect the glomerulus, such as acute glomerulonephritis and lupus nephritis. Once red cells are present in the lumen of the nephron, they clump together to form red cell casts. Red cell casts are probably the most fragile ones in the urinary sediment, which may be why they are rarely observed and why fragments are more often found. When physical conditions indicate that red cell casts may be present, it is imperative that the urine specimen be absolutely fresh and gently treated. The casts may be so fragile that they disintegrate under the microscope as the observer watches.

Red cell casts have a characteristic orange-yellow color caused by hemoglobin, which makes them unlike anything else seen in the urinary sediment (Fig 13–10,E–G). Stain may or may not be useful in the identification of blood casts; however, the casts may have intact red cells, which stain colorless or lavender in a pink matrix. Phase-contrast and interference microscopy are both very useful in detecting red cell casts. The characteristic color is, however, best appreciated with brightfield observation of the unstained sediment.

The number of cells present in the red cell cast is variable. Often only a few intact cells are seen in a hyaline matrix. This may be referred to as a *hyaline red cell cast*. If many cells are clumped together to form the cast, the matrix is often not visible. These casts are more fragile and, unfortunately, more serious from the clinical standpoint.

Red cell casts are often divided into two types: (1) red blood cell casts and (2) blood or blood (hemoglobin) pigment casts. It is also possible to see mixed casts which are a combination of both types. The red blood cell cast contains at least some recognizable red cells. They may be present in a generally hyaline matrix, or appear as a solid mass of conglutinated red cells with little or no matrix between the packed cells. The blood or blood (hemoglobin) pigment cast shows a homogeneous matrix with no cell margins or recognizable red cells. Both types of casts have a characteristic orange-yellow color. The red blood cells within casts may disintegrate, like the cells in epithelial or white cell casts, to form blood pigment casts. The blood or blood pigment cast is then analogous to the waxy cast. In any case, the occurrence of red cells within a cast, regardless of the number of cells, represents a serious situation. When red blood cells are found in the urinary sediment, in conjunction with red cell casts of any sort, renal (usually glomerular) involvement is indicated.

Granular Casts

The granules seen in granular casts may be the result of breakdown of cells within the cast or the renal tubule, or aggregates of plasma proteins including fibrinogen, immune complexes, and globulins in a Tamm-Horsfall matrix. Once all the cells have become granules, it is impossible to say for sure what sort of cell was originally present in the renal tubule. Such a distinction is useful, as red cell casts indicate glomerular injury, epithelial cell casts indicate renal tubular damage, and white cell casts indicate interstitial inflammation or infection. Often casts are seen that are basically granular but show some cells in transition to granules. When cells are present they should be identified if possible. Once again, phase-contrast and interference microscopy are helpful in this distinction, as is cytocentrifugation. The end product of this disintegration is the waxy cast, a finding that represents a serious pathologic condition.

The size of the granules within the granular cast varies; they become progressively smaller as the cells disintegrate. The number of granules also varies, and casts range from those that are completely filled with granules to those that are basically hyaline and contain only a few granules. Such granules may have been present in the renal tubule and trapped in a protein matrix as the cast was formed. Although granular casts are sometimes reported as coarsely or finely granular, the term *granular* is sufficient (see Fig 13–9,E–H). The distinction between coarsely and finely granular is subjective, but relatively easily made. If the cast has a definite hyaline matrix with only a few granules, it is reported as hyaline. When large numbers of granules are present, it is described as granular.

Coarsely Granular Casts.—These casts appear to contain degenerated cells in the form of large granules. They tend to be darker, shorter, and more irregular in outline than finely granular casts. The darker color and larger granules make them easier to find than either hyaline or finely granular casts. They stain with dark-purple granules in a purple matrix. Fat may be present in these casts showing as refractive globules that do not stain.

Finely Granular Casts.—These casts look much like hyaline casts; however, the presence of fine granules makes them more distinctive and easier to find. When viewed with phase-contrast or interference microscopy, hyaline casts generally show a fine granulation. They are usually grayish or pale yellow in the unstained sediment and stain with fine dark-purple granules in a pale-pink or pale-purple matrix. Fat globules may also be found, appearing as highly refractive globules that do not stain.

Waxy Casts

Waxy casts resemble hyaline casts and may be mistaken for them. They are much more significant clinically. The waxy cast is homogeneous, like the hyaline cast, but it is yellowish and more refractive with sharper outlines. It appears hard whereas the hyaline cast has a delicate appearance. Waxy casts tend to be wider than hyaline casts (they are described as broad casts or broad waxy casts) and usually have irregular broken ends and fissures or cracks in their sides (see Fig 13–11). Fairly long forms are also seen. Phase-contrast and interference microscopy and staining are useful in the examination of waxy casts. They generally stain with greater intensity than hyaline casts, making them easier to visualize.

Waxy casts are felt to be the final step in the disintegration of cellular casts and are especially serious since they imply renal stasis. They are associated with severe chronic renal disease and renal amyloidosis, and are seen only rarely and in small numbers in acute renal diseases.

Fatty Casts

The importance and probable mechanism of formation of fatty casts have been discussed along with oval fat bodies and fat globules. These three structures are often seen together in the same urine specimen, along with extremely large amounts of protein (greater than 2,000 mg/dL) and the pale foamy appearance of the specimen associated with the nephrotic syndrome. They are serious because they represent fatty degeneration and desquamation of the renal tubular epithelium. They are also seen in diabetes mellitus with renal degeneration and in toxic renal poisoning as from ethylene glycol or mercury.

Fatty casts, as the name implies, contain droplets of fat. These droplets are highly refractile under the microscope (Fig 13–12). Although phase-contrast and interference microscopy are useful, the characteristic refractile appearance of fat droplets might be better appreciated with the brightfield microscope. If the droplets are neutral fat or triglyceride, they will stain bright orange or red with Sudan or oil red O stains. If cholesterol is present, they will show a Maltese cross pattern with polarized light. When stained with Sternheimer-Malbin stain, the cast matrix will stain, but the refractile fat globules will not.

Fatty casts may be seen as a protein matrix almost completely filled with fat globules, or as fat globules contained within a basically hyaline, cellular, or granular cast. In addition to free fat globules, intact oval fat bodies may be seen within the cast matrix; these are sometimes referred to as *oval fat body casts.*

Other Casts

Various other structures that may be found in the urinary sediment may rarely be incorporated into the protein matrix of a cast. *Pigmented casts* may be seen including hemoglobin (already described), myoglobin, bilirubin, and other drugs such as phenazopyridine. *Hemosiderin casts* contain granules of hemosiderin. *Crystal casts,* which contain urates, calcium oxalate, or sulfonamides, have also been seen. These must not be mistaken for crystals adhering to strands of mucus, however. Rather, the protein matrix must be visualized in a true crystal cast. *Bacteria casts* have also been described.

Structures Confused With Casts

Mucous Threads.—The refractive index of mucous threads is similar to that of hyaline casts; however, the former are long ribbonlike strands with undefined edges and pointed or split ends. They also appear to have longitudinal striations. They are most apparent, and cause the most confusion with phase-contrast or interference

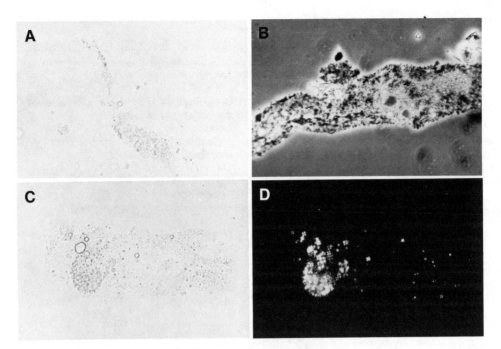

FIG 13–12.
Fatty casts in the urinary sediment. **A,** fatty cast, unstained, ×400. **B,** fatty (oval fat body) cast, phase-contrast microscopy, stained with Sudan III, ×400. **C,** fatty cast with oval fat body inclusion, unstained, ×400. **D,** fatty cast, same field as **C,** showing Maltese cross formation of cholesterol with polarized light, ×400.

microscopy. They are often seen together with hyaline casts. Although difficult to distinguish, hyaline casts are generally more formed or structured (Fig 13–9,A–D).

Rolled Squamous Epithelial Cells.—These may be mistaken for casts when they have rolled into a cigar shape. However, they have pointed ends rather than rounded ones and are shorter, and a single round nucleus may be discovered with careful focusing.

Disposable Diaper Fibers.—These fibers are easily confused with waxy casts, appearing almost identically highly refractile with blunt ends (see Fig 13–16,F). They may be seen in urine specimens from infants, or from geriatric patients or other adults who must use diapers. Unlike waxy casts, diaper fibers are rarely accompanied by other pathologic findings, especially proteinuria. The use of polarizing microscopy may be useful. Waxy casts do not polarize light. Diaper fibers do.

Other Structures.—Bits of *hair* or *threads* of material fibers are also mistaken for casts by the beginner. However, these are extremely refractive structures that have nothing in common with the appearance of protein microscopically. Likewise, *scratches* on the glass slide or coverglass may be mistaken for casts at first. Again, they are much too definite and obvious to be important. Finally, *hyphae of molds* are sometimes mistaken for hyaline casts (see Fig 13–7). This is similar to mistaking yeast for red cells. Hyphae are much more refractive and are jointed and branching, as may be observed on closer examination.

Crystals and Amorphous Material

Clinical Significance

Crystals and amorphous precipitates of certain chemicals make up what has been called the unorganized urinary sediment. These materials are obvious under the microscope. Because they are so striking, there is a natural tendency to pay considerable attention to them, but they are the most insignificant part of the urinary sediment and deserve little attention. In the past, great emphasis was placed on the identification of these materials. However, it is generally preferable to search carefully for more pathologic constituents and note only briefly the occurrence of crystals.

Most urine specimens contain some crystalline material when voided. As urine specimens stand, especially when refrigerated, most become cloudy because of the precipitation of amorphous material and crystals. The student should learn to identify normal crystals and amorphous materials, however, for the following reasons: First, if they are abundant they will obscure such important structures as red blood cells, white blood cells, and casts. The more important structures must be searched for with extreme care when crystals and amorphous materials are present. The use of a stain, such as the Sternheimer-Malbin stain, may be especially useful in this case. Second, the precipitation of certain crystals will accompany kidney stone formation (**lithiasis**). This is one reason for the attention that was formerly given to urinary crystals. Finally, substances such as cystine, leucine, and tyrosine may crystallize in urine and indicate serious metabolic or inherited disorders. Administration of sulfonamide drugs may cause the formation of sulfonamide crystals, especially in acidic urine. The formation of sulfonamide crystals within the kidney may result in blockage of renal output and severe renal damage. This problem was greater when sulfonamide drugs were first introduced. Drugs that are currently used are more soluble, thus less likely to precipitate. However, crystals are occasionally seen when high doses are given.

Normal crystals should be identified and reported merely as a few, moderate, or many per high-power field (×400 magnification). Microscopic examination is sufficient; they do not require chemical tests. **Abnormal crystals** should be reported by enumerating according to the scale criteria given in Procedure 13–13, Microscopic Examination of the Urinary Sediment (and Table 13–5). They cannot be reported on the basis of microscopic evidence alone, but require confirmatory chemical tests. The identification of normal urinary crystals and amorphous material is further simplified by the fact that they occur in either acidic or alkaline urine. Therefore the pH of the urine should always be known when the microscopic examination is made. It must be remembered that it is the shape, rather than the size, that is characteristic of crystals. See summary of normal and abnormal crystals in Table 13–8.

TABLE 13–8.

Crystals Found in the Urinary Sediment

Normal crystals of acid urine
Amorphous urates
Uric acid
Calcium oxalate (also seen in alkaline urine)
Normal crystals of alkaline urine
Amorphous phosphates
Triple phosphates
Ammonium biurate
Calcium phosphate
Calcium carbonate
Calcium oxalate
Abnormal urinary crystals of metabolic origin
Cystine
Tyrosine
Leucine
Cholesterol
Abnormal urinary crystals of iatrogenic origin
Sulfonamides
Ampicillin
Radiographic media

Normal Crystals Seen in Acidic Urine

Amorphous Urates.—This is the amorphous material found in urine of an acid pH. Chemically, amorphous urates are the sodium salts of uric acid. *Amorphous* means without shape or form. The urates show a characteristic yellowish-red shapeless granulation (Fig 13–13,A). When present in sufficient numbers, they form a characteristic fluffy pink precipitate referred to as *brick dust*. Amorphous urates tend to precipitate out of urine that is highly concentrated, as in dehydration and fever. Such urine specimens are typically highly colored (dark amber) and show large amounts of fluffy pink precipitate. Although of an alarming appearance to the patient, such specimens are of little concern clinically. Amorphous urates will change to uric acid when acidified with uric acid. They will dissolve when warmed to 60° C and when treated with dilute alkali.

Uric Acid.—These crystals have a variety of shapes and colors. Typically they are yellow or reddish-brown, much like the chemically related amorphous urates. The typical shape is the whetstone. Other shapes include rhombic plates or prisms, somewhat oval forms with pointed ends ("lemon-shaped"), wedges, rosettes, and irregular plates (Fig 13–13,B–F). They are usually recog-

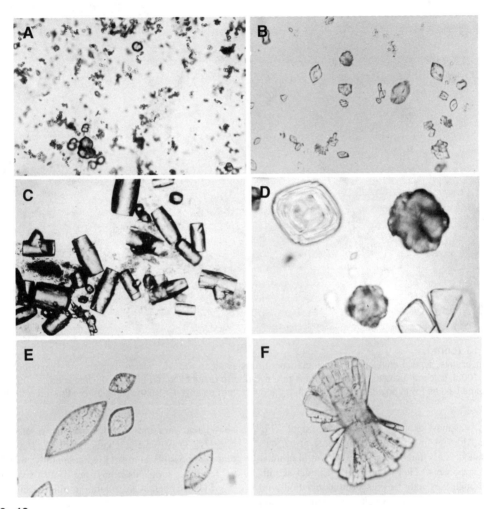

FIG 13–13.
Normal crystals seen in acidic urine. **A,** amorphous urates, stained with Sedistain, ×400. **B,** uric acid crystals, lemon-shaped, unstained, ×400. **C,** barrel-shaped uric acid crystals with amorphous urates, unstained, ×100. **D,** laminated uric acid crystals, unstained, ×640. **E,** large lemon-shaped uric acid crystals, unstained, ×400. **F,** uric acid crystal, unstained, ×400.

nized by color, but some, especially the rhombic plates, may appear colorless. Unusual crystals in urine of an acid pH are generally forms of uric acid.

Uric acid crystals are commonly seen in urine specimens, especially after the specimen has been standing. Amorphous urates and uric acid may be associated with gout or stone formation, besides chronic renal disease and certain malignancies such as leukemias, especially after chemotherapy. However, their presence in urine is not diagnostic of these conditions. A hexagonal form of

uric acid may be mistaken for cystine crystals, which are abnormal and important to detect.

Calcium Oxalate.—Calcium oxalate crystals have a characteristic "envelope" appearance. They vary somewhat in size but are typically small, colorless, glistening octahedrons (see Fig 13–13,G). Less frequently they may appear in a dumbbell shape or an ovoid shape which may resemble red blood cells (Fig 13–13,H,I). Unlike

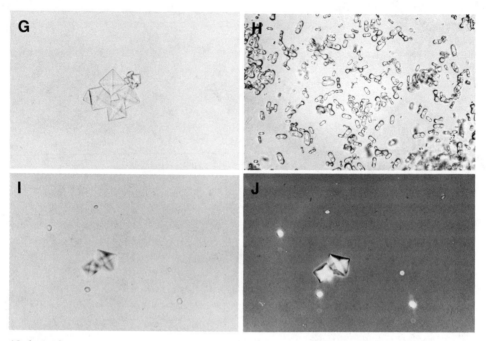

FIG 13–13 (cont.).
G, calcium oxalate, typical envelope shape (octahedral), unstained, ×400. **H,** calcium oxalate, rare dumbbell form, unstained, ×100. **I,** calcium oxalate, typical form plus rare ovoid form resembling red blood cell. Unstained, ×400. **J,** calcium oxalate: same field as **I** with polarized light. Note that the ovoid form polarizes, distinguishing it from the red cell. Unstained, ×400.

red cells, calcium oxalate will polarize light (Fig 13–13,J). Although most common in acidic urine, calcium oxalate crystals may also be seen in neutral or alkaline urine specimens. They are of little clinical significance, although they may be present in association with stone formation, as calcium oxalate is the most common constituent found in kidney stones.

Normal Crystals Seen in Alkaline Urine

Amorphous Phosphates.—The amorphous material found in alkaline urine is amorphous phosphate. Generally, the phosphates give a finer or more lacy precipitate than the amorphous urates and are colorless (Fig 13–14,A). Phosphates are the most common cause of turbidity in alkaline urine and are seen as a fine white precipitate microscopically. They do not dissolve when heated but are soluble in acetic acid and dilute hydrochloric acid.

Triple Phosphates.—Triple (ammonium magnesium) phosphates are colorless crystals and commonly show great variation in size, from tiny to relatively huge crystals. They have a characteristic "coffin-lid" shape that is impossible to miss. Less commonly, they occur in a fernlike form as they go into solution (Fig 13–14,B–E). They are soluble in dilute acetic acid.

Ammonium Biurate.—This ammonium salt is the alkaline counterpart of uric acid and amorphous urates in urine. The crystals are spherical with radial or concentric striations and long prismatic spicules, resembling thorn apples (Fig 13–14,E,F). They are yellow and may be mistaken for some forms of the sulfonamide drugs that may precipitate out of urine. Sulfa crystals are usually seen in acidic urine, however. Ammonium biurates are often present in old urine specimens, especially those that contain unusual sediment constituents and have been retained for teaching purposes. They are much less frequently seen in fresh urine collections. They are soluble at 60° C with acetic acid and in strong alkali. They will convert to uric acid with concentrated hydrochloric acid or acetic acid.

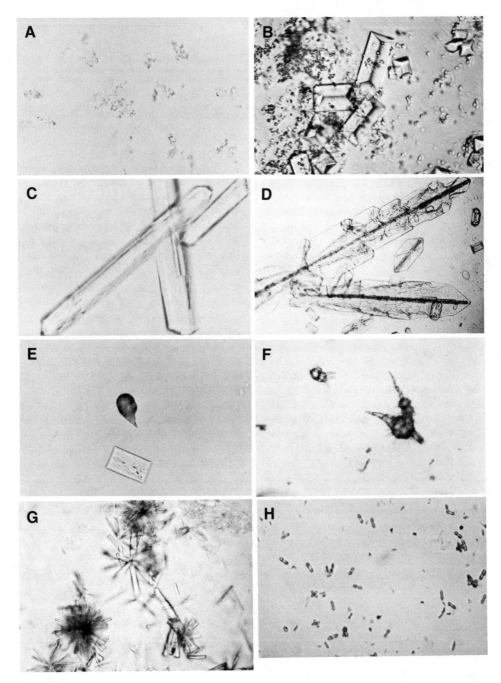

FIG 13–14.

Normal crystals seen in alkaline urine. **A,** amorphous phosphate, unstained, ×400. **B,** triple phosphate, typical coffin-lid form, plus amorphous phosphates, unstained, ×400. **C,** triple phosphate, unstained, ×400. **D,** triple phosphate crystals going into solution. Smaller, more typical forms are also present. Unstained, ×400. **E,** ammonium biurate and triple phosphate, (dissolving), unstained, ×400. **F,** ammonium biurate, thorn apple form, unstained, ×400. **G,** calcium phosphate, most typical form, unstained, ×400. **H,** calcium carbonate, tiny dumbbell form, unstained, ×400.

Calcium Phosphate.—Calcium phosphate crystals are colorless. They may appear as flat plates (which are often mistaken for epithelial cells) or as slender wedges that occur singly or in rosettes (Fig 13–14,G) and may be mistaken for certain sulfonamide crystals. They are slightly soluble in dilute acetic acid and soluble in dilute hydrochloric acid.

Calcium Carbonate.—Calcium carbonate crystals are tiny, colorless granules that typically occur in pairs ("dumbbells") but may occur also singly (Fig 13–14,H). Because they are so small, calcium carbonate crystals represent part of the amorphous material seen in normal alkaline urine specimens. They are soluble in acetic acid with effervescence.

Abnormal Urinary Crystals

All of the abnormal crystals described in the following paragraphs are seen in urine specimens of an acid pH. Normal crystals of urine may be reported on the basis of microscopic examination alone. Abnormal crystals should not be reported without confirmatory chemical tests. The following description of abnormal crystals is superficial. If the occurrence of such crystals is suspected, a more detailed text must be consulted for microscopic appearance and confirmatory chemical procedures.

Abnormal crystals may be further classified as metabolic or iatrogenic (see Table 13–8). Metabolic crystals are present in certain disease states or inherited conditions, while iatrogenic crystals are the result of treatment. Of the following, cystine, tyrosine, leucine, and cholesterol are abnormal crystals of metabolic origin which have pathologic significance, while the sulfonamides, ampicillin, and radiographic media are of iatrogenic origin.

Cystine.—Cystine crystals are colorless, refractile, hexagonal plates which are often laminated (Fig 13–15,A). They may be seen in the urine of patients with the hereditary condition cystinuria, an amino acid disorder. This is serious as these patients are apt to form cystine stones which may lead to kidney damage. The stones may be mistaken for a form of uric acid crystal which is also hexagonal. The presence of cystine should be confirmed with the cyanide-nitroprusside reaction. Cystine is reduced to cysteine by sodium cyanide. The free sulfhydryl groups which result react with nitroprusside to give a red-purple color. Cystine crystals are most

insoluble in acid pH. They are soluble in alkali (especially ammonia) and dilute hydrochloric acid. They are insoluble in boiling water, acetic acid, alcohol, and ether. They are soluble in water and in pH less than 2 and greater than 8.

Tyrosine.—Tyrosine crystals may be present as the result of inherited amino acid disorders and severe liver disease. They are rare and appear as fine needles arranged in sheaves, which appear black as the microscope is focused (Fig 13–15,B). They occur in urine of an acid pH. Tyrosine is soluble in alkali and dilute mineral acid. They are relatively heat-soluble but insoluble in alcohol and ether. They are confirmed with the nitrosonaphthol test.

Leucine.—Leucine crystals are yellow, oily-looking spheres with radial and concentric striations. They are of metabolic origin and extremely rare. Leucine and tyrosine crystals usually appear together and are associated with severe liver disease. Leucine is found in urine of an acid pH.

Cholesterol.—Cholesterol crystals are another crystal of metabolic origin found in urine of an acid pH. They are extremely rare. Cholesterol crystals are large, flat, hexagonal plates with one or more corners notched out (Fig 13–15,C). Crystals of radiographic media (such as meglumine diatrizoate) are fairly commonly found after intravenous radiographic studies. They are morphologically similar to cholesterol, but they are associated with a very high specific gravity (greater than 1.035) and a false-positive, delayed sulfosalicylic acid test for protein. They should not be mistaken for cholesterol (see Fig 13–15,G,H). If present, crystals of cholesterol should be associated with other findings such as free fat, oval fat bodies, or fatty casts. They are more likely to be seen in urine specimens which have been retained and refrigerated. They are very soluble in chloroform, ether, and hot alcohol.

Sulfonamides.—Although a crystal of iatrogenic origin, sulfonamide crystals are important pathologically. Sulfonamide crystals have various forms depending on the form of the drug. They are most insoluble at an acid pH. They include the following (Fig 13–15,D–F).

1. Sulfanilamide is rarely seen. It occurs as large, colorless needles, frequently in sheaves or rosettes.

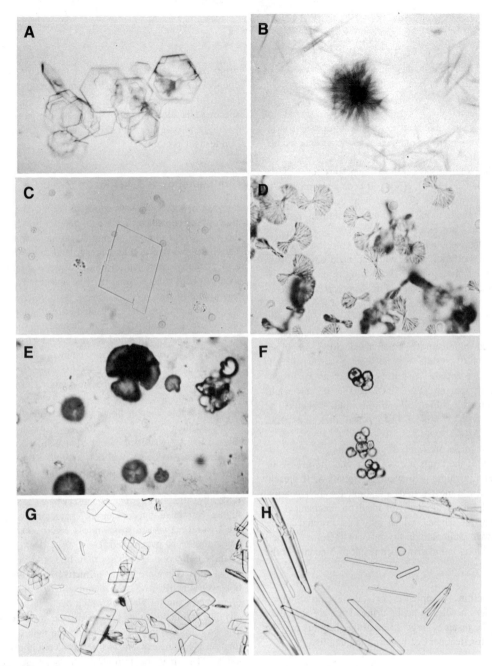

FIG 13-15.
Abnormal crystals in the urinary sediment. **A,** cystine, unstained, ×640. **B,** tyrosine, unstained, ×400. **C,** cholesterol plate (extremely rare). Fat and red cells are also present. Unstained, ×400. **D,** sulfonamide crystals (sulfadiazine). Red cells are also present. Unstained, ×400. **E,** sulfonamide crystals (sulfamethoxazole), unstained, ×400. **F,** sulfonamide crystals (sulfamethoxazole). Note similarity to ammonium biurate. Unstained, ×400. **G,** radiographic contrast media (meglumine diatrizoate). Note similarity to cholesterol. However, a large number of crystals and no other signs of lipid are present. Unstained, ×640. **H,** crystals of radiographic contrast media from false-positive sulfosalicylic acid protein test, unstained, ×400.

2. Sulfapyridine occurs as colorless arrowheads or whetstones, also as brown needles in large conglomerate masses or rosettes.

3. Sulfathiazole occurs as brownish shocks of wheat with central binding or rosettes with radial striations, also as colorless diamond and hexagonal plates, sometimes in rosettes.

4. Sulfadiazine is the most dangerous form of the drug in urine (see Fig 13–15,D). It occurs as colorless to greenish brown shocks of wheat with eccentric binding and rosettes with radial striations, sometimes covered with needlelike processes.

5. Sulfaguanidine appears as colorless needles grouped as shocks of wheat with eccentric binding, also as rectangular plates with slight bulging in the long axis.

6. Sulfamethylthiazole occurs as colorless to greenish brown needles clumped in the shape of a fan.

7. Sulfamethoxazole, supplied in combination with trimethoprim (Bactrim, Septra), is the most commonly encountered sulfonamide. When these drugs are given in high dosage, crystals may be seen in the urine. Sulfamethoxazole appears as dense brown spears or irregular divided spheres (Fig 13–15,E,F). If suspected, sulfamethoxazole, like all sulfonamides, should be confirmed with a clinical history and then the diazo reaction.

Sulfonamides are rarely found in urine, as more soluble forms of the drugs are available and the pH of the urine is kept alkaline to prevent precipitation. If present they represent a most serious situation, for their precipitation in the renal tubules will result in mechanical destruction of the tubules, which may lead to renal failure or shutdown. Sulfonamide crystals are therefore associated with blood in the urine as a result of bleeding in the renal tubules.

Ampicillin.—Ampicillin crystals appear as long thin colorless needles in acidic urine. They are seen only rarely as the result of large doses of the drug, as may be necessary for treatment of bacterial meningitis.

Radiographic Contrast Media.—Crystals of compounds such as meglumine diatrizoate (Renografin) used for diagnostic x-ray procedures may be precipitated in the urine as flat, four-sided plates, or long thin rectangles (Fig 13–15,G,H). They are not abnormal crystals in the sense of the others described in this section, since they are not metabolic products nor do they harm the patient. Rather, they may be regarded as a contaminant in the

urine of iatrogenic origin and do not require chemical confirmation. However, these crystals should not be mistaken for cholesterol. When they are present the urine specimen is cloudy, has a high specific gravity (over 1.035), and may show a delayed false-positive precipitation test for protein.

Contaminants and Artifacts

Many objects and structures in the urinary sediment are contaminants or artifacts, and distract the attention of the observer from the important urinary constituents. These are the objects that students tend to see first when a microscopic examination of the urine is attempted. It seems to be a general rule that if an object is easy to see, it is unimportant.

Contaminating substances and artifacts that are often present in the urinary sediment include *cotton threads, hair, wool fibers,* and *wood fibers* (Fig 13–16,E). These are fairly common and easy to recognize. When wooden applicator sticks are used to mix the urinary sediment, wood fibers are common contaminants. These are *not* casts.

Disposable diaper fibers are particularly troublesome in their resemblance to waxy casts (see Fig 13–16,F). As described earlier, diaper fibers will polarize light but waxy casts will not, and other findings associated with casts, such as proteinuria, are absent.

Scratches on the coverglass are often mistaken for casts by the inexperienced observer. Their regular, highly refractive appearance is characteristic. *Bubbles* are also refractive and structureless and soon accepted as something to be overlooked. *Oil droplets* from lubricants or dirty collection containers may be confused with red blood cells. They are highly refractive and structureless, however (Fig 13–16,C). Contaminating oil must be distinguished from fat globules which occur in lipuria, usually in conjunction with fatty casts and oval fat bodies. The use of polarizing filters is helpful in making this distinction. Granules of *starch* are also common contaminants. They may be introduced from surgical gloves. Starch granules, along with other common contaminants, also pose a problem in that they are doubly refractive, showing a Maltese cross pattern when examined with polarized light. In this case, observation with brightfield illumination clearly differentiates starch from fat globules containing esters of cholesterol (Fig 13–16,A,B). Crystals of talc are also common urinary contaminants and should be recognized as such and then ignored. Like-

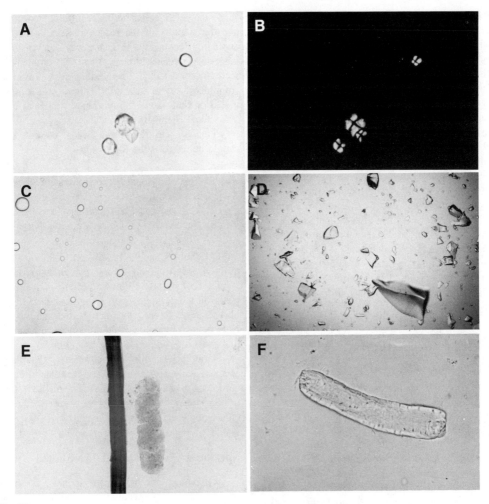

FIG 13–16.
Contaminants in the urinary sediment. **A,** starch granules. Note typical appearance with brightfield illumination, unlike fat. Unstained, ×400. **B,** starch granules, same field as **A** with polarized light. Note typical Maltese cross formation and similarity to globules of cholesterol as seen in Figures 13–6,J and 13–12,D. **C,** immersion oil, unstained, ×500. **D,** glass fragments from coverglass, unstained, ×125. **E,** fiber *(left)* and waxy cast *(right),* stained with Sedistain, ×400. **F,** diaper fiber. Note similarity to waxy casts in Figure 13–11,D. Unstained, ×400.

wise, fragments of glass should not be mistaken for crystals (see Fig 13–16,D).

QUALITY ASSURANCE

The urinalysis laboratory, like all departments of the clinical laboratory, requires a quality assurance program to ensure that results are meaningful for the physician and the patient. The use of multiple reagent strips generally ensures rapid and reliable screening of all specimens for a greater range of abnormal constituents than was possible before they came into routine use. However, the principle of each test and its limitations and possible sources of interference and error must be understood. It is necessary to know which tests can be used only to screen for the presence or absence of a substance and which tests yield semiquantitative results. The necessity for and performance of confirmatory methods must be understood and employed. Tests must be performed in a technically correct manner and the reagent strips and tablets must be stored properly so that they react as they are designed to. The latter is ensured by the use of control specimens.

The quality assurance program begins with adequate and consistent record-keeping. All procedures that are performed must be described in a procedure manual. This should include information regarding controls for the analyte in question, expected values, information regarding confirmatory testing, test principles for each procedure, and current product inserts. In addition, a record of lot number and expiration date of each container of reagent strips should be kept, along with control values. Information must also be recorded along with patient results. This includes time and date of collection, the lot number of the products used in testing the specimen, control solution results, and the initials of the person performing the test.

Control Solutions and Records

Control solutions must be used each day by each shift of workers. They are particularly necessary in the urinalysis laboratory because the least trained and most inexperienced personnel continue to be placed in this important department.

Several quality control products are commercially available and suitable for use in the laboratory. Most are obtained in lyophilized form (freeze-dried human urine) and require reconstitution before use. Positive and negative controls are available, and both should be used in the routine testing program. The products are assayed for expected results with commonly used reagent strips and methods. The assayed values that are available for a product will be a factor in determining which product is used by a laboratory.

Urinalysis control solutions may be used both as a check on the urinalysis reagents and procedures, and as a means of evaluating the ability of the laboratory personnel to correctly perform and interpret the tests. New bottles of reagent strips and tablets should be tested when they are first opened. All previously opened bottles of reagent strips and tablets should be tested at the beginning of each shift. Controls should be included whenever new reagents are used. Control solutions should be employed that check for both false-negative and false-positive re-

sults, the relative sensitivity at different concentrations, and the stability of the reagents. Results should be recorded or documented in such a way as to ensure that the laboratory remains in control and that problems are corrected when detected. The notation system used will vary from laboratory to laboratory; control results may be tabulated on daily and weekly graphs similar to those used for clinical chemistry analyses.

One system describing when control specimens should be tested is the following:

1. Test all opened bottles of reagent strips or tablets each morning.
2. Test each new bottle on opening.
3. Record data on the record sheet daily.

All bottles should be covered tightly when not in use. Directions given by the manufacturer for storage should be carefully followed. If any discoloration appears on the reagent strips or tablets, discard the bottle immediately. Record the date bottles are first opened. Note the expiration date and do not use any product after that date.

Urinometers and refractometers should also be checked daily for accuracy and the data should be recorded in an acceptable manner. The method of checking urinometers and refractometers was described under Specific Gravity earlier in this chapter.

Specimen Collection and Handling

Of course, the best quality control system will be useless if the urine specimen is not collected and handled in an acceptable manner, before and after reaching the urinalysis laboratory, or if it is mislabeled. Such mistakes remain the most frequent cause of error in routine urinalysis. One method of at least partial control of handling or specimen errors is to include blind controls or blind duplicates in the daily collection of urine specimens to be analyzed.

Inspection of Results and Correlation of Findings

Probably the oldest and still most useful tool in quality control of urinalysis is a final inspection of all the results that make up the urinalysis before they are reported to the physician or placed on the patient's laboratory record. Correlation of expected findings has been discussed throughout this section whenever applicable. To correctly inspect the laboratory record for correlated results, the worker must know the limitations of the tests and the reason for their use. Physical properties, chemical test results, and constituents seen in the urinary sediment should be correlated. Some of the expected results, from a visual inspection of the report form, are listed below.

Correlation of Urinalysis Findings
Example A

Physical appearance: red or a variation of red (smoky, pink, orange, brown, or black)
pH: acid or alkaline
Protein: positive or negative
Blood: positive (unless there is ascorbic acid interference)
Sediment: red blood cells if caused by blood, red cell casts (or a variation such as granular casts) if caused by glomerular disease
Suspect: red blood cells, hemoglobin, myoglobin

Example B

Physical appearance: dark amber with fluffy pink precipitate (brick dust)
pH: acid
Specific gravity: relatively high
Chemical tests: variable
Sediment: amorphous urates, uric acid
Suspect: concentrated normal urine

Example C

Physical appearance: cloudy, white
Specific gravity: greater than 1.035 by urinometer or refractometer
Protein: delayed positive protein precipitation test
Sediment: unusual crystals of radiographic media
Suspect: contamination with radiographic media

Example D

Physical appearance: cloudy, white
pH: alkaline
Specific gravity: may be low (variable)
Protein: positive or negative
Blood: positive or negative
Nitrites: positive or negative
Leukocyte esterase: positive or negative
Sediment: amorphous phosphates (most often), bacteria, white cells (neutrophils), epithelial cells (renal to squamous), casts (cellular, granular, waxy, hyaline)
Suspect: normal alkaline urine, lower urinary tract infection, or upper urinary tract infection

---

Example E

Physical appearance: pale, foamy
Specific gravity: low
Protein: very high (>2,000 mg/dL)
Sediment: oval fat bodies, fatty casts, free fat
Suspect: nephrotic syndrome

Example F

Physical appearance: pale, greenish
pH: acid
Specific gravity: high by refractometer or urinometer; normal or low by reagent strip
Protein: positive or negative
Glucose: positive
Ketones: positive
Sediment: yeast may be present
Suspect: diabetes mellitus

Example G

Physical appearance: vivid yellow-brown, green-brown, orange-red, or dark amber
Bilirubin: positive
Urobilinogen: positive or negative
Sediment: may show bile-stained casts or cells
Suspect: jaundice

General Rule

Whenever protein is present, the sediment should be carefully inspected for the presence of casts.

BIBLIOGRAPHY

Becan-McBride K, Ross D: *Essentials for the Small Laboratory and Physician's Office.* St Louis, Mosby–Year Book, Inc, 1988.

Bradley M, Schumann GB: Examination of urine, in Henry, JB (ed): *Todd, Sanford, Davidsohn Clinical Diagnosis and Management by Laboratory Methods,* ed 17. Philadelphia, WB Saunders Co, 1984, pp 380–458.

CAP Surveys Manual, Section II. Appendix II: Glossary of Terms for Urine Sediment and Clinical Microscopy. College of American Pathologists, Northfield, Ill, 1990.

Csako G: Causes, consequences and recognition of false-positive reactions for ketones. *Clin Chem* 1990; 36:7.

Factors Affecting Urine Chemistry Tests, Elkhart, Ind, Ames Division, Miles Laboratories, Inc, 1982.

Freeman JA, Beeler MF: *Laboratory Medicine/Urinalysis and Medical Microscopy,* ed 2. Philadelphia, Lea & Febiger, 1983.

Graff L: *A Handbook of Routine Urinalysis.* Philadelphia, JB Lippincott Co, 1983.

Haber MH: *Urine Casts: Their Microscopy and Clinical Significance,* ed 2. Chicago, American Society of Clinical Pathologists, 1976.

Haber MH: *A Primer of Microscopic Urinalysis.* Fountain Valley, Calif, ICL Scientific, 1978.

Haber MH: *Urinary Sediment: A Textbook Atlas.* Chicago, American Society of Clinical Pathologists, 1981.

Hansten PD: *Drug Interactions,* ed 6, Philadelphia, Lea & Febiger, 1989.

Instructions for Use and Care of the AO TS Meter and Concentrimeter (Goldberg Refractometers). Buffalo, Scientific Instruments Division, American Optical Corp, May 1973.

Kark RM, Lawrence JR, Pollak VE, et al: *A Primer of Urinalysis,* ed 2. New York, Hoeber Medical Division, Harper & Row, 1963.

Lippman RW: *Urine and the Urinary Sediment,* ed 2. Springfield, Ill, Charles C Thomas, Publisher, 1957.

Mahon CR, Smith LA: Standardization of the urine microscopic examination. *Clin Lab Sci* 1990; 3:328.

Modern Urine Chemistry Application of Urine Chemistry and Microscopic Examination in Health and Disease, Elkhardt, Ind, Ames Division, Miles Laboratories, Inc, 1987.

Physician's Office Laboratory Guidelines, Tentative Guidelines. Villanova, Pa, National Committee for Clinical Laboratory Standards, 1989; 9(4) POL1-T.

Physician's Office Laboratory Procedure Manual, Tentative Guidelines. Villanova, Pa, National Committee for Clinical Laboratory Standards, 1989; 9(5) POL2-T.

Raphael SS, et al: *Lynch's Medical Laboratory Technology,* ed 3, vol 1. Philadelphia, WB Saunders Co, 1976.

Ross D, Neely A: *Textbook of Urinalysis and Body Fluids.* Norwalk, Conn, Appleton-Century-Crofts, 1986.

Rutecki GJ, Goldsmith C, Schreiner GE: Characterization of proteins in urinary casts. *N Engl J Med* 1971; 284:19.

Schreiner GE: *Urinary Sediments,* New York, Medical Communications, Inc, 1969.

Schumann GB: *Urine Sediment Examination.* Baltimore, Williams & Wilkins Co, 1980.

Schumann GB, Schumann JL: *A Manual of Cytodiagnostic Urinalysis.* Salt Lake City, Cytodiagnostics Co, 1984.

Schumann GB, Schumann JL: *Cytodiagnostic Urinalysis Urine Sediment Entities Transparencies and Explanatory Text.* Salt Lake City, Cytodiagnostics Co, 1984.

Schumann GB, Schweitzer SC: Examination of urine, in Kaplan LA, Pesce AJ (eds): *Clinical Chemistry Theory, Analysis, and Correlation,* ed 2. St Louis, Mosby–Year Book, Inc, 1989, pp 820–849.

Schumann GB, Schweitzer SC: Examination of urine, in Henry, JB (ed): *Clinical Diagnosis and Management by Laboratory Methods,* ed 18. Philadelphia, WB Saunders Co, 1991, pp 387–444.

Schumann GB, Weiss MA: *Atlas of Renal and Urinary Tract Cytology and Its Histopathologic Bases.* Philadelphia, JB Lippincott Co, 1981.

Schweitzer SS, Schumann JL, Schumann GB: Quality assurance guidelines for the urinalysis laboratory. *J Med Technol* 1986; 3:11.

Stamey TA, Kindrachuk RW: *Urinary Sediment and Urinalysis: A Practical Guide for the Health Science Professional.* Philadelphia, WB Saunders Co, 1985.

Sternheimer R, Malbin B: Clinical recognition of pyelonephritis with a new stain for urinary sediments. *Am J Med* 1951; 2:312.

Strasinger SK: *Urinalysis and Body Fluids,* ed 2. Philadelphia, FA Davis Co, 1989.

Urinalysis Today, Indianapolis, Boehringer Mannheim Diagnostics, 1987.

Watson CJ, Bossenmaier I, Cardinal R: Acute intermittent porphyria urinary porphobilinogen and other Ehrlich reactors in diagnosis. *JAMA* 1961; 175:1087–1091.

14 Examination of Extravascular Fluids

Key Terms	
Birefringence	Pericardial fluid
Cerebrospinal fluid	Peritoneal fluid
Compensated polarized light	Pleural fluid
Cytocentrifugation	Synovial fluid
Effusion	Serous fluids
Extravascular fluids	Transudates
Exudate	Ultrafiltrate of plasma
Hansel's stain	Xanthochromia
Hyaluronate (hyaluronic acid)	

Extravascular fluids (body cavity fluids other than blood or urine) are examined in various divisions of the clinical laboratory, depending on the nature of the test requested. Cell counts are routinely done on most body fluids, and for this reason the specimen is often sent directly to the hematology laboratory after collection (see Chapter 2, Collecting and Processing Laboratory Specimens). The extravascular fluids are termed **pleural** (around the lungs), **pericardial** (around the heart), **peritoneal** (around the abdominal and pelvic cavities), **synovial** (around the joints), and **cerebrospinal** (around the brain and spinal cord). Each of these fluids is handled in special ways. Analyses of synovial fluid and cerebrospinal fluid are discussed separately. The examination of the other body fluids **(serous fluids)** is discussed in general terms.

Several general observations are made for all body fluids. Cell counts and specific gravities are usually determined. Cytocentrifuged slides or smears are made and, after staining with Wright's stain, are examined microscopically. Protein is measured and clot formation is observed. For other tests ordered, the specimen is sent to a particular division, such as chemistry, microbiology, immunology, or cytology. (See Chapters 10, 16, and 17.)

CEREBROSPINAL FLUID

The usual examination of the cerebrospinal fluid (CSF) specimen includes several observations. Abnormal color, the presence of turbidity, and clot formation are noted. The examination includes cell counts, morphologic examination, chemical analysis, Gram's stain, and cultures. CSF is a clear, lymphlike, sterile, extravascular fluid that circulates in the ventricles of the brain, the subarachnoid spaces, and the spinal cord. The normal adult has from 90 to 150 mL of spinal fluid, and the newborn infant between 10 and 60 mL. Spinal fluid has four main functions: it is a mechanical buffer that prevents trauma, it regulates the volume of the intracranial contents, it is a nutrient medium of the central nervous system and it is an excretory channel for metabolic products of the CNS.

Whenever a spinal tap (lumbar puncture) is performed, it is done for serious reasons, for it involves potential harm to the patient. The procedure is done by a physician.

Indications for lumbar puncture include the following: the diagnosis of meningitis—bacterial, fungal, mycobacterial, and amebic; the diagnosis of hemorrhage—subarachnoid, intracerebral, and cerebral infarct; the diagnosis of neurologic disease such as multiple sclerosis, demyelinating disorders, and the Guillain-Barré syndrome; the diagnosis and evaluation of suspected malignancy such as leukemia, lymphoma, and metastatic carcinoma; and for the introduction of drugs, radiographic contrast media, and anesthetics.

The greatest risk of lumbar puncture involves paralysis or death due to tonsillar herniation in patients with increased intracranial pressure. There is also a risk of infection from the procedure.

CSF differs from serous and synovial fluids because of the selective permeability of the membranes and adjacent tissues containing it. This is referred to as the *blood-brain barrier*. As a result, the CSF is not an ultrafiltrate of plasma. Rather, there is active transport between the blood, CSF, and brain, in both directions, giving differing concentrations of substances in each.

Many drugs do not enter the spinal fluid from the blood. Electrolytes such as sodium, magnesium, and chloride are more concentrated in spinal fluid than in plasma or plasma ultrafiltrates, while bicarbonate, glucose, and urea are less concentrated in spinal fluid. Protein enters the spinal fluid in very small amounts. Very few cells are found in normal spinal fluid.

Collection of Cerebrospinal Fluid

There is a certain risk to the patient in the procedure for obtaining a specimen of spinal fluid; hence such specimens must be handled with the utmost care. In practice, three sterile tubes containing about 5 mL each are collected during the spinal tap. These tubes are numbered in sequence of collection and immediately brought to the laboratory. It is important that any cell count or glucose determinations be done as soon as possible after collection to prevent deterioration of cells and glucose. Like other body fluids, spinal fluid is potentially infectious, and must always be collected and handled using universal precautions. These specimens may be highly contagious and should be treated with extreme care.

The three or four tubes that are sequentially collected and labeled in order of collection are generally dispersed and utilized for analysis (after gross examination of all tubes) as follows:

Tube 1.   Chemical and serologic tests.
Tube 2.   Microbiology.
Tube 3.   Cell counts. This is least likely to contain cells introduced by the puncture procedure itself.
Tube 4.   Microbiology (optional). Least likely to contain skin contaminants.

Excess fluid from any of these tubes should not be discarded until there is no further use for it.

Routine Examination of Cerebrospinal Fluid

Gross Appearance

All tubes collected by lumbar puncture are evaluated as to gross appearance. Normal spinal fluid is crys-

tal-clear. It looks like distilled water. Color and clarity is noted by holding the sample beside a tube of water against a clean white paper or a printed page.

Turbidity.—Slight haziness in the specimen indicates a white cell count of 200 to 500/μL and turbidity indicates a white cell count of over 500/μL.

Turbidity in spinal fluid may result from the presence of large numbers of leukocytes, as previously discussed, or from bacteria, increased protein, or lipid. If radiographic contrast media have been injected, the CSF will appear oily, and when mixed, turbid. This artifactual turbidity is not reported.

Clots.—In addition to the gross observations of turbidity and color, the spinal fluid should be examined for clotting. Clotting may occur from increased fibrinogen resulting from a traumatic tap. Rarely, clotting may be associated with subarachnoid block, or meningitis.

Color (traumatic tap vs. hemorrhage).—Bloody fluid can result from a traumatic tap. If blood in a specimen results from this, the successive collection tubes will show less bloody fluid, eventually becoming clear. If blood in a specimen is caused by a subarachnoid hemorrhage, the color of the fluid will look the same in all the collection tubes. In addition, subarachnoid bleeding is indicated by the presence of **xanthochromia**. Xanthochromia is the presence of a pale pink to orange or yellow color in the supernatant CSF. It is the result of the release of hemoglobin from hemolyzed red blood cells which begins 1 to 4 hours after hemorrhage. Pale-pink or pale-orange xanthochromia due to oxyhemoglobin peaks in 24 to 36 hours and gradually disappears in 4 to 8 days. Because hemolysis of red cells will occur in vitro as well as in vivo, the examination for xanthochromia must be done within 1 hour of collection or false-positive results will be obtained. When the hemorrhage is old, the supernatant fluid will show yellow xanthochromia. The yellow color is caused by bilirubin, formed from hemoglobin from the lysed red blood cells. This appears about 12 hours after a bleeding episode, peaks in 2 to 4 days, and gradually disappears in 2 to 4 weeks. When the CSF protein level is elevated over 150 mg/dL, a yellow color may also be seen.

Finally, subarachnoid bleeding is associated with the microscopic observation of *erythrophagia*, which is the ingestion of red cells by macrophages in the CSF.

Red and White Blood Cell Counts

Unlike cell counts on blood, cell counts on CSF (as is the case with all body fluids) are usually performed by manual methods (Procedures 14–1 and 14–2). Although electronic cell counts have been described they are not generally used. The instruments are not standardized for the low cell counts generally seen in body fluids. Problems also occur owing to the viscosity of body (especially joint) fluids, the variation in cell size (especially when tumor cells are present), and background debris which is generally higher than cell counts.

Since these fluids are often contaminated by pathogenic microorganisms, special procedures and equipment are employed to prevent contamination. Semiautomatic micropipettes may be substituted for traditional Thoma red and white cell pipettes, and disposable counting chambers may be employed.

If the spinal fluid appears clear, cell counts may be performed in a hemocytometer counting chamber without using diluting fluid. Cell counts should be done as soon as possible after the specimen is obtained because cells lyse on prolonged standing and the counts become invalid. Counts should be done within 30 minutes of collection.

Normally there are no red cells in CSF. The normal white cell count in CSF is 0 to 8/μL. More than 10/μL is considered abnormal. A predominance of polynuclear cells usually indicates a bacterial infection, while the presence of many mononuclear cells indicates a viral infection.

Morphologic Examination

When the cell count is over 30 white cells per microliter, a differential cell count is done. This may be done on a smear made from the centrifuged spinal fluid sediment, by recovery with a filtration or sedimentation method, or preferably on a cytocentrifuged preparation.

Cytocentrifugation.—This technique requires the use of a special cytocentrifuge such as the Cytospin (Shandon Inc., Pittsburgh, PA). It is a slow centrifugation method which gives better cell yield and morphologic preservation than does ordinary centrifugation. It is relatively easy to learn and to perform and gives an excellent yield with a small amount of sample. The sample is slowly centrifuged from 200 to 1,000 rpm for 5 to 10 minutes. During centrifugation, the fluid portion of the specimen is absorbed into a filter paper and the cellular portion is concentrated in a circle 6 mm in diameter on a

---

Procedure 14–1. Cerebrospinal Fluid Red Cell Count

1. Insert a disposable Pasteur pipette directly into the well-mixed specimen. Carefully mount both sides of a clean counting chamber (hemocytometer).
2. With the low-power ($\times 10$) objective, quickly scan both ruled areas of the hemocytometer to determine whether red cells are present and to get a rough idea of their concentration.
3. With the high-power ($\times 40$) objective, count the red cells in 10 mm^2. Count five squares on each side, using the four corner squares and the center square.
4. Red cells will appear small, round, and yellowish. Their outline is usually smooth, although they may occasionally appear crenated. The percentage of crenated cells had been reported as a measure of subarachnoid hemorrhage, but this is no longer considered a useful distinction.
5. If the number of red cells is fairly high (over 200 cells per ten squares) count fewer squares and adjust the calculations accordingly.
6. If the fluid is extremely bloody, it may be necessary to dilute it volumetrically with saline or some other isotonic diluent. It is preferable to count the undiluted fluid in fewer than ten squares, if possible. Adjust the calculations if dilution is necessary.
7. Calculate the number of cells per liter as follows:

Total cells counted $\times$ dilution factor
$$\times \text{ volume factor} = \text{cells/}\mu\text{L (mm}^3)$$
$$= \text{cells} \times 10^6/\text{L}$$

Example: If ten squares are counted, the volume counted is 1 μL (10 mm^2 $\times$ 0.1 mm) and if the fluid was not diluted, there is no dilution factor. Therefore, the number of cells counted in ten squares is equal to the number of cells per microliter, or $\times$ 10^6/L.

8. Decontaminate the hemocytometer by placing it in a Petri dish and flooding it with disinfectant solution. Allow the disinfectant to remain on the hemocytometer for at least five minutes, then rinse it well with 70% alcohol and clean it.

Procedure 14-2. Cerebrospinal Fluid White Cell Count

1. Rinse a disposable Pasteur pipette with glacial acetic acid, drain it carefully, wipe the outside completely dry with gauze, and touch the tip of the pipette to the gauze to remove any excess acid. It is very important that no glacial acetic acid be left on the outside of the pipette because it would contaminate the spinal fluid specimen when the pipette is placed in it.
2. Place the pipette in the well-mixed CSF sample and allow the pipette to fill to about 1 in. of its length. Tilt the CSF tube slightly, if necessary, to allow filling by capillary action. Place a finger over the clean end of the pipette and remove it from the sample.
3. Mix the spinal fluid with the acid coating the pipette by placing the pipette in a horizontal position and removing your finger from the end of the pipette. Rotate or twist the pipette to mix the CSF and acid together. Be careful not to allow any of the fluid to drip from the pipette.
4. Mount the acidified CSF on both sides of a clean hemocytometer. Wait for 3 to 5 minutes to allow time for red cell hemolysis.
5. With the low-power (×10) objective, quickly scan both ruled areas of the hemocytometer to determine whether white cells are present, and to get a rough idea of their concentration. The white cell nuclei will appear as dark, refractile structures surrounded by a halo of cytoplasm.
6. Using the low-power (×10) objective, count the white cells in 10 mm², 5 mm² mm on each side of the hemocytometer using the four corner squares and the center square.
7. Do a chamber differential as the white cells are counted by classifying each white cell seen as polynuclear or mononuclear. This chamber differential is inaccurate and a differential cell count on a stained preparation is preferred.
   a. To classify cells, change from the low-power (×10) to the high-power (×40) objective.
   b. Polynuclear white cells have a segmented or twisted, irregular nucleus, and a moderate amount of cytoplasm. They are usually neutrophils.
   c. Mononuclear white cells have a round grainy nucleus, and usually a smaller amount of cytoplasm. They may be lymphocytes, monocytes, or other nucleated cells.
8. If it appears that the number of white cells is over 200 cells per ten squares, count fewer squares and adjust your calculations accordingly.
9. Calculate the white cell count in cells per microliter as described in Procedure 14-1.
10. Decontaminate and clean the hemocytometer as described in Procedure 14-1.

---

microscope slide. The cytocentrifuged preparation (often called a Cytospin) is stained with Wright's stain or with a variety of stains for hematologic or cytologic studies.

Smears From Centrifuged Spinal Fluid Sediment.—These may be used when a cytocentrifuge is not available. The spinal fluid is centrifuged for 5 minutes at 3,000 rpm. The supernatant is removed and the sediment is used to prepare smears on glass slides. The smears are dried rapidly and stained with Wright's stain. Recovery of cells is not as good as with other techniques and the cells tend to be distorted or damaged.

Other Concentration Techniques.—These include special sedimentation methods and membrane filter techniques. These are more time-consuming and expensive than cytocentrifugation and require more technical expertise.

Differential Cell Count.—Exactly 100 white cells are counted and classified and the percentage of each cell type is reported. Depending on the method of preparation, morphologic identification may be difficult. In some cases, cells can only be identified as polynuclear or mononuclear. With other preparation techniques (such as Cytospins) identification is more specific. Any of the cells found in blood may be seen in CSF including neutrophils, lymphocytes, monocytes, eosinophils, and basophils. In addition, cells that originate in the CNS may be seen. These include ependymal, choroidal, and pia-arachnoid mesothelial (PAM) cells. If any tumor cells or unusual cells are encountered, the specimen should be referred for cytologic examination.

Chemistry Tests

Several chemical determinations can be done on spinal fluid. The same chemical constituents are generally found in CSF and plasma, but because of the blood-brain barrier and selective filtration, normal CSF values are different from plasma values. Abnormal CSF values may result from alterations in the permeability of the blood-brain barrier, or from production or metabolism by neural cells in various pathologic conditions. There are relatively few important CSF chemical findings. Some of the more routine analyses will be described.

Protein.—Protein tests and protein electrophoresis are common and of diagnostic significance for a variety of conditions and disease states. Protein fractions are generally the same as in plasma, but the ratios vary. The normal CSF protein varies with methodology and site of collection, with a reference range of 12 to 60 mg/dL. Increased CSF protein levels are the most common pathologic finding, and are seen with meningitis, hemorrhage, and multiple sclerosis. Low values are associated with leakage of fluid from the CNS. Electrophoresis has replaced the colloidal gold test for the evaluation of spinal fluid protein fractions.

Glucose.—The glucose level in spinal fluid is about 60% to 80% than in blood, but the amounts may vary. Both levels should be measured simultaneously, as it is the difference between these values that is clinically significant. Bacteria and cells utilize glucose. The glucose level in spinal fluid is especially reduced in bacterial meningitis, but *not* in viral meningitis, primary brain tumor, or vascular accidents. It is low in metastatic tumor and insulin shock, and elevated in diabetic coma.

Lactate.—Determination of lactate levels in CSF are used in the diagnosis and management of meningitis. Elevation over 25 mg/dL is seen in bacterial, fungal, and tubercular meningitis and is more consistent than a depression in glucose levels. The elevated serum lactate levels remain during initial treatment, but a fall indicates successful treatment. However, increased lactate levels occur in oxygen deprivation and are seen in any condition in which oxygen flow to the brain is decreased.

Glutamine.—The presence of increased CSF glutamine is an indirect measure of the presence of excess ammonia in the CSF. Glutamine is produced by brain cells as a way of removing toxic ammonia from the CNS by combining ammonia and α-ketoglutarate. Increased levels of blood and CSF ammonia are seen in some liver disorders. Measurement of glutamine is preferable to ammonia as it is a more stable compound.

Lactic Dehydrogenase.—The various isoenzymes of lactic dehydrogenase (LD) are used to help diagnose meningitis by helping to confirm the presence of neutrophils or lymphocytes, and by indicating destruction of brain tissue.

Other Tests.—Tests for bilirubin and chloride are less commonly done. The chloride level in spinal fluid is normally higher than in blood, and determinations should be done simultaneously. Spinal fluid levels of other electrolytes are normally lower than blood levels but tend to rise during inflammation.

Microbiological Examination

Gram's stains and culture are done. Spinal fluid specimens are normally sterile. Gram's stains are most useful in the diagnosis of acute bacterial meningitis, as the organisms can actually be seen in the Gram's-stained specimen. Tuberculosis and cryptococcus infections may also be detected with microscopic examination of the CSF.

Serology Tests

The VDRL test is a well-known serologic test for syphilis that is done on spinal fluid. However, it may be negative in 40% to 50% of cases. The fluorescent treponemal antibody absorption (FTA-ABS) test is more sensitive but less specific.

SYNOVIAL FLUID

Synovial fluid is the fluid contained in joints. Synovial membranes line the joints, bursae, and tendon sheaths.

Normal synovial fluid is an ultrafiltrate of plasma with the addition of a high-molecular-weight mucopolysaccharide called **hyaluronate** or **hyaluronic acid.** The presence of hyaluronate differentiates synovial fluid from other serous fluids and spinal fluid. It is responsible for the normal viscosity of synovial fluid which serves to lubricate the joints so that they move freely. Hyaluronate is secreted by the synovial fluid cells (synoviocytes) which line the joint cavity. This normal viscosity is responsible for some difficulties in the examination of synovial fluid, especially in performing cell counts.

Normal Synovial Fluid

Normal synovial fluid is straw-colored and viscous, resembling uncooked egg white. The word *synovial* comes from *syn,* with, and *ovi,* egg. About 1 mL of synovial fluid is present in each large joint, such as the knee, ankle, hip, elbow, wrist, and shoulder.

In normal synovial fluid the white cell count is low, less than 200/μL, and the majority of the white cells are mononuclear with less than 25% neutrophils. Red cells and crystals are normally absent and the fluid is sterile. Since the fluid is an **ultrafiltrate of plasma,** normal synovial fluid has essentially the same chemical composition as plasma without the larger protein molecules. A small amount of protein is secreted by the synovial cells, resulting in less than 3 g/dL total protein.

Aspiration and Analysis

The aspiration and analysis of synovial fluid may be done to determine the cause of joint disease, especially when accompanied by an abnormal accumulation of fluid in the joint **(effusion).** The joint disease (arthritis) might be crystal-induced, degenerative, inflammatory, or infectious. Morphologic analysis for cells and crystals together with Gram's stain and culture will help in the differentiation. Aspiration is also done with effusions of unknown etiology, and with pain or decreased joint mobility. Effusion of synovial fluid is usually present clinically before aspiration, and therefore it is often possible to aspirate 10 to 20 mL of the fluid for laboratory examination, although the volume (which is normally about 1 mL) may be extremely small, so that the laboratory receives only a drop of fluid which is contained in the aspiration syringe.

In the management of joint disorders, the differential diagnosis is essential so that the correct treatment can be instituted. The analysis of synovial fluid can be invaluable in this diagnosis. It can give an immediate diagnosis in some disorders, and provide valuable information concerning other diseases of the joints. If fluid volume or resources are limited, the most important aspects of analysis are an examination for crystals with **compensated polarized light** microscopy, and microbiological study.

Classification of Synovial Fluid in Joint Disease

The differential diagnosis of diseased synovial fluid usually classifies the fluid as noninflammatory, inflammatory, infectious, crystal-induced, or hemorrhagic. Although there is an overlap of disease states in this grouping, it is helpful.

Noninflammatory synovial fluid is seen in degenerative joint disease, such as osteoarthritis, traumatic arthritis, and neurogenic joint disease. The fluid is usually clear and viscous; the white blood cell (WBC) count is less than 2,000/μL, less than 25% of which are neutrophils. The glucose and protein contents are approximately the same as in normal synovial fluid. Collagen fibrils or cartilage fragments may be seen, especially with phase microscopy.

Inflammatory effusions are associated with immunologic disease such as rheumatoid and lupus arthritis. The fluid is cloudy, yellow, has low viscosity, and has a moderately high white cell count (2,000–20,000/μL) with over 50% neutrophils. The glucose content is normal and the protein content is high. The fluid may form spontaneous fibrin clots.

Infectious effusions suggest a bacterial infection. The fluid is generally cloudy and has low viscosity. The fluid may be yellow, green, or milky. The white cell count is very high, 500 to 200,000/μL with over 90% neutrophils. The glucose content is characteristically very low. The protein content is high and fibrin clot formation is common. Most infections are bacterial. *Staphylococcus aureus* and *Neisseria gonorrhoeae* are the most common infecting agents, although streptococci, *Haemophilus,* tuberculosis, fungi, or anaerobic bacteria are also seen. The most common type of organism found varies with the age of the patient.

Crystal-induced effusions are seen in gout and pseudogout. The fluid is yellow or turbid, has a fairly high, but variable, white cell count (500–200,000/μL) with an increased percentage of neutrophils (up to 90%). Crystals of monosodium urate are seen with gout, and calcium pyrophosphate dihydrate crystals with pseudogout. They are recognized by morphology and appearance when examined by polarized microscopy with the addition of a full-wave compensator.

Hemorrhagic effusions are characterized by the presence of red blood cells from bleeding or hemorrhage in the joint. This may be the result of traumatic injury, such as fracture or tumor. Coagulation deficiencies, such as hemophilia, and treatment with anticoagulants may also result in hemorrhagic effusions.

Collection of Synovial Fluid

Synovial fluid is collected by needle aspiration, called *arthrocentesis*. It is done by experienced persons under strictly sterile conditions. The fluid is collected with a disposable needle and plastic syringe, to avoid contamination with confusing birefringent material.

The fluid should be collected both anticoagulated and unanticoagulated. Ideally the fluid should be divided into three parts. (1) a sterile tube for microbiological examination, (2) a tube with sodium heparin or liquid ethylenediaminetetraacetic acid (EDTA) for microscopic examination, and (3) a plain tube (without anticoagulant) for clot formation, gross appearance, and chemical and immunologic procedures. Oxalate, powdered EDTA, and lithium heparin anticoagulants should not be used, as they may appear as confusing crystals in the crystal analysis. This is especially true when only a small volume of fluid is aspirated, giving an excess of anticoagulant, which may crystallize.

Normal synovial fluid does not clot, and therefore an anticoagulant is unnecessary. However, infectious and crystal-induced fluids tend to form fibrin clots making an anticoagulant necessary for adequate cell counts and an even distribution of cells and crystals for morphologic analysis. There is some disagreement as to whether anticoagulated or plain tubes should be used for analysis of crystals. A decision may be necessary on an individual basis. Ideally, both tubes would be made available so that if artifactual anticoagulant crystals are suspected, the plain clot tube could be examined.

Although an anticoagulant will prevent the formation of fibrin clots, it will not affect viscosity. Therefore, if the fluid is highly viscous it can be incubated for several hours with a 0.5% solution of hyaluronidase in phosphate buffer to break down the hyaluronidate. This reduces the viscosity, making the fluid easier to pipette and count.

Routine Examination of Synovial Fluid

The routine examination of synovial fluid should include the following: (1) gross appearance (color, clarity and viscosity); (2) microbiological studies; (3) WBC and differential cell counts; (4) polarizing microscopy for crystals; (5) other tests, as necessary. The most important tests are the microbiological studies, especially Gram's stain, and crystal analysis. If the quantity of aspirated fluid is limited, these should be done first.

Gross Appearance

The first step in the analysis of synovial fluid is to observe the specimen for color and clarity. The noninflammatory fluid is usually clear. To test for clarity, read newspaper print through a test tube containing the specimen. As the cell and protein content increases, or crystals precipitate, the turbidity increases, and the print becomes more difficult to read.

In a traumatic tap of the joint, blood will be seen in the collection tubes in an uneven distribution, which diminishes as the aspiration continues. It may also be seen as an uneven distribution with streaks of blood in the aspiration syringe. A truly bloody fluid is uniform in color, and does not clot. Xanthochromia in the supernatant fluid indicates bleeding in the joint, but is difficult to evaluate because the fluid is normally yellow. A dark-red or dark-brown supernatant is evidence of joint bleeding rather than a traumatic tap.

Viscosity

This is most easily evaluated at the time of arthrocentesis by allowing the synovial fluid to drop from the end of the needle. Normally, synovial fluid will form a string 4 to 6 cm in length. If it breaks before it reaches 3 cm in length, the viscosity is lower than normal. Inflammatory fluids contain enzymes that break down hyaluronic acid. Anything that decreases the hyaluronic acid content of synovial fluid lowers its viscosity.

Viscosity has been evaluated in the laboratory by means of the *mucin clot test*. However, this test is of questionable value as results rarely change the diagnosis and are essentially the same as with the string test for viscosity. Therefore, it is no longer recommended as part of the routine synovial fluid analysis.

The mucin clot test is based on the polymerization of hyaluronic acid. To perform the mucin clot test, synovial fluid is added drop by drop to dilute acetic acid. The resulting clot may fragment easily, indicating inflammatory fluid, or may remain firm, indicating noninflammatory fluid. Clots are graded as good, fair, poor, and very poor. Good clots do not break up easily when they are agitated, and they are surrounded by clear solution. A soft clot in turbid solution is graded as fair. A poor clot breaks up easily when agitated, ending up in small pieces, and is surrounded by a cloudy solution. If no clot forms and there are only flakes in a cloudy suspension, this is graded as very poor.

Viscosity can also be assessed by merely tipping the unanticoagulated collection tube and noting whether the fluid appears thick (viscous) or watery (thin).

Red and White Blood Cell Counts

The appearance of a drop of synovial fluid under an ordinary light microscope can be helpful in estimating the cell counts initially and in demonstrating the presence of crystals. The presence of only a few white cells per high-power ($\times 40$) field suggests a noninflammatory disorder. A large number of white cells would indicate inflammatory or infected synovial fluid. The total WBC count and differential count are very important in diagnosis. When cells are counted in other fluids, such as blood, the usual diluting fluid is dilute acetic acid. This cannot be used with synovial fluid because it may cause mucin clotting. Instead, a solution of saline containing methylene blue is used. If it is necessary to lyse red blood cells, either hypotonic saline or saponinized saline can be used as a diluent. The undiluted synovial fluid, or, if necessary, suitably diluted fluid, is mounted in a hemocytometer and counted as described for CSF counts. Since acetic acid cannot be used as a diluent, both red and white cells are enumerated at the same time. This is most easily accomplished, using a phase-contrast rather than a brightfield microscope.

Cell counts below $200/\mu L$ with less than 25% polymorphonuclear cells and no red cells are normally observed in synovial fluid. Monocytes, lymphocytes, and macrophages are seen. A low white cell count ($200-2,000/\mu L$) with predominantly mononuclear cells suggests a noninflammatory joint fluid, while a high white cell count suggests inflammation and a very high white cell count with a high proportion of polymorphonuclear cells strongly suggests infection.

Morphologic Examination

As with CSF, cytocentrifuged preparations of the synovial fluid are preferred for the morphologic examination and white cell differential. The procedure is gener-

ally as described for CSF. Slides should be prepared as soon as possible after collection to prevent distortion and degeneration of cells. Digestion with hyaluronidase may be necessary with highly viscous fluids. If increased neutrophils are present, they are especially prone to disintegration, making them difficult to recognize.

If a cytocentrifuge is not available, smears are made as for CSF from normally centrifuged sediment. They should be thin, as hyaluronic acid will distort the cells. Smears are sometimes prepared from the fluid at the time of aspiration. The smears are air-dried and stained with Wright's stain.

Lupus erythematosus (LE) cells may be found in stained slides from patients with systemic lupus erythematosus and occasionally in fluid from patients with rheumatoid arthritis. The in vivo formation of LE cells in synovial fluid probably results from trauma to the white cells.

Eosinophilia may be seen in metastatic carcinoma to the synovium, acute rheumatic fever, and rheumatoid arthritis. It is also associated with parasitic infections, Lyme disease, and following arthrography and radiation therapy.

Microscopic Examination for Crystals

Brightfield or Phase-Contrast Microscopic Examination.—A drop of unclotted synovial fluid is first examined with an ordinary brightfield or, preferably, a phase-contrast microscope. The drop is placed on a slide and a coverglass applied as is done for the examination of urinary sediment (see Chapter 13). In order to avoid confusion from extraneous particles that might polarize, it is recommended that slides and coverglasses be cleaned with alcohol and carefully dried with gauze or lens paper just prior to examination. It has also been recommended that the coverglass be immediately sealed with clear fingernail polish to reduce drying from evaporation. If nail polish is used, the slide should be allowed to dry for 15 minutes before examination to prevent damage to the objective. An unsealed preparation can be examined during this waiting period if desired. Any crystals at the junction of the nail polish and synovial fluid should be ignored.

Needle-shaped, intracellular urate crystals (sodium acid urate) seen in a simple wet preparation of synovial fluid are characteristic of gouty arthritis (Fig 14–1). Pseudogout, a crystal-deposition disease distinct from gout, is demonstrated by the presence of rhomboid calcium pyrophosphate dihydrate (Fig 14–2). Cholesterol

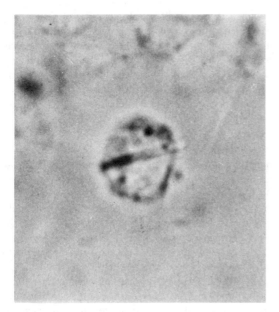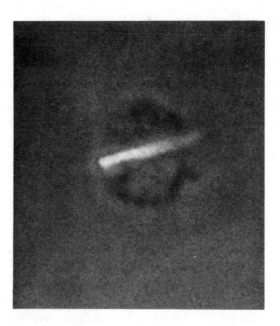

FIG 14–1.
Monosodium urate crystals in synovial fluid. **A,** neutrophil with crystal morphologically resembling monosodium urate, typical of gouty arthritis. Unstained wet preparation, brightfield illumination. **B,** same field as **A** with polarized light, showing a strongly birefringent, needle-shaped crystal.

crystals are seen in synovial fluid from persons with rheumatoid arthritis and not in normal synovial fluid. They are flat, clear, rhombic crystals with one corner punched out.

Lipid crystals showing a Maltese cross formation with polarized light have also been reported as causing acute arthritis. Crystals of hydroxyapatite have also been

reported as causing apatite gout. They are too small to be seen with ordinary microscopy. Clumps of these crystals may, however, be seen as spherical microaggregates. Finally, crystals of calcium oxalate may occur in oxalate gout, in patients with chronic renal dialysis or very rare primary oxalosis.

Other crystals may be present in the synovial fluid

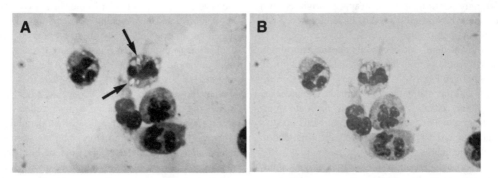

FIG 14–2.
Calcium pyrophosphate dihydrate crystals in synovial fluid. **A,** neutrophil showing several chunky crystals, morphologically resembling *CPPD,* characteristic of pseudogout. Cytocentrifuged preparation, Wright's stain, brightfield illumination. **B,** same field as **A** with polarized light showing weakly birefringent, small chunky intracellular crystals.

which are iatrogenic or extraneous. Starch might be introduced from gloves. These show a Maltese cross pattern that might be confused with lipid droplets of cholesterol. If the joint has been treated with corticosteroids, crystals may be seen which resemble both monosodium urate (MSU) and calcium pyrophosphate dihydrate (CPPD). The crystals are generally extracellular and show numbers significantly greater than is typical of MSU or CPPD, but identification without the clinical history is very difficult. Other substances which might be present and confusing are collagen fibrils, fibrin strands, and fragments of cartilage.

Polarized Light.—More definitive microscopic identification of crystals in synovial fluid can be made with the use of polarized light (see Chapter 3). A polarizing microscope with a first-order red compensator (quartz compensator) is used. To set up the microscope, a polarizing filter (referred to as a polarizer) is placed between the light source (bulb) and the specimen. A second polarizing filter (referred to as an analyzer) is placed between the objective and the eyepiece (either at some point in the microscope tube or in the eyepiece). One of the polarizing filters (usually the polarizer) is rotated until the two are at right angles to each other. This is seen as the extinction of light through the microscope (one sees a black field as all light waves are canceled when the filters are at right angles to each other).

Certain objects or crystals have the ability to rotate or polarize light so they are visible when viewed through crossed polarizing filters. This property is called **birefringence,** and objects are termed weakly or strongly birefringent depending on how completely they polarize light. Strongly birefringent crystals appear bright (white) against a dark background; weakly birefringent crystals appear less bright.

In synovial fluid, MSU crystals appear as strongly birefringent needle or rod-shaped crystals from 1 to 30 μm in length (see Fig 14–1). They may be intra- or extracellular, and this distinction is recorded. The presence of intracellular crystals is characteristic of acute gout. Crystals from a tophus may be quite large. MSU crystals are found in almost 100% of acute gouty arthritis, and in 75% of chronic gout.

CPPD crystals are also found in synovial fluid. These crystals are weakly birefringent, rod-shaped, rectangular, or rhomboid (see Fig 14–2). Occasionally they are needle-shaped. They may be very short and chunky, varying from 1 to 20 μm in length and up to about 4 μm

in width. These crystals are characteristic of pseudogout (also referred to as pyrophosphate gout or calcium pyrophosphate dihydrate crystal–deposition disease) as seen in patients with degenerative arthritis, and in arthritides associated with hypothyroidism, hyperparathyroidism, hemochromatosis, and other conditions. Symptoms of pseudogout resemble gout, rheumatoid arthritis, and osteoarthritis.

Compensated Polarized Light.—Crystals of monosodium urate and calcium pyrophosphate dihydrate that have been identified by polarized light are further identified by adding a first-order red compensator. Morphology and intensity of birefringence, although helpful, are not sufficient in separating these crystals.

Birefringent crystals have different properties when viewed with polarized light with the addition of a first-order red compensator. When the compensator is in place, the background appears magenta, rather than black. The compensator may be inserted either above the analyzer or the polarizer. It is inserted in such a manner that the axis of slow vibration of the compensator (referred to as the slow wave) is at an angle of 45 degrees to the crossed polarizers. In determining the type of crystal in question, the direction of the slow wave must be known. Crystals are identified by observation of the color of the long axis of the crystal in its relationship or orientation to the direction of the slow wave.

Crystals of MSU and CPPD have opposite characteristics when viewed with compensated polarized light. Crystals of MSU appear yellow when the long axis of the crystal lies parallel to the slow wave of the red compensator. These crystals appear blue when the long axis of the crystal lies perpendicular to the slow wave. This may be demonstrated by looking for crystals in the fluid which are so oriented, or by observing a crystal in a parallel orientation and then repositioning the slow wave at right angles to its original position. Alternatively, if the microscope has a rotating stage, the stage may be moved so that the crystal is rotated 90 degrees. In the case of MSU, the crystal will change from a yellow to a blue color. Crystals that appear yellow when parallel and blue when perpendicular to the slow wave are termed negatively birefringent. That is, the sign of birefringence is negative. The term *negative* should be avoided in reporting findings in synovial fluid so that the word is not taken to mean that the crystal in question is absent. Crystals are reported as being present or absent and are identified as to crystal type.

In the case of crystals of CPPD, the crystal appears blue when the long axis of the crystal is parallel to the direction of the slow wave. The same crystal will appear yellow when it lies perpendicular to the slow wave, which can be demonstrated as described above. The sign of birefringence in this case is positive, which is by definition blue when the long axis is parallel to the slow wave. A determination of the type of birefringence with these crystals may be troublesome, as it may be very difficult to determine their long axis, which may be very short, almost square.

An understanding of the polarizing microscope and the principle of birefringence is essential when examining synovial fluid for crystal identification. Although memorization of color patterns is discouraged, a useful mnemonic device is *yellow parallel equals gout.*

When crystals are analyzed with compensated polarized light for the type of birefringence, it is essential to use a control preparation to assure the correct interpretation. Several control preparations are possible. A permanent cytocentrifuged preparation, or a prepared wet preparation of a specimen known to contain MSU crystals may be used. Besides causing confusion when evaluating synovial fluid specimens, the birefringent properties of corticosteroids, which are commonly used to treat joint disease, may be utilized. A suspension of betamethasone acetate corticosteroid is very similar to MSU with compensated light. Either a wet preparation or a more permanent cytocentrifuged preparation may be used. Other forms of corticosteroids are positively birefringent, showing the opposite pattern when viewed with compensated polarized light.

Microbiological Examination

Pathogenic organisms can be identified by use of Gram's stain and by culturing the synovial fluid. Cultures for suspected bacteria or mycobacterial or fungal infections are an essential part of the synovial fluid analysis. Immediate bedside inoculation of the sample onto chocolate agar and the use of special media for the propagation of gonococcal organisms are suggested. Gonococcal arthritis is a joint disease that is sometimes difficult to diagnose unless special techniques and care are used.

Chemistry Tests

Glucose.—The determination of glucose in the synovial fluid is valuable when infectious diseases are suspected. For example, when the glucose level is signifi-

cantly lower in synovial fluid than in serum or plasma, infection of the joint is suggested. Samples of the patient's synovial fluid and blood must be obtained at the same time for a comparison of the two values to be valid.

Protein.—Total synovial protein is increased in several conditions. With inflammatory joint disease, such as rheumatoid arthritis, the total protein level approaches that of plasma. Normally it is about one-third of the plasma value. Values are also increased in gout and infectious arthritis.

Other Tests.—These include LD, uric acid, and lactate determinations.

Immunologic Tests

The synovial fluid normally contains a lower immunoglobulin concentration than plasma. This is not the case in rheumatoid arthritis where the level of immunoglobulin is about equal to plasma, which suggests production of immunoglobulins in the affected joint.

Rheumatoid factor has been reported in the synovial fluid as well as in the serum of patients with rheumatoid arthritis. The presence of rheumatoid factor in the synovial fluid but not in the serum can be helpful in the diagnosis of this disease. Other immunologic tests include antinuclear antibodies, which are associated with systemic lupus erythematosus, and the demonstration of decreased complement levels.

SEROUS FLUIDS (PLEURAL, PERICARDIAL, AND PERITONEAL)

Serous fluids are the fluids contained within the closed cavities of the body. These cavities are lined by a contiguous membrane which forms a double layer of mesothelial cells, called the *serous membrane*. The cavities are the pleural (around the lungs), pericardial (around the heart), and peritoneal (around the abdominal and pelvic organs) cavities. A small amount of serous fluid fills the space between the two layers and serves to lubricate the surfaces of these membranes as they move against each other. The fluids are ultrafiltrates of plasma, which are continuously formed and reabsorbed, leaving only a very small volume within the cavities. An increased volume of any of these fluids is referred to as an *effusion*.

Transudates and Exudates

Since normal serous fluids are formed as an ultrafiltrate of plasma as it filters through the capillary endothelium, they are **transudates.** Normally, serum protein exerts colloidal osmotic pressure and helps retard movement of fluid into the serous cavity. If plasma protein levels decrease, the colloidal osmotic pressure falls and effusion results as movement of the transudate into the serous cavity increases. The formation is also affected by capillary pressure and permeability.

An increase of serous fluid volume (effusion) will occur in many conditions. In determining the cause of the effusion, it is helpful to determine whether the effusion is a transudate or an **exudate.** In general, the effusion is a transudate as the result of a systemic disease. An example of a transudate includes ascites, an effusion into the peritoneal cavity, which might be caused by liver cirrhosis or congestive heart failure. Transudates may also be thought of as the result of a mechanical disorder.

Exudates are usually effusions which result from conditions that directly affect the membranes lining the serous cavity. These are inflammatory conditions, which include infections and malignancies.

Although it may be difficult to determine whether an effusion is a transudate or an exudate, the distinction is important from a practical standpoint. If the effusion is a transudate, further testing is generally unnecessary. However, if it is an exudate, further testing is required for diagnosis and treatment. If infection is suspected, Gram's stain and culture are indicated while suspected malignancies might require cytologic tests and biopsy.

Serous effusions have been classified as transudates and exudates on the basis of the amount of protein present and the specific gravity. Effusions with a specific gravity less than 1.015 and a total protein content under 3 g/dL are considered transudates, while those with a specific gravity over 1.015 and total protein over over 3 g/dL are exudates. Unfortunately there is a good deal of overlap in separating the effusions. A more reliable method of separating transudates and exudates is the simultaneous measurement of the fluid and serum for protein and LD. Appearance of the fluid, cell counts, and spontaneous clotting are also useful in the differentiation.

Collection

Serous fluids are collected under strictly antiseptic conditions. The aspiration may be for diagnostic purposes or for mechanical reasons to prevent inhibition of the actions of the lungs or heart. A pleural effusion may compress the lungs, a pericardial effusion may cause cardiac tamponade, and ascites (peritoneal effusion) may elevate the diaphragm compressing the lungs.

At least three anticoagulated tubes of fluid are generally collected and used as follows: (1) An EDTA tube for gross appearance, cell counts, morphology, and differential; (2) a sterile heparinized tube for Gram's stain and culture; and (3) a suitably anticoagulated tube for chemical analysis.

Additional tubes or the entire collection with a suitable preservative is collected for cytologic examination for tumor cells. Sequentially collected tubes are observed for a possible traumatic tap.

Description of Individual Serous Fluids

Pleural Fluid

Normally, there is about 1 to 10 mL of pleural fluid moistening the pleural surfaces. It surrounds the lungs and lines the walls of the thoracic cavity. If inflammation occurs, the plasma protein level drops, congestive heart failure is present, or if there is decreased lymphatic drainage, there can be an abnormal accumulation of pleural fluid.

Pericardial Fluid

The pericardial space enclosing the heart normally contains about 25 to 50 mL of a clear, strawcolored ultrafiltrate of plasma, called pericardial fluid. This fluid forms continually and is reabsorbed by the nearby lymph vessels (lymphatics), leaving a small but constant volume. When an abnormal accumulation of pericardial fluid occurs, it fills up the space around the heart and can mechanically inhibit the normal action of the heart. In this case, immediate aspiration of the excess fluid is indicated.

Peritoneal Fluid

Normally less than 100 mL of the clear, straw-colored fluid is present in the peritoneal cavity (the abdominal and pelvic cavities). An abnormal accumulation of the fluid is indicated by severe abdominal pain and may be caused by a ruptured abdominal organ, hemorrhage resulting from trauma, postoperative complications, or an unknown cause. If this occurs, the excess fluid is aspirated. The presence of such an accumulation must always be considered in the light of other findings.

Routine Examination of Serous Fluids

The routine examination of serous fluids generally includes an observation of gross appearance, cell counts, morphology and differential, Gram's stain, and culture. Certain chemical analyses, and cytologic examination for tumor cells and tumor markers are performed when indicated.

Gross Appearance

Normal serous fluid is pale and straw-colored. This is the color seen in a transudate. Turbidity increases as the amount of cells and debris increases. An abnormally colored fluid may appear milky (chylous or pseudochylous), cloudy, or bloody on gross observation. A cloudy serous fluid is often associated with an inflammatory reaction, either bacterial or viral. Blood-tinged fluid can be seen as a result of a traumatic tap, and grossly bloody fluid can be seen when an organ such as the spleen or liver or a blood vessel has ruptured. Bloody fluids are also seen in malignant disease states, after myocardial infarction, in tuberculosis, in rheumatoid arthritis, and in systemic lupus erythematosus.

Clotting

To observe the ability of the serous fluid to clot, the specimen must be collected in a plain tube with no anticoagulant. Ability of the fluid to clot indicates a substantial inflammatory reaction.

Red and White Blood Cell Counts

Cell counts are done on well-mixed anticoagulated serous fluid in a hemocytometer. The fluid may be undiluted or diluted as indicated by the cell count. The procedure is essentially the same as that described for CSF red and white cell counts. If significant protein is present, acetic acid cannot be used as a diluent for white cell counts, owing to the precipitation of protein. In this case, saline may be used as a diluent and the red and white cell counts are done simultaneously. The use of phase microscopy is helpful in performing these counts. As with CSF cell counts, 10 mm^2 are generally counted with the undiluted fluid. Results are reported as the number of cells per microliter (or liter).

Leukocyte counts over 500/μL are usually clinically significant. If there is a predominance of neutrophils (polynuclear cells), bacterial inflammation is suspected. A predominance of lymphocytes suggests viral infection, tuberculosis, lymphoma, or malignancy. Leukocyte counts over 1,000/μL are associated with exudates.

Red cell counts of more than 10,000/μL may be seen as effusion with malignancies, infarcts, and trauma.

Morphologic Examination and White Cell Differential

This is essentially the same as described for CSF. Once again, slides prepared by cytocentrifugation are preferred to smears prepared after normal centrifugation. Slides are generally stained with Wright's stain and a differential cell count is done. The white cells generally resemble those seen in peripheral blood with the addition of mesothelial lining cells. Generally 300 cells are counted and differentiated as to percentage of each cell type seen. If any malignant tumor cells are seen or appear to be present, the slide must be referred to a pathologist or qualified cytotechnologist.

Specific Gravity

The specific gravity of the serous fluids may be determined by refractometer, as described in Chapter 13.

Microbiologic Examination

This will include Gram's stain and culture on all body effusions of unknown etiology (see Chapter 16).

Chemical Analysis

Protein.—Total protein is measured in the fluid and the plasma. The level and the ratio are helpful in distinguishing an exudate from a transudate. Protein electrophoresis is used in some cases.

Lactate Dehydrogenase.—LD is also measured in the fluid and plasma. The level and ratio, together with the total protein levels and ratios, are used to distinguish an exudate from a transudate.

Glucose.—In bacterial infections, serous fluids have a lower concentration of glucose than does blood. Glucose determinations on serous fluids should be accompanied by a simultaneous blood glucose collection. Fasting levels are preferred.

Other Tests.—Determinations of amylase, lipase, other enzymes, ammonia, and lipids, among others, are also done in various conditions.

NASAL SMEARS FOR EOSINOPHILS

Persons with an allergic reaction show a distinct increase in the number of eosinophilic cells in a differential count on a smear of the nasal discharge. Smears may be made directly from the nostril by using a swab or from material blown into waxed paper by the patient or aspirated with a soft rubber bulb (Procedure 14–3). The nasal material is spread as thinly as possible on a glass slide and air-dried, and the slide is stained with Wright's stain, **Hansel's stain,** or eosin and methylene blue. The eosinophils contain bright-red granules and are easily recognized under the oil-immersion (×100) objective.

An increase in the number of eosinophils normally indicates that the patient may be in an allergic state rather than having an infection of some kind.

Examination of the nasal smear for eosinophils is simple and useful. It can indicate whether a patient's upper respiratory tract involvement is caused by an allergy (hay fever) or a nasal infection, which may be viral or bacterial.

The procedure for staining nasal smears with eosin and methylene blue stain is more-time consuming than Hansel's stain. However, since Hansel's stain may be difficult to obtain, an alternative method is included here (Procedure 14–4).

Reagents

1. *Eosin stain.* Dissolve 1.8 g eosin Y in 360 mL acetone-free methyl alcohol.
2. *Methylene blue stain.* Dissolve 1.8 g methylene blue in 360 mL acetone-free methyl alcohol.
3. *Absolute ethyl alcohol.*

Procedure 14–3. Nasal Smear for Eosinophils With Hansel's Stain

1. After the smear has been air-dried, it is covered with Hansel's stain for 30 seconds (Hansel's stain is available from Lide Laboratories, Inc., St. Louis, MO). The time may be increased for thick mucous secretions.
2. Distilled water is added to take up the stain and the mixture is allowed to remain on the smear for another 30 seconds.
3. The slide is then tilted to pour off the stain. Any excess is removed by flooding with distilled water.
4. With the slide tilted, 95% ethyl alcohol or 75% methyl alcohol is dropped over the stained smear to decolorize it. Care should be taken to not use too much alcohol, for the cytoplasm of the neutrophils may be excessively decolorized and will appear pink. This could cause confusion in looking for eosinophils.
5. The slide is carefully air-dried.
6. Alternatively, Wright's stain may be used for staining nasal smears.

Procedure 14–4. Staining Nasal Smears With Eosin and Methylene Blue Stain

1. Allow the slide to air-dry.
2. Flood the slide with eosin stain for 1 minute.
3. Layer deionized water over the stain and allow to remain for 1 minute.
4. Tilt the slide to pour off the stain and decolorize with absolute ethyl alcohol.
5. Flood the slide with methylene blue and allow to stain for 10 seconds.
6. Layer deionized water over the methylene blue and allow to remain for 10 seconds.
7. Rinse slide with deionized water.
8. Decolorize with absolute ethyl alcohol.
9. Rinse again with deionized water.
10. Allow to air-dry.

Interpretation of the Nasal Smear

Both of the stains described can also be used to stain cytocentrifuged preparations of urinary sediment for the presence of eosinophils. In the case of urinary sediment, the presence of any eosinophils would be consid-

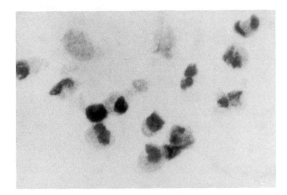

FIG 14–3.
Eosinophils in nasal smear. Eosin and methylene blue stain, brightfield illumination, ×1,000.

ered abnormal. The stained smear is examined first under low power and then with the oil-immersion (×100) objective. Eosinophils may be recognized by their red cytoplasm and large, deep red granules. The nucleus is stained blue (Fig 14–3). Normally, the nasal smear contains mucus with scattered neutrophils, mononuclear cells, and occasional epithelial cells. If neutrophilia is pronounced, infection is probably present, especially if bacteria are present in large numbers. Eosinophilia is positive evidence of nasal allergy. However, there can be a mixture of infection and allergy.

One method of evaluating the nasal smear is based on enumerating the eosinophils seen in four representative fields. If 10% or more eosinophils are seen in any of the four fields, nasal allergy is presumed to be present.

BIBLIOGRAPHY

Becan-McBride K, Ross D: *Essentials for the Small Laboratory and Physician's Office.* St Louis, Mosby–Year Book, Inc, 1988.

Germain BF: *Synovial Fluid Analysis in the Diagnosis of Diseases of the Joints,* New Orleans, The Upjohn Co, 1976.

Kjeldsberg CR, Knight JA: *Body Fluids. Laboratory Examination of Amniotic, Cerebrospinal, Seminal, Serous and Synovial Fluids: A Textbook Atlas,* ed 2. Chicago, American Society of Clinical Pathologists Press, 1986.

Krieg AF, Kjeldsberg CR: Cerebrospinal fluid and other body fluids, in Henry JB (ed): *Clinical Diagnosis and Management by Laboratory Methods,* ed 18. Philadelphia, WB Saunders Co, 1991, pp 445–473.

Litt M: Eosinophils and antigen-antibody reactions. *Ann NY Acad Sci* 1964; 116:964.

Ross D, Neely A: *Textbook of Urinalysis and Body Fluids,* Norwalk, Conn, Appleton-Century-Crofts, 1986.

Strasinger SK: *Urinalysis and Body Fluids,* ed 2. Philadelphia, FA Davis Co, 1989.

15 Examination of the Feces

Key Terms	
Acholic stool	Melena
Apt test	Occult blood
Gum guaiac	Peroxidase
Malabsorption	Steatorrhea
Meconium	Stercobilin

Several useful diagnostic laboratory procedures are performed on fecal or stool specimens. The gross appearance of the feces is helpful in diagnosing certain disease states and indicating further laboratory testing.

The most often tested fecal substance utilizes a screening test for the presence of **occult** (hidden) **blood.** These tests are routinely performed as part of mass screening for colorectal cancer. Besides the detection of colorectal cancer, tests for blood are used to detect gastrointestinal bleeding in general. It is necessary to determine whether the presence of blood is caused by carcinoma, ulcers, or some other nonmalignant process.

The existence of **malabsorption** is indicated by the presence of increased amounts of fat, termed **steatorrhea.** This is most easily detected by microscopic analysis for fat and fibers. Additional tests are used to determine the cause of steatorrhea and to differentiate pancreatic disease from other forms of malabsorption.

Microscopic examination for ova and parasites is common in many geographic locations and uncommon in others. A cellophane tape collection method is used for the detection of pinworm (see Chpater 16). The general identification of ova and parasites is not discussed in this book.

Microbiological examination of the feces for *Salmonella* and *Shigella* sp. and Gram's staining for staphylococcal overgrowth are also commonly done on fecal specimens. When mucus is noted in the gross examination, tests for fecal neutrophils may also be indicated.

Additional tests include a test for pH and reducing sugars in suspected intolerance to certain sugars, and an **Apt test** for maternal hemoglobin ingestion in newborn infants.

The gross examination, tests for occult blood, and microscopic examination for fat are described in detail in this chapter.

COLLECTION

Specimens should be collected and submitted to the laboratory in labeled, clean containers. These may be made of plastic-covered cardboard, glass, or preferably plastic jars with screw caps, of a type often used for urine collections. Specimens for occult blood are commonly collected by the patient at home and a portion applied to the test slide which is then submitted to the laboratory for testing. Paint cans are commonly used for 3-day collections for quantitative fecal fat. The specimen must be collected without being contaminated by urine, and the amount depends on the test to be done.

The patient must be properly instructed about the manner in which the specimen is to be collected. These directions should be given orally and in writing (see also Chapter 2).

A well-cleaned and rinsed bedpan is a convenient collection container. Partially cut plastic bags, opened and taped to the toilet seat, are also suitable. If the specimen is to be rescued from the toilet bowl, it is important that it not be contaminated with strong cleaners and oxidizing agents. One of the commercially available tests for occult blood comes with a tissue which is floated on the surface of the toilet bowl, and flushed once the specimen is sampled. The sample may be transferred to the collection container with wooden tongue depressors or cardboard. It is important that the patient be instructed not to contaminate the outside of the container. They should also be instructed not to overfill the container. Accumulation of gas, which is common, may result in an explosive release of the specimen.

GROSS EXAMINATION

Normal Findings

A soft but formed stool specimen is normally seen. The amount varies greatly, depending on the individual and his or her eating habits. Persons on strictly vegetarian diets normally excrete greater amounts of feces than those on diets with a high meat content. With this in mind, the amounts excreted are normally about 100 to 250 g/day.

The normal color of the stool specimen is brown. This color is caused by **stercobilin,** a pigment derived from bilirubin after conversion to urobilin. The formation of the normal color requires bacterial oxidation to take place in the colon. Without bacteria (a situation that may occur when patients are on antibiotic therapy) the stool loses its normal brown color. The normal color is also influenced by diet.

The newborn infant passes meconium, a viscid, elastic, greenish-black material composed of amniotic fluid, biliary and intestinal secretions, and epithelial cells. In the first days after birth (neonatal period) the stool is normally soft and yellow because of the presence of unchanged bilirubin. As the child becomes older, the stools become brown and formed as solid foods are introduced and milk is decreased in the diet.

Abnormal Findings

The following are noted in the gross examination of the feces: the quantity, the shape or form, the consistency, and the color.

Yellow to Yellow-Green Color

This color is seen in diarrhea, or when the normal bacterial flora is not present in the bowel, as in antibiotic therapy.

Acholic Stool: Clay- or Putty-Colored

This is the generally colorless, chalky-appearing specimen that results when bile salts or bilirubin is lacking in the gut so that stercobilin is not formed. It is characteristic of obstructive jaundice, as seen in cases of gallstones in the common bile duct or carcinoma of the head of the pancreas.

Frothy, With Gray or Yellow Color

These are bulky, foul-smelling specimens which have a greasy appearance. They contain large quantities of gas and fat. This increased fat, known as *steatorrhea,* is seen in pancreatic disease including cystic fibrosis and other malabsorption syndromes. The specimens also have a tendency to float on water owing to the increased gas and fat content. However, this phenomenon is not diagnostic of malabsorption; it may also be seen in healthy persons.

Gray Color

This may be seen after a barium enema or barium meal, which is used for diagnostic radiographic procedures. It appears much like the acholic stool specimen, but is not pathologic.

Tarry or Black Color

Bleeding from the upper gastrointestinal tract characteristically produces the dark, tarry stools of frank **melena.** The intensity of the color depends on the rate of passage through the gastrointestinal tract. The longer the transit time, the darker the color. About 50 to 75 mL of bleeding in the upper gastrointestinal tract is necessary to produce a dark color. If the color persists for 2 to 3 days,

substantial bleeding is indicated. This may be from the esophagus, stomach, or duodenum.

Occasionally, dark specimens may be seen after the ingestion of iron or charcoal.

Red Color

A bloody red color will be seen in cases of bleeding from the lower gastrointestinal tract, or from a massive bleeding episode in the upper gastrointestinal tract with an increased transit time. The ingestion of excessive amounts of anticoagulants, salicylates, steroids, phenylbutazone, rauwolfia derivatives, and indomethacin may cause gastrointestinal bleeding which may be seen as dark or frankly bloody specimens.

Certain persons will also produce a red-colored stool specimen after the ingestion of beets. This is an initially alarming, but benign condition. A bright-red color may be seen after intravenous injection of Bromsulphalein dye (BSP) which is used in liver function tests. These colors should not be confused with blood.

Blood Streaks

Streaks of obvious blood on the exterior of the specimen are associated with diseases of the lower rectum and anus, such as hemorrhoids.

Mucus and Pus

These may be seen macroscopically in strings or sometimes in balls. Mucus in the feces is seen in inflammatory conditions such as colitis, as are blood and pus. They may also indicate a bowel tumor. Pus is seen in diseases such as ulcerative colitis and bacillary dysentery.

Parasites

Adult roundworms or segments of tapeworms may be seen macroscopically in the feces.

FECAL (OCCULT) BLOOD

Clinical Significance

Tests for hemoglobin in fecal specimens are often referred to as tests for *occult blood.* This is because hemoglobin may be present in the feces, as evidenced by positive chemical tests for blood, and yet not be detected by the naked eye. In other words, occult blood is hidden blood and requires a chemical test for its detection. Occasionally there will be enough blood in the feces to produce a tarry-black or even bloody specimen. However, even bloody specimens should be tested chemically for occult blood. In such cases the outer portion is avoided and the central portion of the formed stool is sampled. The detection of occult blood in the feces is important in determining the cause of hypochromic anemias resulting from chronic loss of blood and in detecting ulcerative or neoplastic diseases of the gastrointestinal system. Blood in the feces may result from bleeding anywhere along the gastrointestinal tract, from the mouth to the anus.

Tests for occult blood are especially useful for the early detection and treatment of colorectal cancer. Such tests are useful for over half of all cancers (excluding skin) are from the gastrointestinal tract. Early detection results in good survival. Persons over age 50 years are commonly screened annually for occult blood. They sample their own stool specimens for three consecutive collections, apply a thin film to the test slides, and mail to the laboratory for testing. Dietary considerations are important to avoid false-positive results, and special instructions are generally included with the test slides. It is now rare for the laboratory to receive the actual fecal specimen to be tested for occult blood.

Bleeding at any point in the gastrointestinal system representing as little as 2 mL of blood lost daily may be detected by the tests for occult blood. However, false-negative results occur for unknown reasons, possibly because of inhibitors in the feces.

Implications of both false-positive and false-negative tests are important clinically. Early diagnosis and treatment of serious disease might be missed with false-negative results, resulting in poor prognosis and death. Positive results are serious, as any positive results require extensive further testing to determine the cause of bleeding, or to rule out false-positive reactions. Further testing is both unpleasant for the patient and expensive.

Principle and Specificity

Numerous tests have been described for the detection of hemoglobin (or blood) in both urine and feces. Most of these tests are based on the same general principles and reaction. They all make use of **peroxidase** activity in the heme portion of the hemoglobin molecule.

Most tests now use **gum guaiac,** a phenolic compound that produces a blue color when oxidized. Other reagents which are or have been used for the detection of hemoglobin include benzidine, and *o*-toluidine. However, both benzidine and *o*-toluidine are carcinogenic and rarely used.

All of the tests described require the presence of hydrogen peroxide or a suitable precursor. The peroxidase activity of the hemoglobin molecule results in the liberation of oxygen from hydrogen peroxide (H_2O_2), and the released oxygen oxidizes gum guaiac, benzidine, or *o*-toluidine to colored oxidation products, which are usually blue or green. These reactions are summarized below:

$$\text{Hemoglobin} + H_2O_2 \xrightarrow{\text{peroxidase}} \text{oxygen}$$

$$\text{Oxygen} + \text{reduced form of chromogen} \longrightarrow \text{blue or green oxidation products}$$

The reagents vary in sensitivity. *Ortho*-toluidine is generally reported to be the most sensitive, benzidine less sensitive, and gum guaiac the least sensitive. In general, the more sensitive a test is to hemoglobin, the less reliable it is, since it will be more likely to detect interfering substances. For this reason, gum guaiac has been considered the most reliable indicator and *o*-toluidine the least reliable. The gum guaiac test is the one most often used as a screening test for occult blood in feces.

Interfering Substances and Dietary Considerations

Several interfering substances may give false-positive results for occult blood. These include those of dietary origin with peroxidase activity, especially myoglobin and hemoglobin in red meat. Vegetable peroxidase, as found in horseradish, can also cause positive results. Several foods have been identified as causing erroneous reactions. These include turnips, broccoli, bananas, black grapes, pears, plums, and melons. Cooking generally destroys these peroxidases, and therefore patients are generally instructed to eat only cooked foods. White cells and bacteria also have peroxidase activity which might result in false-positive reactions. Various drugs, including aspirin and aspirin-containing preparations and iron compounds, are known to increase gastrointestinal bleeding. Vitamin C and other oxidants may give false-negative results.

Patients are generally instructed to eat no beef and lamb (including processed meats and liver) for 3 days before collecting the first specimen and to remain on this diet through the collection of three successive samples. They may eat well-cooked pork, poultry, and fish. They are also instructed to avoid raw fruits and vegetables, especially melons, radishes, turnips, and horseradish. Cooked fruits and vegetables are, however, acceptable. Ingestion of high-fiber foods, such as whole-wheat bread, bran cereal, and popcorn, is encouraged. The ingestion of over 250 mg/day of vitamin C is to be avoided as it may cause false-negative results. Aspirin and other nonsteroidal anti-inflammatory drugs should be avoided for 7 days prior to and during the test period.

Guaiac Slide Test for Occult Blood

Various commercial tests have been developed to test for the presence of hemoglobin in the feces. At least eight guaiac-based tests for occult blood are available commercially. The Hemoccult II (SmithKline Diagnostics, Sunnyvale, CA), which seems to have the lowest rate of false-positive results, is described here (Procedure 15–1). Other tests are similar. In all cases, the manufacturer's directions should be followed.

Hemoccult II is available as a slide test which contains filter paper uniformly impregnated with gum guaiac. The specimen is applied in a thin film in each of two boxes on the front side of the slide. This may be done by the patient or the laboratory. The specimen is applied with a wooden applicator which is supplied with the test kit. The kit includes dietary information for the patient and instructions for collecting the specimen.

The American Cancer Society recommends that two samples from three consecutive specimens be collected for colorectal screening. Therefore, test kits are usually supplied to patients in groups of three slides. The patient is instructed to allow the test slides to dry overnight, and then return to the physician or laboratory. If the slides are to be mailed, they must be placed in an approved US Postal Service mailing pouch. They may not be mailed in a standard paper envelope.

When the slides are received in the laboratory, the specimen is tested on the back (opposite side) of the test slide. When the perforated window on the back of the slide is opened, two specimen windows plus positive and negative performance monitor areas (controls) are revealed. If the specimen is applied in the laboratory, it must air-dry before the developer solution is applied so as to increase the sensitivity of the test.

The developer solution is a stabilized mixture of hydrogen peroxide and denatured alcohol which is supplied with the test. Only reagent supplied with the test slides can be used for color development. When the fecal specimen containing occult blood is applied to the guaiac-impregnated test paper, peroxidase in the specimen comes in contact with the guaiac. When the developing solution is then applied to the test paper, a reaction between the guaiac and peroxidase results in formation of a blue color.

The reaction requires that blood cells be hemolyzed for proper release of peroxidase. This usually takes place within the gastrointestinal tract. If whole, undiluted blood is applied to the test paper, the red cells may not hemolyze and the reaction may be weak or atypical. The test is significantly more sensitive to the presence of occult blood if the specimen is allow to dry on the slide before the developing solution is applied. The American Cancer Society recommends that slides be tested within 6 days of preparation, and that the slides not be rehydrated. They also recommend that a single positive smear be considered a positive test result, even in the absence of dietary restriction.

FECAL FAT (MICROSCOPIC EXAMINATION)

Clinical Significance

The appearance of fecal specimens with steatorrhea has already been described. The microscopic examination of a random stool specimen for the presence of increased amounts of fat can be used as a screening procedure for the detection of steatorrhea associated with malabsorption (Procedure 15–2).

This qualitative assessment of the presence or absence of steatorrhea is done microscopically after treating the specimen with Sudan dyes or oil red O. The number and size of stained fat globules are noted. Some fat is present in normal feces. Over 50 to 60 globules of fat over 4 μm in diameter is, however, considered abnormal. This is equivalent to over 5 g of fat excretion in 24 hours.

Fecal fat is composed of neutral fats, fatty acids, and soaps, each of which takes on a characteristic appearance when stained with Sudan dyes. Since fats are

---

Procedure 15–1. Testing for Occult Blood With Hemoccult II

Application of Specimen to Hemoccult II Slide

1. Collect a small amount of fecal specimen on one end of the applicator stick provided. Apply a thin smear inside box A of the front of the slide.
2. Collect a second sample from a different part of the stool using the same applicator. Apply a thin smear inside box B.
3. Close the cover flap, and allow the slide to air-dry.

Color Development

1. Open the perforated window on the back of the slide.
2. Apply two drops of the peroxide solution (developer) to guaiac paper directly over each smear.
3. Read the results between 30 and 60 seconds. Any trace of blue on or at the edge of the fecal smear is positive.
4. Develop on slide performance monitor areas (controls): Apply one drop only of the peroxide solution between the positive and negative performance areas. Always test the specimen, and read and interpret the results *before* developing the controls. A blue color from the positive control might spread into the specimen and cause confusion or a false-positive reaction. Read the results within 10 seconds. A blue color will appear in the positive, and no color in the negative performance monitor area if the slides and developer are reacting according to product specifications.

Interpretation

Any trace of blue color is positive whether the intensity of color development is weak or strong. Reagent paper that has turned blue or blue-green before use should be discarded. If discolored test paper has been used by the patient, the test should be repeated if there is any question in interpretation.

---

normally present in the feces, the observations should be interpreted with caution. The presence of a large amount of neutral fat may indicate that the patient has had mineral or castor oil, or used rectal suppositories.

The presence of increased fat in the feces indicates malabsorption for which there are numerous causes. These include maldigestion as seen in pancreatic disease, small-bowel disease with loss of absorptive surface, increased excretion caused by various drugs, and motility disorders. Once steatorrhea is established, determination of the cause requires other laboratory tests. To confirm the presence and extent of steatorrhea, quantitative measurement of fecal fat on a 3-day collection of the stool may be done.

Stools from some patients with *pancreatic disease* show a marked increase in neutral fat because of the absence of pancreatic lipase, which is necessary for fat digestion. This is often seen in children with cystic fibrosis and is confirmed with a sweat chloride test. A positive qualitative fecal fat examination has been used as an early indication of rejection after pancreas transplant.

Excess fat may also appear in feces when normal lipase is present when there is a rapid transit time through the intestine. This is seen with diarrhea, certain diseases of the small bowel, or surgical removal of part of the intestine.

Qualitative Fecal Fat Procedure

The patient should eat a diet containing at least 60 g/day of fat for 2 to 3 days prior to the test. Mineral oil and suppositories and vaginal, rectal, or perineal creams and ointments should be avoided. The specimen should be placed in a plastic container with a screw cap. Waxy containers are not suitable.

Reagents

1. Ethanol (95% by volume).
2. Saturated solution of Sudan III in ethanol.
3. Glacial acetic acid (36% by volume).

Total Fat Procedure

Soaps and other fat combinations including triglycerides are dissociated as free fatty acids by the addition of 36% glacial acetic acid and heat. This converts the neutral fats and soaps to fatty acids and melts the fatty acids, causing them to form droplets, which stain strongly with Sudan III. The slide is examined while it is warm. After acidification and heat, up to 100 stained droplets of fat ranging from 1 to 4 μm in diameter may normally be seen per high-power ($\times$40) field.

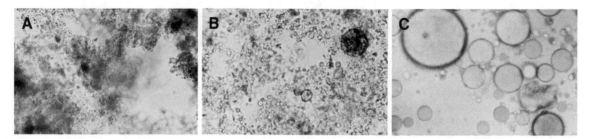

FIG 15–1.
Qualitative fecal fat. **A,** normal fecal fat. **B,** increased fecal fat, over 50 fat globules per high-power field, over 4 μm in diameter. **C,** dramatically increased fecal fat from a patient without a pancreas, before transplantation. All slides stained with Sudan III, original magnification ×400.

Procedure 15–2.—Microscopic Examination for Neutral Fat (Triglyceride)

Procedure

1. Place a small amount of thoroughly mixed feces on a glass slide.
2. Add two or three drops of water to the sample and mix thoroughly with an applicator stick. If the specimen is liquid, omit the water.
3. Add two drops of 95% ethanol and mix thoroughly.
4. Add about three drops of Sudan III reagent.
5. Mix with the edge of a coverglass.
6. Apply a coverglass to the preparation and let stand for 5 minutes.
7. Examine for yellow-orange to red refractive globules of fat under the microscope, using the high-power (×40) objective. Globules of fat tend to collect at the edge of the coverglass.

Interpretation

Fatty acids are lightly staining flakes or needle-like crystals, which do not stain and may be missed. Soaps do not stain but appear as well-defined amorphous flakes or rounded masses of coarse crystals. Neutral fats appear as large yellow, orange, or red droplets.

Normally, fewer than 50 small droplets of fat ranging from 1 to 4 μm in diameter are seen in each high-power (×40) field (Fig 15–1). With steatorrhea both the size and quantity of fat globules are increased. Over 50 to 60 globules of fat over 4 μm in diameter indicates steatorrhea (see Fig 15–1).

Microscopic Examination for Fibers

The feces may also be examined microscopically for the presence of fibers. Muscle fibers from undigested meat are recognized by their cross-striations and yellow-brown color. Plant material is commonly seen as large starch granules, curled fibers, and woody fragments.

Undigested food particles are commonly seen, and their presence depends on many factors such as the extent of cooking of the food and the transit time through the gastrointestinal tract. The presence of fibers is therefore difficult to interpret. In adults, large numbers of undigested meat fibers are excreted when there is pancreatic disease or carcinoma of the head of the pancreas. In children, such fibers may accompany diarrhea or steatorrhea.

BIBLIOGRAPHY

Bradley GM: Fecal analysis much more than an unpleasant necessity. *Diagn Med* 1980; March/April:64–74.

Freeman JA, Beeler MF: *Laboratory Medicine/ Urinalysis and Medical Microscopy,* ed 2. Philadelphia, Lea & Febiger, 1983.

Kao YS, Liu FJ: Laboratory diagnosis of gastrointestinal tract and exocrine pancreatic disorders, in Henry JB (ed): *Clinical Diagnosis and Management by Laboratory Methods,* ed 18. Philadelphia, WB Saunders Co, 1991, pp 519–549.

Strasinger SK: *Urinalysis and Body Fluids,* ed 2. Philadelphia, FA Davis Co, 1989.

16 Microbiology

+--+
| ***Key Terms*** |

| Acid-fast stain   Inoculating loop or needle |
| Aerobes   Microorganisms |
| Anaerobes   Minimal inhibitory concentration (MIC) |
| Autoclave   Mycology |
| Bacteriuria   Parasitology |
| Biochemical properties and reactions   Petri dish or plate |
| Colony-forming units (CFU) of bacteria   Pure culture |
| Culture medium   Quantitative urine culture methods |
| Decontamination   Rapid streptococcal antigen detection |
| Differential stains   Sensitivity to antimicrobial agents |
| Fluorescent antibody (FA) techniques   Simple stain |
| Gram's staining reaction   Streak plate |
| Genitourinary tract specimens   Throat swab |
| Group A β-hemolytic streptococci   Virology |
+--+

Microbiology involves the study of organisms so small that they cannot be seen with the naked eye. They can be observed only with a microscope. For most routine studies the brightfield microscope is used, and the organism appears dark against a bright background. Other optical systems that are sometimes used in microbiology are the darkfield, phase-contrast, ultraviolet, fluorescent, and electron microscopes.

Microorganisms, or microbes, are distributed throughout nature and interact in human and other life cycles. For example, certain bacteria are normal constituents of the human intestinal tract. These microorganisms benefit from this association, for they derive essential food materials from the host. The host also benefits, for the microorganisms synthesize and aid in the digestion of vitamins that are essential for human life. The life cycle in general involves the bacterial breakdown of dead plants and animals into simpler substances, which can be utilized by green plants to make foodstuffs that are utilized by higher animals. Some plant microorganisms that inhabit the digestive tracts of ruminants, such as cows, are essential for the digestion of cellulose, which is the major foodstuff of these animals.

Although microorganisms are generally beneficial and essential for life, some are harmful to their hosts. These are disease-producing, or *pathogenic,* microorgan-

isms. The discussion in this chapter is concerned with pathogenic microorganisms.

The pathogenic microorganisms include living organisms of both the plant and animal kingdoms. The only true microbes of the animal kingdom are the *protozoa,* which are single-celled animals, classified as parasites in this chapter. Most of the protozoa are harmless, but some may be pathogenic. The protozoa are further subdivided into amebas, ciliates, flagellates, and sporozoa. An example of a disease resulting from protozoa is amebic dysentery, which is caused by a specific protozoan ameba.

Certain pathogenic worms are often included in the field of microbiology, although they are not microorganisms (see under Tests for Parasites). Examples of worms that cause disease are the tapeworm *Taenia solium,* the fluke *Fasciolopsis buski,* and the roundworm *Strongyloides stercoralis.* An even higher class of parasitic animals, the arthropods, are included in microbiology in some instances. These organisms themselves rarely cause disease; however, they serve as vectors in certain microbial infections. Some insects are essential in one stage of the life cycle of true microorganisms that cause malaria. Also, some ticks are bloodsucking parasites themselves.

Several different groups of microorganisms are studied in the microbiology laboratory, including bacteria, viruses, rickettsiae, fungi, protozoa, and other parasites, and algae. Organisms in each of these groups can cause disease. Medical microbiology is concerned with identifying pathogens and developing effective ways to eliminate or control them.

The field of medical microbiology is generally divided into areas of specialization, depending on the type of microorganism being studied. For example, the study of bacteria is called *bacteriology,* the study of viruses *virology,* the study of fungi *mycology,* the study of rickettsiae *rickettsiology,* and the study of algae *phycology.* In addition, certain parasites are also studied in many microbiology departments; the study of parasites is called *parasitology.*

In this chapter the discussion deals more with bacteriology than with any other area of microbiology. However, it is possible to apply the skills learned in dealing with bacteria to the other areas. As in other divisions of the medical laboratory, if the basic skills are understood and learned well, many other specific tests and procedures can easily be done. The routine procedures, such as initial media inoculation, handling of media, and staining of slides, are extremely important for the final identification process. Techniques involved in the growth (culture) and identification of various pathogenic bacteria are also discussed in this chapter.

CLASSIFICATION OF MICROORGANISMS

In discussing microorganisms, it is necessary to touch on the method by which living things are classified. By using biological classification methods, it is possible for the laboratory microbiologist to systematically identify microbes. This classification system provides a relatively simple method for placing microbes into categories according to their morphologic and biochemical properties.

In the terminology of biological classification, the word *species* is frequently used. It is the basic unit of the biological world. The species category is based on reproduction: members of the same species are able to mate successfully and produce others of their kind. The *genus* is the next larger classification. The microbes studied in the medical laboratory will have two Latin names, the genus name (often abbreviated) and the species name. These Latin names are printed in italics. The same genus can include several different species, all of which differ

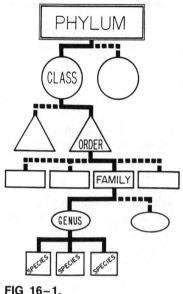

FIG 16–1.
Biological classification system.

somewhat from one another. For example, the genus *Haemophilus* includes several species. Depending on the species, the organisms cause different diseases in humans. *Haemophilus influenzae* type b is a pathogen that causes acute respiratory tract infections and can lead to meningitis, and *Haemophilus parainfluenzae* and *Haemophilus aphrophilus* are both a cause of subacute endocarditis. Other species of this genus can cause different human diseases.

Continuing up the classification system, microbes that have common characteristics are grouped into successively larger categories. Similar genera are grouped into *families,* related families are classified as an *order,* related orders make up a *class,* and classes with common characteristics constitute a *phylum* (Fig 16–1).

In the opinion of Haeckel, in 1866, microorganisms were neither plant nor animal, but belonged to a new kingdom, called Protista.* The kingdom Protista encompassed bacteria, fungi, protozoa, and algae. Bacteria make up the most numerous group in the Protista kingdom. In another opinion, the majority of pathogenic microorganisms belong to the plant kingdom, which includes the fungi and simpler organisms. The systematic classification of these organisms is complex. Fungi are

*Murray P, Drew WL, Kobayashi GS, et al: *Medical Microbiology.* St Louis, Mosby–Year Book, Inc, 1990, p 3.

simple colorless plants that are further subdivided into the molds, yeasts, and bacteria. Microorganisms more simple than bacteria include pleuropneumonia and pleuropneumonia-like organisms, rickettsiae, and viruses.

PROTECTION OF LABORATORY PERSONNEL AND DECONTAMINATION AND STERILIZATION OF MATERIALS

All clinical laboratories have procedures in place that must be followed for the general protection of the workers (see Chapter 1). Since the material to be examined in the microbiology laboratory may contain dangerous pathogens, it is necessary to protect the microbiologist from these also.

Microbiology laboratories pose an additional hazard to those of blood and body fluid specimens themselves (involving the universal precautions policies). Potentially hazardous infectious cultures of pathogenic agents are necessarily prevalent in this laboratory and require extra precautionary measures. Laboratorians who engage in microbiology work and who routinely handle these agents must pay special attention to all measures employed by the laboratory for their protection and safety. Protection from infection from pathogenic microbiological agents requires specific additional safety practices.

Safety Practices in the Microbiology Laboratory

Access to this laboratory should be limited to those persons who understand the potential risk involved in simply being in this area. Some high-risk work can be done in a separate area from the main microbiology laboratory, where access is strictly limited.

The air-handling system of the microbiology laboratory should operate to move air from low-risk areas to high-risk areas and not the reverse. Air should ideally not be recirculated after it has been in this area. If special procedures are done that generate aerosols that are infectious, a biological safety cabinet should be in place. Several diseases may be contracted by inhalation of the infectious particles—tularemia, tuberculosis, brucellosis, histoplasmosis, and legionnaires' disease, to name a few. There are several processes carried out in microbiological studies that can create aerosols. Techniques like mincing, vortexing, and preparation of direct smears have been known to produce aerosol droplets. These procedures should be carried out in a biological safety cabinet (see under Protection From Aerosols in Chapter 1).

Protective laboratory clothing, such as laboratory coats, should always be worn while in the laboratory. These coats should be removed before leaving the laboratory (see under Barrier Precautions in Chapter 1).

Any material that has become contaminated with an infectious agent must be decontaminated before final disposal. All such materials must first be placed into biohazard containers, clearly marked as such. These materials include media that have been inoculated, along with any remaining patient specimens. The biohazard bags or containers are then disposed of in the way established by the health care facility. Any sharp objects, needles, blades, and so forth, must be placed in special puncture-resistant sharps containers for disposal prior to decontamination. The actual decontamination can take place by several means. Some of the more common are by steam sterilization as in an autoclave, or by incineration or burning.

Nothing should ever be put into the mouth in the laboratory. Smoking, eating, or drinking in the laboratory is absolutely prohibited, as these are ideal modes of infection. Personal objects should not be placed on the work area, as they may become contaminated with pathogens.

The work area should be cleaned with a phenolic compound or bleach before and after use each day. A mild disinfectant or diluted solution of bleach is used primarily for cleaning. Diluted bleach is a very effective decontaminant against viral agents and is the antiseptic of choice for laboratories where viral studies are done. There are commercially available decontaminants which are used in some laboratories. It is also important to keep the laboratory free of dust, for this can be the cause of infection by dangerous pathogens.

All specimen containers must be transported to the laboratory in plastic, leakproof, sealed bags. The outside surface of the container should not be contaminated with any of the specimen contents.

It is essential that strict adherence to the policies of universal precautions be maintained (see Universal Precautions in Chapter 1). One important aspect of this is the conscientious use of barrier precautions, the most common barrier being the use of gloves while handling patient specimens and for any work done in the microbiology laboratory. Gloves must be worn at all times during laboratory procedures dealing with all specimens and microbiological work. Gloves should be changed after specimen processing, the hands washed, and clean gloves put on again. Clean gloves should be used at any point when known contamination has taken place.

The use of needles and syringes should be limited to only those situations when they are essential.

The hands should be washed thoroughly with soap before leaving the microbiology laboratory. They must also be washed in case of contamination. The microbiologist should not work with uncovered open cuts or broken skin. These should be covered with a bandage or some suitable material before putting on gloves.

If open flame burners are used in the laboratory to sterilize the inoculating "loops" and needles, special caution must be taken. Fire hazards may be minimized by turning off burners whenever they are not in use. In addition, burners should be kept away from material that is flammable. When inoculating loops or needles are flamed in a flame burner, care must be taken to prevent splattering of material during the process (Fig 16–2). These burners should be housed in a protective container to prevent accidental burns. An alternative to using the open flame burner is the incinerator burner.

If any reusable equipment becomes contaminated during a laboratory procedure, prompt **decontamination** must be initiated. Decontamination is an ongoing process in the microbiology laboratory.

These are only a few general rules for working in the microbiology laboratory. Specific laboratories will have additional rules, which are established for the safety of the personnel.

Decontamination and Sterilization Techniques

Since microorganisms are so widely distributed in nature, it is essential that sterile media be used to grow pure cultures of bacteria. In general, all equipment and glassware and all media used in the microbiology laboratory must be absolutely sterile to ensure the preparation of pure cultures of microorganisms. Media in which microorganisms have been cultured or anything contaminated by infected material must be decontaminated or sterilized. It must also be decontaminated or sterilized or placed in special biohazard discard bags, before being discarded in order to prevent infection of those responsible for its removal.

Sterilization refers to the killing or destruction of all

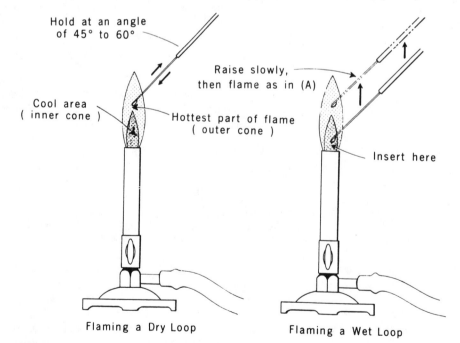

FIG 16–2.
Flaming of wet and dry inoculating loops.

microorganisms. There are various ways in which it may be achieved. In general, physical means such as heat or filtration and chemical means such as oxidation are involved.

Use of Bleach or Antiseptic Agents

If the work area is actually contaminated, a strong disinfectant such as 5% phenol or 5% bleach (hypochlorite) solution must be used. For example, if a culture is dropped or spilled, a bleach solution should be poured over the contaminated area, covered with paper towels, and let stand for at least 15 minutes. Then the contaminated material must be removed and placed in an appropriate container for discard of biohazardous materials.

Use of Heat or Burning

The effect of heat on organisms is generally known, and heat is a widely used and efficient physical means of sterilization. Heat may be employed in the form of *dry heat* or *moist heat*. Dry heat destroys bacteria by oxidation, while moist heat works through the coagulation of protein. Except for burning or incineration, sterilization by moist heat is generally more rapid. However, the type of sterilization method that is used will depend on the nature of the material being treated, since many materials are destroyed by burning and many are harmed by the application of moist heat. Sterilization by dry heat includes burning and the use of hot air. Sterilization by moist heat includes the use of boiling water, "live" steam (steam at atmospheric pressure), and steam under pressure.

Burning is an especially useful means of sterilization in various steps in the culture and identification of microorganisms. Infected material from the original specimen, material from isolated colonies, and material from liquid cultures are usually manipulated by means of a transfer needle or inoculating loop. These needles and loops are made of inert metals such as platinum or suitable alloys such as Nichrome. They are unharmed when held in an open flame burner or an incinerator burner and are decontaminated or sterilized in this manner. Therefore, when material is to be transferred, the inoculating loop or wire is flamed until it glows, cooled to room temperature by waiting approximately 30 seconds, and then reflamed after use to sterilize it. The open flame burner (Bunsen burner) or incinerator burner is a commonly used piece of equipment in the microbiology laboratory (see also under Special Techniques for Microbiological Studies).

Use of Dry Air

Sterilization by dry heat is achieved by use of a *dry-air* chamber that is similar to an oven. The material must be kept at a temperature between 150 and 160°C for at least 1 hour. To be sterilized in this time the material must be a good heat conductor. This method is most useful for materials that are destroyed by moist heat. Sterilization by dry heat is used for pipettes and other glassware in the microbiology laboratory, when nondisposable types are used.

Use of Moist Heat

Moist-heat sterilization by *boiling water* is convenient because it requires little special equipment. Boiling in water for 5 minutes is sufficient to kill all vegetative forms of bacteria. Unfortunately, certain species of bacteria of the genus *Bacillus* have the ability to form spores under unfavorable conditions, but return to normal when favorable conditions return. Since spores are highly resistant forms of bacteria, they pose a great problem in decontamination or sterilization. To kill spores by boiling in water generally requires 1 to 2 hours, although certain spores have been known to survive 16 hours of boiling. For this reason, certain chemicals may be added to the water to achieve more rapid sterilization by boiling. For example, 1 g/dL sodium carbonate makes the destruction of spores more rapid and also prevents rusting of certain metals sterilized in this manner. To achieve more rapid sterilization, 2% to 5% carbolic acid (phenol) may be used; this will usually kill anthrax spores in 10 to 15 minutes.

For sterilization by *live steam,* or steam at atmospheric pressure, an Arnold sterilizer is usually employed, although makeshift apparatus may be devised from kitchen equipment. A modification of sterilization by live steam that is sometimes required in the microbiology laboratory is fractional sterilization, or tyndallization. This method is required for materials or media that cannot tolerate high temperature and high pressure. However, live steam does not kill spores. To achieve the destruction of spores, the material to be sterilized is exposed to live steam for 15 to 30 minutes on three successive days. The vegetative cells that are present are killed by the first exposure to steam, and the exposed material is then incubated until the next day. During this time, spores develop into vegetative cells, which are killed by the next exposure to steam. The third exposure ensures sterility. This method, however, can be used only if the material to be sterilized is conducive to bacterial growth.

It is especially useful for sterilizing liquid culture media, but is not effective for material such as glassware.

Use of the Autoclave (Steam Under Pressure)

The most effective means of sterilization with moist heat involves the use of *steam under pressure,* and a special device called an **autoclave.** It is the method of choice for any material that can fit in the apparatus and is not injured by moisture, high temperature, and high pressure. Some equipment is sterilized in this manner, as are some infected materials that are to be discarded.

Several types of autoclaves are available. Basically, the device is a heavy metal chamber with a door or lid that can be fastened to withstand the internal steam pressure, a pressure gauge, a safety valve, and a temperature gauge. The steam may be supplied by boiling water in the chamber or from heating pipes. Whatever type of autoclave is used, it is essential that *all* the air be displaced from the chamber by steam before the system is sealed. If this is not done, the chamber will contain unsaturated steam, which is a mixture of dry heat and moist heat and is significantly less efficient in achieving complete sterilization.

The exact details of operation of the autoclave may be found in the operating instructions provided with the autoclave. The material is exposed to pure steam in the autoclave at 121°C for 15 to 20 minutes. This temperature is achieved by applying pressure. Generally, 15 lb above atmospheric pressure is required to reach 121°C. This time and temperature will kill all forms of bacterial life, including spores. The temperature of steam in an autoclave at 15-lb gauge pressure at sea level is 121.3°C. Temperature chart recorders must be used for documentation of autoclave maintenance.

It is strongly recommended that the efficiency of the autoclave be checked regularly. This may be conveniently done by one of several methods, using biological or chemical indicators. Commercial test kits provide sealed glass ampules containing a standardized spore suspension of *Bacillus stearothermophilus,* culture medium, and indicator. The ampule is autoclaved and exposed, incubated, and read. An unheated ampule is included as a positive control. The spores of *B. stearothermophilus* are destroyed when exposed to 121°C for 15 minutes. An alternative to ampules is the use of strips impregnated with the *B. stearothermophilus* spores which can also be used to monitor sterilization.

Use of Filtration

In the preparation of certain media that are used in microbiology, none of the preceding methods of sterilization is applicable, since they result in deterioration of the media. In these cases, some other means such as filtration through sintered Pyrex (unglazed porcelain), infusorial earth, compressed asbestos, or membranes may be necessary.

SPECIMENS FOR MICROBIOLOGICAL EXAMINATION

When a patient has certain disease symptoms, the physician will often want to identify the causative agent if a microbiological infection is suspected. The physician should alert the laboratory to possible suspected organisms or tentative diagnoses. Positive identification of the causative agent is important in the correct treatment of the patient. Therefore, the physician will send appropriate specimens to the laboratory. All specimens must include their site of origin (as "wound" culture, sputum, etc.) In the case of a possible kidney or urinary tract infection, a urine specimen will be collected for bacterial analysis. If the patient has a sore throat, the throat will be swabbed, and this will be submitted for analysis. Possible dysentery will require the examination of stool specimens, while the examination of infected wounds will require swabs or appropriate material from the area of infection. Other sites of infection from which swabs or material is submitted to the laboratory for culture and identification include the blood; various body fluids; cervix; urethra; vagina; ear; endometrium; eye; spinal, ventricular, or subdural fluid; bronchi or trachea (sputum material); and various tissues (see also Chapter 2).

Types of Microbiology Specimens Collected

Sputum

When a specimen of sputum is collected, the patient must cooperate fully to ensure that a proper specimen is obtained. Sputum is usually collected in the morning, and it should be sent to the laboratory and processed immediately. Deep coughing will usually bring up a good sputum specimen. It is necessary to avoid collecting nasal or salivary fluids. A wide-mouthed sterile container is best used for collecting this type of specimen.

Urine

The collection of urine for microbiological studies also requires the cooperation of the patient. A midstream sample, usually the first morning specimen, is suitable for culture, provided care has been taken to clean the urethral area before the collection (see also Chapter 2). A sterile container must be used for the collection. When a patient is too ill or cannot void properly, a specimen is obtained by catheterization. This is not done unless necessary, however. The specimen should be sent to the laboratory for immediate processing.

Blood

A blood sample for culture is extremely useful, as normal blood is sterile and should not contain any microorganisms. Special blood-collecting equipment is used. Sterile collecting bottles containing the proper nutrient broth media, blood-collecting sets with needles and tubing that allows the blood to flow into the collecting bottle, as well as the proper skin-cleaning equipment, are necessary to ensure a properly collected blood specimen for culture. Special care must be taken to clean the venipuncture site carefully before puncture to avoid possible contamination of the blood sample.

Cerebrospinal Fluid

Spinal fluid is collected only by a physician. Rapid handling of spinal fluid samples in the laboratory is extremely important, since some of the organisms associated with meningitis quickly "self-destruct" after collection. Spinal fluid is collected by lumbar puncture into sterile tubes. The tubes are sent to the laboratory immediately for various studies.

Swabs of Various Fluids

Swabs are used to collect cultures from various openings of the body, such as the nose, throat, mouth, vagina, anus, and wounds. These swabs must be collected carefully and placed in the proper transport media before they are taken to the laboratory for processing. It has been found that certain organisms survive longer when polyester rather than cotton swabs are used.

Feces

Feces normally contain large numbers of bacteria, and a specimen of feces is usually cultured to isolate certain types of pathogenic organisms. Feces are usually collected early in the day and should be cultured immediately. Swabs of the rectal area are also commonly used.

Specimen Requirements for Culture

There are certain possible sources of infection of each area from which material may be submitted for examination. The microbiologist must be aware of the types of infective agents that may be responsible for a disease and test for these accordingly. Likewise, for each source of infected material there is a certain set of tests that must be performed to discover the cause of infection.

When material is submitted to the microbiology laboratory for culture and identification, certain procedures are the responsibility of the people actually collecting the specimen. This is rarely done by the laboratory personnel. However, it is the responsibility of the laboratory to inform the hospital staff of correct procedures for collecting microbiological specimens and to provide suitable containers for this purpose. The following are general considerations for the collection of specimens.

The treatment of a disease or infection often involves the use of antibiotics or other agents that destroy various pathogens. The antibiotics are often administered before the causative agent is identified, since such identification takes 1 day or more while the patient requires immediate treatment. However, culture of the causative agent will often be impossible once antibiotics have been administered. Therefore, the appropriate specimen should be obtained before antibiotics are administered.

It is important to remember that material should be collected for culture from the location where the suspected organism is most likely to be found. An example of this is the culture of specimens from draining lesions containing coagulase-positive staphylococci. This type of specimen should also be collected with as little external contamination as possible.

Another factor that contributes to the successful isolation of the causative agent is the stage of the disease during which the specimen is collected. Enteric pathogens are found in much greater numbers in the acute stage of certain diarrheal intestinal infections, and are therefore more likely to be isolated from specimens obtained at this stage. Viruses causing meningitis are isolated from cerebrospinal fluid with greater frequency when the fluid is obtained at the onset of the disease. It is important that the physician understand the necessity of collecting microbiological specimens at the correct time, as well as in the proper manner.

The physician should inform the laboratory of the source of the material to be examined and of the tentative diagnosis. This information will help to ensure that the correct medium is inoculated with the specimen and will aid in the correct identification of the pathogen.

Specimen Containers

Correct identification of a causative agent requires isolation and growth of a **pure culture** of that organism in the laboratory. To do this, the original specimen must be collected in a sterile container and not contaminated at any stage in its subsequent transfer to or isolation in the laboratory. The microbiology laboratory should provide sterile containers to the patient care unit or physician with specific information about the type of container to be used for various types of specimens and about the manner of collection. It is also important, for the protection of the laboratory personnel and anyone else handling the specimen, that the specimen be placed entirely within the appropriate container and not allowed to contaminate the outside. Proper transport procedure must be followed. Microbiology specimens often contain dangerous pathogens that could infect anyone coming in contact with the infected material.

The container holding the specimen should neither contribute its own microbial flora nor increase or decrease the original flora contained in the specimen. A variety of containers have been manufactured for collecting microbiology specimens. Most are disposable. One of the most useful pieces of collecting equipment is a wooden applicator stick tipped with cotton, calcium alginate, or polyester. Applicator sticks tipped with the appropriate fiber, packaged in a capped sterile tube, are available commercially. These sticks may be used for the collection of material from the throat, nose, eye, or ear; from wounds and sites of operation; from urogenital orifices; and from the rectum. In many instances, another tube containing sterile broth is included with these units, and when the specimen has been collected on the swab it is immediately placed in the broth tube to prevent drying out. The whole unit is properly labeled and promptly sent to the laboratory.

Many innovations have been made in sterile, disposable culture units of various types. To prolong the survival of microorganisms that have been collected, transport media can be used. This is especially desirable when a significant delay occurs between collection and culturing. Swabs of infectious material can be prevented from drying out by immersion in broth or another holding medium until culture is done. If the suspected organism is an anaerobe, conventional transport tubes should not be used. The crucial factor in the successful final culturing of anaerobic (oxygen-sensitive) organisms is the transport of the original specimen. Atmospheric oxygen, which kills such organisms, must be kept out until the specimen has been processed anaerobically by the laboratory. Special double-stoppered collection tubes containing oxygen-free carbon dioxide or nitrogen can be used. The specimen is injected through the rubber stopper, avoiding the introduction of air. If only a swab can be obtained, the swab should be one that has been prepared in a special "gassed-out" tube and then transported to the laboratory in a rubber-stoppered tube partially filled with an anaerobic medium (see under Oxygen Requirements: Aerobes and Anaerobes).

Handling Laboratory Specimens

Most pathogenic organisms are not greatly affected by small changes in temperature, but they are generally susceptible to drying out. Certain bacteria, however, such as meningococci in cerebrospinal fluid, are susceptible to low temperatures and require immediate culturing. Most pathogenic organisms are preserved by refrigeration if immediate culturing cannot be done. Refrigeration will also prevent overgrowth of other organisms that are present, which could make the isolation of the significant microbe more difficult. Refrigeration is particularly effective for specimens of urine, feces, sputum, and material on swabs from a variety of sources. It is not effective for anaerobic organisms from wound cultures; these specimens should be kept at room temperature until cultured. Still other specimens require freezing to preserve the organism. It is important that those working in the microbiology laboratory understand thoroughly the factors that affect the survival of the organisms being handled. Only when the specimens are properly collected and properly handled initially by the laboratory will the final results of the culturing methods be valid.

Once the specimen has been placed in the appropriate container, it should be delivered to the laboratory immediately and not allowed to stand at the patient care unit. Although many organisms remain alive for long periods after collection, some are extremely fastidious outside the host and require rapid inoculation into a suitable culture medium in order to be detected. In fact, some organisms are so fragile that arrangements must be made to take a special culture medium to the patient so that the material can be placed directly on it. Some pathogens will be obscured by the rapid and overwhelming growth of other organisms that are normally present in the material to be cultured. For example, fecal samples normally contain several types of bacteria that will obscure the detection of such pathogens as *Shigella* if the specimen is not delivered to the laboratory and plated onto a suitable medium soon after collection.

When the specimen reaches the laboratory, it is not always possible to inoculate the correct culture medium immediately. Most specimens may be stored under refrigeration at 4 to 6°C until the culture medium can be inoculated. With certain microorganisms, however, the medium must be inoculated immediately, and it is the responsibility of the laboratory personnel to know which organisms require immediate inoculation.

SPECIAL TECHNIQUES FOR MICROBIOLOGICAL STUDIES

Microbiologists use special techniques and equipment to isolate and grow pure cultures of microorganisms free of contamination by other microorganisms that are present everywhere. Such techniques and equipment include the inoculating needle or loop, the Bunsen burner, tube cultures, Petri dish cultures, slides, and stains. See also Smear Preparation and Stains Used in Microbiology.

Inoculating Needle and Loop

Probably the most important tool of the microbiologist is the inoculating needle or loop (Procedure 16–1). Disposable and reusable types are used. Disposable inoculating loops are made of plastic and are meant to be discarded after use. The classic reusable type may be either a straight wire or a wire with a loop at one end inserted into a suitable holder. The wire is usually platinum or an alloy, such as Nichrome, that can be heated to glowing without being harmed and returned to room temperature fairly rapidly. An object that can be safely heated until it is red is sterilized almost instantaneously. The needle or loop is used to transfer microorganisms from one medium to another or from a culture to a microscope slide. Because it can be sterilized quickly, it can be used repeatedly for this purpose. When a transfer is to be made, the needle or loop is sterilized in a flame, used to perform the transfer, then resterilized before it is set aside. The procedure for sterilizing the inoculating loop by flaming is as follows (see also Fig 16–2).

Procedure 16–1. Flaming the Inoculating Loop or Needle

1. Hold the inoculating loop between the thumb and index finger. This leaves the three outer fingers free to remove tops from test tubes or culture plates.
2. Push the loop into the upper flame of the Bunsen burner at an angle of about 45 to 60 degrees. (Observe the special technique described below if the loop is wet.) Continue heating until the entire loop is red hot. Then briefly flame the hub of the loop holder. An incinerator burner can also be used for this step.
3. Allow the loop to cool to room temperature before using. If used hot, it will kill the organism under study.

A flame normally has two parts: the outer part is the *outer cone,* and within this part, extending down to the base or origin of the flame, is the *inner cone.* The hottest part of the flame is the upper portion, above the top of the inner cone. The inner cone at the base of the flame is cool. If an inoculating needle or loop filled with bacteria is inserted into the hottest part of the flame, a small amount of steam will form. This will result in explosive sputtering of the material to the desk top, hands, and clothing of the worker. This is extremely dangerous, as the bacteria are often still viable when this occurs and can produce infection. To prevent this, an alternative method of flaming must be followed. If the needle or loop is wet, it must be first inserted into the cool inner cone at the base of the flame. It is then slowly raised through the inner cone and finally flamed in the hottest part of the flame. The needle or loop must always be flamed before it is set aside.

Transfer From Tube Culture Using an Inoculating Needle

Microorganisms are commonly grown and maintained in presterilized test tubes that contain a liquid or liquefiable solid medium and have been covered with loose-fitting metal caps or screw caps. In general, the cap is removed with and held in the hand holding the inoculating needle. The lip of the tube is flamed before and after entry to prevent contamination of the culture. The transfer is performed with a sterilized inoculating needle.

Tube Cultures

If the medium is to be used in test tubes, it is usually dispensed and autoclaved in the tubes. If liquefiable solid medium is to be used in slant tubes, it is dispensed in the liquid state into test tubes, autoclaved, and then allowed to harden while set at an angle (Fig 16–3).

Petri Plate Cultures

The **Petri dish or plate** is often used for culture. It is a shallow glass or plastic plate with a loose-fitting cover of the same material, shape, and depth as the dish but slightly larger in diameter. The deep cover prevents contamination of the dish. Petri dishes are used for liquefiable solid media. The medium is poured into the dish, allowed to harden, covered, and stored in an inverted position in order to prevent condensation on its surface. The plates are also stored in an inverted position after inoculation; they are labeled on the back of the portion of the plate in which the medium is contained. Plates of liquefiable solid media may be used as streak plates or as pour plates.

Streak Plates

Streak plates are prepared by streaking material across the surface of the hardened medium contained in a Petri dish. Streaking is especially useful for isolating individual colonies originating from a single bacterial cell (Fig 16–4). These isolated colonies may then be transferred to another medium. Thus, pure cultures may be prepared from mixtures of bacteria. Characteristics of isolated colonies may also be observed on streak plates.

The technique of streaking a plate will vary from laboratory to laboratory and even within a particular laboratory, depending on the source of material and the characteristics of the microorganism under investigation. It should be remembered that the streak plate is used primarily as a means of obtaining isolated colonies of microorganisms (see Throat Cultures and Genitourinary Cultures under Culturing Common Specimens). The aim is therefore to inoculate successively smaller quantities of material onto the medium, so that at one point the organisms are plated thinly enough to allow the growth of individual isolated colonies.

If a swab is submitted for culture, it may be used to make the inoculation onto the medium, instead of an inoculating loop (see Throat Culture under Culturing Common Specimens).

There are certain important things to remember when using the plate culture method. Plates should be perfectly dry before use, or the organism will tend to spread; this will hinder the formation of individual colonies. When a loop is used to inoculate the plate, it should be held lightly and not dug into the medium.

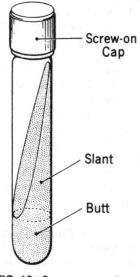

FIG 16–3.
Slant tube, showing slant and butt.

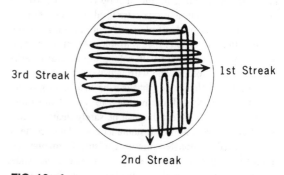

FIG 16–4.
Preparation of a streak plate.

In general, a small and sometimes measured amount of material is streaked onto the periphery at one side of the plate. Streaking is achieved by drawing the inoculating loop across the surface of the medium in a zigzag motion. The first streak is continued across approximately half the plate. The plate is then turned 90 degrees and streaked again, beginning at the periphery, overlapping the previously inoculated area once or twice. The second streak is continued across half the plate. Finally, the plate is turned 90 degrees once again and streaked a third time, beginning at the periphery, drawing the loop through the second streak once, and continuing across the remaining quarter of the plate (see Fig 16–4). The isolated colonies will generally be found in the third area of streaking.

Sometimes the needle must be flamed between each streak as well as before and after inoculation. Sheep blood agar plates are often cut one or more times with the inoculating loop at the conclusion of streaking in the third or first area of streaking, or in both, in order to observe hemolysis reactions of certain bacteria.

Pour Plates

Pour plates represent another manner of inoculating culture media in Petri dishes. They are less commonly used than streak plates. Pour plates are generally used to determine the number of viable organisms in a liquid—particularly in testing such liquids as milk and water for bacterial contamination.

In using the pour plate, one generally first dilutes the specimen serially to achieve isolation of colonies. The diluted specimen is then inoculated into a liquefiable solid medium that is in the liquid state. The medium and inoculum may be mixed in a test tube or in the plate itself, depending on the technique being used. Thorough mixing must be achieved in any case. When the medium has been inoculated at the appropriate temperature for the desired length of time, it is allowed to harden. Plates are then observed for growth and the colonies are counted to obtain an estimate of the concentration of microorganisms in the original specimen. The use of pour plates rather than streak plates provides at least partially anaerobic conditions in the deeper layers of the plate, facilitating the culture of anaerobic microorganisms. As with streak plates, colonies may be observed on the pour plate itself or introduced into additional media in order to obtain pure cultures or observe growth on differential media.

USING MICROBIOLOGY TO DIAGNOSE DISEASE

For the microbiologist to correctly identify the causative agent of an infection, several tests must be carried out. These tests involve a general knowledge of microorganisms and their mode of action. The field of microbiology is too extensive to be covered in this textbook. This section therefore deals only with the laboratory aspects of the subject. The identification of most microorganisms involves microscopic observations, culture studies, and biochemical tests. In the laboratory, bacteria are classified into groups based on two major microscopic observations: (1) the Gram's staining reaction of the bacteria and (2) the shape or morphology of the bacteria, i.e., round (cocci), rod-shaped (bacilli), or spiral-shaped (spirilla), and culture studies including morphologic characteristics, the oxygen requirements of the bacteria (whether they require oxygen for growth **[aerobes]** or grow without oxygen **[anaerobes]** and patterns of biochemical reactions.

Microscopic Observation

One necessary step in the identification of a particular species of bacteria involves morphologic observation under the microscope. Since bacteria are so small and have refractive indices approximately equal to that of glass, a stain must be used to accentuate the microorganisms.

If bacteria are placed on a glass slide and observed under the microscope, they appear as transparent, colorless structures and may be homogeneous or granular. They have a refractive index close to that of glass, and therefore should be stained to be made more visible. Various staining procedures may be used, depending on the information desired. To observe gross morphologic features, a simple stain such as crystal violet, fuchsin, methylene blue, or safranin may be used. However, the most widely used stain in the bacteriology laboratory is Gram's stain, which differentiates bacteria as gram-positive or gram-negative, besides showing gross morphologic features. Other stains include **acid-fast stain,** capsule stains, flagella stains, stains for metachromatic granules, spore stains, relief stains, and stains for spirochetes, rickettsiae, yeast, and fungi.

Properly prepared and stained preparations of specimens may give excellent clues to the media to be inoculated or the further examinations to be done. Preliminary reports on the results of Gram's staining of spinal fluid, urethral smears, and sputum, for example, can be of great value to the physician in the treatment of the patient.

When preparing a smear, it is essential to use only clean slides. The material is spread thinly but evenly over the appropriate area of the slide, using an inoculating loop. This material may be from a suspension of bacteria in a liquid medium, a colony on a solid medium, or a patient specimen. The smear is allowed to dry and then heat-fixed by passing it rapidly through a flame (see under Smear Preparation and Stains Used in Microbiology).

Several staining procedures are used in the microbiology laboratory. Gram's stain is most likely to yield valuable information and should be done in all cases when a staining procedure is indicated. Gram's stains are also used routinely for the examination of cultures to determine purity and for identification. Gram's stains are usually examined with an ordinary light microscope. The use of different microscopy techniques is also important in certain microbiological assays. One such technique is that utilizing fluorescence microscopy.

Fluorescence Microscopy

Fluorescent antibody (FA) techniques are used in many laboratories and are replacing some of the older serologic methods for the identification of certain microorganisms. It is possible to pretreat certain antibodies with fluorescent dye and then react them with bacteria specific for the complementary antigen. The antibody-antigen complex is fluorescent and can be observed under the microscope. In fluorescence microscopy, the specimen is self-illuminating and a light image is observed against a dark background. A special darkfield fluorescence microscope is used (see under Other Types of Microscopes [Illumination Systems], in Chapter 3). Group A beta hemolytic streptococci may be identified on pure cultures isolated from throat swabs from patients with acute pharyngitis (strep throat), and there is a rapid method for detecting human influenza virus infection by utilizing nasal smears. In some cases, FA techniques completely replace time-consuming culture methods. In others, preliminary identification of microorganisms by FA methods may be followed by culture confirmation.

Gram's Staining Reaction

Differential staining methods are very useful in microbiology, for in addition to showing gross morphologic features, they serve to differentiate bacteria or divide them into useful groups. Two of the most widely used differential stains are the Gram's stain and the acid-fast stain.

Gram's stain is particularly useful in bacteriology. There are several modifications of the method, but it generally involves the primary stain crystal violet; the addition of iodine, which serves as a mordant; decolorization with an alcohol-acetone solution; and counterstaining with a secondary stain such as safranin. (A mordant is a substance that combines with a particular dye, forming an insoluble complex, or "lake," and fixing the color in the substance dyed.) This staining method divides bacteria into two broad groups. Bacteria that stain *purple* as a result of retention of the crystal violet–iodine complex are termed *gram-positive*. Bacteria that stain *red* from the counterstain are termed *gram-negative*. Differentiation into these categories is particularly helpful in determining the subsequent tests and means of culture for eventual identification of the bacteria. It is also a guide to treatment of the patient, for certain antibiotics are generally effective against gram-positive bacteria, while gram-negative bacteria are not as susceptible to their action. The procedure for preparation of slides and for Gram's stain is included under Smear Preparation and Stains Used in Microbiology.

Morphology of Bacteria

Bacteria are a form of fungus. Fungi are the colorless plants—that is, plants that do not contain chlorophyll. More specifically, bacteria are fungi belonging to the class Schizomycetes, which also includes related forms of the group Protophyta, the primitive plants.

Each species of bacteria has a characteristic shape, which is one of three basic shapes. Spherical or round bacteria are *cocci,* straight rod-shaped ones are *bacilli,* and spiral rod-shaped ones are *spirilla*. Most bacteria are either cocci or bacilli, the bacilli being the most numerous.

There are certain variations of the three basic shapes, such as club-shaped bacilli and bacilli with square ends. The particular species may be further classified according to whether the cells normally occur singly, in diploids or pairs, in chains, or in clusters. The prefix *diplo-* describes bacteria that occur as pairs of cells, *strepto* describes bacteria occurring as chains of cells, and *staphylo-* refers to irregular clumps or clusters of bacterial cells.

Although bacteria can be seen under the ordinary compound light microscope, they are extremely small structures. They are normally observed under oil immersion with an ×100 objective, giving a total magnification of ×1,000 when the ×10 ocular is used. Bacteria are measured in micrometers (1 μm = $\frac{1}{1,000}$ millimeter or about $\frac{1}{25,000}$ in.). There is a good deal of variation in size among bacteria. Cocci may range from 0.15 to 2.0 μm in diameter, although most pathogens measure 0.8 to 1.2 μm. The bacilli show an even greater size variation. *H. influenzae* is a very small rod, about 0.5 μm long by 0.2 μm wide. *Bacillus anthracis* is a relatively large rod, 5 to 10 μm long and 1 to 3 μm wide. For comparison, a red blood cell is approximately 7 μm in diameter.

Each bacterium has four distinct morphologic parts: the protoplasm, cytoplasmic membrane, cell wall, and capsule. Different stains may be used to accentuate these parts. Other morphologic structures have been discovered by means of the electron microscope.

The morphologic character of a bacterium is useful for identifying it. One should determine its general shape (sphere, straight rod, or spiral rod), its Gram's-staining reaction, and its association with other bacterial cells (single, in chains, or in clusters). However, these and other morphologic characteristics only rarely lead to the final identification of the bacterium. For the final identification it is necessary to know the cultural characteristics of the bacterium. This is discussed later in this section.

Each bacterium is a single cell and, like most cells, it possesses cytoplasm surrounded by a cell membrane, which in turn is surrounded by a cell wall. Some bacteria also have other external structures, such as flagella or capsules. Some typical organelles found within a single bacterium are the nucleus, ribosomes, vacuoles, and granules. Another important organelle contained within the cytoplasm is the spore. Bacteria can manufacture a slimy gelatinous layer around the cell wall, and this layer of slime often becomes an integral part of the bacterial cell structure called a capsule. If special staining techniques are used, the capsule may be seen more easily. The presence or absence of a capsule is used clinically to help identify the microorganism.

The most significant external structures of bacteria are flagella—long, threadlike structures anchored within the cell wall and cell membrane. The whiplike motion of the flagella enables the bacterial cell to move. Flagella vary in their number and position on the bacteria, and this pattern is also helpful in identifying the species.

The cytoplasm of bacteria contains a variety of granules, many of which can be identified by special staining procedures. Some bacteria have spores, or endospores, in their cytoplasm. Spores are able to survive under extremely unfavorable conditions, even when the active or vegetative bacterial cell dies. Thus, spore-forming bacteria can survive conditions that would kill non-spore-forming bacteria.

Bacterial Culture Studies

This step in the identification of microorganisms requires growing and isolating the suspected organism. A pure culture of the organism taken from the patient specimen must be obtained. Bacteria from patient specimens are almost always isolated by streaking on the surface of a culture medium in a culture plate or Petri dish. A suitable medium will allow a single bacterial cell to grow into a colony. Various culturing methods enable the microbiologist to separate individual cells on the media and eventually allow them to grow into separate colonies.

It is important that the streaking be done properly to provide the best opportunity for isolation of the bacterial colonies. When isolated colonies are grown, a portion of the pure culture may be picked up for identification. There are several ways in which a plate may be streaked to ensure the appearance of isolated colonies on incubation. One method is illustrated in Figure 16–4. Special streaking methods are used for certain types of specimens (see Special Techniques for Microbiology studies above).

Other culture studies include the use of agar slants for maintenance of cultures or for certain biochemical studies, semisolid media for motility or biochemical studies, and broth media for maintenance or biochemical studies (see under Culture Media). Many (but not all) microorganisms may be grown in the laboratory away from their natural habitat. To grow microorganisms artificially, it is necessary to provide the proper nutrients and growth conditions. The growth of microorganisms on artificial material is referred to as *culture* of the microorganism, and the mixture of nutrients on which the microorganism is grown is the **culture medium.**

Bacteria are grown in or on specially prepared culture media, although future trends in clinical microbiology are pointing toward more use of non-growth-dependent methods. The isolation and identification of viable pathogenic organisms on culture media is still the gold standard for diagnosis of infectious disease processes. Specimens are plated and inoculated on several different growth media, depending on the etiologic agent that is suspected. Choosing appropriate culture media is essen-

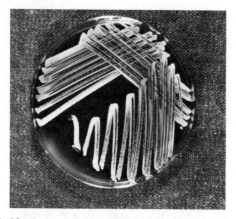

FIG 16–5.
Culture plate with bacterial growth after 24 hours. (From Becan-McBride K, Ross DL: *Essentials for the Small Laboratory and Physician's Office.* St Louis, Mosby–Year Book, Inc, 1988, p 344. Used by permission.)

tial for the isolation, growth, and final identification of pathogenic organisms. There is a certain amount of time needed for any final identification using the common culture and testing procedures—usually about 2 days. Most bacteria will be seen growing on culture media within 24 hours (see Fig 16–5).

Oxygen Requirements: Aerobes and Anaerobes

Some microorganisms require an atmosphere containing oxygen for growth; they are called *aerobes* or *aerobic organisms*. Others are able to derive oxygen from their food sources and are actually inhibited by atmospheric oxygen. To culture these *anaerobes* or *anaerobic organisms,* atmospheric oxygen must be excluded. There are also organisms with oxygen requirements between those of the obligate aerobes and obligate anaerobes. *Facultative anaerobes* are able to grow under either aerobic or anaerobic conditions. *Microaerophilic organisms* grow best under conditions of low oxygen tension and are inhibited by high oxygen tension.

Anaerobic conditions may be produced in the laboratory in a number of ways, including displacement of air by carbon dioxide, use of special media such as thioglycolate broth, or inoculation into the deeper layers of solid media (see also under Oxygen, Requirements for Culture Media).

Anaerobic Culture Methods.—Most of the common pathogenic bacteria are aerobic and grow well in the presence of oxygen. Some pathogenic organisms are incapable of growth in oxygen and are classified as anaerobic organisms. All specimens for anaerobic studies must be cultured as soon as possible after collection to avoid loss of viability. Special methods are required for the isolation and study of anaerobic bacteria.

The techniques for culturing anaerobic organisms are essentially of three types, involving the use of (1) media containing reducing substances that eliminate oxygen, (2) media and methods by which oxygen can be excluded, and (3) anaerobic jars, plates, and incubators from which oxygen can be removed and replaced by hydrogen or nitrogen.

One of the most useful media for growing anaerobic organisms is thioglycolate broth. It contains sodium thioglycolate, which absorbs oxygen from the medium. It can be used to study and identify anaerobes, but is generally not very satisfactory for the isolation of cultures. For isolation, it is desirable to streak plates of blood agar, infusion agar, or thioglycolate agar. When the plates have been streaked, they are placed in an anaerobic jar or other special container and the oxygen is removed (Fig 16–6).

Prereduced media are commercially available. They appear to be very practical and reliable for the isolation of anaerobic bacteria.

Types of Culture Media

By studying the cultural characteristics of a particular bacterium, certain growth patterns may be seen and the presumptive species identification may be made. The types of culture media vary greatly. They may be prepared in liquid or solid form. Most are in a solid medium form and may be prepared in a flat, circular dish called a *Petri dish* or plate. When the specimen is placed on the medium in the plate, it is said to be *inoculated.* A tube of solid medium can be prepared as a *stab* or a *slant.* In a slant culture, of the surface of the medium is inclined at an angle (Fig 16–7), and an **inoculating loop or needle** is used to place the specimen on the surface of the medium. A tube of medium can also be inoculated by stabbing or passing through the medium with an inoculating needle, thus leaving the specimen behind in the medium. A tube prepared in this way is referred to as a *stab tube.* In a stab culture the surface of the medium is perpendicular to the sides of the test tube (see Fig 16–7). Tubes containing liquid broth media can also be inoculated with

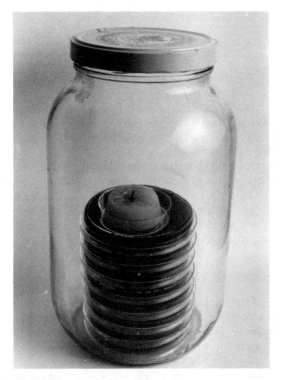

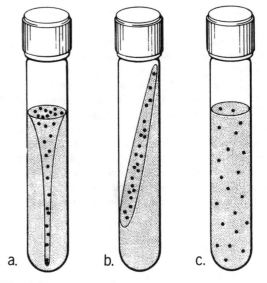

FIG 16–7.
Examples of types of culture media in tubes: *(a)* Stab culture tube. *(b)* Slant culture tube. *(c)* Liquid broth culture tube.

FIG 16–6.
Anaerobic candle jar for culture of anaerobic organisms. (From Baron EJ, Finegold SM: *Bailey and Scott's Diagnostic Microbiology,* ed 8. St Louis, Mosby–Year Book, Inc, 1990, p 53. Used by permission.)

bacteria by using an inoculating loop or needle (see Fig 16–7).

Most microbiologists can now purchase the majority of materials needed for culture, identification, and susceptibility testing of pathogenic microorganisms. In the past, much of the media was prepared by the laboratory. The commercial production of testing materials for microbiologic use has simplified much of what used to be a time-consuming effort by the laboratory personnel. Much of the microbiologic culture media is purchased already in Petri plate form but some is in the form of a dehydrated powder which must be reconstituted. If media must be prepared, it must be prepared in clean glassware, following the manufacturer's directions carefully. If the media is to be sterilized in an autoclave, the container is capped. Safety precautions should be taken when using the autoclave for this purpose.

Many hundreds of types of media are available for culture purposes. Some are used as part of routine culture protocol and others are only used rarely. Descriptions of available media can be found in the Difco (Difco Laboratories, Inc., Detroit, MI), Scott (Scott Laboratories, Inc., Fiskeville, RI), and BBL (Baltimore Biological Laboratories) (Becton-Dickinson Microbiology Systems, Cockeysville, MD.) manuals.

Colony Characteristics of Bacterial Cultures

When inoculated onto suitable semisolid or solid nutrient media with the proper temperature and moisture, bacteria rapidly multiply and form macroscopic colonies. Under ideal conditions, the growth of a microbial cell is a geometric progression with time. For example, a single bacterium such as *Escherichia coli,* having a generation time of 20 minutes, would produce 2.2×10^{43} cells in 48 hours. Certain limiting factors come into play that ultimately terminate growth, however. A culture that is a closed system will eventually stop growing as a result of exhaustion of essential nutrients, accumulation of toxic products, or development of an unfavorable pH.

The type of culture medium used—liquid or solid—can affect the appearance or growth of the colonies. In liquid media bacterial growth does not have a characteristic appearance, and organisms cannot be separated from "mixed cultures." By contrast, on solid media the appearance of a culture is extremely useful in initially differentiating the colony type and pure cultures can be isolated.

Bacteria multiply by binary fission, or division into two equal parts. Macroscopic bacterial colonies form in 24 to 48 hours. The colonies originate from individual cells, although each colony is a mass of individual cells, each of which functions independently. Different species of bacteria form colonies that differ in appearance; therefore, colony appearance is useful in identifying the species of bacteria. Colony characteristics that are observed for the purpose of identification include the following:

1. Bacteria without slime capsules produce colonies that appear dry and rough.
2. Bacteria with slime capsules produce colonies that appear smooth and shiny.
3. Bacteria may possess a pigment that gives a characteristic color (e.g., white, red, yellow, or orange) to the colony.
4. Bacteria may spread from the original colony, which indicates that they are motile. Nonmotile bacteria remain in discrete colonies.

Bacterial colonies should be observed for their relative size, shape, elevation, texture, marginal appearance, and color. This information, in addition to morphologic appearance under the microscope, various staining reactions such as with Gram's stain and results of biochemical tests performed, helps in the eventual identification of a particular species of bacteria.

Growth of a Pure Culture

Specimens for microbiological analysis must be collected in sterile containers because the identification of microorganisms generally requires isolation and growth of a pure culture of bacteria. A bacterium placed on a suitable culture medium will multiply until an isolated colony of bacteria is formed. It is assumed that each colony of bacteria originates from a single cell. In culturing bacteria in the laboratory, the infected material is treated in such a way that single bacterial cells are separated on the culture medium and allowed to grow into isolated colonies. Material from a single isolated colony is then further inoculated onto additional media, so that several colonies will appear, all arising from a single bacterium.

The growth of several colonies originating from a single colony, and hence a single cell, is what is meant by a *pure culture.*

Temperature of Incubation for Routine Cultures

Human pathogens generally multiply best at temperatures close to those of the host. Most often, therefore, only two incubators are necessary for a routine microbiology laboratory—one set at 35°C, close to the normal human internal body temperature, and one set at 30°C, the temperature of the surface of the body. Most incubations are carried out at 35°C. The temperature of the incubators must be periodically monitored as part of the maintenance documentation required by quality assurance programs.

Biochemical Tests

Many bacteria cannot be identified on the basis of microscopic or cultural studies alone. The **biochemical properties and reactions** of bacteria form the basis for an important series of identification procedures. Biochemical identification has been used increasingly and is an important function of the microbiology laboratory. Biochemical tests rely on bacterial physiology and the end products produced in reactions of bacterial cells. Important biochemical reactions involve oxidation and fermentation, starch hydrolysis, hydrogen sulfide production, urea hydrolysis, and tryptophan hydrolysis. In each biochemical procedure, the unknown bacterium causes a change of some type in the medium, to which a specific test substance has been added. The change may be indicated by the formation of gas or by the formation of color. In some media a pH indicator is used—for instance, when an acid is produced during fermentation. Some bacteria can break down starch in the medium, and iodine is used to test for the presence or absence of starch. Metabolism of the amino acid tryptophan can produce *indole,* which can be detected by a color change in another indicator. Biochemical tests may be done individually, or they may be incorporated into culture media.

Some biochemical tests can be performed directly on colonies seen growing on primary culture plates. Some of these are rapid tests taking only minutes and others take a few hours of incubation for results to be seen. Use of information gained from the results of biochemical tests can place an organism into a further division, together with colony characteristics, and morphologic and microscopic information. In this way, a tentative or preliminary identification can be made which is often valuable diagnostic information needed in cases of serious infectious processes.

Modifications of the traditional biochemical tests have been made to facilitate inoculation of media, shorten the incubation time, automate procedures, or in some way make the identification of species based on reaction patterns easier to do.

In some modifications, a heavy suspension of organism being tested is inoculated on a small volume of media. Some commercial suppliers prepare reagent-impregnated paper disks or filter paper strips that are used along with small volumes of water (elution process) or saline to produce the desired test substrate. Tablets are also available which can be added to water to produce the substrate needed. This type of substrate is useful for differentiating two similar species that differ in only one characteristic.

There are also multitest systems in which conventional biochemicals are prepared in microdilution trays. Some of these substrate products are shipped in a frozen state and stored frozen until needed. They must be thawed prior to inoculation and require overnight incubation as conventional biochemicals need. Some substrate products are provided in a dried state in a tray. These products are rehydrated with a suspension of the organism during inoculation.

There have been many innovations devised commercially to include the traditional biochemical tests. Biochemicals have been placed in trays, tubes, and other holding devices. Many different substrates are included in wells in a single test tray. The suspension of the organism being tested is inoculated into the plastic wells, the tray incubated, and the organism allowed to mix with the various substrates. In many instances, results are available after 4 hours of incubation. Some of the more traditional biochemical tests are now described.

Catalase Test

In this test, the enzyme catalase breaks down hydrogen peroxide into oxygen and water. The test is usually performed on a glass slide. If a small amount of an organism that produces catalase is added to hydrogen peroxide, bubbles of oxygen are seen immediately. The oxygen bubbles represent the gaseous product of the enzyme's activity occurring in this reaction. This test is commonly used to differentiate streptococci from staphylococci. Staphylococci are catalase-positive and will produce copious bubbles. Streptococci do not produce catalase and consequently are catalase-negative producing no visible bubbling of the hydrogen peroxide reagent.

Coagulase Test

The clumping factor test (coagulase test) is cell-associated and binds plasma fibrinogen causing agglutination of the organisms by binding them together by means of aggregated fibrinogen. Detection of a positive test is seen by observation of clumping of cells. The coagulase test is used primarily to identify isolates of *Staphylococci aureus*, an important human pathogen. *S. aureus* is almost always coagulase-positive. Immediate visible aggregation will be seen when coagulase plasma reagent is mixed with coagulase-positive organisms, usually resulting in the complete clearing of the suspension background. Coagulase-negative organisms will retain the smooth, milky appearance of the original suspension. A control is always included with this test. A specific immunologic agglutination test for *S. aureus* has supplanted the coagulase test in many laboratories.

Spot Indole Test

Organisms that produce the enzyme tryptophanase can degrade the amino acid tryptophan to yield indole as one end product. Indole can be detected by its ability to combine with certain aldehydes to form a colored compound. Indole reagent, containing the indicator aldehyde, is added to a filter paper in the bottom of a Petri dish. The reagent should saturate the filter paper. A portion of the isolated colony to be tested is rubbed onto the filter paper. Indole-positive organisms will result in the rapid development of a blue color on the filter paper if the indicator aldehyde is paradimethylaminocinnamaldehyde. This test can be used to differentiate swarming *Proteus* species from one another and as a presumptive identification of *Escherichia coli*. Positive organisms such as *E. coli* will give a blue-green color on the filter paper and negative organisms remain colorless.

Bile Solubility Test

Some organisms contain an active autocatalytic enzyme that will lyse the organism's own cell wall during cell division. Upon the addition of a bile salt, such as sodium deoxycholate, these organisms rapidly autolyze. When a drop of bile salt detergent reagent is added to isolated colonies of *Streptococcus pneumoniae* on a blood agar or chocolate agar plate, there will be visible dissolution of the colony within 30 minutes after exposure to the test reagent. Species of *Str. pneumoniae* result in a positive reaction which is the disappearance of the suspected colony leaving a flat area. Other streptococcal species will not be affected by the addition of the bile salt reagent.

Spot Oxidase Test

Organisms which produce the enzyme cytochrome oxidase are able to oxidize the test reagent tetramethyl-*p*-phenylenediamine dihydrochloride (Kovac's reagent) forming a colored end product. A dark-purple end product will be visible when an organism producing the enzyme is added to filter paper that has been impregnated with the reagent substrate. The test is primarily done to presumptively identify *Neisseria* species and to initially characterize gram-negative bacilli. *Neisseria* species, oxidase-positive organisms, will turn the filter paper a dark purple within 10 seconds. Oxidase-negative organisms will remain colorless or keep the color of the original colony within 10 seconds.

Rapid Urease Test

Organisms that produce the enzyme urease are able to hydrolyze urea-releasing ammonia as an end product. The production of ammonia changes the alkalinity, thus causing the pH indicator phenol red to change from yellow to red. This test can be used to screen lactose-negative colonies on differential media which have been plated with a stool specimen, thereby assisting in the differentiation of the pathogenic *Salmonella* and *Shigella* species, which are urease-negative, from the urease-positive nonpathogens. Commercial urease testing supplies are available with reagent-impregnated swabs that are rubbed across the colony to be tested—this being done directly on the culture plate. Another method uses a urea broth which is inoculated with a heavy suspension of the organism to be tested. The observance of a color change from that of pale straw or yellow to a red color identifies the presence of a urease-positive organism, such as *Proteus* species.

Rapid Carbohydrate Fermentation Reaction Test

Different bacteria ferment different carbohydrates (sugars), producing lactic acid. The ability of microorganisms to ferment certain carbohydrates often serves to identify them. Tubes for these tests contain peptone broth in addition to a solution of the sugar in question. The medium also contains a pH indicator, phenol red, which is red in alkaline solutions and yellow in acid solutions.

In the carbohydrate fermentation tests, carbohydrates are metabolized by certain organisms with subsequent changes in pH. The pH indicator in the peptone broth tubes is phenol red, which changes from red to yellow in the presence of positive organisms. One portion of the broth should be retained without carbohydrate to serve as a control. This control tube should remain red after the incubation period. The presence of buffers controls the pH change and the use of a heavy amount of inoculum allows rapid detection of the positive reaction. The broth tubes are incubated for up to 4 hours and should be observed periodically for any color change.

If a microorganism ferments the sugar into which it has been inoculated, it produces lactic acid from the sugar and therefore lowers the pH of the medium. This change of pH is indicated by a color change of the phenol red indicator from red to yellow. Hence, the formation of a yellow color indicates fermentation of the sugar, or a positive reaction. Growth may occur in sugar tubes without the production of lactic acid (i.e., without fermentation). There will be no color change in this case. The sugars used most in the identification of bacteria are glucose, maltose, fructose, and sucrose.

SMEAR PREPARATION AND STAINS USED IN MICROBIOLOGY

There is some merit in studying unstained preparations of bacteria, as bacterial motility may be observed in this way. Most bacteria can be observed unstained with the ordinary light microscope. Spirochetes, however, are so feebly refractive that it is necessary to use darkfield illumination or phase-contrast microscopy.

Smear Preparation

To stain bacteria, the material to be examined is spread thin on a glass microscope slide and allowed to dry. The film should be thin enough so that individual bacteria can be seen. If the material to be examined is a liquid, such as a broth culture, it may be transferred by means of a sterile, cooled inoculating loop and spread directly on the dry slide. If it is taken from an isolated colony on a Petri plate or other dry material, a drop of sterile water must first be placed on the slide and the material added and mixed by using the sterile, cooled inoculating loop or needle.

If the specimen to be stained is on a single swab obtained directly from the patient, culture media must be inoculated first and then the swab rolled onto the surface of the dry, clean glass slide. Slides are not sterile and thus are prepared last, after all other culture media are inoculated.

All slides prepared must be labeled with all patient identification information. It is sometimes helpful to draw a circle on the back side of the slide under the area where the specimen has been placed on the slide, using a wax pencil, so it may be more easily examined after staining.

After the material has air-dried completely, it must be *fixed* to the slide—that is, hardened and preserved for microbiological study. The fixing process prevents many of the bacterial cells from washing off the slide in subsequent staining operations. Fixation is achieved by simply passing the back of the microscope slide through the burner flame two or three times. The film side of the slide must not be exposed to heat, and the bottom of the slide must not be so hot that it cannot be held against the back of the hand. This heating coagulates the bacterial protein, causing cells to adhere to the slide. However, the air-drying and fixation do not necessarily kill all the bacterial cells on the slide, and to prevent accidental infection the slides must be handled carefully and placed in biohazard containers for glass and discarded appropriately.

Staining Techniques

Biological staining is the microscopic procedure most commonly used in microbiology to identify a particular bacterial species. Stains are chemical substances that contain colored dyes. Certain bacterial structures have affinities for particular dyes. It is common to use commercially prepared stains. These are usually purchased in a ready-to-use state. Actual methods will vary from manufacturer to manufacturer so the directions included with the stains must be followed carefully. Special stains are useful for showing the morphology of bacteria and specific structures such as capsules, flagella, spores, and granules. **Simple stains** such as methylene blue or more complex **differential stains** are used to show special cellular details. One commonly used differential stain is Gram's stain. The way bacteria react to this stain depends on the chemical composition of the cell wall.

Simple Stains

Simple staining procedures employing crystal violet, fuchsin, methylene blue, or safranin have only limited use in the microbiology laboratory. These are termed *simple* stains because only one stain is used and all structures present are stained the same color. They accentuate the otherwise colorless bacterial cell, but that is about all. When a simple stain is used, organisms should be observed for size, shape, and uniformity of staining. The procedure for using one simple stain in microbiology, the methylene blue stain, appears in Procedure 16–2.

Procedure 16–2. Staining With Methylene Blue

1. Spread a thin film of material on the clean microscope slide; air-dry and heat-fix. Place the slide on the staining rack.
2. Flood the surface of the slide with methylene blue staining solution. Allow the stain to remain on the slide for 2 minutes.
3. Wash the slide gently with running water to remove excess stain.
4. Allow the slide to air dry.
5. Examine the smear with the oil-immersion microscope lens, noting the size, shape, and uniformity of staining of the microorganisms present.

Differential Stains

Differential stains are used to show specific cellular details not shown when using a simple stain. The most commonly used differential stain is Gram's stain (see also Gram's Staining Reaction under Using Microbiology to Diagnose Disease).

Gram's Stain.—Gram's stain is used to differentiate various types of bacteria which have similar morphologic features. When bacteria are exposed to a solution of crystal violet stain, a purple-blue color, in combination with an iodine dye complex, and then washed with alcohol (or acetone-alcohol), some organisms retain the purple color and others are decolorized. The organisms that retain the purple color are called gram-positive and those that lose this purple color when washed with alcohol are called gram-negative. Another dye of a contrasting color is used as a counterstain. Safranin is a red dye, is used in Gram's stain as a counterstain, and colors the gram-negative organisms red, making them visible.

One method of Gram's staining (basically the Hucker modification) is described in Procedure 16–3. Reagents may be commercially prepared or prepared as follows:

Reagents

1. *Crystal violet stain.*
   a. Stock crystal violet. Dissolve 20 g of crystal violet 85% dye in 100 mL of 95% ethanol.
   b. Stock oxalate solution. Dissolve 1 g of ammonium oxalate in 100 mL of distilled water.
   c. Working solution. Dilute the stock crystal violet solution 1:10 with distilled water. Mix this with 4 volumes of stock oxalate solution. Store in a glass-stoppered bottle.
2. *Gram iodine solution.* Dissolve 1 g of iodine crystals and 2 g of potassium iodide in 5 mL of distilled water. Add to this 240 mL of distilled water and 60 mL of a 5% aqueous solution of

---

Procedure 16–3. Staining With Rapid Gram's Stain

1. Flood the heat-fixed slide with crystal violet stain and wait 10 seconds.
2. Pour off the stain and rinse with the iodine solution.
3. Cover with the iodine solution and wait for 10 seconds.
4. Rinse with running water, shaking off the excess.
5. Decolorize quickly with the alcohol-acetone solution, or with 95% alcohol if the alcohol-acetone decolorization proves to be too rapid. Continue until no more color is extracted by the solvent. This usually takes 10 to 20 seconds, but take care not to decolorize the film too much.
6. Flood with safranin for 10 seconds.
7. Rinse with water, then allow to air-dry.

---

sodium bicarbonate. Mix well and store in an amber glass bottle.
3. *Alcohol-acetone decolorizer.* Mix 250 mL of 95% ethanol with 250 mL of acetone. Store in a glass-stoppered bottle.
4. *Safranin counterstain.*
   a. Stock safranin. Dissolve 2.5 g of safranin stain in 100 mL of 95% ethanol.
   b. Working safranin. Dilute stock safranin 1:5 or 1:10 with distilled water. Store in a glass-stoppered bottle.

In the first step, all organisms present are stained violet by the primary stain, crystal violet. The iodine added in the second and third steps forms a crystal violet–iodine complex, which is fixed or retained in gram-positive but not in gram-negative organisms. The mechanism involved in the retention of this complex in gram-positive but not gram-negative organisms is not completely understood, but it reflects significant differences between the two groups.

The fifth step, decolorization with a mixture of acetone and alcohol, removes all color from gram-negative organisms but does not affect gram-positive ones, which remain purple. Since the gram-negative organisms are colorless after the fifth step, they are counterstained in the sixth step with the red secondary stain safranin so that they can be visualized under the microscope.

If a slide were observed under the microscope after each step of the Gram's staining process, the following results would be noted. After steps 1, 2, and 3, all organisms would be colored purple. After step 5, gram-positive organisms would appear purple, and gram-negative organisms would be colorless. After step 6, all gram-positive organisms would appear purple and all gram-negative organisms red.

Acid-fast Stain.—Acid-fast stain is used mainly to detect organisms that cause tuberculosis and leprosy. These organisms are extremely difficult to stain by ordinary methods because of their highly resistant fatty (or lipid) cell membranes. Once stained, they retain the dye color and decolorization is difficult, even with an acid-alcohol solution—hence the term acid-fast bacteria. Other bacteria are easily decolorized by the acid-alcohol reagent.

The Ziehl-Neelsen acid-fast method uses carbolfuchsin as the primary stain, heat as the mordant, a mixture of hydrochloric acid and alcohol as the decolorizer, and methylene blue as the counterstain. The Kinyoun acid-fast method uses a slightly different carbolfuchsin preparation and Tergitol 7 as the mordant (Procedure 16–4). After the first step, all bacteria present on the slide appear red. Following decolorization with acid-alcohol reagent, the acid-fast bacteria appear red and all other bacteria are colorless. After counterstaining with methylene blue, the acid-fast bacteria appear red and all other cells appear blue.

The Kinyoun carbolfuchsin method may be performed using commercially prepared stains or by preparing them as follows:

Reagents

1. *Kinyoun carbolfuchsin stain.* Dissolve 4 g of basic fuchsin in 20 mL of 95% ethanol. Add 100 mL of distilled water slowly while shaking the preparation. Melt phenol in a 56°C water bath. Add 8 mL of melted phenol to the stain. To accelerate the staining procedure add one drop of Tergitol 7 to every 30 to 40 mL of the Kinyoun carbolfuchsin stain.

2. *Acid-alcohol reagent.* Add 3 mL of concentrated hydrochloric acid to 97 mL of 95% ethanol.

3. *Counterstain.* Dissolve 0.3 g of methylene blue in 100 mL of distilled water.

Procedure 16–4. Staining for Acid-Fast Organisms Using the Kinyoun Carbolfuchsin Method

1. Flood the heat-fixed smear with Kinyoun's carbolfuchsin stain containing Tergitol 7 for 1 minute.
2. Wash with water.
3. Decolorize by adding acid-alcohol reagent drop by drop with continuous agitation until carbolfuchsin no longer washes off. This requires approximately 2 minutes for smears of average thickness.
4. Wash with water.
5. Counterstain with methylene blue for 20 to 30 seconds.
6. Wash with water and air-dry.

CULTURE MEDIA

The media used in clinical microbiology are generally prepared from precisely measured quantities of known substances that are formulated to give highly repeatable culture results. Media of this type are produced synthetically and consist of the specific amino acids, sugars, salts, vitamins, and minerals needed to ensure the proper growth of certain bacterial species. They are usually produced commercially and used for diagnostic purposes. Commercially prepared media in disposable culture plates or tubes have generally replaced media prepared in the individual laboratory. The National Committee for Clinical Laboratory Standards (NCCLS) has published recommendations to be followed by manufacturers of commercial media. See under Quality Control of Media. Broths are also sometimes used as culture media. They are less well chemically defined and are used mainly to maintain bacterial growth. They are generally not used for identification of bacterial species. Broths are meat extracts of protein materials—either peptone, an intermediate product of protein digestion, or digested protein.

A culture medium may be prepared as a solid, liquid, or semisolid, depending on the bacteriologic studies to be done. Liquid media are well suited for studying the production of a gas, odor, or change in pH. Media in a semisolid or solid form are most useful for the observation of colony size, shape, and color.

Agar is used extensively in the preparation of solid media. It is a seaweed extract that is liquid when heated and solid when cooled. It does not affect bacterial growth and is an excellent base for nutrient media. Agar can be melted and poured into tubes or plates, where it will solidify when cool. The more agar used, the more solid the final medium will become. Plates, slants, and stabs are all prepared with agar as the base.

Requirements for Culture Media

Bacteria, like all living things, have specific requirements to sustain life and to reproduce. The culture requirements for bacteria include a source of nutrients, the proper temperature, an adequate supply of oxygen (or in some cases the absence of oxygen), and the correct pH.

Nutrients

The *proper nutrient elements* must be available as microorganisms differ in their food requirements. Some grow on media containing simple mixtures of inorganic salts, since they are able to synthesize their own organic compounds. Others, especially many pathogens, are very particular and may require complex mixtures of nutrients, including many of the B vitamins and certain amino acids. In general, the culture medium must be able to supply carbon, nitrogen, and inorganic salts. Peptone is used in a variety of culture media as it contains nitrogen in a form (amino acids and simple nitrogen compounds) that can be used by most microorganisms. Certain bacteria require media to which serum, blood, or ascitic fluid has been added. In some media it is advantageous to add carbohydrates, and in some instances salts of calcium, manganese, magnesium, sodium, and potassium are required by the microorganism for growth.

In addition to nutrient sources, dyes or indicators may be added to culture media as a means of detecting metabolic activity by the microorganism or of promoting the growth of some microorganisms by inhibiting the growth of others. Finally, certain microorganisms either require or are enhanced by the presence of growth-promoting vitamin-like substances in the media.

Temperature

All organisms have a minimum *temperature* below which development ceases, an optimum temperature at which growth is maximum or luxuriant, and a maximum temperature above which death occurs. The majority of bacteria grow within the temperature range of 15 to 43°C. However, the pathogens generally have a narrow temperature range with optimum growth at 35°C, and for this reason most cultures are incubated at 35°C. Since the heat of an incubator would promote drying, the incubator should always be equipped with containers of water or some other suitable source of humidity. In addition, most microorganisms grow in the absence of light, and sunlight should be avoided.

Oxygen

Another factor that must be considered in culturing microorganisms is the presence or absence of *oxygen*. Pathogenic organisms are either aerobes, utilizing oxygen for their growth; anaerobes, intolerant to oxygen; or microaerophilic, growing best in an atmosphere of reduced oxygen tension. Aerobes can be incubated in room air. Most clinically significant aerobes are really facultatively anaerobic where they grow under either aerobic or anaerobic conditions.

Specimens originating from sites where an anaerobic agent is suspected are cultured on both aerobic and anaerobic media. Enriched media as well as differential and selective media are inoculated. The enriched and selective media are needed because anaerobes are fastidious and because most anaerobic infections are mixed with aerobic and other anaerobic organisms present also. Inoculated plates are immediately placed in an anaerobic environment for incubation. Jars, chambers, or commercially produced pouches and bags can be used. Cultures are incubated for 48 hours at 35°C. Usually these cultures should not be exposed to any oxygen until after 48 hours of incubation. Colony morphology can change dramatically between 24 and 48 hours. If plates are in a chamber or an anaerobic bag, they can be observed after 24 hours without oxygen exposure (see also Oxygen Requirements: Aerobes and Anaerobes, under Bacterial Culture Studies).

pH

Another factor affecting the growth or culture of microorganisms is the *pH* of the medium. Not only must a culture medium contain the proper nutrients in the correct concentrations, it must have the correct degree of acidity or alkalinity. Most microorganisms prefer culture media that are approximately neutral, although some require a medium that is acid. Most microorganisms grow within a pH range of 3 to 9. Although changes in pH may not actually prevent the growth of a particular organism, its metabolic activities may not be normal if the pH is not optimum.

The pH of media is controlled by use of buffers, or substances that resist changes in hydrogen ion concentration. Buffers are especially useful for microorganisms that produce acid as part of their metabolism. These microorganisms would kill themselves by their own acid production if a suitable buffer were not present. Conversely, some bacteria produce alkaline products such as ammonia, which must also be buffered or the culture would destroy itself. Blood, milk, and seawater are all solutions that are naturally buffered and are therefore useful as culture media. Synthetic media often contain phosphate buffer systems.

Sterile Conditions

To obtain a pure culture of a microorganism, the culture medium must be *sterile*. Not only is sterilization necessary for separation of the inoculated organism, but contamination by other forms may influence or prevent the growth of the desired microorganism. Most culture media are sterilized by use of the autoclave. Commercially prepared media are sterilized and packaged ready for use. Media prepared by the laboratory must be sterilized prior to use. Quantities of media up to 1 L should be autoclaved for 15 minutes at 121°C, and larger volumes may require a longer period. The culture media should be prepared according to directions and then placed in test tubes or Erlenmeyer flasks. These are loosely capped and placed in the autoclave. The test tubes should be autoclaved in racks or baskets, and the flasks should not be more than two thirds full. Oversterilization or prolonged heating must be avoided, as it can change the composition of the medium; it may cause precipitation in agar media or an increase in acidity. Some culture media may be harmed by autoclaving and may have to be sterilized by tyndallization or filtration.

Moisture

All microorganisms require some moisture for growth. Bacteria in general require a high concentration of water in their environment for growth and multiplication. Formation of highly resistant spores by bacteria that are spore formers is stimulated by drying or lack of water. Water is required for the metabolic reactions that take place in the bacterial cell and is the means of supplying nutrients to and removing waste products from the cell. Water is an integral part of the organism's protoplasm and accounts for much of the weight of the bacterial cell.

The amount of moisture in culture media varies. A medium may be used as a liquid, solid, liquefiable solid, or semisolid. Liquid media, or *broths*, may be converted to solid media by adding whole egg, egg white, or blood serum and heating until the mixture coagulates. Alternatively, potatoes may be used as a solid medium.

Liquefiable solid media are prepared by adding gelatin, which is a protein with a low melting point, or agar-agar, which is a complex carbohydrate prepared by adding certain seaweeds to a liquid medium such as nutrient broth. Agar-agar is superior to gelatin for this type of medium. It melts just before boiling, solidifies just above body temperature, and is digested by only a few bacteria. Gelatin has a lower melting point than agar-agar, many organisms do not develop satisfactorily at temperatures below its melting point, and many organisms liquefy gelatin. When gelatin is added to a broth,

the medium too is referred to as a *gelatin*. For example, a mixture of gelatin and nutrient broth is called *nutrient gelatin*. Similarly, a mixture of agar-agar and nutrient broth would be called *nutrient agar*.

Semisolid media are prepared in much the same way as the liquefiable solid media. However, a much smaller amount of agar-agar is added.

Storage

Culture media must be protected from *external contamination*. Media and cultures in Petri dishes are protected from external contamination by the design of the dish. Test tubes and flasks may be covered with screw caps or loosely fitting metal or autoclavable plastic covers. The cover must not be too tight or too loose, and it must protect the lip of the container from contamination by dust. Screw caps must be used with care, for they may result in anaerobic or partially anaerobic conditions. Cotton plugs are useful because they prevent the entrance of foreign microorganisms and debris while admitting sterile filtered air, which is necessary for the growth of aerobic microorganisms. Cotton plugs can be a fire hazard, however, and should be used carefully if near a flame. Polyurethane foam plugs are becoming more popular, as they do not pose a fire hazard or tend to fall out of test tubes that have been entered repeatedly, both of which are problems with cotton plugs.

Media are generally stored under refrigeration (4°C) to prevent deterioration and dehydration. Certain media require special storage, but such information will be provided with the media. In general, a medium should be allowed to warm up to room temperature before it is inoculated, or microorganisms may be destroyed.

Classification of Media

Although culture as well as morphologic characteristics are essential in the identification of bacteria, additional determinations are often necessary. Culture media may be simply supportive or employed to give additional information. In this context media are classified as selective, differential, or enrichment media.

Supportive Media

Supportive media contain nutrients that allow most nonfastidious organisms to grow at their normal rate. These media do not give one organism any growth advantage over another. The organism's own metabolism affects the progress of its growth.

Selective Media

Selective media are semisolid plating media prepared by adding dyes, antibiotics, or other chemical compounds to certain media. These substances selectively inhibit the growth of certain microorganisms and permit the growth of others. Selective media are used for fecal and sputum specimens, where many normally occurring bacteria could obscure the presence of the pathogenic material. The normally occurring bacteria are selectively inhibited so that the pathogens can be seen if they are present.

Enrichment Media

Enrichment media permit one organism to grow rapidly while inhibiting the growth of other organisms. Enrichment media are especially useful in the isolation of *Salmonella* or *Shigella* from stool cultures, which contain several bacteria—the *normal intestinal flora*—that are so numerous that they would obscure the growth of the pathogens. Therefore, cultures of stool specimens for pathogens normally include an enrichment medium that inhibits the normal intestinal flora and promotes the growth of the pathogens that must be identified. Subculture to a solid plating medium from the enrichment broth must be made to obtain isolated colonies for final identification.

Differential Media

Differential media contain dyes, indicators, or other constituents that give colonies of particular organisms distinctive and easily recognizable characteristics. The final identification of an organism often involves isolation on a suitable culture medium and then the characteristic reaction or growth on a differential medium. Such a characteristic reaction constitutes a confirmatory test for the microorganism.

Quality Control of Media

The NCCLS has developed recommendations for use of abbreviated quality control testing for media that have been commercially prepared where, in the process of preparation, the manufacturer has followed these recommendations. If the manufacturer has followed the NCCLS recommendations, it has been found that the performance of their media is consistent and adequate and that these media do not require further testing in the local laboratory as to quality.

There are some commercially prepared media which must be tested in the local laboratory before use. The NCCLS has identified the media that need quality control testing on a local basis. For this purpose, there are quality control organisms which can be purchased along with their expected results. The relevant NCCLS publication, *Quality Assurance for Commerically Prepared Microbiological Culture Media, Approved Standard* (see Bibliography), should be consulted for this information. All media prepared in the laboratory must be tested before being used for routine culture. Clones of stock organisms for which the media are intended are used for testing the media for quality.

Commonly Used Types of Media

The eventual identification of a particular microorganism requires its culture on various media (selective, enrichment, or differential). There is no one system that is universally employed in the identification of pathogens (see also Biochemical Tests).

Trypticase Soy Broth (Tryp Broth)

Tryp broth is a very good general-purpose medium. Almost everything grows well in it. All tryp broths contain dextrose, some type of peptone, inorganic salts, and water. Most cultures are inoculated into tryp broth to maintain the growth of *all* organisms in the specimen. A small amount of agar is added to the medium to make it thicker, but not enough to solidify it. This permits the growth of some anaerobic organisms, since oxygen does not diffuse to the bottom of the medium if agar is added.

Thioglycolate Broth (Thio Broth)

Thio broth is used particularly for the cultivation of anaerobic organisms. It contains thioglycolic acid (sodium thioglycolate) and agar to encourage anaerobic growth. The medium is in a reduced state, and contains the indicator resazurin, which turns pink if the medium is oxidized. If more than one-third of the medium is pink, it contains too much oxygen for anaerobic growth. The oxygen can be driven off by heating the tube of medium. All cultures in which an anaerobic organism is suspected are inoculated into thio broth.

Sheep Blood Agar (SB or BA)

This medium supports the growth of most ordinary bacteria. It is therefore used for primary plating and for subculturing. It is a good general medium for the growth of pathogens, since the blood adds many of the accessory substances that pathogens require. Most pathogens can be recognized on sheep blood. The medium is also useful in distinguishing different types of streptococci by their ability to hemolyze the red blood cells present in the medium. They are differentiated as follows: alpha streptococci—green hemolysis; beta streptococci—clear hemolysis; gamma streptococci—no hemolysis.

Rabbit Blood Agar (RB)

This medium consists of 5% fresh sterile rabbit blood in nutrient agar. It is the primary medium for nose and throat cultures of material taken from pediatric patients or when *Haemophilus* infection is suspected. It is used for the isolation of *H. influenzae,* since it contains the X and V growth factors required by this organism. RB is rarely used for other cultures because it produces too diffuse hemolysis.

Eosin–Methylene Blue Agar (EMB), Levine's

This medium promotes the growth of gram-negative organisms and inhibits that of gram-positive organisms. In addition, many gram-negative organisms have a characteristic appearance on EMB. Lactose fermenters produce acid, which precipitates the two dyes (eosin, giving a metallic sheen to *E. coli* and methylene blue, inhibiting gram-positive organisms) and gives colonies of the lactose-positive organisms a purple center. Urine cultures are inoculated onto EMB plates as well as sheep blood agar, since many urinary tract infections are caused by gram-negative rods. MacConkey agar can be used in place of EMB.

MacConkey Agar (Mac)

Mac is a differential medium used in the primary plating of routine cultures (urine in particular). The medium should be lightly inoculated. Crystal violet is included to inhibit the growth of gram-positive organisms, and bile salts are present to inhibit nonpathogenic gram-negative organisms. The medium is used in the diagnosis of dysentery, typhoid, and paratyphoid bacteria, which do not ferment lactose. Colonies of organisms that do ferment lactose are red in this medium because the lactic acid that results from fermentation reacts with the bile salts, with subsequent absorption of neutral red. Neutral red is an acid-base indicator (red indicates an acid reaction, yellow an alkaline reaction). Therefore, the pathogens that do not ferment lactose are seen as yellow or colorless colonies on this medium.

Mac medium is sometimes used in place of EMB, since it tends to inhibit the spread of *Proteus* species more than EMB does.

Phenylethyl Alcohol Agar (PEA)

This is essentially sheep blood agar with phenylethyl alcohol added. The medium inhibits the growth of gram-negative organisms except *Pseudomonas aeruginosa*. It allows growth of gram-positive organisms and permits their identification and separation, even when they are mixed with gram-negative organisms. If *P. aeruginosa* is present in a mixed culture and isolation of gram-positive organisms is desired, the culture is mixed with ether and then streaked onto the PEA plate, since ether destroys *Pseudomonas*. Hemolysis cannot be observed on the PEA plate.

Chocolate Agar (Choc)

Choc is prepared by adding blood to a nutrient base medium at 75 to 80°C. The heat denatures proteins in the blood, causing the blood to coagulate and turn brown. This gives a richer medium than ordinary blood agar providing a higher moisture content required by some fastidious organisms and is used in the cultivation of the pathogenic *Neisseria* species. These organisms cause gonorrhea and meningitis and are difficult to grow. They require an atmosphere of 10% carbon dioxide in addition to the special medium. The medium also supplies the special growth requirements for *H. influenzae.*

Thayer-Martin Agar (Modified Thayer-Martin, Martin-Lewis Agar, Transgrow Agar)

This is a selective medium for *Neisseria gonorrhoeae* and *Neisseria meningitidis*. It is a modification of Choc, containing hemoglobin along with the various nutrients from the lysed red cells. It contains various antibiotics present to inhibit the growth of other types of bacteria and fungi.

Salmonella-Shigella Agar (SS)

SS is a highly selective medium that is very inhibitory to coliforms and gram-positive organisms. Brilliant green is present to inhibit the gram-positive organisms. It is used along with Mac in routine stool cultures. The medium should be heavily inoculated. It is designed to isolate the *Salmonella* and *Shigella* species in the presence of other gram-negative organisms. It can also differentiate lactose-fermenting from non-lactose-fermenting strains. Colonies of lactose fermenters are red and those of nonfermenters are yellowish or colorless. Neutral red is an acid-base indicator. Organisms that produce hydrogen sulfide show black centers on this medium.

Sabouraud Agar With Chloramphenicol (SAB)

This medium promotes the growth of fungi while inhibiting bacterial growth. It has a low pH and high osmotic pressure. It should always be incubated at room temperature. Chloramphenicol is included to inhibit gram-positive and gram-negative organisms. Cyclohex-imide (Acta-Dione) may be included to inhibit nonpathogenic fungi.

Selenite Broth

This is an enrichment medium used for stool cultures. The medium inhibits the growth of gram-positive organisms and coliform bacilli (gram-negative organisms that are part of the normal intestinal flora), while favoring and therefore isolating *Shigella* and *Salmonella,* the causative agents of dysentery and typhoid fever, respectively. The medium suppresses growth of organisms other than *Shigella* and *Salmonella* for 12 to 18 hours. After this time coliforms and streptococci (enterococci) grow rapidly. Therefore, after 18 hours of incubation, cultures grown in selenite broth must be subcultured onto a MacConkey plate or other suitable differential medium. Selenite broth is most effective under reduced oxygen tension. Therefore, it is dispensed into tubes to a depth of 2 in. The broth should be inoculated heavily with fecal material—an amount about the size of a pea.

Urea Agar (Christensen's)

This is an enrichment agar slant that is used to test the ability of a microorganism to utilize urea as its only source of nitrogen. To do this, the organism must produce the enzyme urease. Breakdown of urea by the action of urease results in the production of ammonia, which raises the pH of the medium, as indicated by a color change of the phenol red indicator to red. The organism is streaked onto the slant only. The butt is *not* stabbed. Some organisms give a red color in only the slant; others color both the butt and the slant.

Tests for urease production may also be done on urea broth, which contains a buffered urea solution and phenol red indicator.

Triple Sugar Iron Agar (TSIA)Slants

TSIA slants are slant tubes having a lump, or butt, of medium at the bottom and a slant above (see Fig 16–3). It is essential that the slants be inoculated with a pure culture. Therefore, a single, well-isolated colony should be used for the inoculum. The medium is inoculated by streaking the slant and then stabbing the butt with a straight inoculating needle.

The medium is especially useful as a first step in the identification of gram-negative rods. It is used to test the ability of gram-negative rods to ferment dextrose, sucrose, and lactose, and to produce hydrogen sulfide (H_2S). Fermentation of sugars is accompanied by acid production, which is indicated by a change in the color of the phenol red indicator from red to yellow (yellow in acid pH and red in alkaline pH). Ferrous ammonium sulfate is present. This is black in the presence of hydrogen sulfide. Production of hydrogen sulfide is therefore indicated by the formation of a black color as hydrogen sulfide combines with ferrous ammonium sulfate. Splitting of the agar in the butt indicates gas production.

Since a variety of reactions occur in the TSIA slants, there must be a scheme for observing and recording these reactions. Reactions in the slant and butt are recorded as acid (A) or alkaline (Alk) and the production of hydrogen sulfide (H_2S) and gas (G) is noted. An acid reaction is indicated by the presence of a yellow color, and an alkaline reaction by a red color. No reaction would be recorded as NR. Various observations and interpretations are shown in Table 16–1.

As indicated, failure of the organism to ferment any of the three sugars results in an Alk/Alk reaction (or no reaction), indicated by a red slant and butt. An Alk/A reaction (red slant and yellow butt) results when only dextrose is fermented. Organisms fermenting only dextrose will initially give an A/A reaction, or yellow slant and butt. However, the small amount of dextrose present is used up as the incubation continues. The slant is under aerobic conditions and reverts to alkaline (or red) in 18 to 24 hours. In the butt, however, anaerobic conditions exist, there is no reversion to alkaline pH, and the acid (or yellow) reaction remains.

An A/A reaction (yellow slant and butt) results when dextrose and lactose or sucrose or both are fermented. The medium contains ten times more lactose and sucrose than dextrose. Therefore, organisms fermenting lactose or sucrose or both do not use up the sugars except after very prolonged incubation. Fermentation of sucrose or lactose is indicated by acid (yellow) conditions in both the slant and the butt. However, with pro-

TABLE 16-1.

Observations of Triple Sugar Iron Agar (TSIA)

Notation	Color Change	Metabolic Change
A/A	Yellow slant, yellow butt	Dextrose fermented, lactose *or* sucrose *or* both fermented
Alk/A	Red slant, yellow butt	Dextrose fermented, lactose and sucrose not fermented
Alk/Alk or NR	Red slant, red butt	None of the three sugars fermented, or no reaction
H₂S	Black in butt	H₂S production
G	Splitting of agar in butt	Gas production

longed incubation (48–72 hours), lactose and sucrose may also be used up, and formerly acid reactions may revert to alkaline. Therefore, the time of incubation is critical. The time recommended to obtain typical reactions is 18 hours.

There are other media that are similar to TSIA. One such medium is Kligler's iron agar (KIA). This medium differs in that it tests fermentation of only dextrose and lactose. Sucrose is not included.

Simmons Citrate Agar

Simmons citrate is also an agar slant. It is not a nutrient agar, but contains simple inorganic salts. It is used to test the ability of the organism to utilize sodium citrate as its sole source of carbon and monoammonium phosphate as its sole source of nitrogen. The medium also contains the indicator bromothymol blue to indicate growth. Bromothymol blue is green (the color of the uninoculated medium) when the organism is not growing and turns blue when it is. Therefore, a positive reaction is observed as a change of the color of the medium from green to blue. This medium is important in separating different types of gram-negative rods.

Tryptophan Broth and Peptone Water (Indole Medium)

This is a culture medium which can be used for the *indole test*. Tryptophan is an amino acid. The ability of bacteria to split indole from the tryptophan molecule is highly diagnostic. If a microorganism growing in peptone water with tryptophan has produced indole, the addition of Kovac's reagent to the culture results in a red color. Therefore, a positive test for indole production is the production of a red color after addition of Kovac's reagent. The indole test is useful in the identification of gram-negative rods.

Clark-Lubs Broth

Clark-Lubs medium is important as the culture medium for two differential tests, the methyl red test and the Voges-Proskauer test, used in the identification of gram-negative rods.

Bordet-Gengou Agar (BG)

This is a special plate used in the diagnosis of whooping cough, caused by *Bordetella pertussis*. Colonies of the organism have a special diagnostic appearance on this medium. Penicillin may also be added to the medium to inhibit growth of the normal bacterial flora. However, certain strains of *B. pertussis* are also inhibited by penicillin, so two BG plates should be inoculated, one with and one without penicillin.

CULTURING COMMON SPECIMENS

Urine Cultures

Cultures are done on urine to diagnose bacterial infections of the urinary tract (bladder, ureter, kidney, and urethra). Urinary tract infections (UTI) are of two main types—cystitis, an infection of the bladder, and pyelonephritis, an infection of the renal parenchyma (kidney).

Collecting the Specimen

The urine specimen for culture must be collected in a clinically reliable manner; proper cleaning of the collection site, especially for females, is very important.

The clean-catch, midstream urine sample collection is the one utilizing the least invasive technique and, consequently, the one most commonly used (see also Specimens for Microbiological Examination; and Collecting Urine Specimens, in Chapter 2).

The specimen must be collected into a sterile container and if not cultured immediately in the laboratory, must be refrigerated to prevent bacterial growth. Urine is normally sterile within the bladder but is easily contaminated during the collection process if caution is not used in cleaning the collection site. **Quantitative urine culture methods** are needed to differentiate true **bacteriuria** (bacteria in the urine) from contamination. The classic criterion of infection is the presence of greater than 100,000 **colony-forming units (CFU) of bacteria** per milliliter of urine. If a quantitative culture results in a colony count between 10,000 and 100,000 CFU/mL urine, a repeat culture is done on a fresh urine specimen to confirm the result. The quantitation of polymorphonuclear neutrophils present in the urine, in conjunction with the results of the urine culture, increases the diagnostic value of both tests.

Methods for Detection of Bacteriuria

Rapid Screening Test Strips.—Rapid screening test strips have been developed to test for bacteriuria. Nitrite tests have been incorporated into reagent strips used in many laboratories for routine urine analysis (see Chapter 13). Common organisms that cause urinary tract infections, such as species of *Enterobacter, Escherichia, Proteus, Klebsiella,* and *Pseudomonas,* contain enzymes that reduce nitrate in the urine to nitrite (see Nitrite in Chapter 13.) Organisms must contain the reductase enzyme necessary to carry out this process.

The use of rapid screening test strips for bacteriuria are most useful when the test for nitrite is combined with that for leukocyte esterase. Chemical test strips are available which combine nitrite and leukocyte esterase tests. Multiple reagent test strips also are available which contain tests for these constituents. Test strips for leukocyte esterase utilize a diazo reaction which is specific for esterase. Leukocyte esterase is an enzyme present in the primary or azurophilic granules of granulocytes such as neutrophils. Since neutrophils are generally increased in a urinary tract infection, the presence of leukocyte esterase in the urine is an indicator of infection (see Leukocyte Esterase in Chapter 13). The absence of leukocyte esterase does not rule out a urinary tract infection, however. The finding of nitrite-positive and leukocyte esterase–positive

urine using chemical screening tests is helpful in detecting bacteriuria, especially in combination with the presence of bacteria and white cells in the urine sediment. To identify the organism causing the infection, Gram's stain and a quantitative urine culture can be done.

Commercial Screening Systems.—Automated methods have been developed to screen urines rapidly for bacteriuria. One such device is the Bac-T-Screen system (Marion Laboratories, Inc., Kansas City, MO), which employs a filter paper detection method screening out negative urine specimens in about 2 minutes. With this system, a measured amount of the urine sample is drawn by suction through a paper filter. Bacteria and other particles such as white blood cells adhere to the filter paper. A stain is passed through the filter paper giving a color, the depth of which depends on the number and type of stainable particles. The filter paper is manually inserted into a photometric device on the instrument which compares the unknown filter paper color to that of a standard. The filter paper can also be examined visually and if the color is less than that of the control, the testing can be stopped at this point as it is considered to be negative. The Bac-T-Screen system has shown excellent correlation with the clinical diagnoses of urinary tract infections.*

Nonculture Methods: Gram's Stain and Polymorphonuclear Neutrophil Enumeration.—If a screening test is positive, a Gram's stain should be done on the well-mixed urine sample. One drop of uncentrifuged urine is placed on a glass slide, allowed to air-dry and then stained with Gram's stain. The stained smear is examined microscopically using the oil-immersion objective. If at least one organism per field (after examining at least 20 fields) is seen, this correlates with a significant bacteriuria of greater than 100,000 CFU/mL urine.† If three or more morphologic types of bacteria are detected, the urine is contaminated with distal urethral or perianal bacteria and another specimen must be collected.

In an uncentrifuged urine specimen, polymorphonuclear neutrophils (PMNs) may be enumerated. The pres-

*Baron EJ, Tyburski M, Almon R, et al: Visual and clinical analysis of Bac-T-Screen urine screen results. *J Clin Microbiol* 1988; 26:2382.

†Washington JA II, White CM, Laganiere M, et al: Detection of significant bacteriuria by microscopic examination of urine. *Lab Med* 1981; 12:294.

ence of more than 8 PMNs per microliter correlates well with an excretion rate of more than 400,000 PMNs being excreted into the urine per hour, which is a good indicator of the presence of infection. This test is best done by using a hemocytometer. Since it requires extra time to perform, it is not commonly done by most laboratories. The standard PMN enumeration done as part of a routine urinalysis does not correlate well with either the PMN excretion rate or the presence of infection.

Quantitative Methods.—Quantitative methods must be used to determine the number of colony-forming units of organism per milliliter of urine specimen and cultures done to identify the pathogenic organism present. The traditional streak plate culture method is done in many laboratories and commercial dip culture methods are used by some.

Streak Plate for Quantitative Urine Culture.—

A streak plate method for quantitating the growth of microorganisms in the urine is commonly used in many hospital laboratories (Procedure 16–5). A special standardized inoculating loop, holding 0.001 mL of urine or fluid, is used to transfer the well-mixed specimen to the culture plate and to streak the plate. Care must be taken

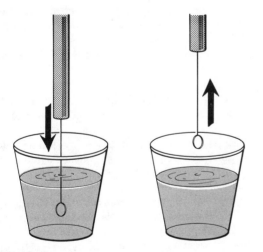

FIG 16–8.
Method for inserting a calibrated loop into urine to ensure that the proper amount of specimen will adhere to the loop. (From Baron EJ, Finegold SM: *Bailey and Scott's Diagnostic Microbiology*, ed 8. St Louis, Mosby–Year Book, Inc, 1990, p 260. Used by permission.)

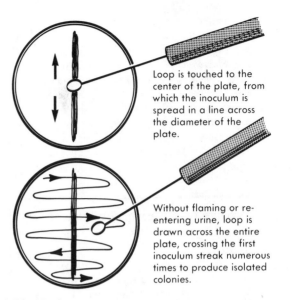

Loop is touched to the center of the plate, from which the inoculum is spread in a line across the diameter of the plate.

Without flaming or re-entering urine, loop is drawn across the entire plate, crossing the first inoculum streak numerous times to produce isolated colonies.

FIG 16–9.
Method for streaking a loopful of urine with a calibrated inoculating loop to produce isolated colonies and countable colony-forming units of organisms. (From Baron EJ, Finegold SM: *Bailey and Scott's Diagnostic Microbiology*, ed 8. St Louis, Mosby–Year Book, Inc, 1990, p 260. Used by permission.)

in obtaining the specimen with the calibrated loop (Fig 16–8). In common practice, a general medium such as SB and a selective medium such as Mac or EMB are streaked with the urine specimen. This is done in such a way that the drop of urine is spread as uniformly as possible on the plate (Figs 16–9 and 16–10). After streaking and incubation, the number of colonies seen is multiplied by 1,000 to give the number of colonies in 1 mL of urine. The blood agar plate gives a total colony count, as most common organisms grow on it. The selective medium indicates whether gram-negative rods (and some in-

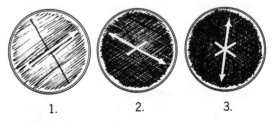

1. 2. 3.

FIG 16–10.
Streak plate for quantitative urine culture.

hibited gram-positive organisms) are present. The EMB and Mac media also indicate whether the organisms are lactose-positive or lactose-negative. *E. coli, Klebsiella* sp., and *Enterobacter* sp. are lactose fermenters that show pink colonies, whereas *Proteus* sp. and *Pseudomonas* sp. are lactose-negative (do not ferment lactose) and show yellowish colonies. *Proteus* sp. may also be recognized on blood agar by its spreading growth. Gram-positive organisms such as staphylococci and streptococci (enterococcus) grow well on blood agar but are inhibited on EMB or Mac medium.

Procedure 16–5. Quantitative Urine Streak Plate

1. In streaking the urine for a quantitative colony count, the urine must first be mixed well.
2. The calibrated inoculating loop is flamed, cooled, and dipped into the bubble-free surface of the specimen (see Fig 16–8).
3. The loopful of urine is streaked undiluted over the surface of the SB and EMB or Mac plates (see Fig 6–10). After streaking the SB plate, three or four small cuts are made in the agar to check for hemolysis.
4. The culture plates should be incubated at 35 to 37°C in an inverted position for 18 to 24 hours.
5. Interpret results.

Interpreting Results of Quantitative Urine Cultures.—Normal urine is sterile. Plates that show no growth may be discarded and reported as no growth. Bacteriuria is considered clinically significant when laboratory findings show the presence of 100,000 (10^5) or more bacteria colonies per milliliter of urine specimen. After the incubation period, the number of colonies growing on the plates are counted and multiplied by 1,000 (if 0.001 mL urine has been plated) to determine the number of microorganisms per milliliter of original urine specimen. A count of 100,000 CFU/mL urine indicates a UTI in asymptomatic patients. A count of 1,000 CFU/mL urine may be significant for a UTI in a symptomatic patient. Therefore, it is important to combine the results of colony counts with the clinical information available.

The growth characteristics of the colonies on the plates are also observed. As discussed previously, the

EMB or Mac plates are observed for presumptive identification of gram-negative organisms and growth on the SB plates noted. Any cultural observations should agree with the results of Gram's stain. Further biochemical tests can be done to identify the suspected organism.

Dip Cultures Used for Bacteriuria.—Several commercial dip culture products are available for urine. These products vary somewhat, but in general consist of a slide or paddle covered on both sides with combinations of culture media. The dip slide is dipped into a freshly voided urine specimen. If bacteria are present in the specimen, some of the organisms will adhere to the surfaces of the slide. The dip cultures are incubated for an appropriate length of time and checked for colony growth. These products can give satisfactory quantitation if they have been properly inoculated. Some of these systems seem to be more accurate for either negative specimens or specimens that contain more than 100,000 CFU/mL urine. The manufacturer's directions must always be carefully followed.

Throat Cultures

Throat cultures are done primarily to diagnose group A β-hemolytic streptococcal *(Streptococcus pyogenes)* sore throat (strep throat). Sore throats caused by this streptococcal organism, the major throat pathogen, must be identified and treated because, if untreated, rheumatic fever and glomerulonephritis can follow this infection in some patients.

Collecting the Specimen

The proper collection of the sample is important. A sterile swab is used to collect the specimen. Throat cultures are done by swabbing the rear pharyngeal wall and the tonsillar area (see also Throat Culture Collection, in Chapter 2). The swab used to collect the specimen must be transported quickly to the laboratory for plating. Transport media can be used to sustain the swab if transport to the laboratory must be delayed. These media will allow survival of suspected streptococcal organisms for 24 to 48 hours at 4°C. Culture of the throat swab specimen is traditionally done by using SB plates.

Methods of Detection of Group A β-Hemolytic Streptococci

The traditional culture using blood agar plates continues to be used by many laboratories (Procedure

16–6). Several nonculture methods are also used, their advantage being that results are obtained much more rapidly.

Procedure 16–6. Plating Throat Cultures

1. Using the **throat swab** obtained from the patient, cultures are made by rolling the swab onto one edge of an SB plate, being certain to get as much of the specimen off onto the plate as possible.
2. The inoculating loop is flamed and used to streak the plate out from the inoculated area, as shown in Figure 16–11. The streaking is done so as to isolate the bacterial colonies as much as possible. Three or four cuts should then be made into the agar to check for hemolysis.
3. After 18 to 24 hours of incubation, throat culture plates should be examined for pathogens. If pathogens are present, appropriate subculturing is done for their final identification.

Interpreting Results of Throat Culture Plates.

—After suitable incubation has taken place, the colony morphology and hemolytic appearance on the blood agar plates is used in the identification of streptococci. Streptococci typically appear as translucent to milky, circular, small colonies.

After incubation, hemolysis can be observed. This

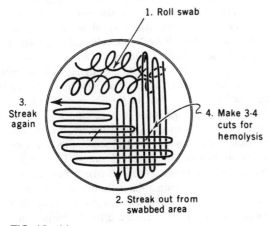

1. Roll swab

3. Streak again

4. Make 3-4 cuts for hemolysis

2. Streak out from swabbed area

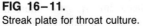

FIG 16–11.
Streak plate for throat culture.

phenomenon is useful in distinguishing different types of streptococci by their ability to hemolyze the red cells present in the medium. Hemolysis is of three types, depending on the type of streptococci: (1) alpha hemolysis (produced by alpha streptococci) appears macroscopically as a green discoloration of the medium surrounding the colony, (2) gamma hemolysis macroscopically shows "no hemolysis" (gamma streptococci do not produce hemolysis), and (3) beta hemolysis (produced by beta streptococci) appears macroscopically as a clear zone surrounding the surface colonies or the stabs in the blood agar representing complete hemolysis.

Since throat cultures are done primarily to detect the presence of the Lancefield **group A β-hemolytic streptococci,** plates are read with this organism in mind. Other pathogens may sometimes be clinically significant.

Normal throat cultures show a predominance of α-hemolytic streptococci and commensal *Neisseria* sp. Other organisms also constitute normal flora. If pathogens are not present, the result should be reported as normal flora.

A bacitracin filter paper disk can be placed directly on the area of initial inoculation and after an overnight incubation period, presumptive identification of *Str. pyogenes* can be made. All group A and a small percentage of group B streptococci are susceptible to the bacitracin. Since the bacitracin test is recommended to be used with a pure culture, traditionally with a subculture made from the primary culture as described previously, it should only be used for *presumptive* identification when used on the primary culture plate. Final identification requires use of a pure culture of the organism isolated from the specimen. Identification of group A streptococci is shown by a zone of growth inhibition around the disk after the plate has been incubated for 18 to 24 hours.

An alternative test utilizes direct antigen detection which is carried out on an isolated β-hemolytic colony appearing after overnight incubation on selective agar. One such medium is Strep Selective Agar. This medium suppresses the growth of almost all normal throat flora and β-hemolytic streptococci except for groups A and B.

Subculturing and Use of Bacitracin Test.

—To identify the group A β-hemolytic streptococci from other β-hemolytic streptococci, the use of the bacitracin test is recommended. With a sterile inoculating loop, a single presumptive colony of group A β-hemolytic streptococci is picked from the plate and streaked completely onto a segment of a new blood agar plate. A bacitracin disk (with 0.04 unit bacitracin) is placed in the center of the inoculated area aseptically and the plate incubated overnight. A zone of inhibition of growth around the disk is indicative of bacitracin susceptibility and should be reported as "group A streptococci by bacitracin."

Rapid Detection Methods: Nonculture Techniques.

—There are numerous commercial products available for the rapid detection of group A β-hemolytic streptococcal throat infections. Instead of waiting for an overnight incubation period for culture plate methods, these results are available within a much shorter time— 15 to 30 minutes. These **rapid streptococcal antigen detection** systems use enzyme-linked immunosorbent assays (ELISA) or latex or coagglutination techniques. Many of these products are based primarily on a latex slide agglutination test for the direct detection of the group A streptococcal antigen taken from the specimen on the throat swab itself. The streptococcal antigen is extracted from the swab and mixed with specific antibody-coated latex beads resulting in a visible agglutination which occurs within a few minutes indicating the presence or absence of the bacterial infection. Specific procedures will vary with the product and the manufacturer's directions must always be followed carefully for optimal results. One such commercial product is Detect-A-Strep (Antibodies, Inc., Davis, CA).

In the Detect-A-Strep test, extraction reagents extract the group A carbohydrate antigen from the streptococcal cell walls while the organisms are still on the swab. The reaction is stopped and neutralized with an additional reagent, preparing the mixture for the latex agglutination step. A specific antibody-coated latex suspension, along with a control latex suspension, is tested for the presence of the specific group A carbohydrate. A positive test for the presence of the group A streptococci is seen as visible agglutination in the specific antibody-coated suspension when compared with the milky smoothness of the control suspension. It is important to include a test using the positive control antigen which is provided with the Detect-A-Strep kit.

Most laboratory comparisons of conventional culture methods and rapid testing methods have shown good sensitivity (>90%) and excellent specificity (>97%). If results are positive using rapid testing methods, it is sufficient reason to begin antibiotic therapy as the rapid test is very specific for the group A β-hemolytic streptococcal infection. In many instances, a negative rapid test result is confirmed with a culture plate method to account for possible false-negative results using the rapid testing method.

Genitourinary Cultures

Microbiological examination of **genitourinary tract specimens** is done primarily to detect *N. gonorrhoeae* for the diagnosis of gonorrhea and to detect *Chlamydia trachomatis* for the detection of chlamydial infections. Chlamydial infections have surpassed the number of gonorrheal infections as the most prevalent sexually transmitted disease in the United States. Other microorganisms which can cause vaginitis in females include *Gardnerella* and *Modiluncas*. *Trichomonas vaginalis*, a parasite, is a commonly recognized sexually transmitted organism and can be recognized in a wet mount of vaginal secretions. See also Tests for Parasites (Parasitology). Fungal infections are common also and can often be the cause of vaginitis in women, especially women who are on antibiotic therapy which inhibits the growth of the normal vaginal bacterial flora. A common fungal infection is caused by *Candida albicans*. See also Tests for Fungi (Mycology). Herpes simplex virus is another frequent cause of genitourinary infections.

Collecting the Specimen

It is essential that genitourinary tract specimens, usually from the vaginal cervix or inflamed perineal areas in women and the anterior urethra in men, be appropriately collected in order that the organisms may be detected. Specimens must be handled carefully to avoid any contamination with other viable infectious material.

For detecting chlamydial organisms, it is important that columnar epithelial cells are collected along with the vaginal secretion as the organism resides in the cells. Vaginal smears or cultures must be collected with the swab inserted well into the vagina. The outer lips of the labia must be held apart so that the swab does not touch them. An endocervical specimen is necessary for suspected gonorrheal infections and requires the use of a speculum. Lubricants should not be used as some of these are toxic to the microorganisms. Urethral smears from men are done by collecting the urethral discharge from the penis using a swab and rolling the collected specimen onto a microscope slide. Special loop swabs are available for collection into the distal urethra if the discharge is minimal. The swab is inoculated directly onto culture medium and a smear made for Gram's stain. Genitourinary specimens must be transported immediately to the laboratory and culturing done without delay or appropriate storage precautions followed.

There are commercially available transport systems for transit and storage of genitourinary tract specimens which enhance the survival of the organisms, if present. Kits are available which contain collection swabs and transport tubes containing specially formulated stabilizing media.

Methods of Detection

The physician must alert the laboratory to the probable organisms causing the infection so the identification process can be initiated using the appropriate culture media and assay protocol.

Gonorrheal Infections.—When *N. gonorrhoeae* is suspected, a special agar medium and carbon dioxide atmosphere for incubation is required for optimal recovery from the clinical specimen being tested. Various supplemental media can also be inoculated. Thayer-Martin agar is a selective medium for *N. gonorrhoeae*. It contains various antibiotics to inhibit the growth of other types of bacteria and fungi. Chocolate agar is also a support medium for *N. gonorrhoeae* but it does not inhibit the growth of normal flora because it does not contain the antibiotics. There are special media kits available which contain Thayer-Martin agar on one side and choc on the other. Some systems have self-generating carbon dioxide that will provide the anaerobic atmosphere necessary for

growth of the gonococcal organisms. Otherwise, classic candle jars or other anaerobic incubation is used. Appropriate inoculation of the medium is important. The swab should be rolled over the surface of the medium in a W or Z pattern (Fig 16–12) and incubation begun as quickly as possible.

After 24 to 48 hours of incubation on Thayer-Martin and choc, colonies of *N. gonorrhoeae* appear small, gray, translucent, and shiny. A Gram's stain should be made of one of these colonies and if the organism is *N. gonorrhoeae,* the characteristic gram-negative diplococci ("coffee-bean" appearance) will be observed. In addition, the biochemical oxidase test should be performed for presumptive identification purposes (see under Biochemical Tests). Only when the Gram's stain results, the appearance of the colony on Thayer-Martin and choc, and an oxidase-positive biochemical reaction all support *N. gonorrhoeae* can the laboratory report indicate "presumptive *N. gonorrhoeae.*" Other testing can be done on the isolates to detect penicillin-resistant strains of the organism. The culture plates should be maintained for at least 72 hours before sending out a negative result. There are latex agglutination, coagglutination, or carbohydrate utilization tests which can be used as additional confirmatory tests for this organism. Several manufacturers have developed kits for this purpose.

Chlamydial Infections.—Infection with *C. trachomatis* is a prevalent sexually transmitted disease in the United States. It is important that the specimen be collected properly from the appropriate site using a

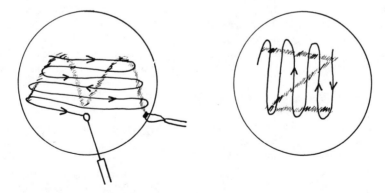

FIG 16–12.
Method for streaking genital specimens. Two appropriate inoculation methods for *Neisseria gonorrhoeae*. The swab should be rolled over the plate in a W or Z pattern, followed by cross-streaking with a sterile inoculating loop. (From Becan-McBride K, Ross DL: *Essentials for the Small Laboratory and Physician's Office.* St Louis, Mosby–Year Book, Inc, 1988, p 370. Used by permission.)

scraping technique or by vigorously rubbing against the involved site to dislodge the necessary cells. The organism resides in columnar epithelial cells and not in squamous epithelial cells or other inflammatory cells. The specimen must be transported to the laboratory immediately. *C. trachomatis* is a fastidious organism that must be grown in protected conditions.

The gold standard for identification of the chlamydial organism is cell culture and staining for the typical intracytoplasmic inclusion bodies present in the cells. Nonculture methods include direct fluorescent antibody studies using monoclonal antisera and an ELISA test. These are direct tests that give relatively rapid results and are very sensitive. A negative nonculture test result does not rule out the presence of chlamydial infection.

Blood Cultures

Blood is normally sterile. The careful and expeditious detection of bloodborne pathogens is a very important function of the microbiology laboratory. Bacteremia (bacteria in the blood) can be a serious consequence of an infectious disease. Positive blood cultures can help provide a clinical diagnosis. Bacteria can be detected in the blood in the absence of disease, especially after dental extractions or any instance where there has been a loss of integrity of the capillary endothelial cells. Septicemia or sepsis indicates a situation in which the bacteria or a toxin produced by the bacteria is causing harm to the host (patient).

Collecting the Specimen

When blood is obtained for culture, it is critical that extra care be taken to clean the skin at the venipuncture site in a special way to prevent any contamination from skin organisms present. The medium into which the blood is drawn is of the enrichment type which encourages the growth and multiplication of all organisms present, even stray bacterial contaminants.

If the blood to be cultured is not drawn directly into the culture medium, it must be collected with an anticoagulant. The best anticoagulant is sodium polyanethol sulfonate (SPS, or Liquoid).

Culture Media for Blood

The basic culture media for blood contain both a nutrient broth and an anticoagulant. Most commercially available blood culture media contain tryp broth, brain-heart infusion agar, peptone supplement, or thio broth. A common ratio of 1:10, blood to medium, is found to be convenient for most laboratories.

For optimal recovery of bloodborne pathogens, the use of two different bottles of blood culture media is recommended. One is vented for aerobic organism growth and the other is not vented, allowing growth of most facultative and some anaerobic organisms.

Processing the Blood Cultures: Traditional Method

Blind subcultures are made after the first 6 to 12 hours of incubation and the bottles are reincubated for 7 days. The blood culture bottles are examined visually at least once a day for 7 days. Growth of organisms is indicated by hemolysis of red blood cells, gas bubbles in the medium, turbidity, or appearance of small colonies in the broth, on the surface of the red cell layer, or sometimes along the walls of the bottle. Microscopic examination of the positive broth culture medium using phase microscopy is done to reveal details of cellular morphology and motility. If no organisms are seen microscopically, subcultures are performed anyway.

Subcultures of positive blood cultures are done to a variety of media types so the growth of most organisms, anaerobes included, can be supported. All isolates from blood cultures should be stored for an indefinite period, preferably by freezing at −70°C in skim milk.

Automated Blood Culture Systems

One automated system, Bactec (Johnston Laboratories, Towson, MD), allows a more rapid detection time for many pathogens, provides the ability to monitor growth without visual inspection or subcultures, automatically handles large numbers of blood culture bottles, and provides an antimicrobial-removal additive to the media.

ANTIBIOTIC SUSCEPTIBILITY TESTS

One of the important functions of the medical microbiology laboratory is to assist the physician in identifying and treating diseases caused by microbes. Therefore, in addition to identification of the infecting organism, it is sometimes necessary to determine the isolated organism's **sensitivity to antimicrobial agents,** or antibiotics. Sensitivity in this context is the ability of the antibiotic to inhibit the growth of the microorganism. The organism is said to be resistant to the antibiotic if the antibiotic does not inhibit the growth of the organism. Patterns of sensitivity and resistance are constantly changing. Many microorganisms, including bacteria and some fungi, have developed resistance even to the newest antibiotics. Since the pattern of resistance and susceptibility is unpredictable, it is necessary to test isolated pathogenic organisms needing antibiotic therapy against the appropriate antimicrobial agents. When choosing an appropriate antimicrobial agent, the one with the most activity against the pathogen, the least toxicity to the host, the least impact on the normal flora, the appropriate pharmacologic considerations, and the least expensive should be selected to attain a more certain outcome for the treatment of the patient's infectious process. A very important service of the laboratory is to test the isolated organisms for susceptibility to antimicrobial agents. To a large extent, the laboratory report showing susceptibility or resistance to a particular antibiotic determines whether the agent is used or withdrawn.

In doing tests for antibiotic sensitivity, the laboratory must maintain a high level of accuracy in the testing procedures, there must be a high degree of reproducibility of results, and there must be a good correlation between the results and the clinical response of the patient.

The lowest concentration of the antimicrobial agent that will inhibit the growth of the organism being tested, as detected by the lack of visual turbidity, matching that of a negative control included with the test, is known as the **minimal inhibitory concentration (MIC).** There are many factors which must be considered in choosing the specific antimicrobial agent, the MIC being one important consideration.

Minimal Inhibitory Concentration vs. Minimal Bactericidal Concentration

The ability of the antimicrobial agent to inhibit the multiplication of the organism is measured by the MIC. Since it is a measure of organism inhibitory status, it is possible that when the antimicrobial agent is removed, the organism could begin once again to grow. In this case, the antimicrobial agent is called bacteriostatic or inhibitory. Sometimes, for certain infections, it is necessary to determine the ability of the agent to actually kill the organism. To determine the ability of the antimicro-

bial agent to kill the organism, a bactericidal activity test can be performed, using a modification of the broth dilution susceptibility testing method. A minimal bactericidal concentration (MBC) is then determined.

Methods Used to Determine Antimicrobial Susceptibility

Susceptibility and resistance are functions of the site of the infection, the microorganism itself, and the antimicrobial agent being considered. By using a standard method, the microbiology laboratory can produce consistent results to aid the physician in his or her therapeutic choice. The organism inoculated into the test medium, whether using a macro- or a microdilution method, is usually 1×10^6 CFU/mL. The organism being tested is inoculated into a broth medium. The number of organisms can be determined in different ways. One practical method is to compare the turbidity of the test liquid medium to that of a standard that represents a known number of bacteria in suspension. Chemical solutions of standard turbidity have been prepared using barium sulfate. Tubes with varying concentrations of this chemical were developed by McFarland to approximate numbers of bacteria in solutions of equal turbidity, as determined by doing colony counts in a counting chamber.*

Various methods are used to determine the susceptibility of a microorganism to an antibiotic. Some methods involve dilution tests, such as broth tube dilution or agar plate dilution. Another commonly used method is the agar diffusion test, employing antibiotic-impregnated disks.

It is important to remember that any in vitro test for antibiotic sensitivity is an artificial measurement and will give only an estimate of the effectiveness of the agent against the microorganism. The only absolute test of antibiotic sensitivity is the clinical response of the patient to the dosage of the antibiotic.

The classic method for testing the susceptibility of microorganisms is that of the broth dilution method yielding a quantitative result for the amount of antimicrobial agent needed to inhibit the growth of a specific microorganism. The NCCLS has published the complete

*See *Performance Standards for Antimicrobial Disk Susceptibility Test, Approved Standard,* ed. 4. Villanova, Pa, National Committee for Clinical Laboratory Standards, 1990; M2-A4.

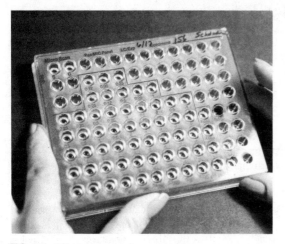

FIG 16–13.
Plastic microdilution tray used for microbroth dilution antibiotic susceptibility testing. Antimicrobial agents are arranged in linear arrays of serial twofold dilutions. (From Baron EJ, Finegold SM: *Bailey and Scott's Diagnostic Microbiology,* ed 8. St Louis, Mosby–Year Book, Inc, 1990, p 180. Used by permission.)

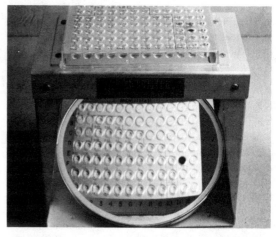

FIG 16–14.
Reading microbroth dilution results using a magnifying mirror reader. (From Baron EJ, Finegold SM: *Bailey and Scott's Diagnostic Microbiology,* ed 8. St Louis, Mosby–Year Book, Inc, 1990, p 180. Used by permission.)

protocol for performing this method.* The adaptation of the broth dilution methods to a microbroth method is used by many laboratories because it saves time for the laboratorian doing the test and it uses micro amounts of reagents.

Microdilution Method

The microdilution method utilizes plastic microdilution trays and is used in many laboratories to give MIC results as part of the routine protocol for microbiology laboratory tests. Most laboratories purchase the microdilution trays commercially. These have been prepared with the wells each holding a consistent, controlled micro amount of the various antimicrobial agents, along with the necessary controls for growth and sterility tests (Fig 16–13). They have been prepared under strict quality control standards and assure the laboratory of consistent performance when used according to the manufacturer's directions. The plates can be read manually by viewing them on a light box or read from the bottom us-

*Methods for Dilution Antimicrobial Susceptibility Tests for Bacteria That Grow Aerobically, Approved Standard, ed. 2. Villanova, Pa, National Committee for Clinical Laboratory Standards, 1990; M7-A2.

ing a mirror reader (Fig 16–14). Automated readers are also available.

Some microdilution systems are prepared and shipped in a frozen state. These are stored frozen until needed by the laboratory and must be thawed before use. These systems are easy to inoculate and usually include a disposable inoculating device which allows a single inoculation of all the wells on the plate simultaneously. Another type of system consists of dried or lyophilized antimicrobial agents requiring reconstitution before use.

Bacterial Disk Diffusion Method

Methods utilizing disks impregnated with various antimicrobial agents placed on an agar culture plate inoculated with the organism to be tested were used extensively before microdilution methodology. The antimicrobial agent on the disk would diffuse into the medium in a circle around the disk, inhibiting the growth of the organism wherever the concentration of the agent was sufficient. Large zones of inhibition were an indication of more antimicrobial activity or greater diffusibility of the drug, or both (Fig 16–15). An area in which there was no zone indicated complete resistance to the drug. Using this method, several drug agents could be tested against one organism isolate at the same time. This method was

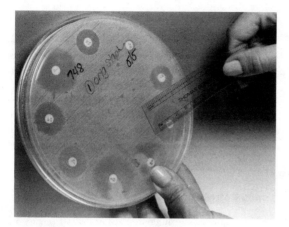

FIG 16–15.
Measuring zones of inhibition on a disk diffusion suscepti-
bility test plate. (From Baron EJ, Finegold SM: *Bailey and
Scott's Diagnostic Microbiology,* ed 8. St Louis,
Mosby–Year Book, Inc, 1990, p 181. Used by permission.)

first described by Bondi et al. in 1947.* In 1966, Bauer
et al. standardized the method and correlated it with
MICs.† They introduced standardized filter paper disks
and enabled this method to be one that yielded qualitative results that correlated well with results obtained by
MIC tests. This agar disk diffusion method continues to
be used by many laboratories as it is less expensive than
the commercial microdilution method and standardization is not difficult. The results can be correlated directly
with MIC values, but clinical interpretation of this
method depends on performing the test in the proper
way.

Disks are commercially available for this method,
and a special disk dispenser is used to distribute the appropriate disks on the inoculated plate. The plate is incubated overnight and observed the following morning.
There will be a zone of growth inhibition around the disk
containing the agent to which the organism is *susceptible,* whereas the organism will grow up to and under the
periphery of the disks containing agents to which it is *resistant.* Much work has been done to standardize the disk

*Bondi A, Spaulding EH, Smith ED, et al: A routine
method for the rapid determination of susceptibility to penicillin and other antibiotics. *Am J Med Sci* 1947; 214:221–225.

†Bauer AW, Kirby WWM, Sherris JC, et al: Antibiotic
susceptibility testing by a standardized single disc method. *Am
J Clin Pathol* 1966; 45:493–496.

procedure, and one modification used in many laboratories is that of Bauer and Kirby et al.

The disk diffusion method is subject to Food and
Drug Administration requirements, which cover standardization of media, formula, pH, agar depth, inoculum
density, temperature, zone sizes, interpretative tables,
and reference strains of bacteria for controls.

Disk Agar Diffusion Method (Bauer et al.)
Selection of Media for Plating.—For antibiotic
sensitivity testing, the Mueller-Hinton (MH) agar plate is
used. MH agar can be purchased commercially. The
plates should be stored in the refrigerator until used and
checked periodically for signs of water loss by evaporation. Plates can be saved longer by wrapping them in
polystyrene and keeping them refrigerated.

Handling and Storage of Disks.—Disks for
antibiotic susceptibility testing are usually supplied in
separate containers with a suitable desiccant to prevent
deterioration. Most antibiotic disks should be refrigerated
until used, but some require freezing to maintain their
potency. The manufacturer's instructions for storage and
handling should be followed. All disks must be discarded
on their expiration date.

Preparation of Inoculum.—A tube of tryp broth
(5 mL) is inoculated with a pure culture of the organism
to be tested and is incubated at 35°C for 4 hours or until
the culture is visibly cloudy. This method is suitable only
for fast-growing organisms. The turbidity of the test organism is compared with that of a McFarland barium sulfate standard. The standard must be vigorously mixed
before use. The turbidity of the broth culture may be adjusted, if necessary, by diluting it with uninoculated
broth in another tube. If the 4-hour broth tube does not
have enough growth, it can be reincubated until adequate
growth is observed. MH plates should be inoculated
within 15 minutes of standardizing the broth.

***Inoculation of the Mueller-Hinton Agar
Plate.***—A sterile swab is dipped into the standardized
broth culture (mixed well), and any excess fluid is removed from the swab by squeezing it on the side of the
tube. The swab is streaked across the plate in much the
same way as the quantitative urine culture plate (see Fig
16–10). While the MH plate is being streaked, the same
swab is used to inoculate an SB plate to check for purity.

All organisms being tested should be inoculated onto their respective plates before any disks are applied. Plates should be labeled with the patient's name, type of specimen, organism, and date. They should be allowed to dry for at least 3 minutes before the disks are applied.

Application of Disks.—The appropriate disks are applied to all the plates, using a disk dispenser if one is available. Special disk dispensers are available with different combinations of antibiotic-impregnated disks. Each disk should be firmly pressed down onto the surface of the agar with a flamed and cooled forceps to ensure complete contact with the agar. The disks should be distributed so that they are no closer than 15 mm to the edge of the Petri dish and so that no two disks are closer than 24 mm from center to center. Once a disk has been placed it should not be moved, as some diffusion of the antibiotic occurs almost immediately. The plates are incubated at 35°C for 18 hours.

Reading of Results.—After incubation, the diameters of the zones of inhibition are measured with a caliper or a zone reader and recorded to the nearest whole millimeter (see Fig 16–15). Susceptibility of the organism to the antibiotic is demonstrated by a clear zone of growth inhibition around the disk. Within the limitations of the test, the diameter of the inhibition zone is a measure of the relative susceptibility to a particular antibiotic. The diameters are compared with a sensitivity table for each antibiotic to see whether the organism is sensitive, intermediate, or resistant to that particular antibiotic. These results are reported to the physician. The term *susceptible* or *sensitive* implies that an infection caused by the strain tested may be expected to respond favorably to the particular antibiotic. Resistant strains, on the other hand, are not inhibited completely by the usual therapeutic concentration of the antibiotic.

QUALITY CONTROL IN THE MICROBIOLOGY LABORATORY

Quality control is necessary in microbiology as in the other areas of the laboratory. The development of quality control for microbiology is comparatively recent, however.

Control of Equipment

Equipment used in the microbiology laboratory can be easily controlled—for example, by monitoring the temperatures, daily or weekly, of incubators, refrigerators, water baths, freezers, and autoclaves. All monitoring data must be recorded as part of the laboratory's ongoing quality assurance program. Also, every laboratory handling biological material must have a safety hood and biological safety cabinets for handling certain specimens and organisms.

Control of Media

Most media are purchased ready-made from media companies. They are generally of high quality and provide good batch-to-batch consistency of results. Commercially prepared media must be stored and used in accord with manufacturers' directions and must be used within the specified expiration date. Quality control measures are followed strictly during manufacture of commercial media if NCCLS recommendations are followed (see Quality Control of Media under Culture Media). If media are prepared by the laboratory, strict controls must be employed in the preparation. The best way to control the quality of media is by *performance testing*—checking the media with cultures of known stock microorganisms. Control strains of bacteria are available commercially.

Control of Reagents and Antisera

New batches of reagents can be tested by using known positive and negative culture controls. Reagents should be dated when they are prepared, as are reagents in other areas of the laboratory. New reagents should be tested with known control cultures. Gram's-staining reagents are best checked by staining and examining slides prepared with known suspensions of gram-negative and gram-positive organisms.

Control of Antimicrobial Tests

Laboratories must periodically monitor their performance of methods used for antimicrobial testing. Control strains of common organisms are available for this purpose. The commercially available microdilution broth plates contain their own controls—some for sterility of the plate itself and others for growth. It is always important to carefully follow directions supplied with commercial products used.

Control of Specimens and Specimen Collection

If proper controls are not placed on the collection of patient specimens and on the procedures for handling these specimens in the laboratory, the identification of pathogens is not very meaningful and quality assurance is not being practiced. Strict controls of collection techniques must be enforced and repeat collections must be made if the circumstances demand it.

TESTS FOR VIRUSES (VIROLOGY)

There is a broad range of viruses responsible for human diseases, but only a few are recovered with any frequency in the clinical laboratory. Common viral diseases include herpes or rubella (German measles). Some specific syndromes can be caused by several different viruses. Pneumonia, for example, can be caused by respiratory syncytial virus (RSV), adenovirus, and influenza and parainfluenza viruses. Viral respiratory infections are especially common and affect persons of all ages. Laboratories must have highly specialized procedures to study viral infectious agents and for this reason most viral tests are not performed in the routine microbiology laboratory. Commonly, viral infections are detected in the clinical laboratory by performing specific serologic antibody titers and noting the rise in the titer which occurs during the disease process.

Unlike bacteria, viruses can only reproduce within cells. Other cells must provide them with the necessary requirements for their reproduction. Viral replication within cells can lead to a local spread which can result in viremia or virus in the bloodstream.

Specimens for Viral Studies

As for other tests, it is important that specimens submitted to the laboratory for viral studies be collected properly. General specimens for viral tests include throat swabs, nasopharynx swabs, stool, cerebrospinal fluid, urine, skin lesions, biopsy material, and blood for culture or for serologic tests. In general, specimens should not be frozen and should be collected as early in the course of the patient's illness as possible. It is always important to review the specimen requirements for the particular test being ordered, however. Certain specimens are more relevant to a disease than others. For example, in respiratory syndromes, it is generally only necessary to collect a throat or nasopharyngeal specimen; stool and urine specimens would not yield useful relevant information about the disease. Most specimens are collected as for bacteriologic culture. Blood for serologic studies should be collected in a serum tube, the blood allowed to clot, and the serum removed. For some serologic tests for viral syndromes, it is necessary to collect a specimen during the acute phase of the disease and, if a virus is not isolated, another specimen is collected at least 7 days after the acute specimen—a convalescent specimen. Serologic tests are used to diagnose viral diseases such as rubella, rubeola, hepatitis, and arbovirus encephalitis. Specimens for viral studies must be transported to the laboratory as soon as possible. The shorter the interval between collection and arrival of the specimen in the laboratory, the better the chance that the viral agent can be isolated. If it is feasible to do so, specimens other than blood, feces, and tissue should be inoculated into culture tubes at the patient's bedside.

Virology Testing Techniques

Microscopic examination of the viral specimen directly for presence of characteristic viral inclusions is the most readily available rapid technique. Viral inclusions will be intracellular and may represent aggregates of virus within an infected cell or may be abnormal accumulations of cellular materials as a result of viral-induced disruption in the cell's metabolism. Use of the Papanicolaou stain can show those inclusions in single cells or in aggregates of cells. Cytologic studies are used to detect inclusion bodies in cases of herpes simplex or cytomegalovirus infections. Culture of the cells is a much more sensitive technique, however.

Virus-infected specimens can be studied by using FA assays for detection of the viral antigen. These examinations may be performed directly on tissues or exudates using specific fluorescein-labeled viral antibody. Indirect immunofluorescence (IF) staining of certain specimens can be a rapid, highly reliable method to detect antigens from a number of viruses, including influenza, parainfluenza, mumps, RSV, measles, rubella, rabies, herpes simplex virus (HSV), varicella-zoster virus (VZV), and cytomegalovirus (CMV). When this testing technique is used, strict criteria for patterns of fluorescence must be applied and the proper use of controls employed. When this protocol is followed, the specificity of the testing method is high.

ELISA provides a technique for detection of viral antigens in fluid specimens. ELISA testing is quite sensitive and the equipment is relatively simple.

For the viral agents that are difficult to isolate in culture, such as hepatitis A and B, rubella, and measles, serologic testing has been a primary diagnostic procedure. Many serologic tests have been adapted to demonstrate antibody response or to identify a particular viral agent. These types of tests include complement fixation (CF), neutralization, hemagglutination inhibition (HI), and indirect fluorescent antibody (IFA) tests.

Viruses grow outside the host only in tissue or cell cultures. These media are made up of layers of living cells growing on the surface of a solid matrix, as on the inside of a glass tube or on the bottom of a plastic flask (see Fig 16–16). Viruses are grown in the laboratory on cell cultures of two cell types: primary cell lines and continuous cell lines. Fresh tissue, such as monkey or human embryonic kidney, is cut up, treated with a proteolytic agent, trypsin, which breaks the tissue up into individual cells, and the cells are seeded into a flask or tube containing a supportive growth medium. The cells attach themselves to the bottom of the container and multiply until they reach a single layer called a *monolayer of confluent growth*. Normal cells are inhibited from growing on top of each other. Primary cells such as fibroblasts, derived from human foreskin tissue, appear spindle-shaped. Other primary cells, such as those derived from kidney tissue, are more irregular. Primary cell lines carry the same number of chromosomes as the tissue from which they are derived (diploid) and will multiply for about only 50 generations before they begin to die off. If cells are obtained from a cancerous tissue, as from a human epithelial cell cancer, they will continue to multiply indefinitely in a cell culture and contain alterations in the number of chromosomes they possess (aneuploid). These cell lines are called *continuous cell lines*. Commercial cell cultures and media are available and facilitate the laboratory's work of isolating the viral agent. Two kinds of media are used for viral culture—growth and maintenance. Growth media are designed to support rapid cell growth while maintenance media are used to keep cells in a steady state of metabolism. The usual volume of specimen inoculated into a single tissue culture tube is 0.25 mL. Inoculated tissue culture tubes are incubated at 35°C and microscopically examined daily for cytopathogenic effect (CPE) for a period of 10 to 14 days. The monolayer is examined, a monolayer being the confluent layer of tissue culture cells one cell thick. Quantification is noted according to the percentage of the monolayer exhibiting the CPE. The CPE criteria will vary according to the viral agent being isolated. Confirmation tests are done for many of the isolates.

TESTS FOR FUNGI (MYCOLOGY)

Characteristics of Fungi

Fungi include both yeasts and molds and differ significantly from bacteria. The fungi that are seen in the clinical laboratory can be separated into two groups based on the macroscopic appearance of the colonies formed. Yeasts produce moist, opaque, creamy, or pasty colonies on culture media whereas molds produce fluffy, cottony, woolly, or powdery colonies. Molds are filamentous fungi.

Yeasts are one-celled organisms that multiply by budding. Most yeasts usually appear similar under the microscope and differentiation of the various genera microscopically is difficult. Molds have a basic structure that is made up of tubelike projections called *hyphae*. As hyphae grow, they intertwine to form a loose network

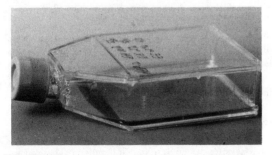

FIG 16–16.
Tissue culture flask used for maintaining cell lines. (From Baron EJ, Finegold SM: *Bailey and Scott's Diagnostic Microbiology,* ed 8. St Louis, Mosby–Year Book, Inc, 1990, p 98. Used by permission.)

called a *mycelium*. Certain types of mycelium can be recognized microscopically which can assist in their early identification.

Fungi as a Source of Infection

Fungi are well recognized as a cause of infection and the testing of specimens for fungi should be provided by the microbiology laboratory. Fungi normally live a nonpathogenic existence in nature, enriched by decaying nitrogenous material. Humans become infected with fungi through accidental exposure by inhalation of spores or by their introduction into tissue through trauma. Any alteration in the immunologic status of the host can result in infection by fungi that are normally nonpathogenic. Fungal infections can occur in persons with diabetes, other debilitating diseases, or in persons with impaired immunologic function resulting from drug therapies using corticosteroids or antimetabolites. In recent years, there have been more fungal infections in immunocompromised patients. Fungi are not communicable in the usual person-to-person or animal-to-person transfer.

To provide a sufficient mycologic service (the study of fungi), the microbiology laboratory should include the direct examination of clinical specimens and information about the proper collection, culturing, and transportation of these specimens to a reference laboratory, if needed. In the mycology laboratory, identification of yeasts is an important service.

Collection of Specimens for Fungal Studies

The selection and collection techniques used for specimens to be used for fungal studies is directly related to the diagnosis of fungal infections. It is extremely important that specimens be collected properly from the proper sites in order that the fungi be recovered. Overgrowth with contaminating bacteria is common, some fungi being slow-growing. For this reason it is important that the specimens for fungal studies be transported to the laboratory as soon as possible. After reaching the laboratory, these specimens should be microscopically examined directly and cultured immediately to ensure the recovery of the suspected fungal organism from the specimen. Mold cultures should be handled in a class II biological safety cabinet to prevent aerosol dissemination of fungal elements. Yeast cultures can be handled on a regular bench top with no extra protection other than the usual common safety measures.

Direct Microscopic Examination of Fungi

Examination of the specimen microscopically is an important part of the microbiology laboratory's fungal examination. It provides a rapid method which in some cases leads to a tentative immediate diagnosis. This process can often provide the first microbiological evidence of fungal etiology in patients with suspected fungal infections. There are several stains which can be used for this purpose.

Acid-fast Stain
This stain is used to detect mycobacteria but can also detect *Nocardia* (see also Smear Preparation and Stains Used in Microbiology).

Calcofluor White Stain
This can be mixed with potassium hydroxide (KOH), another stain traditionally used for fungal smears. It detects the presence of fungi rapidly (in 1 minute) by use of bright fluorescence. This method requires a fluorescence microscope but fungi exhibit an intense easily recognizable fluorescence.

Gram's Stain
This is the stain commonly used for most clinical microbiological specimens. It also will detect most fungi, if present in the specimen (see also Smear Preparation and Stains Used in Microbiology).

Potassium Hydroxide
This has been the traditionally recommended stain for fungi. This reagent clears the specimen, making the fungi more easily visible. A drop of specimen is mixed with a drop of 10% KOH, a coverglass is applied, and the specimen is scanned using the low-power objective for fungal elements. If the specimen is extremely viscous, an overnight incubation of the wet-mounted slide in a humidified chamber may be necessary. If the slide appears cloudy, warming may help to clear it for viewing the fungi.

Culture Media

There are a number of different culture media used for fungi. Laboratories will differ in the media chosen for fungal culture. Sabouraud dextrose medium favors growth of fungi over bacteria and is recommended for primary isolation of dermatophytes, with the addition of the antimicrobial agents cycloheximide and chloramphenicol. Sabhi medium is a combination of equal parts of Sabouraud dextrose agar and brain-heart infusion agar and has proved to be useful for isolation of clinically significant fungi, particularly from specimens also containing bacteria, such as sputum specimens. Most specimens for fungal identification are also contaminated with bacteria and other rapidly growing fungi. For this reason, it is important that antibacterial and antifungal agents be included in the culture medium. Some fungi require the presence of blood in the medium. Because of these needs, fungal specimens are usually cultured on a battery of various culture media.

Culture dishes or screw-capped culture tubes are used for satisfactory recovery of fungi. Fungal cultures are incubated at room temperature or preferably at 30°C for 30 days before being reported as negative. During the incubation period, cultures should be examined at least three times weekly.

Methods for Detection of Fungi

Because there has been an increase in the number of yeast infections, primarily in immunocompromised patients, there is an increased need for the rapid detection of these infecting organisms. Numerous species of *Candida* and other yeasts have been identified. Rapid manual biochemical screening tests are used by some laboratories and commercially available yeast identification systems have provided others with standardized identification procedures.

Biochemical tests include a rapid urease test used to screen urease-producing yeasts, and a rapid nitrate reductase test (see also Biochemical Tests under Using Microbiology to Diagnose Disease). An alternative to this rapid test is the use of Christensen's urea agar which requires incubation (see also Urea Agar (Christensen's) under Culture Media).

Another test done to specifically identify *C. albicans* is the germ-tube test. This test depends on *C. albicans* being able to produce germ tubes from their yeast cells when placed in a liquid nutrient environment and

incubated at 35°C for 3 hours. A *germ-tube* is defined as an appendage that is one-half the width and three to four times the length of the yeast cell from which it arises.

Commercially available yeast identification systems are also in common use by many laboratories. These methods are, for the most part, rapid and the results are available within 72 hours. These systems utilize a large data base of information based on thousands of yeast biotypes and consider a number of variations and reaction patterns when presenting the result. One method utilizes a number of biochemical tests whose reactions are monitored by various indicator systems after addition of a reagent to certain substrates. This system is designed to give an identification within 4 hours. Some systems take longer for the final identification process. In general, these commercial identification systems are easy to use, easy to interpret, and relatively inexpensive when compared with the conventional testing methods.

TESTS FOR PARASITES (PARASITOLOGY)

Human parasitic infections occur worldwide, although more of these problems arise in tropical areas. Because many persons have lived or traveled in these tropical areas, and because there has been a great influx of refugee populations into the United States, many organisms endemic elsewhere are being seen in people now living in this country. Still another consideration is the number of immunocompromised patients who are very much at risk for certain parasitic infections.

Parasites as a Source of Infection

Human parasites belong to five main groups. These are the Protozoa (amebas, flagellates, ciliates, sporozoans, etc.); the Platyhelminthes, or flatworms; the Acanthocephala, or thorny-headed worms; the Nematoda, or roundworms; and the Arthropoda (insects, spiders, mites, and ticks). Parasitic infections are usually diagnosed by detecting and identifying the ova (parasite eggs), larvae (immature form) or adults of some types of parasites, usually the helminths, and the cysts (inactive stage) or trophozoites (motile forms) of others, usually the protozoa. The identification of the various types of parasitic organisms depends on morphologic criteria.

There are also various immunologic tests now available to detect parasitic infections. It is important that the infecting parasitic organism be identified specifically because treatment is dependent on the type of parasite found and its site of infestation. Any identification process first depends on correct specimen collection and adequate fixation. Specimens for parasitic identification include stool, urine, blood, sputum, and tissue biopsies.

Collection of Specimens for Parasite Identification

Specimens for parasite identification come primarily from the intestinal tract as fecal specimens, from the urogenital tract as a vaginal or urethral discharge or as a prostatic secretion, from sputum, cerebrospinal fluid, or biopsy material from other body tissues. Each specimen has unique morphologic criteria for the particular parasites inhabiting the area. There are excellent resource textbooks and other references which contain the specific morphologic criteria needed to correctly identify the more common parasites. Some suggested references for this purpose are:

1. Beaver PC, Jung RC, and Copp EW: *Clinical Parasitology,* ed. 9. Philadelphia, Lea & Febiger, 1984.
2. Committee on Education, American Society of Parasitology: Procedures suggested for use in examination of clinical specimens for parasitic infection. *J Parasitol* 1977; 63:959.
3. Garcia LS, Bruckner DA: *Diagnostic Medical Parasitology.* New York, Elsevier, 1988.

Common Parasites Detected

Trichomonas vaginalis

This is a parasite that can inhabit the urogenital system of both males and females. It is considered a pathogenic parasite. The motile trophozoite stage is found in freshly voided urine of both sexes, in prostatic secretions and in vaginal wet preparations. The diagnosis is usually made by observation of the motile trophozoite in the fresh urine, in vaginal fluid, and in prostatic fluid. The parasites are observed to move with a jerky and undulating motion. Trophozoites cannot be seen in old urine specimens or dry vaginal specimens or prostatic secretions because they are dead in this type of specimen. For

this reason, proper specimen collection and immediate transportation to the laboratory for analysis is very important in the identification process (See also Chapter 13).

Intestinal Ova and Parasites

Specimens for ova and parasite studies must be preserved or fixed immediately. A pH indicator is also added to confirm an approximate pH of 7. Most commercial collection kits for this test contain the appropriate preservative and pH indicator. The preservative-fixative for specimens to be tested for ova and parasites is formalin or polyvinyl alcohol. It is important to be aware of possible collection problems, such as that collection of ova and parasite stool specimens should be done prior to radiologic studies using barium sulfate since excess of the barium crystalline materials interferes with the detection of the parasites for up to a week after the use of barium. Other interfering substances are mineral oil, bismuth, some antidiarrheal preparations, antimalarials, and some antibiotics. Contamination with urine should also be avoided. For a routine examination for parasites prior to any treatment, a minimum of three specimens should be collected. If amebiasis is suspected, a series of six specimens should be collected. Many parasitic organisms do not appear in specimens in consistent numbers on a daily basis; thus many procedures call for the collection of stool specimens on alternate days. A series of three specimens should be collected within no more than 10 days and a series of six within no more than 14 days.

The microscopic identification of intestinal protozoa and helminth ova is based on recognition of specific morphologic characteristics. When doing these studies, it is imperative that a good microscope, with a good light source, be used. The microscope should be equipped with a calibrated ocular micrometer to measure the size of the ova and parasites seen.

Wet mounts of the specimen are observed directly to detect motile trophozoite stages of the protozoa. It is not sufficient to identify these protozoa by only using the direct wet mount preparation. Permanent stained smears should also be examined to confirm the identification of the parasitic organism.

After examination of the wet preparation is complete, a drop of iodine can be placed at the edge of the coverslip. This stained preparation will assist in the identification of protozoan cysts that stain with iodine. These will be seen as cysts with yellow-gold cytoplasm, brown glycogen material, and paler refractile nuclei. There are other stains available which are used to reveal nuclear detail in the trophozoite stages of the protozoa.

Pinworm (Enterobius vermicularis)

This parasite is very common in children worldwide. It is a roundworm whose adult female migrates from the anus during the night, depositing her eggs in the perianal region. Most laboratories use the cellophane tape method to make the diagnosis.

To identify pinworm, the specimen must be collected using a particular technique. The cellophane tape method is commonly used and performed in the following way: A piece of clear cellophane tape, held with the sticky side toward the patient, is pressed against the skin across the anal opening using even, thorough pressure. Next, the sticky side of the tape is placed down against the surface of a clear glass slide. The slide should be labeled with the patient's name and any other identifying data. These specimens must be collected first thing in the morning before bathing, defecating, or urinating. Negative findings must be confirmed with more tests done on subsequent days. The microscopic examination is performed by adding a small drop of toluene or xylene under the tape on the slide. This will clear the tape so the ova of the pinworm may be observed. They are ellipsoid (football-shaped) with one slightly flattened side. A known control slide of pinworm ova should be used for comparison purposes.

BIBLIOGRAPHY

Baron EJ, Finegold SM: *Bailey and Scott's Diagnostic Microbiology,* ed 8. St Louis, Mosby–Year Book, Inc, 1990.

Becan-McBride K, Ross DL: *Essentials for the Small Laboratory and Physician's Office.* St Louis, Mosby–Year Book Inc, 1988.

Henry JB (ed): *Clinical Diagnosis and Management by Laboratory Methods,* ed 18. Philadelphia, WB Saunders Co, 1991.

Howard BJ, Klaas J II, Rubin SJ, et al: *Clinical and Pathogenic Microbiology.* St Louis, Mosby–Year Book, Inc, 1987.

Lennette EH, Balows A, Hausler WJ, et al: *Manual of Clinical Microbiology,* ed 4. Washington, DC, American Society for Microbiology, 1985.

Murray PR, Drew WL, Kobauashi GS, et al: *Medical Microbiology.* St Louis, Mosby–Year Book, Inc, 1990.

Physician's Office Laboratory Procedure Manual, Tentative Guidelines, Villanova, Pa, National Committee for Clinical Laboratory Standards, 1989; 9 POL2-T.

Prescott LM, Harley JP, Klein DA: *Microbiology.* Dubuque, IA, William C Brown, 1990.

Quality Assurance for Commercially Prepared Microbiological Culture Media, Approved Standard, Villanova, Pa, National Committee for Clinical Laboratory Standards, 1990; M22-A.

17   Immunology and Serology

Key Terms

Acute and convalescent serum	Heterophil antibodies
Acute phase reactants	Human chorionic gonadotropin (hCG)
Agglutination	Immunologic response
Antibodies	In vitro antigen-antibody reactions
Antibody titer	Latex agglutination procedures
Antigens	Monoclonal antibodies
Complement fixation	Precipitation
Enzyme immunoassay (EIA)	Reagin antibodies
Enzyme-linked immunosorbent assay (ELISA)	Rheumatoid factor (RF)
Flocculation	Serology
Fluorescent antibody (FA) studies	

The body has a unique defense system against foreign substances—the **immunologic response.** The immune system of the human body is extremely complicated and it plays a variety of roles in maintaining health. It serves as a defense against invasion by infectious agents as well as against certain abnormal cells in the body itself that have developed through various mutations. Study of the immune system also includes the autoimmune antibodies that can be produced in response to certain of the body's own cells. The primary function of the immune system is to recognize self from nonself and to defend the body against nonself. Clinical immunology involves the study of **in vitro antigen-antibody reactions.** In clinical immunology tests, there must be a reaction between an antibody and antigen which results in a recordable event. **Serology** is a division of immunology which specializes in detecting and measuring specific antibodies that develop in the *blood* during a response to exposure to a disease-producing antigen. There are several techniques utilized in clinical immunologic and serologic assays. These include precipitation, immunoelectrophoresis, agglutination, complement fixation, cytolysis, neutralization, flocculation, immunodiffusion, enzyme immunoassays, enzyme-linked immunosorbent assays (ELISA), and fluorescent antibody (FA) methods. Determinations of blood groups and Rh factors for persons donating or receiving blood utilize serologic methods (see Chapter 18).

Foreign substances, or antigens, are recognized by lymphoid and plasma cells. Each type of antigen stimulates the production of equally specific antibodies by various body tissues. If an antibody has been formed against a foreign substance, one good way to identify the infecting organism is to identify the antibody produced in response to it. This is the basis for immunologic and serologic determinations. Many years ago researchers in the field of immunology showed that if a known antigen, such as a certain bacterium, is exposed in a test tube to a patient's serum containing antibodies against that antigen, a reaction *(serologic reaction)* will be observed. If the specific antibody is not present in the patient's serum, no reaction will be observed.

Antibodies that have been produced in response to a specific antigenic stimulus can be identified in the serum. The serologic reaction produces an observable change in the mixture in one of several ways. The reaction takes different forms because of variations in the technique being used and the type of antigen being assayed.

ANTIGENS AND ANTIBODIES

Antigens are generally large molecules with molecular weights over 10,000; they are usually proteins. An antigen is generally described as a substance that, when injected into an animal, is recognized as foreign and—provided immunologically active cells are present—provokes an immune reaction. The immune reaction is the production of **antibodies**—substances that protect the body against the antigens. There are times, however, when antibodies are not protective, as in the case of antibody-antigen reactions that cause hay fever, rash, or anaphylactic shock. Antigenicity is not confined to proteins. Certain nonantigenic, nonprotein substances known as *haptens* may bind themselves to protein, and the resulting hapten-protein complex is antigenic.

Some antibodies occur in humans naturally as a result of exposure throughout life to bacteria and plant material, in the form of food, and through inhalation and ingestion. Antibodies can also be produced in response to natural infections, as with pneumonia and typhoid fever organisms, and their production can be artificially stimulated by the injection of antigens in vaccine form. Natural and artificial infections stimulate the production of immune, or protective, antibodies.

Humans are equipped with two strong lines of defense against the invasion of foreign substances. One is a nonspecific resistance to certain diseases that comes about through physiologic and anatomic attributes. The other is the formation of antibodies. Together, these systems work effectively to protect humans throughout life.

PRINCIPLES OF IMMUNOLOGIC AND SEROLOGIC METHODS

Antibodies can be detected by several different techniques or reactions. In some cases, antibodies to an agent may be detected by more than one method, but the different methods may not detect the same antibody.

Agglutination

Agglutination means clumping. In this type of observable reaction, the combination of specific antigens and antibodies results in the formation of visible clumps, which settle out of the solution. Antibodies that form clumps are called *agglutinins* and the associated antigens are called *agglutinogens*. Agglutination occurs only if the antigen is in the form of particles, such as bacteria, red blood cells, latex particles, white blood cells, or any substance that appears cloudy when suspended in saline.

Slide agglutination tests are the easiest to perform and are generally quite sensitive. Reagents for many of these tests are available commercially. Artificial carriers, such as latex particles or treated red blood cells, or biological carriers, such as bacterial cells, can carry antigen on their surface that will bind with antibody that has been produced in response to the specific antigen when it was introduced into the host. Agglutination tests have a wide range of application in the clinical diagnosis of both infectious diseases and in noninfectious immune disorders. There are many commercial agglutination procedures available for use in small laboratories and physicians' office laboratories. These tests can determine many constituents of importance to clinicians and the techniques utilizing agglutination are ideally suited for use in these settings, as well as in large laboratories, to facilitate diagnosis and expedite the overall treatment of the patient. Agglutination tests are also utilized in immunohematologic typing procedures (see Chapter 18).

Mechanisms of Agglutination

Agglutination reactions are influenced by several factors. The first phase of the agglutination reaction is sensitization. This is the physical attachment of the antibody molecule to the antibody and is a reversible reaction subject to certain conditions being present. Physical conditions such as pH, temperature, and length of time of incubation will affect the reaction. The antigen-antibody ratio or the number of antibody molecules in relation to the number of antigen sites per cell is another factor influencing antigen-antibody association reactions.

If the amount of antigen is gradually decreased while the antibody concentration remains constant, a point is reached where large amounts of agglutinate or precipitate appear rapidly. Conversely, when increasing amounts of antigen are added, a point is reached where no agglutinate or precipitate is observed. An excess of antibody is known as the *prozone phenomenon*. This excess of antibody concentration can result in false-negative reactions.

The second phase of the agglutination process is lattice formation. Lattice formation results in the visible aggregation or clumping reaction, necessary for the agglutination technique. To produce this lattice formation, a cross-linking between sensitized particles and antibodies, it is necessary that the cell with the antibody attached to its surface come close enough to another cell to permit the antibody molecules to combine with the antigen receptor sites on a second cell. This bridging action, necessary to lattice formation, takes place slowly.

Direct Bacterial Agglutination

Antibodies produced by the host in response to infection by some bacterial agents can be measured by agglutination tests. In using these tests for bacterial antibody, the specific antibodies produced in the infectious process bind to the surface antigens of the bacterial agent and cause the bacteria to clump together in visible aggregates. A thick suspension of the bacteria is needed for this test. The reaction is called *direct bacterial agglutination*. This type of agglutination reaction can be performed on the surface of glass slides or in test tubes (Fig 17–1). Incubation periods can be included when using test tubes, allowing more antigen and antibody to interact, often making these methods more sensitive. Direct bacterial agglutination tests are used to diagnose diseases in which it is difficult to culture the pathogenic agent in the laboratory. Diseases that are commonly diagnosed using this immunologic assay include tetanus, brucellosis, and tularemia.

Latex Agglutination

Antibody molecules can be artificially bound to the surface of latex beads for **latex agglutination procedures.** The surface of each latex particle can contain many antibody molecules increasing the potential number of exposed antigen-binding sites. If antigen is present in the specimen being tested, such as the C-reactive protein antigen, the antigen will bind to the combining sites of the exposed antibody on the latex bead surface, forming visible cross-linked aggregates of antigen and latex beads (Fig 17–2). In other testing systems, such as that for rubella antibody, the latex particles can be coated with antigen. These specific antigen-coated latex particles and any rubella antibody present in the patient's serum will result in visible clumping of the latex particles. These are called *direct agglutination tests*. Indirect agglutination tests show agglutination when no positive constituent (antibody) is present and produce no agglutination reaction when the constituent is present. Proce-

FIG 17–1.

Agglutination patterns. **Top,** slide agglutination of bacteria with known antisera or known bacteria. A positive reaction is demonstrated by the specimen on the *left,* a negative reaction by the specimen on the *right.* **Bottom,** tube agglutination. A positive reaction is demonstrated by the specimen on the *left,* a negative reaction by the specimen on the *right.* (From Turgeon MJ: *Immunology and Serology in Laboratory Medicine.* St Louis, Mosby–Year Book, Inc, 1990, p 106. Used by permission.)

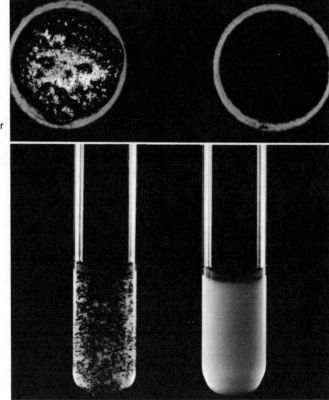

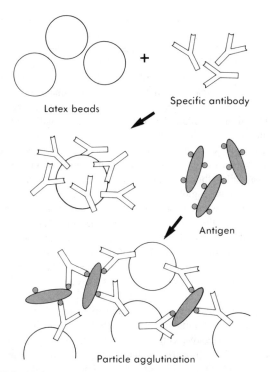

FIG 17–2.

Alignment of antibody molecules bound to the surface of a latex particle and latex agglutination reaction. (From Baron EJ, Finegold SM: *Bailey and Scott's Diagnostic Microbiology,* ed. 8. St Louis, Mosby–Year Book, Inc, 1990, p 128. Used by permission.)

dures utilizing latex agglutination must be performed under strict standardized conditions. Complete systems employing the use of latex or other particle agglutination technology are commercially available for detection of some pathogenic agents. The amount of antigen-antibody binding is influenced by pH, osmolarity, and the ionic concentration of the solution. Other important factors include the time of incubation of the coated particles with the patient's serum (or other source of antibody) and the amount and avidity of the antigen attached to the carrier. It is important that the manufacturer's directions be followed carefully. Immunologic assays employing latex agglutination are used for C-reactive protein, IgG, and IgM rheumatoid factors, cytomegalovirus (CMV), and rubella antibody.

Coagglutination

To enhance the visibility of the agglutination reaction, antibodies are sometimes bound to a particle. This technique is highly specific but may not be as sensitive as the latex agglutination system.

Hemagglutination

Animal red blood cells have been treated for use as carriers of antigen for agglutination tests. These are called indirect or passive agglutination tests because it is not the antigens of the blood cells themselves, but the passively attached antigens that are bound by the antibody. One test commonly performed that utilizes hemagglutination is the microhemagglutination test for antibody to *Treponema pallidum* (MHA-TP). This test is performed on a microtiter plate. Other tests include the hemagglutination treponemal test for syphilis (HATTS), the passive hemagglutination tests for antibody to extracellular antigens of streptococci, and the rubella indirect hemagglutination tests. All of these tests are available commercially.

Precipitation and Flocculation

Precipitation may be defined as the visible result of an antigen-antibody reaction between a soluble antigen and its antiserum (serum containing antibodies). Electrolytes are also needed to bring the process to its desired conclusion, along with the proper pH and temperature of the mixture. Antibodies that react to form precipitates are called *precipitins*. The interaction of a soluble antigen with antibody thus results in the formation of a precipitate, a concentration of fine particles. The observation of a visible **flocculation** or precipitation reaction results because the precipitated product is forced to remain in a particular space within a matrix. The precipitin end product clumps that are formed are visible either macroscopically or microscopically.

Two variations of flocculation tests are used in serologic tests for syphilis. These are the Venereal Disease Research Laboratory (VDRL) and the rapid plasma reagin (RPR) tests. The RPR test is used by many laboratories and is available commercially as a complete testing system, containing positive and negative controls. The RPR test appears to be a more specific screening test for syphilis than the VDRL test.

Precipitin tests have been used historically in the

identification of bacteria, specifically in the classification of streptococci into groups A through K using the grouping methods originated by Lancefield. Serologic typing of the streptococcal cell wall components using the Lancefield precipitin method has classically been used to group these bacteria. Although recent DNA studies have shown that this is not entirely possible, it is still a useful practice in the identification of clinical isolates and therefore in the management of the patient's infection.

Abnormal globulins produced as a result of certain inflammatory diseases can also be identified by precipitin techniques. Certain diseases alter the quantities of some proteins found in the serum, such as immunoglobulin, haptoglobulin, and complement. These increases or decreases are valuable diagnostic tools. Modifications of the precipitin test include the use of counterimmunoelectrophoresis (CIE) or gel diffusion detection of antigen-antibody reactions.

Fluorescent Antibody Techniques

Antigen-antibody complexes formed can also be demonstrated by means of **fluorescent antibody (FA) studies.** In using this method, antibody against insoluble or particulate antigen, such as bacteria or cellular materials, may be detected. In using the FA technique, antibody is labeled with fluorescein isothiocyanate (FITC), a fluorescent compound that has an affinity for proteins. A conjugate is formed when the fluorescein compound forms a complex with the proteins and this conjugate is then able to react with antibody-specific antigen. Fluorescent techniques are very specific and sensitive. Antibodies may be conjugated to other markers, in addition to the fluorescent dye. An example of this is the use of enzyme-substrate marker systems which are continually being expanded. Systems are available commercially to measure antibodies developed against a number of infectious agents as well as against some self-antigens (detecting the presence of autoimmune antibodies).

Indirect Fluorescent Antibody Tests

Serologic tests widely used for the detection of many types of antibodies apply the concept of indirect fluorescent antibody (IFA) techniques. When the IFA technique is used, the antigen against which the patient makes antibody is fixed to the surface of a clean glass microscope slide. An example of this antigen is that of whole *Toxoplasma* organisms or viruses in infected tissue culture cells. Serum from the patient is added to the slide, covering the area in which the antigen was placed. If the specific antibody in question is present in the serum, the antibody will bind to the specific antigen. To remove any unbound antibody, the slide is washed. In the second part of this process, antihuman globulin which has been conjugated to the fluorescent dye is placed on the slide. The conjugated marker will bind to any antibody already bound to the antigen on the slide. This will serve as a marker for the antibody when the slide is viewed under a fluorescence microscope. The dye marker fluoresces apple green. If antibody is absent, the antihuman globulin dye marker will be removed during the washing procedure and no fluorescence will be seen. The fluorescence does not fade appreciably for a few days if the stained slides are coverslipped using a drop of buffered glycerol and if the slides are kept refrigerated in the dark. It is best to examine the prepared slides immediately after staining, however.

Commercially available systems utilizing fluorescence techniques are widely used in many laboratories. These IFA systems include slides with the antigens, positive and negative control sera, diluent for the patient's sera, and the properly diluted conjugated marker. These IFA techniques, if performed properly, will give extremely specific and sensitive results. Immunofluorescence is used extensively in the detection of autoantibodies and antibodies to tissue and cellular antigens. Antinuclear antibodies (ANAs), a group of circulating immunoglobulins that react with the whole nucleus or nuclear components, are frequently assayed using an IFA technique. Indirect fluorescent studies are commonly done to test for antibodies to *Legionella* species, *Borrelia burgdorferi,* varicella-zoster virus, cytomegalovirus, Epstein-Barr virus, herpes simplex viruses types 1 and 2, rubella virus, *Mycoplasma pneumoniae, T. pallidum,* and several rickettsiae.

Lysis

Some serologic reactions cause the destruction of red blood cells containing antigens. Such reactions are used in blood bank procedures. *Lysis,* or hemolysis of the red cells, is a positive indication that a specific antigen-antibody reaction has taken place. The lysing antibody that causes the reaction is known as a *lysin.* One form of *Streptococcus* produces streptolysin, an antigen that can destroy human or rabbit red blood cells.

Complement Fixation

A valuable but time-consuming and difficult way to detect and quantitate soluble antibody is by **complement fixation** tests. These tests detect soluble antigen by virtue of the availability of complement. Complement is a group of serum proteins that, when present or combined with antigen-antibody complexes, lyse antigen if it consists of bacteria or other cellular material. The antigen-antibody complex binds the complement present, and thus it is no longer available to promote additional antigen-antibody reactions. In the hemolysis of red cells, for example, and in the destruction of bacteria (called bacteriolysis), three elements must be present for the reaction to be observed: antigen, antibody, and complement.

Complement fixation tests involve two stages of reactions (Fig 17–3). The first is a serologic reaction between a test serum and antigen, where complement is adsorbed or bound by the antigen-antibody complex, but no visible lysis occurs. The second occurs when red cells coated with anti–red cell serum are added to the suspension. Failure to observe hemolysis is caused by the fixation of complement in the first step of the reaction. It is primarily the availability of complement in the system that determines whether lysis occurs, and the test thus indicates indirectly the presence or absence of specific antibody.

Complement fixation tests have been used to iden-tify some infectious disorders. A well-known historical example is the Wassermann complement fixation test for syphilis, which is now generally outdated.

Enzyme Immunoassays

Enzyme immunoassays employ the use of enzymes as immunochemical labels in the detection of antigen-antibody reactions. The technology for these techniques is expanding rapidly. Other names for these tests include **enzyme-linked immunosorbent assay (ELISA), enzyme immunoassay (EIA),** and enzyme-multiplied immunoassay (EMIT, Syva Corp., Palo Alto, CA) Enzyme immunoassays can detect extremely small quantities of antigen-antibody reactants. Either an antibody or an antigen conjugate can be labeled with the appropriate enzyme and used in a number of immunologic assays for a variety of antigens or antibodies, respectively. The enzyme with its substrate can detect the presence and quantity of antigen or antibody in the patient specimen. In this technique the conversion of a colorless substrate to a colored product allows for either visual or colorimetric detection.

There are a variety of enzymes that can be used in enzyme immunoassays. The most commonly used enzymes are peroxidase and alkaline phosphatase. In a classic enzyme immunoassay, plastic plates, paddles, or

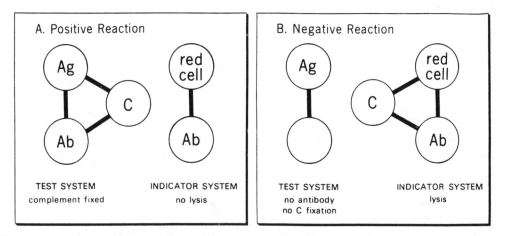

FIG 17–3.
Complement fixation test. Antigen *(Ag)* and antibody *(Ab)* are incubated with complement *(C)*. The indicator system, consisting of red cells coated with antibody, is added. **A,** positive reaction. When antigen and antibody are present in the test system they fix or bind the available complement and none remains to lyse the added indicator cells. **B,** negative reaction. When antigen or antibody is lacking in the test system, complement is available to lyse the sensitized indicator cells.

beads are coated with the antigen. When the patient's serum is added to the antigen, specific antibody present in the serum will react with it. The plate or bead is next incubated with an enzyme-labeled antibody conjugate. If antibody is present, the conjugate reacts with the antigen-antibody complex present. After the addition of a specific chromogenic substrate, the enzyme activity is measured spectrophotometrically.

Enzyme-linked Immunosorbent Assay (ELISA)

This system consists of antibodies that are bound to enzymes that remain able to catalyze a reaction that yields a visually observed end product while still being attached to the antibody. Furthermore, antibody-binding sites remain free to react with their specific antigens. There are several variations of this method—the enzyme tag can be conjugated to either antigen or antibody. These enzyme-conjugated substrates are quite stable and can be stored for relatively long periods of time. The formation of a colored end product can be observed visually or read with a simple photoelectric instrument. The use of monoclonal antibodies has increased the specificity of these testing systems.

Monoclonal Antibodies.—**Monoclonal antibodies** are highly specific and purified antibodies that have been produced from the daughter cells (clones) of a single hybrid cell. They are engineered to bind to a single specific antigen. Since all of the cells are derived from a single cell producing one antibody molecule type, these are called monoclonal antibodies. Monoclonal antibodies have been used successfully in many commercial systems for the detection of infectious agents. In one test used for the rapid detection of a chlamydial infection, a monoclonal antibody to a protein of *Chlamydia trachomatis* is conjugated to a fluorescent dye. When viewed with a fluorescence microscope, the elementary bodies and inclusions present in specimens from patients infected with chlamydiae can be seen.

ELISA "Sandwich" Technology.—One ELISA method involves the use of a sandwich technique. It is utilized in several commercially available testing products. In using the sandwich ELISA technology, the specific antigen is conjugated or fixed to a plastic tube or wall. The patient's serum containing the antibodies is added. A complex is formed with the antibody and its specific antigen in the testing system. Unbound materials are washed away as part of the test procedure. An anti-IgG antibody which has been labeled with an enzyme is added and, after an incubation period, the anti-IgG complexes with the specific antibody if it is present. The enzyme tags commonly used are alkaline phosphatase, glucose oxidase, or peroxidase. After rinsing, a chromogenic substrate is added. The product that is formed by the catalytic action of the enzyme is measured by an observed reaction. The amount of product formed is directly proportional to the amount of antibody in the patient's specimen.

Solid-Phase Immunosorbent Assay.—If the antibody directed toward the agent being assayed is fixed firmly to a solid matrix, either the inside of the wells of a microdilution tray or to the outside of a spherical plastic or metal bead or some other solid matrix, the system is called a solid-phase immunosorbent assay (SPIA).

Western Blot Technology

With this technology, the antigenic proteins or nucleic acids of an organism are separated by gel electrophoresis and transferred or blotted onto membrane filter paper. Antiserum from the patient is allowed to react with the filter paper and, by using labeled anti-antibody detectors, the specific antibody bound to its homologous antigen is detected. That is, if present, the antibodies being sought will bind to the protein or nucleic acid against which they were created. Detection is by use of enzyme-labeled probes or fluorescent markers. Specific assays using the Western blot technology are used to detect antibodies to human immunodeficiency virus (HIV), the causative agent of acquired immunodeficiency syndrome (AIDS). Before an HIV result using a screening enzyme immunoassay is considered positive, the results should be confirmed by the use of at least one additional test. The current standard test for confirming HIV-1 positivity is the Western blot test. The Western blot technique is time-consuming and expensive and has many sources of error.

SPECIMENS FOR SEROLOGY AND IMMUNOLOGY

Immunologic testing is done in many areas of the clinical laboratory—microbiology, chemistry, toxicology, immunology, hematology, surgical pathology, cytopathology, and immunohematology (blood bank), to list a few—and the variety of specimens tested is also great. With the advent of procedures devised to give rapid, accurate results—especially those based on the use of monoclonal antibodies and enzyme immunoassay technology, for example—many clinical constituents of interest to the physician can be determined immunologically. Many types of body fluids can be evaluated using immunologic technology. It is always important to determine the specimen of choice for each procedure being considered. The many commercial kits available for the various assays will state specific specimen requirements and acceptable criteria for collection.

Testing for Antibody Levels

In obtaining specimens for serologic testing, it is important to consider the phase of the disease and the condition of the patient at the time of the specimen collection. This is especially important in assays for diagnosis of infectious diseases. If serum is being tested for antibody levels for a specific infectious organism, generally the blood should be drawn during the acute phase of the illness—when the disease is first discovered or suspected—and another sample drawn during the convalescent phase, usually about 2 weeks later. Accordingly, these samples are called **acute and convalescent serum.** A difference in the amount of antibody present, or the antibody titer, may be noted when the two different samples are tested concurrently. An important concept in any serologic testing is the manifestation of a rise in titer.

Antibody Titer.—The titer is the concentration of the antibody and it is defined as the reciprocal of the highest dilution of the patient's serum in which the antibody is still detectable. That is, the titer is read at the highest dilution of serum that give a reaction with the antigen. An example of reading the titer is: the last tube showing a positive reaction contains a volume of 1 mL and the serum in this tube is 1 part in 1,000 parts; the titer is given as 1,000 units per milliliter. A high titer indicates that there is a relatively high concentration of the antibody present in the serum. For some infections, the titer of antibody rises slowly—months after the acute infection for legionnaires' disease, for example. For most pathogenic infections, an increase in the patient's titer of two doubling dilutions, or from a positive result of 1:8 to a positive result of 1:32 over several weeks, is an in-

dication of a current infection. This is known as a fourfold rise in the antibody titer. To serially dilute a serum specimen, progressive, regular increments of serum are diluted. Most commonly, serial dilutions are "twofold." This means that each dilution is half as concentrated as the preceding one. The total volume is the same in each tube. Titers are usually reported as the reciprocal of the last dilution showing the desired reaction, such as agglutination, lysis, or a change in color.

Types of Specimens Tested

The majority of immunology tests are done on serum. Blood is collected in a plain tube and allowed to clot completely before being centrifuged. Serum should be removed from the clot as soon as possible after processing. Lipemia, hemolysis, or any bacterial contamination can make the specimen unacceptable. Icteric or turbid serum may give valid results for some tests but may interfere with others. Blood specimens should be collected before a meal to avoid the presence of chyle, an emulsion of fat globules that often appears in serum during digestion. Contamination with alkali or acid must be avoided as these substances have a denaturing effect on serum proteins and make the specimens useless for serologic testing. Excessive heat and bacterial contamination are also to be avoided. Heat coagulates the proteins and bacterial growth alters protein molecules. If the test cannot be performed immediately, the serum should be refrigerated. If the testing cannot be done within 72 hours, the serum specimen must be frozen.

For some testing, the serum complement must first be inactivated. To inactivate complement, the tubes of serum are placed in a hot-water bath at 56°C for 30 minutes. If the protein complement is not inactivated it will promote lysis of the red cells and other types of cells and can produce invalid results. Complement is also known to interfere with certain tests for syphilis.

Other specimens include urine for pregnancy tests and for tests for urinary tract infections. It is important that the urine specimen be collected after thoroughly cleaning the external genitalia to prevent contamination for any microbiological assays. Urine for the **human chorionic gonadotropin (hCG)** assay (pregnancy test) must be collected at a suitable time interval after fertilization to allow the concentration of the hCG hormone to rise to a significant detectable level. Any specimen must be collected into a suitable container to prevent changes which could affect the assay results. Proper handling and storage of the specimen until testing is done is essential. Immunologic assays are also done on cerebrospinal fluid, other body fluids, and on swabs of various types of body exudates and discharges. The protocol for each specific assay must be followed for specimen collection requirements and conditions.

COMMON IMMUNOLOGIC AND SEROLOGIC TESTS

As previously discussed, the advent of monoclonal antibody technology has given rise to the development of many new, highly specific and sensitive immunoassays. Classical serologic testing has been an important part of some diagnostic tests in the clinical laboratory for many years. Traditional serologic tests have been done for viral and bacterial diseases. The use of monoclonal antibodies has allowed the identification of specific bacterial and viral proteins and the isolation and characterization of cell surface histocompatibility markers. Monoclonal antibodies should play a significant future role in advancing the knowledge of malignant processes, as more tumor antigens and hormone receptors are identified. In addition, immunologic processes are involved in transplantation technology, including allograft rejection of normal organs. Immunologic testing is employed in tissue typing procedures for organ transplantation. The immune mechanism is currently recognized as a very important factor in diseases across all medical disciplines. Immunologic deficiencies or abnormal immune responses are seen in many types of diseases and disorders.

Among some of the common serologic and immunologic tests that are important in clinical laboratory diagnoses are tests for syphilis; infectious mononucleosis **(heterophil antibodies);** C-reactive protein; streptococcal infections (antistreptolysin O antibodies); cold agglutinins; pregnancy (hCG); rheumatoid arthritis factors; hepatitis, rubella, and herpes simplex viruses; ANAs; thyroid disorder antibodies; and febrile disease antibodies. Some of these tests are discussed separately in this chapter.

Syphilis

Serologic tests are among the most important diagnostic procedures for syphilis. The laboratory results, to-

gether with clinical signs and the patient's history, aid the physician in making the diagnosis. Syphilis tests were some of the first serologic determinations done. They were introduced by Wassermann in 1906, when syphilis was a great threat to humans and many researchers had devoted years to the problem of finding a laboratory diagnosis for syphilis. To many, the terms syphilis and serology have become synonymous.

Syphilis is a sexually transmitted disease that is still a great medical problem. In the United States more than 80,000 cases of syphilis are reported annually. The number of reported cases has continued to rise over the last several years. Early detection and treatment of syphilis are of critical importance to prevent the infection from spreading and doing further harm to the patient.

Adequate diagnosis and treatment are important in all three stages of syphilis. The first stage extends from the initial inoculation with the bacterium, *T. pallidum,* by direct contact (usually sexual) with an infectious lesion, to the formation of the chancre at the initial port of entry. The chancre is a primary lesion that appears 3 to 4 weeks after the initial inoculation. In this first stage, both the blood and the local lesion are infective. The sores often heal by themselves. In the second stage, a rash of the skin and mucous membranes appears. Exudates from the lesion are full of the syphilitic spirochetes. The patient is still highly contagious. Specific antibodies to the spirochete begin to appear about 4 to 6 weeks after the initial inoculation or 1 to 3 weeks after the appearance of the primary sore or chancre. In the third, or latent, stage of the disease, no clinical signs or symptoms are seen; it is recognized only by serologic tests. If the disease goes untreated, severe complications can occur. Complications include cardiovascular problems, central nervous system problems (strokes and seizures), personality changes, and dementia.

In addition to specific antibodies to *T. pallidum,* patients with syphilitic infection respond immunologically by producing a nonspecific reagin antibody-like substance. Serologic tests for syphilis are therefore divided into two categories based on the two types of antibodies present in persons with syphilitic infections: tests for treponemal and nontreponemal antibodies.

Treponemal Antibody Tests
Treponemal antibodies are produced against the antigen of the *T. pallidum* organism itself. Serologic tests for the treponemal antibody include the fluorescent treponemal antibody absorption test (FTA-ABS) and the

MHA-TP *(Microhemagglutination Treponema pallidum)* test. These procedures are used to confirm that a positive nontreponemal test result has been caused by syphilis rather than one of the other biological conditions that can also produce a positive nontreponemal test result. In the FTA-ABS test, the patient's serum is first absorbed with non–*T. pallidum* treponemal antigens to reduce any non-specific cross-reactivity. Then a fluorescein-conjugated antihuman antibody reagent is applied as a marker for specific antitreponemal antibodies in the patient's serum. The test slide is examined for fluorescence intensity us-ing a fluorescence microscope.

Nontreponemal Antibody Tests

Nontreponemal antibodies are also called **reagin antibodies.** These antibodies are produced by the in-fected person against components of their own or other mammalian bodies. Reagin antibodies are almost always produced by persons with syphilis, but can also be pro-duced in other infectious diseases, such as leprosy, tu-berculosis, malaria, measles, chickenpox, infectious mononucleosis, and hepatitis. The reagin antibodies can also be seen in noninfectious disorders such as autoim-mune conditions and rheumatoid disease and in nondis-eases such as pregnancy and old age. The two most widely used tests for nontreponemal antibody are the VDRL test and the RPR test. Both of these tests are based on an agglutination or flocculation reaction in which soluble antigen particles are coalesced to form larger particles that are visible as clumps when aggre-gated by the antibody. These nontreponemal screening tests can be confirmed by another testing method, usually the FTA-ABS test or the MHA-TP test, tests for the presence of specific treponemal antibody.

VDRL Flocculation Test.—This test is performed using cardiolipin-lecithin-cholesterol antigen and heat-in-activated serum from the patient, or with cerebrospinal fluid (Procedure 17–1). It is a tube or a slide test, more commonly the latter. Quality control measures must be employed to ensure reproducible and reliable results from laboratory to laboratory. Technique must be strictly adhered to and standardized reagents must be used to en-sure good results. Positive and negative control sera of predetermined reactivity indicate when corrective action should be taken. Since this tests for nonspecific reagin, antibodies other than those of syphilis may react with the antigen. The test is therefore not 100% specific for syph-ilis, but it is practical, inexpensive, and reproducible. A

positive VDRL test should be confirmed with the FTA-ABS or TP-MHA test.

The reagents necessary for the VDRL flocculation test include buffered saline solution and a stock antigen solution consisting of an alcoholic solution of cardio-lipin, lecithin, and cholesterol. This stock antigen is available commercially in sealed ampules and is made into the working solution by adding buffered saline. The manufacturer's directions must be followed exactly. Pos-itive and negative control sera are available commer-cially.

The special glass slides that are used contain 12 ce-ramic rings in which the suspensions of specimen and re-agents are placed and mixed. An 18-gauge hypodermic needle capable of delivering 60 drops per milliliter is at-tached to a syringe for delivering the antigen suspension. The patient's serum is delivered onto the glass slide from a 0.1- to 0.2-mL pipette calibrated in 0.01-mL divisions, or from a 0.05-mL disposable pipette. A 56°C water bath is used to inactivate the protein complement in the se-rum. A special mechanical rotator is employed to rotate the mixture on the glass slide before reading the results. This serologic rotator is set to revolve at 180 rpm. It fa-cilitates complete and consistent mixing of sample and antigen.

Procedure 17–1. VDRL Flocculation Test

1. Pipette 0.05 mL of the heat-inactivated serum from the patient into one ring of a slide. Pipette control sera in the same manner.
2. Add one drop ($\frac{1}{60}$ mL) of antigen emulsion onto each sample of serum.
3. Rotate slides for 4 minutes at 180 rpm on the ro-tator.
4. Read tests under the microscope immediately af-ter rotation, using the ×10 objective. The anti-gen particles appear as short rods at this magni-fication.
5. Report as follows: nonreactive, no clumping or slight roughness; weakly reactive, small clumps; and reactive, medium to large clumps.

Rapid Plasma Reagin Card Test.—In this test, the patient's serum is mixed with an antigen suspension of a carbon particle cardiolipin antigen on the special dispos-able card provided with the test kit (Procedure 17–2). If the suspension contains reagin, the antibody-like substance present in the serum of persons with syphilis, flocculation occurs with a coagglutination of the carbon particles of antigen. This flocculation appears as black clumps against the white background of the plastic-coated RPR card (Fig 17–4). This reaction is observed and graded macroscopically. Positive reactions are occasionally seen with other infectious conditions or inflammatory states, thus requiring confirmation of all positive results with the qualitative RPR test. Various manufacturers produce RPR kits and the instructions included with the kit must be followed carefully.

One commercial RPR kit is the Macro-Vue RPR Card Test Kit (Hynson, Westcott, & Dunning, Division of Becton Dickinson & Co., Baltimore, MD). The test antigen is similar to that used in the VDRL test, a suspension including cardiolipin, lecithin, cholesterol, choline chloride, and charcoal. The ampule of antigen is stored in the refrigerator and reconstituted according to the manufacturer's directions prior to its use for the test. A plastic dispensing bottle and needle accompany the antigen ampule in the kit. The antigen in the dispensing bottle should be shaken gently before each series of antigen droppings. The antigen should be stored in the refrigerator and allowed to come to room temperature before using it for the test. An 18-gauge dispensing needle that will deliver 60 drops of antigen per milliliter is supplied with the kit. It is important that this needle be held

in a vertical position so the drops will be of the correct, uniform size. Specially coated, plastic cards, each with ten 18-mm circle spots, are used for the test. It is important not to touch the spots with oily fingers as this may cause improper test results. Special Dispenstirs, 0.05 mL per drop, are also included with the kit. These are used for stirring the mixture on the cards. Capillary pipettes of 0.05 mL capacity, or other pipettes which are graduated in 0.01-mL subdivisions, are used to measure the serum and control specimens. Use of a mechanical rotator that will rotate at 100 rpm is suggested, although this test can be hand-rocked when a mechanical device is not avail-

---

Procedure 17–2. Rapid Plasma Reagin (RPR) Card Test

1. Pipette 0.05 mL of unheated serum on an 18-mm circle of the test card. Do not touch the card surface. Pipette control sera in the same manner.
2. Spread the serum in the circle with the Dispenstir or other stirrer to fill the entire circle. Care must be taken to not scratch the surface of the card.
3. Gently shake the antigen dispensing bottle and, holding it in a vertical position, dispense several drops into the dispensing bottle cap to make certain that the needle passage is clear. Add one free-falling drop ($\frac{1}{60}$ mL) of RPR antigen suspension from the needle to each test area of the card containing serum. Do not stir; mixing is accomplished with the mechanical rotator.
4. Place the card on the rotator and rotate for 8 minutes at 100 rpm. Cover the card with a humidifier to prevent evaporation during the rotation process.
5. Observe each specimen immediately in the "wet" state under a high-intensity incandescent lamp or in strong daylight. Observation should be without magnification.
6. Specimens producing questionable results should be retested using a repeat RPR test and with other serologic methods.
7. Report results as: reactive, slight to large agglutination (black clumps); or nonreactive, no agglutination, or very slight roughness (even light-gray color).

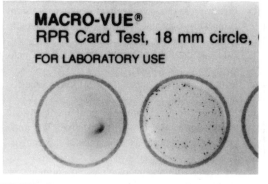

MACRO-VUE®
RPR Card Test, 18 mm circle,
FOR LABORATORY USE

FIG 17–4.
Rapid plasma reagin card test for syphilis. The black clumps against a white background indicate a positive reaction. (Courtesy of Hynson, Westcott, & Dunning, Division of Becton Dickinson and Co, Baltimore MD. Published in Baron EJ, Finegold SM: *Bailey and Scott's Diagnostic Microbiology*, ed 8. St Louis, Mosby–Year Book, Inc, 1990, p 164. Used by permission.)

able. Positive and negative control sera should be tested daily to assure the accuracy of the test antigen reagent. A diagnosis of syphilis cannot be made based solely on a positive RPR card test without clinical signs and symptoms or supportive history. The RPR card screening test should not be used for cerebrospinal fluid specimens.

Antistreptolysin O (ASO) Antibodies

When humans are infected with group A streptococci (Lancefield's classification), extracellular enzymes are produced by the organism. One of the many enzymes produced by group A streptococci, *Streptococcus pyogenes,* is called *streptolysin O.* This enzyme is capable of lysing red blood cells. When the organisms that produce streptolysin O are grown in a special broth culture and the broth is filtered after growth, the filtrates contain streptolysin O. Infection with group A streptococci results in the production of streptolysin O in the body. This acts as an antigen, stimulating the immune mechanism to develop antistreptolysin O (ASO) antibody. Observation of a high titer indicates that the organism is present and is causing disease. The titer can remain elevated weeks to months following the acute disease. Rapid streptococcal antigen tests are discussed under throat cultures in Chapter 16.

When found in large amounts, ASO antibody is useful in diagnosing rheumatic fever, erythema nodosum, and acute glomerulonephritis, which are all diseases resulting from group A streptococci. Thus, ASO levels in serum have become used as evidence of a recent streptococcal infection and are used to follow the course of poststreptococcal disease.

The ASO antibody is a globulin, occurring mostly in the gamma globulin fraction of the serum. It can combine with and fix streptolysin O, neutralizing it in vitro and making it incapable of lysing red cells. The classic titration serologic test used for the detection of ASO relies on several principles: (1) ASO can be specifically fixed with the antigen streptolysin O, inhibiting its hemolytic activity; (2) the amount of ASO can be estimated by serial dilution of the patient's serum in the presence of constant volumes of streptolysin O to the point where there is still complete prevention of hemolysis; and (3) the presence of ASO in the serum is directly related to the production of streptolysin O by the streptococcal bacteria in the infected patient. If no bacteria are present, or if they are eliminated, the ASO titer decreases. It is possible to find significant levels of ASO antibodies in

healthy persons. Titers also vary with age, school-age children commonly having higher titers because of their continual exposure to streptococcal organisms. No normal ASO titer has been established, as there are so many variables. Consequently, the results of ASO titer determinations must be interpreted with caution. A rise in ASO titer of at least 30% over the previous level is generally regarded as a reliable indicator of disease. A single high ASO titer is of little value to the physician because some healthy persons can have high titers.

Patients with complications of streptococcal infections that do not produce or discharge pus (nonsuppurative), such as rheumatic fever and acute glomerulonephritis, usually have a higher incidence of elevated ASO titers and higher numerical titers than patients with uncomplicated streptococcal infections.

Most healthy persons have ASO titers of up to 200 Todd units. Titers of over 200 Todd units are considered abnormal, and titers of 300 or more Todd units may indicate active rheumatic fever or acute glomerulonephritis.

Serologic testing should compare sera from the acute phase with that of the convalescent phase, collected 3 weeks apart. Specimens for the ASO titer test should be collected aseptically, if possible, and the serum stored in a refrigerator until it is tested. If a specimen looks cloudy (contaminated), chylous (fatty), or red-tinged (hemolyzed), it should not be used for this test, as erroneous results will be obtained. Fresh frozen or inactivated sera may be used for the ASO test.

ASO Titration Test

The classic method that has been used routinely for years to measure the ASO titer involves a serial tube dilution technique.* Antigen for the procedure is obtained from the broth of an 18-hour culture of group A streptococci mixed with serial dilutions of the patient's serum and buffer. These mixtures are incubated at 37°C for 15 minutes, and a 5% suspension of human group O or rabbit red blood cells is then added. The tubes are reincubated at 37°C for 45 minutes, centrifuged for 1 minute at 1,500 rpm, and read for hemolysis in the supernatant fluid. The end point, or titer, is the highest serum dilution that gives no hemolysis (that is, in which all the streptolysin O has been inactivated by combination with

---

*Rantz LA, A Randall: Modification of the technique for the determination of the antistreptolysin O titer. *Proc Soc Exp Biol Med* 1945; 59:22.

the ASO). That is, in this test, the ASO is specifically fixed to streptolysin O in vitro, where it neutralizes its hemolytic activity. The titer is reported in Todd units. The value in Todd units for each dilution is the reciprocal of that dilution. Before any results are reported, control sera should be tested and the expected results observed.

Particle Agglutination Test for ASO

Many laboratories have replaced the classic neutralization titration ASO test with the use of a particle agglutination test (Procedure 17–3). These particles can be latex or be coated erythrocytes. The streptozyme test is a particle agglutination test in which erythrocytes are coated with a mixture of streptococcal antigens. It is used as a screening test. Another screening test is the ASO Quicktest Kit (Stanbio Laboratory, Inc., San Antonio, TX) in which a reagent of latex particles coated with streptolysin O is provided. A 0.9% saline solution is also included with the test kit which is used for diluting the serum specimen. The test kit includes a glass slide with six cells. Only the glass slide provided with the kit should be used for this assay. A positive control serum is provided that has a concentration of at least 200 units/mL of ASO and a negative control serum containing less than 100 units/mL is also included with each assay. All test reagents and specimens must be at room temperature prior to beginning the test.

Rubella Infection

Acquired rubella, also known as German measles or 3-day measles, is caused by a virus. It is a highly contagious disease transmitted through respiratory secretions. Before the advent of widespread immunization, this disease was primarily a disease of childhood, although it also affected adults. Contracting the infection or being vaccinated against rubella virus are the only ways of acquiring immunity to this disease. The only proof of immunity is a positive serologic screening test for the rubella antibody. Antibodies appear within a week after infection. After the infection, an elevated titer of antibodies can persist for years or perhaps for life.

It is important to determine the immune status of women of childbearing age and to provide vaccination for those who are not immune. Rubella infection is usually a mild, self-limiting disease with few complications. In pregnant women, rubella infections, can have devastating effects on the fetus, especially in those women in-

---

Procedure 17–3. ASO Quicktest (Rapid Latex Agglutination Test for ASO)

1. Label a 12- × 75-mm test tube for each patient serum to be tested.
2. Pipette 1 mL of the saline solution into each test tube.
3. Using a clean disposable Pasteur pipette for each specimen, add one drop of patient serum to each of the labeled test tubes. Cover the tubes and mix the dilution thoroughly by inverting the tubes several times.
4. Label one division of the six-celled slide for the positive control, negative control, and the patient sera being tested.
5. Pipette 50 μL (0.05 mL) of the control and the patient sera onto the appropriately labeled cells. Clean pipettes must be used for each addition.
6. Add one drop of latex test reagent to each cell. Before being used, the reagent must be mixed by gentle tipping to resuspend the latex particles in the buffer solution. The vial of reagent should not be shaken or agitated. (*Note:* A preservative of sodium azide is added to latex suspension reagents and control specimens. This additive may react with lead and copper plumbing to form highly explosive metal azides. Large volumes of water should be used when flushing any of these products down a drain to prevent the build-up of azide in the plumbing of the sink.)
7. Mix each specimen with a separate, clean applicator stick and spread the mixture evenly over the cell.
8. Rotate the slide for exactly 3 minutes. Examine immediately with a bright direct light source. Prolonged time in reading may give false-positive results.
9. Report results as:

   Positive—agglutination; agglutination indicates 200 units/mL or more of ASO (166 Todd units). Agglutination indicates the presence of antistreptolysin O in the patient's specimen. Positive results should be retested using a quantitative procedure.

   Negative—no agglutination; a negative result is characterized by a lack of visible agglutination and the presence of opaque or slightly granular fluid when compared with the negative control.

fected with the virus during their first trimester. Rubella infection can result in fetal death, miscarriage, or manifestation of a spectrum of congenital defects including encephalitis, deafness, cataracts, bone defects, mental retardation, cardiovascular defects, and hepatomegaly. Women who do not have the antibodies to the rubella virus should be vaccinated before becoming pregnant. Clinical immunology and serology tests can assess the presence of rubella antibodies against the virus. There are several tests available for qualitative and quantitative rubella assays.

Specimens for Antibody Assay

For qualitative antibody assays, a single blood specimen is used. To estimate the immune status of the patient, a single specimen can be used. Any detectable antibody is indicative of immunity and protection against subsequent rubella infections. If a suspected clinical infection or exposure to the virus is being studied, two specimens should be quantitatively assayed: acute phase and convalescent phase. One specimen should be collected within 3 days of the appearance of the rash (clinical symptoms) or at the time of exposure, and the second specimen, the convalescent specimen, collected 7 to 21 days after the onset of the rash or at least 30 days after the exposure, if no clinical symptoms appear. The first specimen collected should be tested in the laboratory as soon as possible and an aliquot frozen for later assay along with the second specimen collected. These specimens should be assayed simultaneously.

Tests for Rubella Antibodies

Historically, the use of hemagglutination inhibition (HAI) antibody tests have been the most frequently used methods of screening for the presence of rubella antibodies. Tests for IgG status are now also done to determine the immune status. Rubella methods vary in sensitivity and specificity when the antibody titers are near the cutoff concentration of a titer of 1:8. There are also latex agglutination procedures, enzyme immunoassays, and FA studies for rubella antibodies. Latex agglutination tests provide a rapid and convenient alternative to the hemagglutination inhibition tests (Procedure 17–4).

In the latex agglutination tests, latex particles are sensitized with soluble rubella antigens from disrupted virus particles that have been inactivated. When the latex reagent is mixed on a dark surface with serum from the patient that contains rubella antibodies, antigen-antibody complexes will form visible clumps. If the antibody is absent or not present in sufficient titer, there will be no agglutination—the latex particles will remain smooth and evenly dispersed. When a qualitative test is performed and a positive reaction is observed, this evidence of rubella antibodies being present in the serum is an indication of a previous infection with the rubella virus. Presumptive immunity can be used to evaluate the immune status of the patient. A single specimen tested determines immunity. It does not provide a serodiagnosis of infection or reinfection.

Heterophil Antibodies in Infectious Mononucleosis

Infectious mononucleosis is an acute infectious disease, viral in origin, that is characterized by clinical symptoms of extreme fatigue, malaise, sore throat, fever, enlarged lymph nodes in the neck, and enlarged spleen. A significant number of cases do not show these classic signs and symptoms. The Epstein-Barr virus (EBV) was first identified in 1964 as the cause of infectious mononucleosis. EBV is a human herpes DNA virus and there are a variety of antigens encoded by this virus. An infection with EBV results in the expression of viral capsid antigen, early antigen, and nuclear antigen, each with their corresponding antibody responses. There are assays for IgM and IgG antibodies to the EBV antigens. These tests are usually performed in virology laboratories or reference laboratories. Antibodies to this virus are produced early in the disease and can also be detected by complement fixation tests and immunofluorescence techniques. Heterophil antibodies are commonly produced in high titer in infectious mononucleosis and are quite easily detected in the laboratory. For this reason, routine tests for the presence of heterophil antibodies are used for the diagnosis of infectious mononucleosis, along with hematologic findings.

Common characteristic laboratory findings for infectious mononucleosis include peripheral blood with abnormal, enlarged lymphocytes with atypical nuclei (see Examination of the Blood Film in Chapter 11) and serum that contains a high titer of heterophil antibodies.

Heterophil Antibodies

Heterophil antibodies are antibodies that appear in cells and fluids of apparently unrelated animals and microorganisms. They are stimulated by one antigen and react with an entirely unrelated surface antigen present on cells from different mammalian species. Heterophil antibodies react with an antigen entirely different from

---

*Procedure 17–4. Rubascan Rubella Card Test**

1. Remove the cap from the bottle of latex agglutination reagent and attach the green hub needle to the tapered fitting.
2. Mark the test card to identify the low-reactive and nonreactive control and all the patient specimens. These test cards must be flat for proper reactions to take place. Care should be taken to not place finger marks in the test areas of the cards. This may transfer oil to the card and be the cause of incorrect results. Each card should be used only once and then discarded.
3. Using a micropipettor, place 25 μL of low-reactive control in one labeled circle of the test card. With clean pipette tips for each measurement, use the same micropipettor to add 25 μL of nonreactive control and the patient sera to be tested to the other labeled circles on the test card. Patient sera are tested undiluted unless other sensitivity levels are needed.
4. Using a new plastic stirrer for each circle, spread each of the specimens or controls to be tested to fill the entire circle.
5. Place the bottle cap over the tip of the needle and carefully mix the latex reagent several times by inversion.
6. While holding the bottle of latex reagent in a vertical position, dispense several drops of antigen into the bottle cap until a drop of uniform size has been formed. Then dispense one free-falling drop of antigen (approximately 15 μL) onto each circle containing serum or control. Care must be taken to avoid contaminating the bottle cap during this step. The antigen in the bottle cap can be returned to the bottle and reused. (*Note:* The latex reagent and controls contain a sodium azide preservative which can react with lead or copper. Azides may form highly corrosive substances. When disposing of these products down laboratory drains, flush with large volumes of water to prevent azide build-up.)
7. Place the card on a rotator and rotate for 8 minutes under a moist humidifying cover to prevent evaporation during this process.
8. Immediately following mechanical rotation, read the card macroscopically in the wet state using a high-intensity incandescent light. Weak agglutination can be differentiated from no agglutination by using brief hand rotation of the card (three or four back-and-forth motions) following the mechanical rotation. Fluorescent lighting is usually not sufficient to read minimally positive agglutination results. Magnification in reading test results is not generally recommended.
9. The reactive control should show visible agglutination and the nonreactive control should demonstrate no agglutination.
10. Report results as:
    Positive reaction—presence of visible agglutination; the presence of antibody in a single patient specimen is indicative of previous exposure and immunity to the rubella virus. Demonstration of any detectable antibody is indicative of immunity and protection against subsequent rubella infection. Quantitative assays must be done to determine the presence of a fourfold increase in rubella antibody titer in paired specimens (acute and convalescent phase collections). A fourfold rise in titer is indicative of a seroconversion, diagnostic of a recent or current infection with rubella virus.
    Negative reaction—no visible agglutination observed.

---

and phylogenetically unrelated to the antigen responsible for their production. An example of one of the earliest heterophil antibodies is that discovered by Forssman in

**Becton Dickinson Microbiology Systems, Cockeysville, MD.

1911. This *Forssman antibody* was formed when an emulsion of guinea pig organs was injected into rabbits. The production of this Forssman antibody in the rabbit was shown to lyse sheep red cells in the presence of complement. Heterophil antibodies are made up of a group of antibodies that cross-react with antibodies

TABLE 17–1.

Comparison of Forssman, Serum Sickness, and Infectious Mononucleosis Antibodies

	Absorbed by	
Antibody	Guinea Pig Kidney	Beef Red Blood Cells
Forssman	Yes	No
Serum sickness	Yes	Yes
Infectious mononucleosis	No	Yes

against any one member of the particular heterophil group.

Heterophil antibodies are present in low titer in the serum of normal persons and are also known as Forssman antibodies. Forssman antibodies resemble the antibodies found in infectious mononucleosis in that they agglutinate sheep red cells, but differ from them in that they are absorbed by an emulsion of guinea pig kidney, which is rich in Forssman antigen, and are not absorbed by beef cells, which are poor in Forssman antigen. In cases of serum sickness, or sensitization to animal (usually horse) serum, a further type of sheep red cell agglutination antibody is found and may be present in high titer. However, this is again distinguished from the antibody of infectious mononucleosis by being absorbed by guinea pig kidney, and from Forssman antibodies by being absorbed by beef red cells. This is summarized in Table 17–1. This comparison was devised by Davidsohn in 1937 and is used today as the basis for presumptive and differential tests.

Tests for Heterophil Antibody

The sheep cell agglutinins of infectious mononucleosis can be distinguished from those of serum sickness and other conditions by means of a differential test, using absorption with guinea pig kidney and beef red cell antigens. The antibody that can be removed by absorption with guinea pig kidney is known as the Forssman antibody, and the guinea pig kidney as the Forssman antigen. The classic sheep red cell agglutination test is carried out in two steps: the presumptive test of Paul and Bunnell, and the differential test of Paul, Bunnell, and Davidsohn. These are the reference tests from which the rapid testing procedures have evolved. Modifications of these classic procedures utilize horse red cells instead of sheep red cells.

Under normal circumstances, rapid screening tests for infectious mononucleosis are done for the presence of heterophil antibodies. Horse red cells are usually used rather than sheep red cells, as they are more sensitive to heterophil antibodies. Persons suffering from infectious mononucleosis begin developing heterophil antibodies shortly after the appearance of the symptoms, usually during the first 2 weeks. Highest titers are found during the second and third weeks of the illness. The titer bears no relationship, however, to the severity of the illness. As a rule, heterophil sheep cell agglutinins appear in only 50% to 80% of cases of infectious mononucleosis, so negative results can be obtained when the disease is present. Negative tests therefore do not rule out the possibility of the disease.

The test for heterophil antibodies is of confirmatory diagnostic importance in cases of infectious mononucleosis with typical clinical and hematologic findings. It is of a deciding diagnostic importance early in the disease when there are unusual clinical findings and hematologic signs, some of which may be caused by complicating factors.

Faster and easier screening tests have been introduced commercially and have replaced the laborious presumptive and differential tests in most laboratories.

The heterophil antibody produced in infectious mononucleosis is IgM and usually appears during the acute phase of the disease. These heterophil antibodies have the following characteristics: they react with horse, ox, and sheep red blood cells; they are absorbed by beef red blood cells; they are not absorbed by guinea pig kidney cells; and they do not react with any of the EBV-specific antigens. These characteristics have enabled the development of several immunologic and serologic tests which are commonly used in the diagnosis of infectious mononucleosis.

Paul-Bunnell Test.—Paul and Bunnell developed their test in 1932 when they first observed that heterophil antibodies developed in persons with infectious mononucleosis.* This test is presumptive, as it indicates only the presence or absence of heterophil antibodies. It does not distinguish between antibodies associated with infectious mononucleosis, serum sickness, or the Forssman antigen. That is, the Paul-Bunnell test is not specific. If the test is negative, however, it does eliminate the need for

---

*Paul JR, Bunnell WW: The presence of heterophile antibodies to infectious mononucleosis. *Am J Med Sci* 1932; 183:90–104.

further testing. In this test, patient serum is mixed with antigen-bearing sheep red blood cells. Sheep cells carry antigens associated with infectious mononucleosis and serum sickness and also the Forssman antigen. Dilutions of the patient serum are mixed with the sheep cells, incubated, centrifuged, and examined macroscopically for agglutination. A positive agglutination reaction is primarily associated with infectious mononucleosis, but as previously stated, the test is not specific.

Davidsohn Modification of the Paul-Bunnell Test.—In 1937, Davidsohn modified the classic Paul-Bunnell test to distinguish the infectious mononucleosis heterophil antibodies from the heterophil antibodies of the Forssman antigen and serum sickness.† This is the classic test for infectious mononucleosis heterophil antibodies and has been used as a basis for the many rapid testing systems which are currently used in many laboratories.

The Davidsohn differential test is dependent on the fact that sheep red blood cells and beef (ox) red blood cells bear some common antigens that are not present on the guinea pig kidney cells. When the patient's serum is exposed to both the guinea pig kidney cells (rich in the Forssman antigen) and beef red blood cells (poor in the Forssman antigen), differential absorption takes place. The guinea pig kidney will absorb or remove any Forssman antibodies present and the beef red cells will absorb or remove any infectious mononucleosis heterophil antibody present. Any absorbed antibodies are removed by centrifugation and the supernatant fluid is tested with the sheep red blood cells. The agglutination patterns are shown in Table 17–1. Positive reactions are recorded only if the differential absorption pattern is typical for the disease. A baseline titer of 1:56 is needed using the preliminary Paul-Bunnell test before this test is performed. In patients with the clinical signs and hematologic features of infectious mononucleosis, a positive Davidsohn differential test establishes the diagnosis.

The sensitivity of this test depends in part on the time after onset of the disease when the specimen is collected and when the test is performed. Peak titers of the heterophil antibody are found during the second and third weeks of the illness. Tests for heterophil antibodies should not be used to follow the clinical course of the disease, as there is a poor correlation between the titer of the infectious mononucleosis antibody and either the stage and severity of the illness or the numbers of atypical lymphocytes seen in the peripheral blood.

In 1968, Lee and Davidsohn found that by using horse red blood cells instead of sheep cells, there was a greater sensitivity in the detection of infectious mononucleosis heterophil antibodies. This adaptation of the classic Davidsohn-Paul-Bunnell test is specific for the disease and has increased the sensitivity. It has also simplified the criterion for a positive test and baseline titers are not needed. The Lee modification has been utilized in the commercially manufactured rapid slide tests for infectious mononucleosis heterophil antibody.*

Rapid Slide Tests.—Rapid slide tests (also called spot tests) have been developed by several manufacturers. Most of these screening tests utilize fine suspensions of guinea pig kidney and beef red cell stromata for the rapid differential absorption, and horse red cells for the sensitive detection of infectious mononucleosis heterophil antibodies. These rapid screening tests are based on the following general principles: (1) the use of horse red cells instead of sheep red cells makes the test more sensitive and thus is especially valuable for low-titer serum found in the early stages of the disease; (2) the unwashed preserved horse red cells remain in a usable condition for at least 3 months and give stronger and quicker agglutination with infectious mononucleosis serum than do horse red cells preserved with formalin; (3) some noninfectious mononucleosis serum also has a high horse agglutinin titer, and therefore serologic tests cannot depend on titers alone; and (4) fine suspensions of guinea pig kidney and of beef red cell stromata give satisfactory instant absorption of antibodies and a clear-cut differentiation between infectious and noninfectious mononucleosis serum.

These tests are done on a slide. The serum from the patient is mixed thoroughly with guinea pig kidney on one square of the slide and with beef red cell stroma on another square. The unwashed horse red cells (preserved) are added immediately to both squares. These reagents are available commercially in the form of test kits. Directions must be followed carefully. Agglutination is observed on both squares of the slide 1 minute after the final mixing. If agglutination is stronger on the square

---

†Davidsohn I: Serologic diagnosis of infectious mononucleosis, *JAMA* 1937; 108:289.

*Lee CL, Davidsohn I, Panczyszyn O: Horse agglutinins in infectious mononucleosis. II. The spot test. *Am J Clin Pathol* 1968; 49:12.

where the guinea pig kidney suspension was mixed with the patient's serum, the test is positive. If it is stronger on the square where the beef red cells were mixed with the patient's serum, the test is considered negative. If the agglutination is equal on both squares, the test is negative. If no agglutination appears on either square, the test is negative. One commercially available test kit utilizing this principle is called Monospot (Ortho Diagnostics, Raritan, N.J.) (Procedure 17–5).

The glass slides used for these rapid screening tests must be carefully cleaned under running water. Use of detergent could cause errors in the results. Most of the widely used immunologic assays for infectious mononu-

cleosis are highly sensitive. It is still necessary, however, to use adequate and proper control programs as the only dependable method of detecting sources of technical errors. When the results are not clear-cut, it is always important to repeat them and to conduct additional serologic tests.

Use of a slide screening test for infectious mononucleosis heterophil antibody is indicated in a patient with the clinical or laboratory evidence of the disease. A positive slide test in a patient with the appropriate clinical signs and symptoms is strong evidence of acute infectious mononucleosis. The slide test is not indicated for screening purposes in an asymptomatic patient.

Procedure 17–5. Monospot* Rapid Slide Test for Infectious Mononucleosis

1. Place the slide on a flat surface under a direct light source.
2. Invert the indicator horse red blood cells to resuspend the cells. Using a clean microcapillary pipette, place 10 lambda of cells on one corner of both squares on the slide. To use the microcapillary pipette, insert the end of the pipette marked with a heavy black line 0.25 in. into the neck of the rubber bulb. Hold the rubber bulb between the thumb and third finger. Tilt the vial of cells and insert the pipette. Allow the pipette to fill to the 20 lambda mark by capillary action. Do not draw the cells into the bulb. To deliver 10 lambda of cells to the slide, place the index finger over the hole in the top of the bulb and squeeze gently until the level of cells in the pipette reaches the first mark. Touch the pipette tip to a corner of square I to release the cells. Repeat the process to deliver the remaining 10 lambda of cells to the corner of square II.
3. Put one drop of thoroughly mixed guinea pig antigen (reagent I) in square I.
4. Put one drop of thoroughly mixed beef red cell stroma (reagent II) in square II.
5. Using a disposable plastic pipette, add one drop of the patient serum or plasma (approximately 0.05 mL) to the center of each square on the slide.
6. Mix the serum (plasma) and the guinea pig antigen in square I at least ten times with a clean wooden applicator stick. Avoid touching the indicator horse red cells in the corner of the square.
7. Mix the serum (plasma) and the beef red cell stroma in square II at least ten times with a clean wooden applicator stick. Avoid touching the indicator horse red cells in the corner of the square.
8. Blend the indicator horse red cells over the entire surface of each square. Use a clean wooden applicator stick for each slide and use no more than ten stirring motions to blend.
9. Start a timer upon completion of the final mixing. Do not move or pick up the slide during the reaction period.
10. Observe for agglutination for no longer than 1 minute after the final mixing.
11. Report results as:
    Positive if the agglutination pattern is stronger on the left side (square I). A positive test result is indicative of the presence of the heterophil antibody specific for infectious mononucleosis. Negative if the agglutination pattern is stronger on the right side (square II). If no agglutination appears on either side (I or II) of the slide, or if the agglutination is equal on both squares of the slide, the test is also negative. (*Note:* Some persons with infectious mononucleosis do not develop detectable heterophil antibody. Specific EBV antibodies can be identified in these cases.)

*Ortho Diagnostics, Raritan, NJ.

Specimens of serum are usually used for these screening tests. The presence of hemolysis in the specimen makes it unsuitable for testing. If testing cannot be done immediately, serum or plasma may be stored at 2 to 8°C for several days after being collected. Capillary specimens can be used by drawing the specimen into capillary tubes, either heparinized or nonheparinized. Enough serum or plasma (0.05 mL is required for the test) can usually be obtained from the use of four capillary tubes (standard 75-mm length) if the patient's hematocrit is less than 50%. The tube is centrifuged and the serum removed after breaking the tubes at the interface between the cells and serum or plasma. Serum from two tubes is needed as the sample required for each side of the slide according to the directions for use.

Before any reagents are used for the test, the reagent cells should be shaken well to provide a homogeneous mixture. The reagents should be used at room temperature.

Control sera should be tested, using both a positive and a negative control specimen, each time a patient specimen is tested.

False-negative slide tests may be obtained in patients with a low heterophil titer. This can occur early in the first 1 or 2 weeks after onset of symptoms. False-negative tests can also be seen in the patient who does not mount a heterophil antibody response to the infection. This can be true especially in young children. The slide test can be repeated at a later date or an EBV titer for IgM can be performed to help establish the diagnosis for these persons.

False-positive tests for heterophil antibody have been reported in cases of CMV infections, leukemia, Hodgkin's disease, Burkitt's lymphoma, rheumatoid arthritis, viral hepatitis, multiple myeloma, and myocardial infarction.

Anti-nuclear Antibody Tests for Systemic Lupus Erythematosus

Anti-nuclear antibody procedures are used as a screening test for systemic lupus erythematosus (SLE), an autoimmune disease of the connective tissue. SLE is a generalized disorder that affects more women than men and expresses itself as an inflammatory condition of the vessels. It usually involves many organ systems—skin, kidney, blood vessels, blood cells, heart, joints, and central nervous system. The primary cause of death in severe cases of SLE results from a pathologic decrease in kidney function. There is no cure for SLE although steroids and immunosuppressive drugs can help control the course of the disease.

Severe immunologic findings are associated with SLE. A striking laboratory finding is the appearance in the serum of numerous globulins with the properties of antibodies that are directed against various cell nuclei. These are known as *antinuclear antibodies* or LE (lupus erythematosus) factor. ANAs are usually IgG, but they may also be IgM or IgA.

The ANA tests have virtually replaced the LE cell test, formerly the classic diagnostic test for SLE. The LE cell is a neutrophil that has ingested a homogeneous globular mass of altered nuclear material. The LE factor present in the blood of persons with SLE has the ability to cause depolymerization of the nuclear chromatin of polymorphonuclear (PMN) leukocytes. The depolymerized material is subsequently phagocytosed, or ingested, by an intact PMN leukocyte, giving rise to the LE cell.

The transformed nuclear material in the white cell attracts phagocytes, usually segmented PMNs and occasionally monocytes. The phagocytes with the ingested nuclear material are the LE cells. Formation of LE cells requires the presence of the LE factor, damaged leukocytes, and normal active leukocytes. In patients with SLE, LE cells are found in the bone marrow and the peripheral blood when the smears are prepared according to specific procedures. A standard method is to mash the blood clot, centrifuge the clot fragments, and make buffy coat smears from the resulting cell suspension.

Antinuclear Antibodies

Antinuclear antibodies are immunoglobulins that react with the whole cell nucleus or nuclear components such as nuclear proteins, DNA, or histones in the tissue of the host. The presence of ANAs is the serologic hallmark of SLE. ANAs are found in other diseases such as scleroderma, polymyositis, rheumatoid arthritis, associated with the use of certain drugs, and in aging persons without disease. Thus the assays for ANAs are not specific for SLE. ANAs are, however, present in more than 95% of persons with SLE. Since the detection of ANAs is not diagnostic of only SLE, their presence cannot confirm the disease. However, the absence of ANAs can be used to help rule out SLE. The significance of the presence of ANAs in a patient's serum must be considered in relation to the patient's age, sex, clinical signs and symptoms, and other laboratory findings. Fluorescent antinuclear antibody (FANA) techniques are commonly used in screening tests for SLE. An indirect fluorescent technique is usually used.

Indirect Immunofluorescent Tests for ANA.—

The use of indirect immunofluorescent tests for ANA is based on the utilization of fluorescein-conjugated antiglobulin. These methods are extremely sensitive. In one assay, the serum specimen is delivered into a well on a microscope slide that contains a mouse liver substrate. Substrates of rat or mouse liver or kidney, or cell-cultured fibroblasts, can also be used as the antigen and are fixed to the slides. If antibody is present in the serum of the patient, the unlabled antibody will attach to the nuclei of the cells in the substrate. After the substrate is washed in buffer, the slide is incubated with fluorescein-labeled goat antihuman immunoglobulin. If the patient antibodies have attached themselves to the nuclear antigens in the substrate, the fluorescein-tagged goat antihuman immunoglobulin will attach to these antibodies. Fluorescence will be seen microscopically using ultraviolet light. The slides should be examined as soon as possible. If immediate examination is not possible, the slides can be stored in the dark at 4°C for up to 48 hours prior to being read.

Several different patterns of fluorescence reactivity are seen depending on whether the ANAs have reacted with the whole nucleus or with nuclear components such as the nuclear proteins, DNA, or histone (a simple protein). This difference in nuclear fluorescence pattern reflects specificity for various diseases. Patterns are described as being diffuse or homogeneous, peripheral, speckled, or nucleolar fluorescence. Nuclear rim (peripheral) patterns correlate with antibody to native DNA and deoxynucleoprotein and bear correlation with SLE, SLE activity, and lupus nephritis. Homogeneous (diffuse) patterns suggest SLE or another connective tissue disorder. Speckled patterns are found in many diseases, including SLE. Nucleolar patterns are seen in patients with progressive systemic sclerosis and Sjögren's syndrome. After ensuring that the results for positive and negative control specimens are giving the expected reactions, the results for the patient are reported. Results from the screening tests are reported as positive or negative. The normal person is expected to give a negative reaction: no green or gold fluorescence is observed. The degree of positive fluorescence may be semiquantitated on a scale of 1+ to 4+. Positive samples give a green-gold fluorescence of a characteristic pattern (homogeneous, peripheral, speckled, or nucleolar).

Rheumatoid Factor

The identification of **rheumatoid factor (RF)** in the serum or synovial fluid of patients with clinical features of rheumatoid arthritis (RA) assists in confirming the diagnosis. Rheumatoid arthritis is a chronic inflammatory disease, primarily affecting the joints and joint tissues. It is generally accepted that immunologic reactions contribute significantly to the pathogenesis of the disease. Rheumatoid factors are autoantibodies that are directed against the Fc fragment of IgG. The serum of most patients with RA have detectable abnormal protein immune complexes. These protein complexes circulate and are known collectively as rheumatoid factor. RF is now generally accepted to be actually a group of immunoglobulins that interact specifically with antigenic determinants on the IgG molecule. Most commonly, RF is associated with either IgG or IgM. RF is present in many persons with RA, but not all. RF can also be present in other diseases, but the highest titers are found in persons with RA. Patients with tuberculosis, bacterial endocarditis, hepatitis, and collagen diseases may also have RF in their serum. RF that appears in chronic diseases virtually disappears when the infectious process is treated with the appropriate therapy; RF that is present in RA persists indefinitely. RF is not found in degenerative joint diseases like osteoarthritis or in gout or infectious joint diseases. The determination of the presence of RF is important in the prognosis and management of RA. High titers of RF are indications of greater amounts of joint destruction, possible increased systemic involvement, and generally more severe disease. RF can also be detected in synovial fluid, but its significance is little more than that of RF in serum.

Tests for Rheumatoid Factor

The tests for RF are based on the reaction between antibodies in the patient's serum (RF), and an antigen derived from gamma globulin. Generally all tests are designed to detect antibodies to immunoglobulins. A latex-coated suspension coated with albumin and chemically bonded with denatured human gamma globulin serves as the antigen in one commonly used test for RF. If RF is present in the serum, macroscopic agglutination will be visible when the latex reagent is mixed with serum. Latex agglutination procedures have a 95% correlation with a clinical diagnosis of probable or definite RA. False-positive tests are possible with other rheumatic diseases such as lupus erythematosus, in chronic infectious dis-

---

*Procedure 17–6. Rheuma-Fac Rheumatoid Arthritis Rapid Slide Test**

1. Prepare a 1:20 dilution of the patient's serum by diluting 0.1 mL of serum with 1.9 mL of diluent which is provided with the kit. The diluent is a glycine-saline buffer reagent with a pH of 8.2 ± 0.1. Mix the serum and diluent completely.
2. Using one of the capillary pipettes provided with the kit, fill approximately two-thirds of the pipette with the diluted serum. Deliver one free-falling drop of the diluted serum from the pipette by holding it perpendicular to the center of one of the oval divisions on the glass slide provided with the kit. It is important that the pipette be held in this perpendicular position in order to provide a drop of the correct size from the pipette.
3. Add one drop of positive control and one drop of negative control to other properly labeled oval divisions on the slide.
4. Mix the latex reagent and add one drop of this reagent to the patient specimens and to each of the controls on the slide. This latex suspension is made up of stabilized polystyrene latex particles coated with human albumin and chemically bonded with denatured human gamma globulin. The reagent should be stored in the refrigerator. It should not be frozen. (*Note:* Sodium azide is used as a preservative in latex suspensions, buffer, and control specimens. Sodium azide may react with lead or copper and form highly explosive metal azides. Large volumes of water should be used when flushing these products down a drain to prevent azide build-up in the plumbing.)
5. Mix each specimen and controls with the latex suspension using a clean applicator stick. All the contents of the mixtures must be spread evenly over the entire area of their respective divisions on the glass slide.
6. Tilt the slide back and forth, slowly and evenly, for 2 minutes.
7. Place the slide on a flat surface and observe immediately for macroscopic agglutination. Use a direct light source.
8. Report results as:

   Positive reaction: visible agglutination of the latex suspension is an indicator of the presence of RF in the specimen. It is recommended that all positive reactions using the slide tests be followed with a quantitation of the titer of RF. False-positive reactions may be observed if the serum specimens are lipemic, hemolyzed, or heavily contaminated with bacteria. Drying artifact may be confused with agglutination if the reaction time is longer than 2 minutes.

   Negative reaction: absence of visible agglutination and the presence of an opaque fluid constitutes a negative reaction. False-negative reactions can occur if undiluted specimens are used for the test. Undiluted specimens can have an antigen excess interfering with the agglutination reaction if there are high levels of C-reactive protein in the serum.

---

eases such as hepatitis, tuberculosis, and syphilis, and in other diseases, such as liver cirrhosis and sarcoidosis. Other RF tests utilize sensitized sheep cells in hemagglutination procedures. The latex agglutination and sheep cell agglutination tests are the most popular of the routine tests used for RF. There are several commercial kits available for assay of RF; some use test tubes and some are rapid slide tests.

Rapid Latex Agglutination Test for RF.—Serum is usually the specimen used for this test. If the test cannot be performed immediately, the specimen should be

*ICL Scientific, Fountain Valley, CA.

refrigerated. If the test cannot be performed within 72 hours, the specimen should be frozen. Frozen serum should be thawed rapidly at 37°C prior to testing. Before the test is done, the specimen should be at room temperature. All reagents used for the rapid slide RF tests must be at room temperature. It is always important to carefully follow all instructions provided with the testing product (Procedure 17–6).

C-Reactive Protein

C-reactive protein (CRP) was first recognized in 1930 as a constituent of the serum of patients with acute pneumonia that formed a precipitate with the C polysaccharide of the pneumococcus. This protein is also found in the serum of persons suffering from acute phases of infections other than pneumonia and in noninfectious inflammatory conditions. It is the basis for several serologic tests that aid in the diagnosis of rheumatic fever and other inflammatory conditions. CRP is not found in clinically significant amounts in normal serum, and it disappears when the inflammatory condition has subsided.

As CRP is found in many infections and in noninfectious diseases, it is nonspecific, and its presence in the blood is a sensitive but nonspecific **acute phase reactant** indicator of infection, inflammation, or tissue damage. The presence of CRP is clinically important even when it cannot be associated with a specific disease. It is consistently found in bacterial infections (particularly the colon-typhoid group), active rheumatic fever, acute myocardial infarction, and widespread malignant diseases, and is commonly found in active rheumatoid arthritis, viral infections, and tuberculosis.

Tests for C-Reactive Protein

Serologic tests for CRP use the serum of the patient and either purified pneumococcal C polysaccharide or anti-CRP serum obtained from rabbits immunized with purified CRP. The tests are divided into several categories depending on the type of procedure employed. There are CRP agglutination tests using latex particles coated with antibodies to human CRP which interact with the patient's serum either on a microscope slide or in a test tube. These tests are known as *latex fixation tests* and are commonly used in many laboratories for CRP assays. Latex fixation tests are very sensitive. Other CRP tests include FA tests and precipitation tests. In addition, some of the precipitation tests are gel tests utilizing electrophoresis or electroimmunodiffusion techniques. There has been new interest shown in the study of CRP owing to its potential as a mediator or modulator of the immune response. Sensitive, specific, rapid tests have been developed for its determination. Even though the significance of CRP is not completely known, it is felt by many that a molecule that is produced in such abundance during the acute inflammatory phase of disease processes must have biological significance. Because CRP is synthesized more rapidly than other acute phase reactants, assays of CRP are considered very useful in suspected inflammatory conditions.

C-Reactive Protein Rapid Latex Agglutination Test.—The ICL CRP kit (ICL Scientific, Fountain Valley, CA) is a rapid latex agglutination test based on the reaction between the serum of the patient containing the CRP antigen and the corresponding antibody coated to the treated surface of latex particles. When antigen is present in the patient's serum, the coated particles enhance the detection of an agglutination reaction. The latex CRP reagent is a suspension of latex particles coated with specific antihuman CRP produced in goats or sheep. A dropper assembly for the reagent is provided in the test kit. Positive and negative control sera should be tested with this reagent to assure accurate results when using the patient's specimen. Controls are provided with the kit and are run with each patient sample. Special glass test slides are provided with the kit. Specimens and all reagents must be at room temperature before testing is started.

C-Reactive Protein Capillary Tube Precipitation Test.—The original method devised by Anderson and McCarty or a modification of it is used.* The method consists of observing and measuring the precipitate formed when CRP antiserum and patient's serum are mixed in a capillary tube. After a period of incubation, the degree of precipitation is observed and recorded for a positive test. A control serum should be included with the test serum. Commercial products are available for this test. A general procedure is given in Procedure 17–8.

Cold Agglutinins

In the early 1940s, agglutinins were discovered in the serum of patients with primary atypical pneumonia which agglutinated red blood cells of all blood groups at 0°C. Because these antibodies reacted only at low temperatures (0–10°C), they were called cold agglutinins. They did not agglutinate the same red cells at 37°C. Cold agglutinins are beta or gamma globulins that react in saline. They are nonspecific in their reactions because they react well with all red cell types. Red cell walls contain lipoid material that acts as an antigen or reactive site for cold agglutinins.

Normal persons can have cold agglutinin titers up to 1:28, but more often a normal titer is approximately

---

*Anderson HC, McCarty M: Determination of the C-reactive protein in the blood as a measure of the disease process in acute rheumatic fever. *Am J Med* 1950; 8:455.

Procedure 17–7. C-Reactive Protein Qualitative Slide Test*

1. Make a 1:5 dilution of the patient serum by pipetting 0.1 mL of serum into a test tube and adding 0.4 mL of the commercially prepared diluent, a glycine-saline buffer solution. Mix well.
2. Using one of the capillary pipettes provided in the kit, fill the pipette with undiluted serum to approximately two-thirds of the pipette length. Holding the pipette perpendicular to the slide, deliver one free-falling drop to the center of one of the oval divisions of the slide.
3. Using a clean capillary pipette provided in the kit, fill the capillary pipette with the diluted serum (1:5) to approximately two-thirds of the pipette length. Holding the pipette perpendicular to the glass slide, deliver one free-falling drop to the center of one of the oval divisions of the slide. (*Note:* The pipettes must be held perpendicular to the slide to deliver the correct and consistent amounts of test serum using the free-falling drop method. Use clean, unused capillary pipettes for each measurement. If a calibrated pipettor is used, adjust the pipettor to deliver 0.05 mL (50 μL) of the specimen.
4. Using the squeeze dropper control vials provided with the kit, add one drop of positive control and one drop of negative control to separate labeled divisions on the test slide.
5. Resuspend the CRP latex reagent by gently mixing until the suspension appears homogeneous. Using the dropper provided, add one drop of the CRP latex reagent to each serum specimen and to each control.
6. Using separate applicator sticks, mix each specimen and each control thoroughly. The contents of the mixtures should be spread evenly over the entire area of their respective divisions on the test slide.
7. Tilt the slide back and forth, slowly and evenly, for 2 minutes. Place the slide on a flat surface and observe immediately for macroscopic agglutination using a direct light source.
8. Report results as:

    Positive: agglutination of the latex suspension indicates the presence of CRP in the specimen at a level equal to or greater than 1.0 ±0.2 mg/dL. A positive reaction is reported when either the undiluted or the 1:5 dilution demonstrates agglutination or when both exhibit agglutination. Agglutination in the 1:5 dilution is indicative of a CRP level greater than 5 mg/dL.

    Negative: the absence of visible agglutination and the presence of opaque fluid indicates a negative reaction. A negative result is reported *only* when both the undiluted and the 1:5 dilution exhibit no visible agglutination.

1:8. They are found regularly in the blood of persons with diseases such as *Mycoplasma pneumoniae* pneumonia, tonsillitis, African trypanosomiasis, and staphylococcemia. High titers are often found in patients who are pregnant or who have cirrhosis of the liver, emboli of the veins or pulmonary system, influenza, or other acute respiratory infections. Transient cold agglutinins are frequently found in persons with infectious mononucleosis.

Special precautions should be taken when drawing the blood specimen for cold agglutinin tests. The syringes and needles, as well as the collecting tubes, should be warmed at 37°C before use in the venipuncture. The specimen should be kept warm submerged in water at 37° C while it is delivered to the laboratory. In testing for cold agglutinins, the blood sample must be kept warm, preferably near 37°C, in a water bath. After the clot has completely retracted, the serum and cells are separated. Centrifugation is not recommended. The serum is removed and used in the test. If the test cannot be done within 2 days, the serum may be frozen.

The serial tube dilution procedure of Horstmann and Tatlock is used, with fresh human group O red cells as the antigen.[†] The tubes are incubated overnight in the refrigerator, and the presence of agglutination is determined before the cells are warmed. All positive tubes are then incubated at 37°C for 30 minutes. If the agglutination is caused by cold agglutinins, it will disappear or disperse on heating, whereas other antibody-mediated agglutination will not. To interpret the results, the titer is observed after incubation in the refrigerator. The titer is

*ICL Scientific, Fountain Valley, CA.

†Horstmann DM, Tatlock H: Cold agglutinin—a diagnostic aid in certain types of primary atypical pneumonia. *JAMA* 1943; 122:369–370.

Procedure 17–8. C-Reactive Protein Capillary Tube Precipitation Test

1. Collect a fasting specimen of blood, allow it to clot, and separate the cells from the serum.
2. Draw up the CRP antiserum about 1.0 to 1.5 cm into the capillary tube. Wipe off the outside of the tube to remove excess antiserum.
3. Place the capillary tube into the patient's serum and draw up a volume equal to the volume of CRP antiserum in the previous step. The patient's serum must be in contact with the antiserum. Air pockets between the patient's serum and the test serum should be avoided.
4. Slowly invert the tube several times and allow the liquid contents to flow back and forth. Thorough mixing is important.
5. Place the tube in a Plasticine block or rack with the large air space toward the bottom. The meniscus of the tube should be above the Plasticine.
6. Leave the tube in an incubator at 37°C for 2 hours, followed by overnight incubation at 4°C.
7. Make a qualitative reading after the 2-hour incubation period by holding the tube between a light source and the eye. The presence of CRP is indicated by a white precipitate in the tube.
8. Make a semiquantitative reading after the overnight incubation by measuring the height of precipitate in the tube in millimeters. Read the amount of precipitation as follows: no precipitation, negative; slight precipitation, trace; 1 mm, 1+; 2 mm, 2+; 3 mm, 3+; and 4 mm or more, 4+.
9. Interpret these results as follows: absence of precipitation, no CRP present; precipitation, CRP present.

---

the highest serum dilution exhibiting 1+ or greater agglutination (1+ is the least amount of visible clumping). A titer of 1:32 to 1:64 in a single specimen from a convalescing patient is significant.

Pregnancy Tests

Immunologic tests are done frequently in the laboratory to detect pregnancy in the early stages. Laboratory tests for pregnancy are based on the fact that during pregnancy, the placenta produces a hormone called chorionic gonadotropin. This hormone rapidly disappears after delivery. Human chorionic gonadotropin (hCG) is also produced in other conditions, as in the presence of a hydatidiform mole, choriocarcinoma, and in malignant teratomas of the ovaries and testes. In pregnancy, hCG is produced by trophoblast cells of the developing placenta. It is a glycoprotein consisting of two subunits, alpha and beta, with a combined molecular weight of about 35,000. hCG appears about 2 days after implantation.

At between the 8th and 10th weeks of gestation, peak production of hCG is attained. After the 10th week of gestation hCG production sharply declines. The rate of excretion of hCG into the urine of a pregnant woman increases rapidly between the 30th and 60th days of pregnancy, with peak levels between the 60th and 70th days of gestation. After this time, the level of hCG decreases slowly with a low level remaining throughout the remainder of the pregnancy. After delivery, the hCG level drops rapidly over a 2- to 3-day period and it is undetectable 2 weeks after delivery. The international reference unit for gonadotropin activity is determined by using a dried urinary gonadotropin standard kept at the World Health Organization in London.

The presence of hCG is usually measured in the urine because a urine sample is easy to obtain. Urinary hCG parallels the rise and fall of the levels in serum. Laboratory tests for pregnancy are generally used to detect hCG no earlier than 10 days after the last missed menstrual period and are used through the first trimester, or to about the 12th week of pregnancy. After the first trimester, the levels of hCG may be undetectable by routine laboratory methods.

The stage of pregnancy has a marked influence on the test results, especially on the incidence of false-negative results. Between the 7th or 8th and 12th weeks of gestation, even a relatively insensitive assay will be almost 100% positive. If the assays are made before the 6th week of gestation, even the most sensitive assay may show an appreciable number of false-negatives. Since the levels of hCG fall after the first trimester, false-negative results may be obtained in an obviously pregnant woman.

The most common reason for a positive test is pregnancy, but greatly increased levels of hCG may be seen in other instances. An increase in the level of hCG after the removal of a hydatidiform mole, for example, would indicate either that the mole was not completely removed, or that it was malignant and is redeveloping. The test for hCG is therefore a valuable tool for purposes other than the confirmation of pregnancy.

A minimum quality control program for hCG assays requires that each assay be done in duplicate, that known negative and positive samples be assayed to check the system, and that tests be done regularly with samples of different, known hCG levels to check the low and high sensitivity of the system.

Early methods for the determination of pregnancy were biological and involved the use of animals. These tests were costly and very time-consuming. Test results were not available for several days, and often the animals had to be sacrificed to carry out the determination. Early biological tests employing animals, usually frogs, toads, rabbits, or rats, were the Aschheim-Zondek test and the Friedman test. The accuracy, economy, and convenience of immunologic tests for pregnancy have made animal tests a thing of the past.

Immunologic pregnancy tests are done in one of several ways. They differ in the carrier for the external source of hCG, which is commonly latex particles or red blood cells. Rapid slide agglutination or test tube agglutination methods or enzyme immunoassays are used. A variety of commercial kits are available for these methods. The kits also include positive and negative controls, sensitized particles, and antiserum.

Specimens for Pregnancy Tests

Most pregnancy tests are routinely performed on urine specimens. A first morning urine specimen is required and it should have a specific gravity of at least 1.015. It should be tested immediately or refrigerated until the test can be performed. Specimens that contain blood and those with heavy proteinuria are likely to cause interference and give false-positive results. Drugs can also contribute to false-positive tests. False-negative results may be obtained if the urine is too dilute (low specific gravity) and it is too early in the pregnancy. Most pregnancy tests give reliable results about 42 days after the onset of the last normal menstrual period and are not reliable after the first trimester of the pregnancy. ELISA tests give a positive reaction with a much lower concentration of hCG and consequently will give positive hCG results earlier in the pregnancy. Urinary hCG levels generally parallel the rise and fall of the serum levels.

Types of Pregnancy Tests

Many of the available commercial tests are slide or tube tests and are based on the inhibition of latex particle

agglutination. They are generally two-stage procedures. The accuracy of the commercial immunologic pregnancy tests depends on several factors. The manufacturer's directions must be followed carefully, the reagents must be properly shipped and stored, and the specimens must be properly collected and delivered promptly to the laboratory for testing. Other important factors are the stage of pregnancy, whether the pregnancy is normal or abnormal, the presence of interfering substances in the urine (including drugs, proteins, and red cells), the sensitivity and specificity of the assay procedure, and the use of quality control programs.

Types of tests include hemagglutination inhibition, latex particle inhibition, direct latex particle agglutination, enzyme immunoassay, sol particle immunoassay, and radioimmunoassay. For the most part, these tests are easy to perform and several of them have been incorporated into home test kits for pregnancy.

Hemagglutination Inhibition.—This test involves a two-stage testing process and can be carried out in a test tube. The hCG in the patient's urine will neutralize anti-hCG antiserum that is added to the sample (an antigen-antibody reaction occurs if hCG is present in the specimen). Red cells coated with hCG are next added to the tube, and the tube is observed for agglutination. If the hCG in the patient's urine has reacted with the anti-hCG in the first stage, no agglutination will be observed in the second stage when the coated red cells are added. Unagglutinated red cells settle in a ring in the bottom of the tube. Agglutinated red cells settle in a button. A positive test for pregnancy is therefore reported when no agglutination is observed in the second stage of the test. A negative test is reported when agglutination occurs in the second stage. This test may be used with both urine and serum samples. For quantitation of hCG, a 24-hour urine specimen is required.

Latex Particle Agglutination Inhibition.—This type of test is based on the interference of hCG in a specimen when it is added to a system of latex particles that have been coated with hCG. As part of the first stage of the test, an anti-hCG serum reagent is mixed with the patient's urine on a slide. For stage 2 of the test, the hCG-coated latex particles are added. If hCG is present in the specimen, it has been neutralized by the anti-hCG and no agglutination is observed. If the patient's urine contains hCG in sufficient quantities (because of pregnancy or another condition previously described), an antigen-antibody reaction has occurred between the patient's hCG and the anti-hCG in the reagent serum, leaving no more anti-hCG to react with the coated latex particles added during the second stage of the test. Therefore, a negative agglutination reaction suggests a positive pregnancy test. Conversely, the absence of hCG in the specimen allows agglutination of the latex particles by the anti-hCG within approximately 2 minutes, the specific reaction time depending on the test kit being used.

The anti-hCG is manufactured by injecting purified hCG into animals (usually rabbits) and allowing the animal to produce the specific antibodies to the hCG in its serum.

Latex Particle Agglutination Test.—In this test, latex particles are coated with anti-hCG antiserum. These are agglutinated when the urine specimen being tested contains hCG. A positive pregnancy test is indicated by the presence of agglutination. This is in contrast to the latex particle inhibition test described above.

Enzyme Immunoassays.—There are several ELISA tests available as a result of monoclonal antibody technology. In these tests two types of monoclonal antibodies are used:

One is an hCG-specific antibody bound to a membrane or other solid support medium. This can be a membrane in a tube or on a disk, for example. The characteristics of nitrocellulose, nylon, or other membrane material can be used to enhance the speed and the sensitivity of ELISA reactions. When there is an absorbent material below the membrane, it can help to pull the liquid reactants through the membrane and help separate components that have not reacted from those that have formed antigen-antibody complexes and have bound to the membrane during the testing process. The washing steps are simplified in this way. When the urine specimen containing hCG is added (or in some instances, plasma, serum, or whole blood can be used), the hCG molecules present are bound to the antibodies on the solid support membrane.

The second monoclonal antibody is an hCG antibody that has been linked to a specific enzyme (alkaline phosphatase). This enzyme-linked antibody is added to the testing system and will bind to a different site on the hCG molecule creating a sandwich of bound antibody-hCG-enzyme-labeled antibody. After an incubation period, any unbound enzyme-labeled antibody is washed free. A chromogenic substrate reagent is next added which undergoes a specific color change in the presence

of the alkaline phosphatase enzyme, indicating the presence of hCG. The color change is often to blue. Variations in these tests include the use of impregnated membranes and strips.

Test results should be reported as "hCG-positive" or "hCG-negative", not as "pregnancy-positive" or "pregnancy-negative" owing to the possibility of a false-positive pregnancy test reaction. False-positive results are less common with the ELISA tests. ELISA tests are very sensitive, giving positive reactions as early as 10 days after conception (before the first missed menses).

---

*Procedure 17–9. hCG in Urine Using Abbott TestPack Plus**

1. Remove the reaction disc from the protective pouch and place on a flat, dry surface.
2. Using the transfer pipette supplied with the kit, dispense three drops of urine specimen into the sample well on the reaction disc. The first morning urine specimen usually contains the highest concentration of hCG and therefore is the specimen of choice—any urine specimen may be tested, however.
3. The test results should be read immediately after the appearance of a red color in the end of assay window. Test results are observed in the result window. Positive results can be observed in as little as 3 minutes but the appearance of a red color in the end of assay window is required for maximum sensitivity or to confirm negative results.
4. Interpret results as follows: a positive (+) sign indicates that the specimen contains elevated levels of hCG—manufacturer's instructions must be followed in regard to specific interpretation details; a negative (−) sign indicates the absence of detectable hCG. This test will detect urine hCG concentrations of 50 mU/mL or greater. Occasionally, specimens containing less than 50 mU/mL may also give a positive result.
5. If a positive (+) or a negative (−) sign fails to appear in the Result Window, or if no color appears in the End of Assay Window, the specimen should be retested.

---

*Abbott Diagnostics, Abbott Park, IL

Abbott TestPack hCG Urine (Abbott Diagnostics, Abbott Park, IL).—By use of the commercial ELISA test kit, TestPack Plus hCG Urine, hCG in urine can be identified (Procedure 17–9). By using a combination of both monoclonal anti-hCG antibodies and polyclonal antibodies, hCG in urine can be identified selectively with a high degree of sensitivity. The urine specimen is allowed to migrate through the membrane in the reaction disc. As it passes through the membrane, it first mobilizes the anti-alpha hCG antibody-coated complex. The urine and antibody-colloid complex move through the immobilized anti-beta hCG antibody capture region and then on to the end of the membrane. The plus (+) and minus (−) sign format gives a clearcut readout for positive or negative specimens. The appearance of the negative (−) sign with a negative specimen gives an added assurance of quality control by demonstrating antibody recognition, assuring that the procedure was performed correctly and that the reagents were chemically active. This becomes a procedural control. If neither a plus or a minus sign appears, the test must be repeated.

If hCG is present at levels of 50 mU/mL or greater, a positive (+) sign will be seen in the result window. If hCG is absent, a negative (−) sign will appear in the result window. The appearance of a red color in the end of assay window assures the user that the test is complete. Quality control samples should be used daily to ensure proper kit performance and samples should be tested according to the established protocol of the laboratory.

It is always essential to follow the manufacturer's instructions carefully. Package inserts will also indicate causes for false-positive or false-negative reactions. This information should be understood in conjunction with the performance of the test.

BIBLIOGRAPHY

Baron EJ, Finegold SM: *Bailey and Scott's Diagnostic Microbiology,* ed. 8. St Louis, Mosby–Year Book, Inc, 1990.

Becan-McBride K, Ross DL: *Essentials for the Small Laboratory and Physician's Office.* St Louis, Mosby–Year Book, Inc, 1988.

Bryant NJ: *Laboratory Immunology and Serology,* ed. 2. Philadelphia, WB Saunders Co, 1986.

Henry JB (ed): *Clinical Diagnosis and Management by Laboratory Methods,* ed, 18. Philadelphia, WB Saunders Co, 1991.

Glossary and Guidelines for Immunodiagnostic Procedures, Reagents, and Reference Materials, Approved Guideline. Villanova, Pa, National Committee for Clinical Laboratory Standards, vol 6, 1986; D11-A.

Physician's Office Laboratory Guidelines, Tentative Guidelines, Villanova, Pa, National Committee for Clinical Laboratory Standards, 1989; 9 POL 1-T.

Turgeon ML: *Immunology and Serology in Laboratory Medicine.* St Louis, Mosby–Year Book, Inc, 1990.

18   Immunohematology

Key Terms	
Agglutination	Genotype
Alleles	Immune response
Antibody	Linked genes (linkage)
Antigens	Phenotype
Antihuman globulin reaction or test	Plasma
Antiserum	Rh immune globulin (RhIG)
Blood transfusion	Rh-negative
Chromosomes	Rh-positive
Compatibility testing	Sensitization
Complement	Serum
Components	Transfusion reactions
Crossmatch	Typing
Derivatives	Unexpected antibodies

The field of immunohematology has advanced rapidly and all indications point to further advancement as techniques in transfusion medicine continue to change. Since 1951, new discoveries have been made at a rapid pace and the nature of the immunologic response to different antigens has been shown to be vastly more complicated than was at first supposed. Before 1951, nine independent blood group systems had been discovered. These important systems and their approximate dates of discovery are ABO (1900), MN (1927), P (1927), Rh (from rhesus) (1939), Lutheran (1945), Kell (1946), Lewis (1946), Duffy (1950), and Kidd (1951). The complexity of the red cell and its antigenic polymorphism seems almost endless, and it is expected that as methodology for studying red cell antigen-antibody reactions improves, the boundaries of knowledge will continue to expand.

The risk of transfusion-transmitted infections such as viral hepatitis and human immunodeficiency virus (HIV) infection has significantly changed the practice of transfusion medicine. These include changes in the manner in which blood is tested before transfusion, the way in which donors are selected, and the nature of the blood component or derivative used for transfusion.

A study of the immunologic reactions of blood cells is critical when therapeutic replacement of blood is necessary. The many possible antigen-antibody reactions that can occur must be anticipated and tested for by the laboratory procedures available in the immunohematology laboratory. In many diseases and health problems, therapeutic administration of blood and blood products is indicated. Severe illness and death are closely associated with loss of blood, which impairs the ability of the circulatory system to deliver adequate amounts of oxygen to the body cells and critically upsets the delicate homeostatic water and acid-base balance of body fluids. Blood loss may be caused by hemorrhage, excessive destruction of red cells, or the body's inability to replenish its own blood supply. In specific instances, administration of whole blood or its components is indicated. The technique of replacing whole blood and its components is known as blood *transfusion*. The procedures involved in collecting, storing, processing, and distributing blood are called *blood banking*. The techniques and procedures involving the study of the immunologic responses of blood cells are called *immunohematology*.

Immunohematology and blood banking are unlike other fields of clinical laboratory investigation. Although accuracy is always important in the laboratory, it is absolutely essential in blood banking. Even the smallest error can directly result in the death of a patient from a hemolytic transfusion reaction. As R. R. Race said, "Blood group tests are different from most laboratory tests used in medicine in a vital way—the reported result must be correct, for the wisest physician cannot protect his patient from the consequences of a blood grouping error."*

This chapter is meant only as a very general introduction to the subject of blood banking. It is definitely not sufficient preparation for work in blood banking laboratories. Specific blood banking procedures are not presented; only principles are discussed. Several excellent texts are available in the field of blood banking; however, most of them seem complex (even unintelligible) to the person who has no background in this area. Probably the best single reference, in a practical sense, is the American Association of Blood Banks *(AABB) Technical Manual.* This indispensable reference will be found in any licensed blood bank and should be consulted by the regular blood bank staff.

To carry out blood banking procedures a thorough knowledge of the principles involved, recognition of the many difficulties that may be encountered, and exactness of technique are essential. Short cuts must never be taken. Everyone working in a particular blood bank must use exactly the same technique. Also, an elaborate system of safeguards must be established and thoroughly understood by all personnel. These are the standard operating procedures which must be established and followed for each blood bank laboratory. These safeguards and checks may seem repetitive but are essential. When an incompatible transfusion reaction occurs, it is usually caused by a breakdown of, or failure to observe, the established system.

Complete, permanent, legible records must be kept of every sequence of the many steps involved in administering a unit of blood. Results and observations are always entered directly on the permanent record and never recopied, as recopying will invariably result in error at some time.

---

*Race RR, in Preface: Dunsford I, Bowley CC (eds): *Techniques in Blood Grouping.* Edinburgh, Oliver & Boyd, Ltd, 1955.

BLOOD

Whole human blood consists of two major portions: solid and liquid. The solid portion consists primarily of the formed elements—red blood cells, white blood cells, and platelets—and makes up about 45% of the total blood volume. The liquid portion consists of the **plasma,** which makes up about 55% of the total volume. The blood volume of normal adults is approximately 5 to 6 L. In blood banking reference is often made to a *unit* of blood. For practical purposes, a unit may be considered about 500 mL.

Infused blood, or blood that is administered by transfusion, must be anticoagulated. However, the portion of blood that is used for blood bank testing procedures such as typing and crossmatching is generally clotted blood. Although **serum** (from clotted blood) is preferred, plasma may be used. If plasma from anticoagulated blood is used, there is a chance that small fibrin clots may be present in the plasma and may be incorrectly interpreted as a positive result. Therefore, laboratory blood bank tests generally employ red cells and serum (the liquid remaining after blood has been allowed to clot), not red cells and plasma. Another important reason for using serum rather than plasma in laboratory testing is that complement activation is usually prevented by an anticoagulant. Most anticoagulants bind calcium, which is necessary for complement integrity. Persons doing blood banking procedures are repeatedly reminded that complement activity occurs in laboratory tests only when serum is used. In the body, plasma does not have the added anticoagulant, and therefore the complement integrity is not lost. Therefore, complement activation occurs as readily in serum in the laboratory as it does in plasma in the body. This is important in the laboratory as several blood group antibodies require complement activation in order for an observable reaction to be seen.

HISTORICAL INTEREST IN TRANSFUSIONS

The importance of blood must have been realized from the earliest times. Early humans must have observed that loss of blood could lead to death. In addition, some primitive groups had rituals in which the blood of one person was given to another; it was thought that in this way various characteristics of the donor could be given to the recipient. The discovery of the circulation of blood by Harvey in 1616 did much to advance interest in blood transfusion. In one early transfusion, attempted by Denis in 1667, lamb's blood was transfused into a man. At first this seemed to benefit the man, who was given a total of three such transfusions. However, after the third transfusion of lamb's blood the man suffered a reaction and died. It was found that it is impossible to transfuse the blood of one species of animal into another, whether from animal to human, human to animal, or animal of one species to animal of another species. Transfusions were also attempted within the same species of animal, from human to human and from one animal to another of the same species. These transfusions seemed to work about half the time, but far too often the result was death.

BLOOD GROUPS

It is now known that the incompatibility of many transfusions was caused by the presence of certain factors which we now know are **antigens** on red cells. Each species of animal, humans included, has certain antigens that are unique to that species and are present on the red cells of all members of that species. If the red cells of sheep, for example, are transfused into a human, an antisheep substance **(antibody)** will be produced in the blood of the human. The antisheep substance will destroy any sheep red cells that are subsequently introduced. This cell destruction is what is meant by an incompatible hemolytic transfusion reaction, and it results in the death of the recipient.

It is also known that certain antigens are common to some, but not all, members of a particular species. If blood containing such antigens is transfused into a recipient whose red cells do not contain that antigen, the recipient will form an antibody that may result in an incompatible transfusion reaction.

So far, this seems rather simple. Why all the difficulty in blood banking? All that is necessary is to find the antigen present on the red cell and transfuse only blood containing that antigen. The principle is correct, but a great number of antigens may be present on one person's red cells. The antigens that are known have been grouped into units referred to as *blood group systems*. Hundreds of blood group systems have been described. A partial list includes

ABO	Kidd	Lutheran	Kell
Rh	P	I	Xg
Lewis	Diego	MNSs	Duffy

More systems are being discovered all the time. The antigens that exist on a person's red cells within a particular blood group system represent that person's type for that system. The number of possible types within one system varies. In the ABO system there are six main types, plus additional types determined by less frequent subgroups. The more complex Rh-Hr system alone has over 100 possible types. Taking all systems and type combinations into account, over 500 billion different types of blood are possible. In essence, each person has a unique blood type.

At this point it would seem that blood transfusion is impossible, since no two persons should have exactly the same type of blood. Fortunately, only certain antigens are likely to give problems in transfusion (i.e., incompatible transfusion reactions), although there is always the possibility that an unknown or untested-for antigen may occur that will result in such a reaction. The antigens most likely to cause reactions are located within the ABO and Rh-Hr systems and must be tested for whenever blood is administered. Other antigens are routinely tested for indirectly through crossmatching and antibody screening techniques. Persons who are given an antigen not present on their red cells may produce an antibody in their plasma that will react with the foreign antigen. This is evidenced by the destruction of the red cell containing the foreign antigen.

INHERITANCE OF BLOOD GROUPS

Genes

All the factors or antigens present on a person's red cells are inherited. Each antigen is controlled by a *gene,* which is the unit of inheritance. In other words, antigens are inherited as genes. If the gene for a particular antigen is present, that antigen will be found on all the red cells.

Chromosomes

Each cell (except for mature red cells) consists of cytoplasm and a nucleus. If the nucleus is observed under the microscope at approximately the time of cell division, several long, threadlike structures will be visible. These structures are referred to as *chromosomes*. Each species has a specific number of chromosomes, and the chromosomes occur in pairs. Humans have 46 chromosomes (23 chromosome pairs). The paired chromosomes are similar in size and shape and have their own distinct functions. A complete set of 23 chromosomes is inherited from each parent. Chromosomes occur in pairs in all cells of the body, except the sex cells (sperm and ovum), which contain 23 single chromosomes.

Gene Location (Linkage)

Since the gene is the unit of inheritance, it must also be located within the nucleus. Genes are exceedingly small particles that, when associated in linear form, make up the chromosome. They are too small to see under the normal brightfield microscope but together are visible as the chromosome. Genes are made up of deoxyribonucleic acid (DNA). Each trait that is inherited is controlled by the presence of a specific gene. The genes responsible for a particular trait always occur at exactly the same point or position on a particular chromosome—this position is referred to as the *locus* of the gene. Research in the field of genetics is continually revealing new information about the location or sequence of genes on the chromosome and about diseases that are genetically inherited or environmentally induced. If genes for different inherited traits are known to be carried on the same chromosome, they are said to be *syntenic*. This term is useful in referring to genes on a single chromosome that are too far apart to display absolute linkage in inheritance. Genes that are located on the same chromosome and are normally inherited together are known as **linked genes.** The closer the loci of the genes, the closer the **linkage** is said to be.

Alleles

Inherited traits are somewhat variable within a species. For example, eye color varies and it is known to be inherited. Therefore, each possible eye color must be the result of a gene for that color. Variants of a gene for a particular trait are referred to as **alleles** for that trait. Since we have only two genes (one pair) for any given trait, our cells will have only two alleles. However, the number of possible alleles for a trait varies. A person who has identical alleles for a trait is said to be *homozygous* for that trait. For example, a person with blue eyes carries two blue-eye genes and is homozygous for blue eyes. A person who has two different alleles for a trait is *heterozygous* for that trait—for example, having a blue-eye gene in addition to a brown-eye gene.

In general, certain alleles may be stronger than, or may mask the presence of, other alleles. In the case of eye color, brown-eye genes mask the presence of blue-eye genes, and are said to be *dominant* over blue-eye genes. Persons who have one brown-eye and one blue-eye gene have eyes that appear brown. Blue-eye genes are then said to be *recessive* in relation to brown-eye genes. One must have two blue-eye genes in order to have blue eyes. However, in blood banking, the various alleles for a particular blood group system are equally dominant, or *codominant*. If the gene is present (and there is a suitable testing solution available), it will be detected.

Phenotypes and Genotypes

Two other genetic terms that are often used in blood banking are **phenotype** and **genotype.** The phenotype is the blood type determined by tests made directly on the blood, even though other antigens may be present. The genotype refers to the actual total genetic pattern for any system. It is usually impossible to determine the complete genotype in the laboratory; this usually requires additional studies, especially family studies.

ANTIGENS AND ANTIBODIES

All blood banking is based on a knowledge of antigens and antibodies. Unfortunately, they cannot be defined simply. In general, an antigen may be thought of as a foreign substance—foreign in the sense that if it is introduced into the body of a person who does not already have the antigen, an antisubstance called an antibody will be produced. The antibody is found in the plasma and other body fluids. It reacts with the foreign antigen in some observable way, and it is specific for the antigen

against which it is formed—that is, it reacts with only its corresponding antigen and no other antigen.

The significance of antigens and antibodies is not limited to blood banking. They are the basis of immunity. Various microorganisms have antigenic properties. Therefore, when introduced into a host, they elicit antibody formation. The antibody formed in response to the foreign antigen (in this case, the microorganisms) protects the person from subsequent infections by that particular organism. For example, a person who has had chickenpox is immune to the disease in the future. The immunity is a function of antibody production by the host. However, immunity is not immediate, as can be seen from the fact that on first infection the person is ill or incapacitated by the disease. Antibodies require about 2 weeks to develop sufficiently, after which subsequent exposure to the antigen will elicit an effective antigen-antibody reaction and therefore protective immunity.

Transfusion Reactions

In blood banking, antibody formation does not result in protective immunity. The blood antigens are present on the red cells, and the antibody is found in the plasma or serum. The antigen-antibody reaction results in the destruction of the antigen-carrying red cell by antibody in the serum of the person receiving the red cells. Clinically the result of this red cell destruction is the transfusion reaction. It may be a hemolytic reaction or decreased red cell survival due to antibodies coating the red cells which are removed by the reticuloendothelial system (RES). The reaction varies from patient to patient, but generally the immediate reaction is characterized by chills, high temperature, pain in the lower back, nausea, vomiting, and shock as indicated by decreased blood pressure and rapid pulse. These first effects of the reaction are rarely fatal; however, the byproducts of red cell destruction pose many problems, primarily severe renal involvement. The patient may eventually die from kidney failure.

Nature of Antigens

Chemically, antigens are usually proteins, although polysaccharides, polypeptides, or polynucleotides may also be antigenic. They are usually large molecules with a molecular weight of 10,000 or more. The specificity of an antigen is related to the chemical composition together with the spatial configuration or arrangement of the amino acids, simple sugars, and fatty acids that make up the chemical composition of the molecule. However, not all antigens are equally antigenic. Some are extremely effective in their ability to cause antibody production, while others are relatively weak and not as likely to result in antibodies. If this were not true, blood could never be transfused. Antigenicity is influenced by several things. These include the molecular size and electrical charge, the solubility, the shape of the molecule, and the biological and chemical composition.

The same blood antigens are found not only on the red cells but also in other body fluids such as urine, saliva, plasma, and gastric juice.

Immune Response

The response to an antigenic stimulus is referred to as an **immune response.** It involves the recognition and elimination of foreign substances by the immune system, a complex interrelated system of tissues and organs which are generally lymphoid. Lymphoid cells (lymphocytes) come from a common stem cell. The lymphocytes are further classified as T and B cells. T cells are lymphocytes that are derived from the thymus or are influenced by thymic hormones. B lymphocytes are derived from the bone marrow and secrete antibodies. (See also Chapter 11.)

An immune response may be *cellular* or *humoral*. A humoral response involves antibodies (proteins produced by B lymphocytes) and the complement system. The cause and effects of the humoral response are the primary concern in immunohematology or blood banking. The cellular or cell-mediated response involves actions of lymphocytes (especially a subset of T lymphocytes) together with plasma cells and macrophages. Taken all together, the immune response is a finely tuned regulatory mechanism which involves B lymphocytes, together with T lymphocytes, and mononuclear phagocytic cells.

Antibody Production

Antibodies are produced in response to foreign antigenic stimuli. For example, persons whose red cells contain group A antigen are unable to form anti-A antibody. However, several factors influence the amount of antibody that will be formed after foreign antigen stimulation.

Antigenic Strength

The stronger the antigen, the greater the antibody response. In blood banking the ABO and D antigens are very strong, whereas such antigens as Lutheran and Kidd are relatively weak.

Number of Antigens

The number of foreign antigens that are introduced at a particular time also influences the amount of antibody production. In general, exposure to only one antigen elicits a stronger antibody response than simultaneous exposure to more than one antigen.

Number of Exposures

The number of exposures to foreign antigen also plays a role in antibody response. Repeated exposures result in greater antibody formation.

Interval Between Exposures

The interval between exposures to a foreign antigen also has a role in antibody formation. A number of exposures repeated rapidly are less likely to result in antibody formation than the same number of exposures spaced over a longer period of time. The quantity of antigen introduced has some effect; however, the number of exposures and the interval between them are more important in terms of antibody production.

Threshold Effect

There is apparently a threshold amount of antigen related to antibody production. If more than this threshold amount of antigen is introduced, the amount of antibody produced is relatively small in proportion to the quantity of antigen. In addition, a large excess of antigen may completely inhibit an antibody response. This is important in blood banking, for a relatively small amount of incompatible blood produces as much antibody as a relatively large amount. The transfusion of any incompatible blood may result in serious sensitization of the patient.

Individual and Age Differences

Finally, there are individual and age differences in antibody formation. Some persons are more prone to form antibodies than others. Newborn infants do not form antibodies but receive them passively from the mother across the placenta. They begin forming gamma globulin and therefore antibody at about 3 months and usually have a normal gamma globulin level by 6 months. This is important when newborn infants are typed for antibodies in the ABO system.

Primary Response

Antibodies are proteins. It is believed that they are synthesized by B lymphocytes or plasma cells from gamma globulin. When a foreign antigen is first introduced, the antibody cannot be detected immediately in the serum or plasma. It is observed about 10 to 14 days after antigenic stimulation, and the titer (concentration) is greatest at about 20 days, after which it gradually decreases.

Secondary Response

A second exposure to the same antigen, however, rapidly results in detectable amounts of antibody in the plasma or serum. There appears to be some sort of memory phenomenon that results in an immediate antibody response on the second or subsequent exposures. This secondary antibody response also produces a higher and longer-lasting titer of antibody. In addition, the antibody is more effective in its reaction with antigen or has better combining properties.

Types of Antibodies

Antibodies are mainly proteins of the gamma globulin type of serum protein. Therefore, they are also referred to as *immunoglobulins* (Ig). When antibodies result from exposure to antigen material from another species, they are referred to as xenoantibodies or *heteroantibodies*. An example of a heteroantibody used in blood banking is Coombs' antihuman globulin (AHG) antisera. When antibodies result from antigenic stimulation within the same species, they are referred to as *alloantibodies* or *isoantibodies*. Blood group antibodies are isoantibodies; these are the antibodies that cause transfusion-related problems.

Five classes of gamma globulin antibodies occur in human body fluids. These are IgA, IgD, IgE, IgG, and IgM. These immunoglobulins differ as to molecular size, carbohydrate content (all are glucoproteins), biological activity, and plasma half-life. The size and relative amount present in serum are shown on Table 18–1.

IgG and IgM are probably the most important of the blood group antibodies. IgG is the predominant immunoglobulin of serum and makes up about 80% of the total.

TABLE 18–1.

Immunoglobulins in Serum or Plasma

Immunoglobulin Type	Molecular Weight (daltons)	Proportion of Total Immunoglobulin
IgA	160,000–500,000	13%
IgD	180,000	1%
IgE	196,000	Trace
IgG	150,000	80%
IgM	900,000	6%

It is the smallest of the immunoglobulins. IgM is the largest of the blood group antibodies and makes up about 6% of the total. IgA is the immunoglobulin component of external secretions, such as saliva. The serum levels of IgA, IgG, and IgM are influenced by a number of factors, including age and race. IgM is the type of antibody that results from primary exposure to foreign antigen. Secondary exposure results in IgG formation. Repeated stimulation results in IgG antibody formation.

IgM is the first type of antibody that the newborn infant is able to form, and it is effectively synthesized at about 9 months. IgG is effectively synthesized at about 3 to 4 years, whereas IgA is not produced until adolescence. IgG is the only type of antibody that is able to cross the placenta. This is important in respect to hemolytic disease of the newborn.

Antibody Structure

All of the immunoglobulins have a similar chemical structural configuration, as shown in Figure 18–1. The common configuration consists of a monomer composed of two identical heavy chains and two identical light chains connected by disulfide bonds or bridges in the hinge region. The chains are polypeptides; the light chains have a molecular weight of approximately 22,500 daltons and the heavy chains range from 50,000 to 75,000 daltons. As shown in Figure 18–1, IgG is a simple monomer while IgM is a pentamer (made up of five monomers). Each monomer has reactive sites capable of combining with corresponding antigens.

The chemical structure of the heavy chains is responsible for the differences in the various classes of antibodies. However, the light chains are of only two types (κ and λ) that are common to all classes of immunoglobulins.

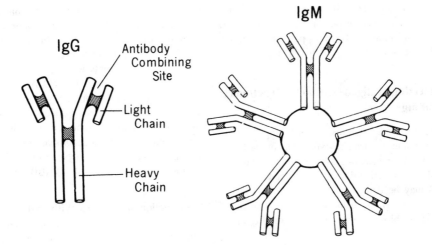

FIG 18–1.
Examples of antibody molecular structure. Two antibody molecules shown to have blood group activity are IgG and IgM. IgG is a simple monomer composed of two heavy chains and two light chains connected by disulfide bonds or bridges. IgM is in the form of a pentamer. Each has reactive sites capable of combining with corresponding antigens.

Monoclonal and Polyclonal Antibodies

Polyclonal antibodies are derived from multiple ancestral clones of antibody-producing cells. Although of a particular specificity, polyclonal antibodies contain a mixture of about two-thirds κ light chains and only one-third λ light chains. Most antibodies found in serum are of the polyclonal type. Polyclonal antibodies recognize a broader range of antigenic determinants than do monoclonal antibodies directed against the same antigen. Polyclonal antibodies are characteristically produced in infectious diseases. In blood banking, the antisera that are used in the Coombs' antiglobulin test, and those used for red cell typing and HLA typing are generally polyclonal antibodies.

Monoclonal antibodies are of a more homogeneous, restricted nature. They are more precise in recognition of the corresponding antigen than the polyclonal antibody directed to the same antigen. They are derived entirely from a single ancestral antibody-forming parent cell. Unlike polyclonal antibodies, monoclonal antibodies of a given specificity are entirely either κ or λ light chains, but not both. Monoclonal antibodies are secreted into the serum in large quantities when associated with malignant proliferations of plasma cells or their precursors, as in multiple myeloma. They may be encountered in blood banking in patients with chronic cold hemagglutinin disease with IgM antibodies directed against red cells.

Monoclonal antisera, produced by hybridization, are utilized in diagnostic testing because of their greater diagnostic precision.

Natural and Immune Antibodies

A different antibody classification in immunohematology includes *natural* and *immune* antibodies. The natural antibody appears to exist without antigenic stimulus, whereas the immune antibody is the result of stimulation by specific blood group antigens. An example of natural antibodies in blood are the anti-A and anti-B antibodies found in the ABO blood group system. In this system, if the red cell lacks the A antigen, anti-A antibody will be found in the serum. If the red cell lacks the B antigen, anti-B antibody will be found in the serum. Hence the name *natural antibody*. Substances very similar to blood group antigens A and B are so widely distributed in nature that the antibody will develop in anyone if the antigen is not present. Certain bacteria and foods may have A- or B-like antigens. The natural anti-A and anti-B antibodies are routinely used in testing for the ABO blood group. (They are saline solution–active and of the IgM type.) There are several other natural IgM blood group antibodies.

Immune antibodies are also referred to as **unexpected antibodies.** They are usually the result of specific antigenic stimulation, and they result from immunization by way of *pregnancy, transfusion,* or *injection of red cells.* Once immunization exists, it is permanent. Immune antibodies are of the IgG, IgA, or IgM type.

Means of Detecting Antigen-Antibody Reactions in Blood Banking

Two terms that are used in discussing biological reactions are in vivo and in vitro. In vivo means in the living body, and in vitro means in glass (or in a laboratory setting). A biological reaction that normally occurs in the body (in vivo) may be demonstrated in vitro, or under laboratory conditions. Blood banking reactions that are used in determining blood groups and compatibility are in vitro reactions.

Antisera

To determine a person's blood type, some sort of substance must be available to show what antigens are present on the red cell. The substance used for this purpose is referred to as an **antiserum** or *antisera.* An antiserum is a prepared and highly purified solution of antibody. It is named on the basis of the antibody it contains. For example, a solution of anti-A antibodies is called *anti-A antiserum.*

Preparation of Antisera.—Most of the antisera that are used in blood banking are prepared commercially and purchased by the blood bank. In general, antiserum is prepared as follows: (1) animals are deliberately inoculated with antigen and the resulting serum, which contains antibody, is purified and standardized for use as an antiserum. (2) Serum is collected from humans who have been sensitized to an antigen through transfusion, pregnancy, or intramuscular injection. (3) Monoclonal antisera are produced by hybridization, a fusion of a single clone of human neoplastic antibody-producing cells with sensitized splenic lymphocytes obtained from a rodent species.

Antisera Requirements.—Antiserum must meet certain requirements to be acceptable for use. It must be specific for the antigen to be detected—that is, specific under the manufacturer's recommended test conditions. It must have a sufficient titer to detect antigen. It must have a certain avidity for, or strength of reaction with, corresponding red cells. It must also be sterile, clear,

provided in a good container with a dropper, and stable. It should be marked with an expiration date and must never be used after this date. In addition, it must be stored at 4° C when not in use.

Exact requirements for antisera are defined by the Food and Drug Administration (FDA) Center for Biologics Evaluation and Research. When commercial antisera are used, the manufacturer's directions must be followed carefully and quality assurance procedures established and documented. For antisera that are produced locally, and unlicensed, there must be records of reactivity and specificity as described in the AABB manual.

Reaction of Antisera With Red Cells.—When antiserum is mixed with red cells, an antigen-antibody reaction may or may not occur. If a reaction does occur, the corresponding antigen must be present on the red cell, and the result is a positive reaction. If a reaction does not occur, the antigen is absent, and the result is negative. A positive reaction with anti-A antiserum demonstrates the presence of A antigen on the red cell, and so on.

In the original definition of antibody, it was stated that antibody resulting from antigenic stimulation will react with the antigen in an observable manner. In blood banking, two types of observable reactions may occur: **agglutination** and *hemolysis.*

Agglutination

Agglutination is clumping, or close association, of red cells caused by a specific antibody or antigen present on the cells. A positive antigen-antibody reaction results in an immediate combination of antibody and antigen on the red cell, followed by the visible agglutination, which takes longer to form. The IgG antibody, for example, is thought to be a somewhat Y-shaped structure with a reactive site at the end of each arm of the Y (see Fig 18–1). Each reactive site is capable of combining with corresponding antigen. Agglutination is thought to be the result of bridging of the red cells by antibody reacting with antigen sites on adjacent red cells. This bridging causes the red cells to stick together. Several such bridges result in visible clumping. The degree of agglutination varies. Very strong agglutination forms a large mass of cells that can be easily seen macroscopically. Less strong agglutination results in correspondingly smaller clumps of cells that can also be seen macroscopically, and finally in clumps of cells that can be seen only microscopically.

The ability to observe all degrees of agglutination requires great care and experience. It is not a simple task, yet it is imperative that the degree of agglutination be detected.

Hemolysis

Hemolysis is the result of lysis, or destruction, of the red cell by a specific antibody. It is probably the third stage in an antigen-antibody reaction and does not occur in all cases. The antibody causes rupture of the cell membrane with release of hemoglobin. The result is a crystal-clear red solution, with no cloudiness since no cells are present. Whenever hemolysis occurs, it is a positive antigen-antibody reaction. However, it may be overlooked and reported as negative, since agglutination is much more common and hemolysis looks much like a negative reaction with no agglutination. In the case of a negative reaction, however, the cells remain in a smooth, cloudy suspension.

It is also possible to have partial hemolysis, when some cells are hemolyzed and others agglutinate. This is particularly difficult to interpret. Misinterpretation of hemolysis is a cause of false-negative results in the blood bank and may end in disaster for the patient.

Role of Complement in Hemolysis

For hemolysis to occur, a substance called complement must be present in the serum being tested. Complement is a complex substance with at least nine components. It is important in blood banking because some antigen-antibody reactions require the presence of complement to be demonstrated in vitro, and although almost all normal sera contain complement when fresh, complement is destroyed by heat. Therefore, to have complement activity, the serum must be either fresh or stored correctly. Complement will remain active if stored for 24 to 48 hours at 4° C or for 2 months at −50° C. If an antibody is to be detected that utilizes complement, it must be provided in the test medium.

Blood Banking Techniques

In summary, the detection of antigen on red cells requires the demonstration of a positive reaction of the cells with a specific solution of antibodies (antiserum). The technique by which the red cell and antiserum are brought together varies widely, depending on a number of factors. The most important factor is the manner of action of the particular antigen-antibody system being

tested for; in other words, knowledge of the antibodies of the blood group system involved is necessary.

In general, blood group tests are performed either on a microscope slide or in test tubes. When test tubes are used, they are 10 × 75 or 12 × 75 mm. Results are seen as agglutination or hemolysis, as described above. Other methods of detecting antigen-antibody reactions include inhibition of agglutination, immunofluorescence, radioimmunoassay, enzyme-linked immunosorbent assay (ELISA), and solid phase red cell adherence tests using indicator red cells. Each of these is described in the AABB manual.

Many factors affect red cell agglutination, which is thought to occur in two stages. The first stage involves the physical attachment of antibody to red cells, and is referred to as **sensitization.** Sensitization is affected by temperature, pH, incubation time, ionic strength, and the antigen-antibody ratio. These factors are influenced by the testing medium which is employed: isotonic saline solution, low-ionic-strength saline, or albumin solution.

The second stage of agglutination involves the formation of bridges between sensitized red cells to form the lattice which is seen as agglutination. Factors which influence this stage include the distance between the cells, the effect of enzymes, and the effect of positively charged molecules such as hexadimethrine (Polybrene).

In all, many factors affect the reactions that are used to detect an antibody-antigen reaction. These include the use of adequate serum and red cells, the concentration of cell suspensions, the testing medium, the temperature and duration of incubation, the use of centrifugation, the use of reagents and glassware, and the reading and interpretation of agglutination reactions.

The correct conditions are essential for reliable tests. Development of correct techniques requires thorough knowledge of all these considerations as well as of the blood groups. The technique will also depend on the brand of antiserum that is used and the manufacturer's directions, which must be followed for accurate results.

THE ABO BLOOD GROUP SYSTEM

The ABO blood group system was first discovered and described in 1900 and 1901 by Karl Landsteiner. By taking the blood of six of his colleagues, separating serum and cells, and mixing each cell suspension with each serum, Landsteiner was able to divide the blood into three groups: A, B, and O. In 1902 the fourth group, AB, was discovered by von Decastello and Struli, two of Landsteiner's pupils.

ABO Phenotypes

The ABO system consists of the blood groups, or phenotypes, A, B, AB, and O. These four groups may be explained by the presence of two antigens (or factors) on the red cell surface, the A antigen and the B antigen. If a person belongs to group A, the A antigen is present on the red cell. Group B persons have B antigen on their cells. Group AB individuals have both A and B, while group O people have neither A nor B.

ABO Genotypes

The antigen present on the red cell is determined by genes on the chromosomes. Three allelic genes can be inherited in the ABO system: the A, B, and O genes. Since each person has two genes for any trait, one from each parent, the following combinations of alleles are possible: AA, AO, AB, BB, BO, and OO. These combinations represent the possible genotypes in the ABO system.

If the A gene is present on the chromosome, A antigen will be present on the red cell. The presence of B gene results in B antigen on the red cell. The presence of O gene results in neither antigen on the red cell.

However, group O individuals have significant H antigen on their red cells, since H is the precursor of A and B antigen.

ABO Typing Procedures

Red Cell Typing for Antigen

In testing blood for the ABO group, a suspension of red cells in saline solution is prepared. This suspension is tested by mixing one portion with a solution of known anti-A antiserum (anti-A antibodies). A second portion is mixed with known anti-B antiserum (anti-B antibodies). The mixtures are then observed for a reaction. A positive reaction is the occurrence of agglutination or hemolysis. A negative reaction is the absence of agglutination or hemolysis. Results may be grouped as follows:

> Group A blood—positive reaction of cells with
> anti-A antiserum

> Group B blood—positive reaction of cells with
> anti-B antiserum
> Group O blood—negative reaction of cells with
> both anti-A and anti-B antiserum
> Group AB blood—positive reaction of cells with
> both anti-A and anti-B antiserum

In these typing reactions, the blood is merely tested for the presence or absence of A and B antigens. No direct test is made for the presence or absence of the *O* gene. This is phenotyping, or typing by means of tests made directly on the blood. Since blood is tested only for the A and B antigens, genotypes *AA* and *AO* will both type as blood group A. Genotypes *BB* and *BO* both contain B antigen and will type as blood group B. Genotype *AB* will type as group AB, since both antigens are present to react with the appropriate antisera. All blood that types as group O must belong to the genotype *OO*, since the blood will not react with either anti-A or anti-B antiserum.

Landsteiner's Rule

As is the case with any blood group system, corresponding antigens and antibodies cannot normally coexist in the same person's blood. In other words, persons who are blood group A cannot form anti-A antibodies and will not have anti-A antibodies in their serum. However, in the ABO system, unlike other blood group systems, if the A or B antigen is lacking on the red cell, the corresponding antibody will be found in the serum. These are the so-called natural antibodies discussed previously. Adults lacking group A antigen will be found to have anti-A antibody in their sera. The sera of adults with red cells lacking B antigen have anti-B antibody. This occurrence of natural anti-A or anti-B antibody when the corresponding antigen is lacking from the red cell is known as *Landsteiner's rule*. It exists only in the ABO system.

Serum Typing for Antibody

These naturally occurring anti-A and anti-B antibodies are important for several reasons, especially for ABO blood grouping in the laboratory. It is essential to avoid giving a blood transfusion to a person whose serum contains an antibody for an antigen present on the transfused red cells. If this occurred, there would be an immediate and severe hemolytic transfusion reaction. It is absolutely essential that the correct ABO blood type be trans-

TABLE 18–2.

ABO Typing Reactions

Blood Group	Antigen on Red Cells	Antibody in Serum	Antigen, Front, or Direct Typing		Antibody, Back, or Indirect Typing		Possible Genotype
			Reaction of Undetermined Cells With Anti-A Antiserum	Reaction of Undetermined Cells With Anti-B Antiserum	Reaction of Undetermined Serum With A_1 Cells	Reaction of Undetermined Serum With B Cells	
A	A	Anti-B	+	−	−	+	*AA, AO*
B	B	Anti-A	−	+	+	−	*BB, BO*
AB	A and B	Neither	+	+	−	−	*AB*
O	Neither	Anti-A and anti-B	−	−	+	+	*OO*

fused, or a severe reaction and death might result. For these reasons, the occurrence of natural anti-A and anti-B antibodies is made use of in the ABO typing procedure. In addition to testing red cells with known antibody, as described, the serum is tested with known group A_1* and group B red cells to determine what antibodies are present. In these tests, serum from the undetermined blood is separated from the cells. One portion of the serum is mixed with red cells known to contain group A_1 antigen. A second portion of serum is mixed with cells known to contain group B antigen. The mixtures are then observed for a positive or negative reaction as evidenced by agglutination or hemolysis. If there is a positive reaction with known group A_1 cells, the serum contains anti-A antibodies. If there is a positive reaction with known group B cells, the serum contains anti-B antibodies. If the serum reacts with both A_1 and B cells, both anti-A and anti-B antibodies are present. If no reaction occurs with either cell type, both antibodies are lacking. Remembering that in the ABO system the serum contains the corresponding antibody for the A or B antigen lacking from the red cell, the results may be grouped as follows:

> Group A blood—positive reaction of serum with group B cells
> Group B blood—positive reaction of serum with group A_1 cells
> Group O blood—positive reaction of serum with both A_1 and B cells

*A_1 is a subgroup of A antigen that will be defined later. For the present it may be considered synonymous with A antigen.

Group AB blood—no reaction with either A_1 or B cells

Summary

Typing reactions that employ undetermined red cells and known antibody or antiserum are referred to as *antigen, cell, direct,* or *front-typing* reactions. Typing reactions that employ undetermined serum and known red cells are referred to as *antibody, serum, indirect,* or *back-typing* reactions. These reactions are summarized in Table 18–2.

When the ABO group is to be determined, both the cells and the serum should be typed as described. The antigen- and antibody-typing results should then be compared to be sure that mistakes have not occurred and that the results are consistent. This is an excellent way to guard against mistakes in ABO grouping. However, in certain instances the antigen- and antibody-typing results show discrepancies.

Natural Antibodies of the ABO System

One cause of cell and serum discrepancies in ABO typing procedures involves the natural antibodies, which are expected to occur in most adults. They cannot be expected to exist in newborn infants, since infants do not normally begin to produce antibodies until they are 3 to 6 months of age. The titer of natural antibodies normally increases gradually through adolescence and then decreases gradually. For this reason, serum-grouping results may also show discrepancies in very elderly patients.

Variation in Titer

It should also be mentioned that there is a variation of the antibody titer in the population. In general, the anti-A titer seems to be higher than the anti-B titer. In the laboratory the antibody titer of serum will only rarely approach the antibody titer of commercially prepared antiserum. For this reason, reactions with cellgrouping tests are generally stronger and easier to read than serum-grouping reactions.

Subgroups

The occurrence of subgroups of group A or group B antigen might also result in discrepancies between cell- and serum-grouping reactions. The classification of blood in the ABO system into groups A, B, AB, and O is an oversimplification. Both group A and group B may be further classified into subgroups. The most important subdivision is that of group A into A_1 and A_2. Both A_1 and A_2 cells react with anti-A antisera. However, anti-A_1 reagent can be prepared from group B human serum or with the lectin of *Dolichos biflores* seeds. This anti-A_1 antibody will react with A_1 cells only. Practically, the subgroups should be kept in mind when there is difficulty in ABO grouping or **compatibility testing.**

H Substance

H substance is a precursor of A and B blood group antigens. Thus, the ABO system is concerned with substances A, B, and H.

Genetically, the ABO system is controlled by at least three sets of genes. We have described one set, the A, A_1, B, and O gene set, which occupies a specific locus or position on corresponding chromosomes.

Another set is described as H and h which are alleles for another locus or position. The H gene is extremely common; over 99.9% of the population inherits the H gene. Very few people carry an h allele, and the hh genotype, called Bombay or O_h is extremely rare. It is a cause of unexpected blood typing reactions, as the cells type as group O. However, the serum of these Bombay individuals reacts strongly with group O red cells, owing to the presence of a potent anti-H antibody. Anti-H antisera are also prepared from the anti-H lectin of *Ulex europeaus*. Anti-H antisera will not agglutinate red cells from Bombay individuals, but will give a strong reaction with group O red cells.

Finally, the Se and se alleles occupy a third locus. The Se and se genes regulate the presence of A, B, and H antigenic material in the body secretions. About 78% of the population has inherited the Se gene (SeSe or Sese). These persons are secretors who have H, A, or B substance produced by their secretory cells. Thus, corresponding H, A, or B substance will be found in the saliva of these persons.

Summary

It is because of the existence of subgroups that A_1 test cells must be used in ABO serum grouping. Subgrouping tests will involve the use, for example, of anti-AB serum, absorbed anti-A serum, and lectins.

It must be stressed that if discrepancies between the results of cell and serum grouping occur, they must be resolved. These problems should be referred to a person with sufficient training and experience in the area of blood banking.

Immune Antibodies of the ABO System

Thus far, only natural anti-A and anti-B antibodies have been discussed. However, anti-A and anti-B antibodies may also be of the immune type. Serum may contain immune antibodies in addition to the natural ones. Natural antibodies are normally found in the serum of adults if the red cell lacks the corresponding antigen, and they probably arise from the inevitable stimulation by ABH substances widely distributed in nature. Immune anti-A or anti-B antibodies result from specific antigenic stimulation. This stimulation may occur through incompatible transfusion, pregnancy, or injection of ABH substances or substances having ABH activity.

Physical and Chemical Properties

Immune and natural antibodies differ in physical and chemical properties and in their serologic behavior. In addition, natural ABO antibodies react best if the red cells are suspended in saline solution and the test is carried out at room temperature or 4° C. Immune antibodies differ in that they react better if cells are suspended in albumin or serum and incubated at 37° C. There are other differences in mode of reaction in the laboratory, and they must be taken into account when the occurrence of an immune-type anti-A or anti-B antibody is suspected or possible—for example, in cases of hemolytic disease of the newborn (HDN) with ABO incompatibility and in screening blood for low titers of anti-A and anti-B.

Size

The natural antibody is a large molecule with a molecular weight of about 900,000, whereas the immune antibody has a molecular weight of about 150,000. Probably because of this size difference, natural antibodies are unable to cross the placental barrier, whereas immune antibodies may cross it. This is important in HDN. Natural antibodies are of the IgM type, whereas immune antibodies are of the IgG type.

Universal Donors and Recipients

One concept that must be discussed in conjunction with the ABO system is that of the "universal donor" and the "universal recipient." These are terms familiar to most people, yet to the blood banker the concept is considered oversimplified and is therefore avoided. The concept is made use of only in cases of extreme emergency.

When blood is to be transfused, there are two questions that must be kept in mind: (1) Does the patient's serum contain an antibody against an antigen on the transfused red cell? and (2) Does the serum to be transfused contain an antibody against an antigen on the patient's red cells? The first situation is the more serious one. It can result in a major reaction and in the death of the patient. This is because all the transfused blood will be destroyed by antibody in the patient's circulatory system, resulting in accumulation of toxic waste products and probably in severe renal failure and death.

The second situation, in which the donor serum contains antibody against the patient's red cells, is not as serious. A minor reaction would occur, because only a small amount of blood compared to the patient's total blood volume is infused. As a result, only a small proportion of the patient's red cells are actually destroyed by donor serum, and this is offset by the benefits of the donor red cells that remain intact and viable.

These transfusion situations are made use of in the concepts of universal donor and recipient. Universal donor blood is group O blood. It is felt that group O red cells can be safely transfused into a person with any ABO blood type, because patient's serum cannot contain an antibody to group O cells. In other words, a major reaction cannot occur. However, group O blood does contain anti-A and anti-B antibodies. Therefore, if it is given to group A persons, a minor reaction can occur with anti-A antibodies. In the case of group B persons, there can be a minor reaction with anti-B antibodies, while the AB person can have a minor reaction with both anti-A and anti-B.

Because these minor reactions can occur, it is preferable that group O blood that is to be used as universal donor blood have most of the plasma removed. This is common practice as whole blood is very rarely transfused. In virtually all cases, the transfusion of red cells, without plasma, is preferable. If this is not possible, the donor blood must be screened with certain additional tests. There is no universally accepted method of screening for "safe" blood for such use. An additional problem is the possible presence of immune anti-A or anti-B antibodies in addition to the natural forms.

In the case of the group AB patient, it is even more dangerous to transfuse group O blood, since both anti-A and anti-B antibodies are present to react with the patient's red cells. For this reason, if group AB blood cannot be secured for transfusion it is preferable to use either group A or group B red cells, rather than group O. The so-called universal recipients are those with group AB blood, since they may be infused with group A, B, or O red cells in emergency situations.

In summary, it should be stressed that ABO type-specific blood should be used whenever possible. Whenever group O blood is used for the A, B, or AB patient and A or B blood for the AB patient, a certain risk does exist. Although screening methods are available to test the titer of anti-A and anti-B, these methods are not perfect, and a severe transfusion reaction may still take place. Transfusion of non-type-specific blood includes situations in which group-specific blood is not available and blood must be transfused, or there may not be enough time to type the patient's blood and test for compatibility, or the patient's blood group cannot be accurately determined. In cases of ABO HDN, group O red cells are generally used. Finally, there may be such unusual circumstances as disasters or military situations in which blood cannot be typed for use before it is transfused.

THE RH BLOOD GROUP SYSTEM

Definition of Rh Factors and Inheritance

Rh Antigens

The Rh blood group system is considerably more complex than the ABO system. Basically, it consists of six related blood group factors, or antigens, C, D, E, c, d, and e, and the corresponding antibodies anti-C, anti-D, anti-E, anti-c, and anti-e (anti-d antibody does not exist). Because of the lack of an anti-d antibody, the existence of d as an antigen is disputed. For this reason, the so-called presence of d should be thought of as the absence of D antigen.

The six antigens that have been defined are not the only antigens in the Rh system, for over 40 variants have been described. To date there are at least 35 related factors in the system. However, C, D, E, c, and e are the most important factors. The weak expression of D antigen, referred to as D^u is also important in blood banking procedures.

Nomenclature

More than one system of nomenclature is used to define the antigens of the Rh-Hr system. There is the Rh system of Wiener, the CDE system of Fisher and Race, and the numerical system of Rosenfield et al. These systems are compared in Table 18–3. The CDE nomenclature is commonly used.

CDE Terminology and Inheritance (Fisher-Race)

The Rh factors that have been discovered on red cells are inherited traits, as are the antigens of the ABO system. However, in the ABO system only three allelic genes could be inherited. In the Rh system, D, C, E, d, c, and e are not all alleles for the same position. Rather, C and c are alleles for the same trait, while D and d are alleles for another chromosome position, as are E and e. The factors are inherited in groups of three, so that a particular chromosome will have one position for the Dd alleles, a second position for the Cc alleles, and a third position for the Ee alleles. In other words, each chromosome carrying the Rh determinants has three closely linked loci for the three related Rh alleles. Everyone has loci for six Rh genes.

Thus, there are three pairs of Rh-Hr factors that are genetically related. Everyone must have at least one of or both of the paired alleles Cc, Dd, and Ee. Since D and d are alleles for the same trait, if D is absent, d must be present, and if d is absent, D must be present. This means that there are three possible combinations of genes for the Dd alleles. A person may possess two D genes, DD, and be homozygous for D. Or a person may possess a D gene and a d gene, Dd, and be heterozygous for D. Finally, the person may possess two d genes, dd, and be homozygous for d. This is also true of the Cc and the Ee alleles: persons may be homozygous or heterozygous for Ee and Cc.

Since the Rh alleles are inherited in groups of three paired factors, and each person has two chromosomes for the Rh factors, each person has a total of six Rh factors. This means that there are eight possible combinations of three factors that can be carried on a particular chromosome. These possible combinations of factors in CDE notation and the corresponding Rh notation, and their approximate frequency are given in Table 18–4. These frequencies are for the white population and differ for other races. They are included to give a general idea of the relative frequencies that might be seen in blood banking. For more definitive frequencies, consult the AABB manual or one of the standard immunohematology textbooks in the Bibliography at the end of this chapter.

One of the eight possible Rh-Hr gene combinations is inherited from each parent, so that the total Rh-Hr genotype for a person would be denoted as CDE/cde or CDe/cDe, and so on. In Wiener's Rh-Hr notation corresponding to the CDE system, the capital letter R refers to the presence of D (Rh_0) antigen, while r refers to the

TABLE 18–3.

Comparative Nomenclature of the Rh Antigens

CDE System (Fisher-Race)	Rh System (Wiener)		Numerical System (Rosenfield et al.)	
D	d	Rh_0	Hr_0	Rh1	
C	c	rh′	hr′	Rh2	Rh4
E	e	rh″	hr″	Rh3	Rh5

TABLE 18–4.

Rh Chromosomes and Approximate Frequency

CDE Notation (Fisher-Race)	Rh-Hr Notation (Wiener)	Approximate Frequency in White Population*
CDe	R^1	Common
cDE	R^2	Common
CDE	R^z	Rare
cDe	R^o	2%
Cde	r′	1%
cdE	r″	1%
CdE	r^y	Very rare
cde	r	Common

*Data from Stratton F, Renton PH: *Practical Blood Grouping.* Springfield, Ill, Charles C Thomas, Publisher, 1958, p 154.

presence of d (Hr_0). The superscript in Wiener's notation refers to the antigens C, c, E, and e.

Thus far, only one theory of Rh-Hr inheritance has been presented here—the theory of Fisher and Race. In this theory the three genes on each chromosome carrying the Rh-Hr determinants are felt to be so closely linked that, in effect, they are inherited as a unit. In other words, the unit of inheritance is considered to be the chromosome rather than the gene in this case. This theory recognizes the existence of six genes, each gene controlling the identical factor in the blood. There is no difference between the gene and the factor.

Rh-Hr Terminology and Inheritance (Wiener)

The other theory of Rh-Hr inheritance is that proposed by Wiener. Weiner differentiated between the genes and the factors that are found in the blood. Wiener felt that there is a single gene on each Rh-Hr chromosome that determines the presence of three factors in the blood. Since there are eight possible combinations of Rh-Hr factors, this theory recognizes eight possible genes. In other words, inheritance of the R^1 gene will result in the presence of C (rh'), D (Rh_0), and e (hr'') antigens on the red cells. A person inheriting an R^1 gene from one parent and an R^z gene from the other would be of genotype R^1/R^z (or *CDe/CDE*), and that person's red cells will contain C (rh'), D (Rh_0), E (rh''), and e (hr'') antigens. Wiener supported his theory of inheritance with the fact that examples of crossovers (mutations resulting from paired chromosomes breaking and recombining) have not been found. In virtually every other case of closely linked inherited traits, crossovers have been found.

In any case, the net effect is the same. People will always have six Rh-Hr factors in their blood. The only real difficulty is that the two theories of inheritance have resulted in more than one system of nomenclature that must be learned by the student.

Historical Background

The discovery of the Rh system was based on work by Landsteiner and Wiener in 1940 and by Levine and Stetson in 1939. A woman who delivered a stillborn fetus was studied by Levine and Stetson. The woman had never received a blood transfusion; however, after delivery she was transfused with her husband's blood. Both the woman and her husband were blood group O. Fol-

lowing transfusion, the woman experienced a severe hemolytic reaction.

Similar transfusion reactions had previously been known to occur following the first transfusion after childbirth, and they did not seem to be associated with the ABO system. Levine and Stetson developed an explanation of their patient's transfusion reaction that has been proved to be correct. They explained the reaction by proposing that the woman's red cells did not contain a "new" antigen. However, the child inherited this new antigen from the father, and the fetal cells containing it found their way into the mother's circulatory system. This resulted in the formation of antibody to the new antigen. Therefore, when the woman was transfused with her husband's blood, her serum contained an antibody to the new antigen contained on her husband's red cells. It was also found that the woman's serum agglutinated not only her husband's red cells but the red cells of 80 of 104 ABO-compatible bloods. Levine and Stetson did not name this new antigen.

The naming of this new factor eventually resulted from studies by Landsteiner and Wiener in 1940. They inoculated rabbits and guinea pigs with the red cells of rhesus monkeys, and found that the resulting rabbit antibody agglutinated the red cells of all rhesus monkeys and, more important, the red cells of about 85% of samples of the white population of New York City. The 85% of the cells that were agglutinated by the anti-rhesus serum were called **Rh-positive**, and the remaining 15% not agglutinated were called **Rh-negative**. Later it was shown that an antibody found in the serum of certain patients who had hemolytic reactions after transfusion of ABO-compatible blood was apparently the same as the antibody in the anti-rhesus serum. It was also found that the antibody contained within the serum of the women studied by Levine and Stetson in 1939 was similar to the antibody in the anti-rhesus serum.

Rh-Positive and Rh-Negative

It is now known that the new antigen described by Levine and Stetson is the D (or Rh_0) antigen. Persons whose red cells contain D antigen either as *D/D* or *D/d* are now termed Rh-positive. They represent approximately 85% of the population. In other words, the antibody responsible for several transfusion reactions is the anti-D (anti-Rh_0) antibody. Persons whose red cells lack the D (Rh_0) antigen are termed *Rh-negative*. Rh-negative persons are then *d/d*. They represent about 15% of the population. (The great majority of Rh-negative persons are *cde/cde*. This genotype is what is meant by a truly Rh-negative person. Other very rare genotypes that are *d/d* must be considered Rh-negative as blood recipients.)

Characteristics of the Rh Antigens

The factors C, D, E, c, and e are all antigenic. This means that they are capable of stimulating the production of antibodies if introduced into the body of a person whose red cells completely lack them. The Rh antigens are permanent inherited characteristics that remain constant throughout life. However, not all the Rh antigens are equally antigenic. The D (Rh$_0$) antigen is the strongest and will generally result in immunization if introduced into a foreign host. For this reason the term *Rh-positive* merely refers to the presence of D antigen without respect to the other Rh factors. The antigenic strength of D also makes it imperative that blood be tested for Rh type before transfusion. Rh-negative persons should not be transfused with Rh-positive (D-positive) blood, for they will certainly develop anti-D antibodies over 80% of the time according to the AABB manual. This would not be lethal at the time of the first transfusion; however, subsequent transfusion with D-positive blood would result in a transfusion reaction. In the case of the woman who was sensitized by an Rh-positive fetus, transfusion with D-positive blood resulted in a hemolytic reaction with the first transfusion.

While D is the most antigenic of the Rh antigens, the other factors (except d) are also antigenic. If strength is considered in terms of antibody frequency, anti-c is most common, followed by anti-E, anti-C, and finally anti-e. Combinations of antibodies in the same blood are also seen.

Weak Expression of D Antigen (D^u)

Not all red cells that contain D antigen react equally well with anti-D blood grouping reagent. Some of these cells may even appear to be D-negative, depending on methodology. This weak reactivity with anti-D sera is refered to as D^u. An explanation is not simple, nor is D^u a single entity. It can be the result of several different genetic circumstances, or result from a position effect on the chromosome. The degree of reactivity results in the terms *high-grade* and *low-grade* D^u. Although typing of red cells for transfusion only tests for the presence of D antigen, donor blood must be tested with techniques that demonstrate D^u. These cells require antiglobulin testing to show agglutination.

Characteristics of the Rh Antibodies

Like all antibodies, the Rh antibodies are made from the gamma globulin portion of the blood plasma. They are specific for the antigen against which they were formed. Unlike the ABO antibodies, all Rh antibodies are immune or unexpected antibodies. There are *no* naturally occurring Rh antibodies. They all result from specific antigenic stimulation, whether by transfusion, pregnancy, or injection of antigen. The lack of natural antibodies in the Rh system is important for several reasons. Practically, it means that antibody typing is impossible in the Rh system. All typing methods in this system depend upon antigen-typing or cell-typing procedures involving unknown antigen and known antiserum.

Rh Typing Procedures

Commercial antiserum is available for the C, D, E, c, and e factors. There is no way of testing for the d factor, since no anti-d antibody has been found. However, routine testing for Rh antigens other than D is not recommended. Antisera other than anti-D may be scarce, and the time and cost involved is unnecessary unless specifically indicated.

Types of Rh Typing Reagents (Antisera)

Two types of Rh antibodies are available commercially. High protein antisera are used for routine D and D^u testing. The sera may be used for slide, rapid tube, or microplate methods. The sera contain 20% to 24% concentrations of protein, and other macromolecular additives accelerate the antigen-antibody reaction. An Rh control supplied by the manufacturer must be used along with high protein antisera and the manufacturer's directions must be followed.

Saline-reactive Rh antisera are also commercially available. These are low protein, saline-reactive antisera that require a test tube method. Saline-reactive antisera are designed to determine the Rh status of red cells that are known or suspected to be giving false or unreliable reactions with reagents containing a high concentration of protein.

High Protein Antisera

It was found that some of the Rh antibodies, although not detectable in saline suspensions of red cells, could be demonstrated if a slightly different technique was used. Rather than saline solution, the cells were suspended in serum or a medium containing sufficient protein. The antibodies that were detectable only when suspended in protein were termed *incomplete,* or *albumin-active,* antibodies, as opposed to the *complete,* or *saline solution–active,* antibodies. Later, another class of antibody was found to be demonstrable only by means of antihuman globulin, or Coombs' reagent. This type of antibody was termed *incomplete univalent.* It is now known that all antibodies have more than one valence (i.e., reactive site), although some are detectable in saline suspension, others require sufficient protein, and still others are demonstrable only by means of the antihuman globulin test.

Commercial antisera of the albumin-active, high protein variety contain IgG-type antibodies. In general, the albumin-active antisera are more avid preparations, and for this reason many of them may be used with either a slide or the test tube technique. In addition, the reaction takes place in less time than with saline solution–active antibody, and the incubation time is shortened. The tube methods with albumin-active antiserum may not even require incubation at 37° C but may produce a reaction at room temperature. In general, Rh antibodies will not react unless the preparation is warmed to (or incubated at) 37° C. Antisera of the incomplete, or albumin-active, variety are labeled "for slide or rapid tube test (or modified tube test)." Again, it is essential to follow the manufacturer's directions.

High Protein Antiserum Control.—There are several causes of false-positive results when high protein antisera are used. For this reason, a high protein control must always be included. There may be spontaneous agglutination of IgG-coated red cells, or there may be factors in the patient's own serum that affect the test which often uses unwashed red cells suspended in the patient's own serum or plasma. Other causes of false-positive results include strong autoagglutinins, abnormal serum protein that causes rouleaux formation, or antibodies against an additive in the reagent itself.

The best control consists of an immunologically inert control reagent, generally the diluent used for manufacturing the particular antiserum. Thus, it is desirable to use the high protein control provided by the same manufacturer as the maker of the antiserum in use.

Low Protein (Saline-Active) Antisera

Antibody of the saline solution–active type is labeled "for saline tube tests." When this preparation is used, reactions must be carried out on saline suspensions of red cells and the test must be performed in a test tube. Slide tests cannot be performed. The first Rh antibodies discovered were active in saline solution.

Anti-C and anti-E antisera (in addition to anti-D) are normally available in a saline solution–active form. Antisera of this type will be labeled "for saline tube tests," and the tests must be performed in test tubes. In general, equal amounts of antiserum and 2% to 4% suspensions of red cells (one or two drops of each) are mixed in 10- × 75- or 12- × 75-mm test tubes and incubated at 37° C for about 1 hour. After incubation, the tubes may be centrifuged. Most blood banking laboratories use a special high speed centrifuge. This centrifuge is set to run at a constant speed and is used to spin serum-cell mixtures before reading. By using this high speed centrifuge, time can be saved and the results of typing tests determined quickly. The results are very carefully read macroscopically by resuspending the cells and tipping the tubes. Negative results are often confirmed by observation under the microscope. The exact technique will vary with different brands of antiserum, and the manufacturer's directions must be followed.

Nature of the Rh Antibody Molecule

The differences in reactivity of antibodies have been found to depend on the length of the antibody molecule. The molecules that are reactive in saline suspensions of cells are of the larger IgM type. Their length is sufficient to cause bridging of adjacent cells in suspension (agglutination). However, red cells in suspension are known to carry an electrical charge, the *zeta potential,* which causes them to repel each other. The IgM-type antibody molecules are so long that they extend beyond the range of the zeta potential and can react with antigenic sites on adjacent cells. Molecules of the smaller IgG type are so short that they do not extend beyond the zeta potential and cannot react with adjacent cells. To demonstrate the existence of IgG molecules by means of agglutination, the repulsion caused by the zeta potential must be overcome or reduced. It can be reduced by suspending the cells in a sufficiently high protein medium (either their own serum or a commercial protein preparation, or both). Other techniques for the demonstration of IgG include high speed centrifugation and enzyme methods.

Typing Blood for Transfusion

When blood is to be transfused, the patient must be tested for the presence or absence of the D (Rh$_0$) antigen. This is because the D factor is so antigenic that most persons who are D-negative (Rh$_0$-negative) or *d/d* may produce an anti-D antibody if transfused with D-positive blood. All persons who are D-negative *(d/d)* must be transfused with Rh-negative or *d/d* blood. Conversely, since d (Hr$_0$) has never been shown to be antigenic, Rh-positive persons may be safely transfused with Rh-negative *(d/d)* blood.

Since the D (Rh$_0$) factor is the most antigenic of the Rh factors, laboratories test only for the presence or absence of this factor and transfuse Rh-positive or Rh-negative blood accordingly. In most cases this is sufficient, since other Rh antibodies are comparatively rare and are tested for indirectly by compatibility testing or antibody screening techniques. If only the D factor is to be tested for, the incomplete, albumin-active, anti-Rh$_0$ (anti-D) antiserum is usually used. Weaker forms of the D antigen (D^u) are not detectable with saline solution–active anti-D antiserum. If only one test is to be performed, the incomplete, albumin-active form of anti-D must be used. Blood that is negative with this test should be further tested for the presence of the D^u variant by means of the antihuman globulin (Coombs') reaction.

Blood is routinely tested for D antigen with both these antisera as a means of checking the accuracy of the test for D antigen. Since all Rh antibodies are immune ones and it is impossible to antibody-type, it is useful to have a means of checking results for the D antigen. The saline and albumin forms of anti-D antiserum should give the same result. The use of albumin-active anti-D allows for the detection of D antigen in a shorter period of time than with saline anti-D. In the case of the D^u variants of the D antigen, only the incomplete form of anti-D antiserum will give positive results. For a more complete explanation of D^u testing, the AABB manual should be consulted.

Typing for Additional Rh Antigens

By performing additional Rh tests, either the complete Rh genotype may be determined positively, or the most probable genotype may be determined by consulting the frequency charts that are available from these typing reactions. This may be useful in determining the probability of occurrence of HDN in mothers negative for a factor that the father is positive for. In this case, both the mother and father are typed and the most probable genotypes are determined to predict the possibility of HDN in their children. The results of tests with these other Rh-typing sera may be used to check the laboratory results by consulting frequency charts. The occurrence of a very infrequent typing reaction will often point to an error in the typing procedure itself.

Conclusion

In summary, the Rh system is considerably more complex than the ABO system. Everyone has six Rh blood group factors but only two ABO blood group factors. One may be either homozygous or heterozygous for the three paired Rh factors, as for the A, B, and O factors. The ABO system has both natural and immune antibodies, while the Rh system has only immune antibodies. In transfusions, ABO type-specific blood should always be given. With the Rh system, blood is routinely tested for only the presence or absence of D antigen and transfused accordingly. However, blood is screened for the presence of unexpected antibodies before transfusion by means of the antihuman globulin test.

Commercial Rh antiserum may be of either the saline solution–active or albumin-active type. The procedure used depends on the form of antiserum employed. Techniques vary with different brands of antiserum.

Experience is invaluable when testing for the Rh factors. Techniques must be mastered and performed with great care. Short cuts must never be taken, and the methods and reasons for them must be thoroughly understood.

THE ANTIHUMAN GLOBULIN REACTION (COOMBS' TEST)

The **antihuman globulin reaction or test** is also referred to as the antiglobulin test (AGT) or the Coombs' test (named for Robin R.A. Coombs who described the use of antihuman globulin for the detection of weak and incomplete Rh antibodies in serum in 1945, along with Mourant and Race).

Different types of antibodies and their laboratory reactions were discussed under Rh Typing Procedures. Antibodies were classified as complete or incomplete depending on their ability to react in saline suspensions of red cells or the requirement for additional techniques, such as the addition of protein to the test medium. This was related to the size of the antibody molecule and its ability to overcome electrical charges on red cells in suspension (the zeta potential). In general, IgM antibodies are large enough to extend beyond the zeta potential and agglutinate red cells in saline suspensions. However, many IgG antibodies are unable to bring about agglutination unless the zeta potential is reduced by such means as adding protein to the red cell suspension. Even after the addition of protein, some IgG antibody molecules will not bring about agglutination. Antibodies that are unable to cause agglutination in any of the laboratory techniques mentioned thus far are detectable by means of the antiglobulin technique. They have been described in the past as incomplete univalent antibodies; however, they are now known to be bivalent in action, although this can only be demonstrated by the antiglobulin technique.

Principle of the Antihuman Globulin Test

The antibodies that are detectable by the antiglobulin technique react with red cells. However, the reaction is not observable in terms of agglutination. The antibodies coat the red cells by reacting with antigenic sites on the cell surfaces. The other arm of the antibody molecule is not able to react with antigen on a second red cell, with resultant bridging and agglutination. To demonstrate the coating of red cells by this incomplete antibody, some sort of reagent must be available to show that the cells have reacted with antibody, as seen in the example in Figure 18–2. It must be remembered that these incomplete antibodies are capable of reacting in the body and, if present, may result in severe transfusion reactions.

In developing a reagent to demonstrate the coating of incomplete antibody on red cells, use is made of the fact that all antibodies are some form of human globulin. The reagent need only be an antibody to human globulin. This is the basis of the antiglobulin, or Coombs', test. The reagent is an antibody to human globulin, or antihuman globulin antibody. This antiglobulin antibody will react with any antibody coating a red cell. Since it is sufficiently long (it is actually an IgM-type antibody), it will react with antibody coating adjacent red cells, and bridging or agglutination of the red cells results.

Preparation and Nature of Antihuman Globulin Reagent

Antihuman globulin reagent is produced commercially by the companies that produce blood group anti-

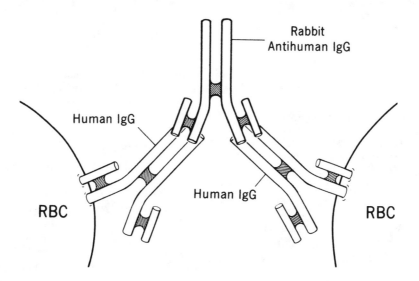

FIG 18–2.
Antiglobulin (Coombs') reaction. Rabbit IgG with anti-human IgG specificity is shown combining or reacting with human IgG on human red blood cells.

sera. The antihuman globulin reagent is prepared by inoculating laboratory animals (usually rabbits) with human serum or a purified globulin fraction of human serum. The laboratory animals produce an antibody to the human globulin, or antihuman globulin antibody. The animal is bled and the serum collected. This serum is purified by various techniques until it is specific for human globulin. The antihuman serum is often prepared in such a way that it reacts with both gamma globulin and complement. The antiglobulin portion of the serum is anti-IgG globulin. However, antibodies other than those of the IgG type must be detected by the antiglobulin test, and it has been found that some of these other antibodies utilize complement in their reaction—they are said to *fix* complement. Antihuman globulin reagent that contains both anti-IgG and anticomplement antibodies is called *polyspecific* antihuman globulin reagent. Current requirements for polyspecific antihuman globulin reagent require antibody to human IgG and the C3d component of human complement. However, the nature of the anti-complement and its inclusion in the antihuman globulin reagent is debatable, and varies. A variety of reagents are available and different types have different uses in the laboratory. These may be polyspecific reagents, or monospecific reagents. Examples of monospecific reagents include anti-IgG with no anticomplement activity or anti-C3d and other complement components with no anti-immunoglobulin activity. These monospecific reagents may be produced as the result of injection of purified fractions of human serum into rabbits, or by the production of murine (mouse) monoclonal antibodies. Monospecific antibodies may be pooled to form polyspecific reagents.

Antihuman Globulin Test Procedures

There are two ways in which the antiglobulin test is performed. These are the *direct* and the *indirect* method. Both tests are essentially the same; only the starting points differ. With the direct test, the starting point is red cells suspected of being coated with antibody. With the indirect test, the starting point is a serum which may contain antibody. With the indirect test, the serum must first be reacted with a suitable red cell indicator, and then the test is carried out as for the direct procedure.

The Direct Antihuman Globulin Test

The direct antihuman globulin test or direct antiglobulin test (DAT) is performed on red cells that are suspected of being coated with antibody. It demonstrates an in vivo antigen-antibody reaction; antibody has coated red cells in the body.

The direct test is used to investigate transfusion reactions, and to diagnose autoimmune hemolytic anemia, HDN, and drug-induced hemolytic anemia.

In performing the test, the cells are first washed meticulously with saline solution to remove all traces of serum (human globulin) from the test medium. Any serum remaining will react with the antihuman globulin reagent, causing false-negative results.

The test is performed in test tubes measuring 10 × 75 or 12 × 75 mm. The cells are washed by completely filling the test tube with a forceful stream of saline solution, resulting in a homogeneous suspension of cells in saline solution. The tube is then centrifuged, and the cells are packed at the bottom of the tube. After centrifuging, the tube is inverted and all the saline solution is decanted in one motion, shaking the tube to remove all saline solution. The tube is then turned upright and shaken to resuspend the cells. The tube must never be covered with the finger or palm of the hand at any stage of mixing, for protein from the skin can inactivate or neutralize the antiglobulin reagent.

The cells are washed with saline solution in this manner at least three times. More washing may be necessary if periodic evaluation of the washing technique shows that three times is not adequate. An alternative way to wash and centrifuge the cells is to use one of the cell-washing centrifuges that are available. These centrifuges can be preset to the desired number of washes and are extremely useful for antiglobulin tests. After the final washing, the saline solution is decanted as completely as possible. The cells are shaken to facilitate resuspension and the antiglobulin reagent is added. The test tube is then incubated and centrifuged as the manufacturer's directions specify, and the results are read macroscopically and microscopically for the presence or absence of agglutination.

The Indirect Antihuman Globulin Test

The indirect antihuman globulin test or indirect antiglobulin test (IAT) is an in vitro test of unknown serum for an antigen-antibody reaction. It tests for antibodies that are freely circulating in the plasma and react with specific antigens on red cells in a test tube. Antibodies may be present in serum when sensitized by transfusion or pregnancy. Patients with autoimmune hemolytic anemia may have free circulating antibody in addition to antibodies coating their red cells. In any case, the indirect test begins a step before the direct method, although it eventually requires the same washing technique and reaction with antihuman globulin reagent.

The indirect antihuman globulin test is the final stage of many antibody detection procedures and has several uses. It is a step in compatibility testing (crossmatching) for transfusion. It is used to detect and identify antibodies in the serum of potential blood donors and transfusion recipients. The demonstration of certain red cell antigens with known antisera, such as Kell typing and D^u testing requires the indirect test. It is also used in the titration of incomplete antibodies.

The indirect test begins with a serum suspected of containing antibodies. The serum is mixed with red cells that contain antigen for the suspected antibody in the serum. The test cells are suspended in saline solution, albumin, or serum (depending on the antibody), mixed with the suspected serum, and incubated for a sufficient period of time for a reaction to occur. Incubation is usually for 15 to 30 minutes at 37° C, but this varies with the antigen-antibody system involved. If the serum contains an antibody for an antigen on the test cells, there will be a reaction—a coating of antibody on the test cells. To demonstrate the reaction, the cells must be washed with saline solution and treated in the same way as in the direct test.

Antibody-Coated Control Cells

One major source of false-negative reactions with the antihuman globulin test is inactive antihuman globulin reagent. The whole vial of antisera may be inactive due to poor storage or contamination by serum globulins. In a given test, the antihuman globulin reagent may be inactive because it has reacted with globulins remaining after inadequate washing of cells. A control which consists of red cells that have been coated with human IgG antibody is used to detect such false-negative reactions. Thus, all tubes which appear to be negative, in both the direct and indirect tests, are reacted with coated control red cells after the final microscopic reading. If the antisera are reactive, agglutination should be seen with the coated control cells. No agglutination after addition of coated control cells indicates inactivation of the antihuman globulin reagent and the total test procedure must be repeated.

Conclusion

Neither the indirect nor the direct antihuman globulin test is specific for any one antibody. They give the same reaction with any antibody contained in human serum. To determine the identity of the antibody responsible for a positive reaction, the antigens present on the red cells must be known. This is done by a process of elimination, using various commercial red cell preparations containing known antigens.

The test is not simple. The reagent is a particularly unstable preparation and must be stored with great care. It is inactivated in several different ways. The AABB manual lists 12 causes of false-negative and 10 causes of false-positive results. All these must be understood before the antihuman globulin test can be performed with reliability. Because of these numerous sources of error, quality assurance procedures must be followed and controls included when the test is performed.

HEMOLYTIC DISEASE OF THE NEWBORN

Pathophysiology

Hemolytic disease of the newborn (HDN), also called *erythroblastosis fetalis,* occurs when a child inherits an antigen for which its mother is negative. The disease most commonly involves factors of the Rh and ABO blood group systems, although it may result from incompatibilities in virtually any blood group system. For this disease to occur, however, the child must be positive for an antigen for which the mother is negative.

This condition develops while the fetus is in the uterus. The mechanism involves sensitization or immunization of the mother to foreign antigen present on her child's red cells. Although the circulatory systems of a mother and her child are separate, and only small molecules such as nutrients can cross the placenta, there can be some seepage of fetal red cells into the mother's circulatory system. This is most likely to occur very late in pregnancy or at the time of birth. If any incompatible fetal red cells do find their way into the mother's circulatory system, she may well develop an antibody to the antigen on them. Once such immunization occurs, it is permanent. The antibody formed by the mother is of the IgG type and it can cross the placenta into the circulatory system of the fetus, where it reacts with corresponding antigen on the red cells of the fetus, with resultant destruction of the cells. HDN is the condition that exists when maternal antibody crosses the placenta and reacts with antigen on fetal red cells. This was the cause of death of the child delivered by the woman studied by Levine and Stetson in 1939, which led to the discovery of the Rh blood group system.

Father heterozygous for D (*D/d*)
Mother homozygous for d (*d/d*)
50% chance of hemolytic disease

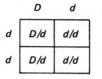

Father homozygous for D (*D/D*)
Mother homozygous for d (*d/d*)
100% chance of hemolytic disease

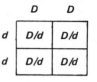

FIG 18–3.
Chance of development of hemolytic disease of the newborn. Chance is based on genotypes for the D factor.

Rh Factors in Hemolytic Disease of the Newborn

HDN most commonly involves the Rh blood group system. It most often involves the D antigen, the mother being negative for D (*d/d*) and the father positive for D. The child inherits this factor from the father and is D-positive (*D/d*). If any of the D-positive red cells of the fetus cross into the mother's circulatory system, she may develop an immune anti-D antibody. This antibody, of the IgG type, crosses the placenta and reacts with the red cells of the fetus. Fortunately, sensitization usually occurs only very late in pregnancy or at the time of delivery, so the first child is rarely affected by HDN. Further, any child who is D-negative cannot be affected by anti-D antibody in the mother's circulatory system. For this reason, genotyping parents in possible cases of HDN is very useful in predicting the chance of occurrence of the disease. For example, if the husband is heterozygous for the D antigen (*D/d*) and the mother is D-negative (*d/d*), chances are that only half the children will inherit the D antigen (Fig 18–3). On the other hand, if the father is homozygous for D (*D/D*), all the children will inherit the D antigen and there is a 100% chance of HDN (see Fig 18–3). (Only children who are D-positive can be affected by the disease, since only they are positive for a factor that the mother is negative for.)

It has been mentioned that the first child is rarely affected by HDN. In fact, fewer than 20% of Rh-negative women actually become immunized during pregnancy. Although a woman can usually have one or two children who are both Rh-positive and encounter no difficulties, her immunization is permanent. Further, once the disease develops in one child, subsequent children positive for the antigen are likely to be affected at least as severely. More important, if a woman has been sensitized before pregnancy as a result of transfusion of incompatible blood or injection of antigenic material, even the first child can be severely affected.

It has been mentioned that the anti-D antibody is the most common cause of HDN. Other antibodies causing this disease include anti-c, anti-K (Kell), anti-E, and even incompatibilities in the ABO system.

Prevention of Rh Immunization (Use of Rh Immune Globulin)

In the 1960s a dramatic decrease in the incidence of HDN was seen following the introduction of **Rh immune globulin (RhIG),** which could prevent immunization to the D antigen during pregnancy. This was an extremely important advance, and the incidence of immunization by pregnancy to the Rh antigen D is very different now. It was found that if RhIG is injected into Rh-negative women who deliver Rh-positive babies within 72 hours of delivery, they are well protected against Rh problems in subsequent pregnancies. The use of RhIG is based on immunosuppression of an Rh-negative mother to prevent immunization (sensitization) by her child's red blood cells. The mother is passively immunized by the administration of RhIG when sensitization by fetal red cells is most likely. This generally occurs at the time of delivery.

About 1 in 10 pregnancies involve an Rh-negative woman and an Rh-positive father. According to the AABB manual, an Rh-negative woman with an Rh-positive infant who is not protected by passive immunization has a 7% to 8% chance of developing anti-D antibodies. When given RhIG post partum, this risk drops to about 1%. This risk is further reduced to 0.1% when RhIG is administered ante partum at 28 to 29 weeks' gestation. It has been found that infants whose mothers have received up to two antepartum doses of RhIG show no adverse effects.

At present, RhIG is injected intramuscularly within 72 hours of delivery in mothers (1) who are D-negative, (2) who have no detectable anti-D antibody, and (3) whose newborn infants are D-positive. Antepartum treatment at 28 weeks' gestation has also been advocated by the American College of Obstetricians and Gynecologists. If so done, a sample of blood obtained immediately prior to treatment should be tested for ABO group, Rh type, antibody screen, and identification of antibody if present.

RhIG is supplied as a sterile, clear 1-mL solution to be injected intramuscularly. It is a concentrated solution (300 μg/mL) of IgG anti-D derived from human plasma. It does not transmit hepatitis or HIV infection.

The anti-D antibody can be detected 12 to 60 hours after the administration of RhIG and is sometimes found for as long as 5 months thereafter. If it is detected 6 months after delivery, active immunization and failure of the RhIG can be assumed. Such failures are infrequent, but they can occur if RhIG is given too late or in too small a dose, or if Rh immunization has already occurred during the pregnancy. Most of the D-positive fetal cells enter the maternal circulation at the time of delivery. The amount of fetal blood present in the maternal circulation is important for the RhIG dosage.

If the amount of Rh-positive fetal red cells entering the mother's circulation is greater than 30 mL of whole blood, the standard dose of RhIG is not enough to prevent anti-D antibody formation. Thus, it is important to determine the presence and amount of fetomaternal hemorrhage. This may be done by use of the rosette test and acid elution or an enzyme-linked antiglobulin test.

The Rosette Test

This is used as a screening test for the detection of large fetomaternal hemorrhage. The test will detect fetomaternal hemorrhage of approximately 10 mL. It uses D-positive indicator red cells to form rosettes around individual D-positive fetal cells that may be present in the maternal circulation. The test gives only qualitative results. For quantitative results, an acid elution test (Kleihauer-Betke) or enzyme-linked antiglobulin test is necessary to determine the amount of the hemorrhage.

Acid Elution Stain (Modified Kleihauer-Betke Method)

This stain is based on the fact that fetal hemoglobin is resistant to acid elution (separation of a substance by extraction) whereas adult hemoglobin is not. That is, when a thin blood smear is exposed to an acid buffer, the adult red cell loses its hemoglobin into the buffer, leaving only the red cell stroma, whereas the fetal red cell is unaffected and retains its hemoglobin. The smears are examined under the microscope after staining and the percentage of fetal cells in the maternal blood is used to calculate the approximate volume of fetal hemorrhage into the maternal circulation. Either clotted blood or anticoagulated blood may be used for this test.

ABO Factors

HDN can also occur as a result of factors in the ABO system. In this case, the mother is usually blood group O and the child inherits the A or B antigen from its father. If this occurs and any fetal cells find their way into the mother's circulation, she develops an immune IgG antibody in addition to her natural IgM anti-A or anti-B antibody. If an immune IgG antibody is produced, it crosses the placenta and reacts with corresponding antigen on the red cells of the fetus. Fortunately, although ABO sensitization may occur fairly often, hemolytic disease caused by ABO incompatibility is less severe and the child may be only mildly affected and require little or no treatment.

Treatment of Hemolytic Disease of the Newborn

When HDN does occur, it varies considerably in severity. In its most severe form, the child is stillborn or aborts early in pregnancy. If the child is alive when born, it may be affected so mildly as to require little treatment, or it may be severely affected by the products of destruction of the red cells and by anemia. The cell destruction results in hemolytic anemia accompanied by abnormal levels of serum bilirubin with the clinical appearance of jaundice. The bilirubin will result in irreversible brain damage if present in sufficient concentration. If the child survives and is not treated adequately, the brain damage will result in severe mental retardation.

Treatment in severe cases of HDN includes blood transfusion. This is referred to as an *exchange transfusion,* for most of the child's blood is replaced with the transfused blood. The exchange transfusion will serve to correct the anemia and remove the abnormal levels of serum bilirubin, thus preventing brain damage.

The type of blood used for transfusion depends on the antibody responsible for the disease. The outstanding consideration is that the blood be negative for the factor against which the antibody has been formed. In other words, the child is given blood that is compatible with the mother. In the case of HDN caused by the formation of anti-D antibody in the mother's serum, the child is transfused with red cells that are specific for its own ABO type but negative for the D antigen. This is because not all of the child's blood is replaced at the time of exchange, and some maternal antibody is left. Therefore, red cells are given that will not react with the remaining antibody yet will not harm the child. In cases of ABO incompatibility that require exchange, the mother is usually group O and the child group A or B. In such cases the child is transfused with group O red cells of the child's Rh type.

In cases of severe HDN, it is sometimes necessary to attempt to treat the fetus before birth. This *intrauterine transfusion* may be necessary to correct severe anemia and prevent death in utero when the risk of early delivery is too great. In such cases, amniocentesis is performed based on maternal antibody titer, obstetric history, and ultrasound. The amniotic fluid is tested for bilirubin level and fetal maturity. If the fetus appears to be severely affected, an intrauterine transfusion may be indicated. In so doing, packed red cells are infused through the fetal abdominal wall into the peritoneum. Direct transfusion into the umbilical vein may also be attempted.

Laboratory Tests in Hemolytic Disease of the Newborn

Many laboratory tests are performed in cases of HDN, on the parents' (primarily the mother's) blood prior to birth and on the child's blood after birth. The first step is to type the mother and father for ABO and Rh during pregnancy to see if HDN can occur. In other words, is the father positive for any factor that the mother is negative for? Depending on the results of genotyping the mother and father, with reference to frequency charts and family studies, the probability of occurrence of the disease can be predicted. The mother's serum is usually screened by means of the indirect antihuman globulin test to see if an antibody exists. If an antibody is found, it is identified and the titer is determined. This titer is rechecked throughout pregnancy as an indication of the possible severity of the disease.

After birth, several tests may be performed on the child's blood, in addition to further tests on the maternal serum. Initially, a sample of umbilical cord blood is tested for ABO group and Rh type, and a direct antihuman globulin test is performed. Some other laboratory tests include hemoglobin determinations, blood smear examination and differential, reticulocyte count, and serum bilirubin determinations on the child's blood.

The decision to perform exchange transfusion will depend on a combination of laboratory results and on the clinical condition of the child. Preparation can and should be made before birth, so that the exchange can be done as soon as possible if necessary.

COMPATIBILITY TESTING AND CROSSMATCHING

Compatibility Testing: Definition and General Considerations

Whenever blood is to be transfused, two considerations must be kept in mind. First, blood must be selected that will not be harmful to the patient or result in a transfusion reaction. Second, blood must be selected that will be of maximum benefit to the patient. For these reasons, whenever blood is to be transfused it must be tested for compatibility between the donor and recipient (patient). Compatibility testing is much more than crossmatching, which is just one part of the testing procedures. Compatibility testing involves a series of tests that must include the following:

1. Correct identification of donor and recipient.
2. A review of the patient's past history and blood bank records for type and the presence of unexpected antibodies.
3. ABO and Rh typing of both donor and recipient.
4. Testing of serum (or plasma) of the donor and recipient for the presence of unexpected antibodies (unexpected antibody screen).
5. Crossmatching of the donor red cells with the patient's serum.

In general, compatibility testing is used to help detect (1) unexpected antibodies in the patient's serum, (2) some ABO incompatibilities, and (3) some errors in labeling, recording, or identifying patients or donors. Unfortunately, compatibility testing is not a perfect or foolproof method that guards against all problems that may arise. The most frequent causes of transfusion of incompatible blood are errors of an organizational, clerical, or technical nature. Although these errors may be detected by means of compatibility testing and the crossmatch, this is not always the case. The laboratory must always work with great care to avoid mistakes of this nature. In addition, although ABO incompatibility may be detected in the crossmatch, not all such errors are found by this method. Correct typing and unexpected antibody screening are also necessary.

Incompatibility in the crossmatching procedure will be discovered only if the patient's serum contains an unexpected antibody to the donor's red cells. Compatibility testing will not prevent immunization if the patient is transfused with foreign antigen. For example, an Rh-negative person who has never been exposed to Rh-positive antigenic material will not show incompatibility if crossmatched with Rh-positive blood, but the person may develop an anti-D antibody. Errors of Rh typing will be detected only if the recipient's serum contains an Rh antibody.

No single crossmatching procedure and antibody screening procedure will detect all unexpected antibodies that may be present in the patient's serum. Even if the blood is found to be compatible, testing procedures will not ensure the normal survival of donor red cells. The blood must be processed and stored correctly.

ABO and Rh Typing of Donor and Recipient

When blood is selected for transfusion, the patient and the donor are tested for ABO type and for the presence or absence of the D (Rh_0) antigen. The ABO group is matched and the Rh type is selected with respect to the D factor. Patients whose cells contain the D antigen are given blood positive for the D factor (Rh-positive blood), while patients who are negative for the D antigen are always given blood that is negative for the D antigen (Rh-negative blood). The other antigens that collectively make up a person's complete blood type are not matched when blood is to be transfused.

Unexpected Antibody Screening

When blood is to be transfused, the patient's serum or plasma must be tested for unexpected antibodies. This is done by testing the patient's serum with a panel (or se-

ries) of group O reagent red cells that are known to contain antigens to the most important clinically significant unexpected antibodies. Antibody screening with reagent red cells is a fairly recent and useful practice in blood banking. It allows for testing of the patient's serum in advance of the actual transfusion, allowing for selection of rare donor blood, when necessary. This prior testing for antibodies will often make it unnecessary to perform an antiglobulin crossmatch, as the serum has already been tested for unexpected antibodies with the antiglobulin procedure.

The group O red cells for antibody screening are available as commercially prepared products. They are supplied in sets of two or three vials, suspended in a preservative solution, and must be refrigerated when not in use. There are federal requirements for antigens that must be present on reagent red cells for antibody screening, and additional antigens are used by various investigators. However, it should be remembered that all antibodies of potential clinical significance cannot be detected by antibody screening.

Crossmatching

As mentioned previously, crossmatching is just part of compatibility testing. There are several different ways to perform the crossmatch. No method is perfect or can even be said to be preferable. In general, there are (1) the saline crossmatch, (2) the high protein crossmatch, (3) the antihuman globulin crossmatch, and (4) the enzyme crossmatch.

Major and Minor Crossmatches

Crossmatches have historically been divided into *major* and *minor* crossmatches. This concept is presently outdated, as the screening of patient and donor serum for unexpected antibodies has generally replaced the minor crossmatch procedure.

The major crossmatch involves testing the patient's serum with the donor's red cells. This is used to detect any unexpected antibodies in the patient's serum that will react with antigens on the donor's red cells. In transfusion, the primary consideration must be what the patient's serum will do to the infused red cells, as destruction of infused red cells will result in a severe transfusion reaction.

The minor crossmatch is just the opposite; it tests the donor's serum with the patient's red cells. It is used to detect the presence of an unexpected antibody in the donor's serum that will react with an antigen on the patient's red cells.

The division into major and minor crossmatches is related to the principles involved in considering group O persons as universal donors and group AB persons as universal recipients. The major crossmatch involves testing the donor's red cells with the patient's serum to detect any antibody in the patient's serum that will react with the donor's red cells. The presence of such antibody in the patient's serum would certainly result in a major transfusion reaction, for all the infused donor cells would be destroyed by the patient's antibodies. Of course, even if the patient's serum did contain an unexpected antibody, it would be detected only if the donor's cells contained the corresponding antigen. For this reason, the patients' serum is screened with group O reagent red cells to detect a greater variety of unexpected antibodies than may be detected by means of a major crossmatch of prospective donors.

The various general types of crossmatches are discussed in the paragraphs that follow, although the exact procedures are not given.

Saline Crossmatch

The saline crossmatch involves mixing serum and a 2% to 4% suspension of cells in saline solution in a test tube. The test tube is first incubated at room temperature, centrifuged, and observed for the presence of agglutination or hemolysis. At this stage ABO incompatibility will be observable, as will incompatibility caused by antibodies of the P, MNSs, Lewis, Lutheran, or Wright systems.

If the test is negative at this point, the test tube is further incubated at 37° C for a sufficient period of time and observed once again. Saline solution–reacting antibodies of the Rh-Hr and Lewis systems will be detected, and antibodies of the P, MNSs, or Kell systems may sometimes react at this stage.

If the saline solution or serum crossmatch is still negative, it may be further tested by means of the antihuman globulin crossmatch.

High Protein (Albumin) Crossmatch

The high protein or albumin crossmatch involves mixing serum with a suspension of red cells in their own serum and then adding a commercial preparation of albumin. (Or, albumin may be added to the saline crossmatch

tubes after initial incubation and observation.) The preparation is mixed, centrifuged, and observed. It is then incubated at 37° C for a sufficient length of time and observed again. The high protein crossmatch will detect most Rh antibodies, including some that are not detected by the saline solution method. The preparation may also be further tested by the antihuman globulin test.

Antihuman Globulin Crossmatch

The antihuman globulin crossmatch may be an extension of either the saline or the albumin crossmatch. After incubation of either type at 37° C, the cells are thoroughly washed with saline solution, as described for the direct and indirect antihuman globulin tests. The antihuman globulin serum is added and the test carried out as recommended by the manufacturer. This is an indirect test between the patient and prospective donor. The crossmatch will detect almost all Rh antibodies. In addition, it may be the only means of detecting some antibodies, especially in the Duffy, Kidd, and Kell blood group systems.

Enzyme Crossmatches

There are also crossmatching procedures that make use of enzyme preparations such as bromelin, ficin, papain, and trypsin. They may detect some Rh antibodies not found by other methods, but may not detect some antibodies of the MNSs, Kell, and Duffy systems. This type of crossmatch is rarely done in the immunohematology laboratory.

Other Crossmatching Techniques

As in typing procedures, there are several other techniques which may be applied to crossmatching and antibody screening. Low-ionic-strength salt solution may be used rather than albumin to ensure the formation of antigen-antibody complexes. Hexadimethrine has been used as a rapid and sensitive crossmatch method. It is useful in detecting ABO incompatibility when the patient has demonstrated a negative antibody screen. Microplate methods for antibody detection using low-ionic-strength salt solution are also used to screen large numbers of sera for unexpected antibodies. A technique which uses polyethylene glycol is also used for antibody detection and identification. This may be used as a supplement to more conventional methods when weak reactions are encountered.

Summary

A well-defined compatibility testing regimen is required whenever blood is to be transfused. Unfortunately, there is no one ideal method to guarantee that all mistakes or incompatibilities have been discovered. If an incompatibility is discovered at any point, its cause must be determined. This determination is far beyond the scope of this brief outline of compatibility testing. There are numerous technical problems that may be encountered which have not been described. Yet, if compatibility testing has been performed with care, with strict adherence to the procedures established by the particular blood bank, transfusion of blood can be a relatively safe procedure of tremendous benefit to the patient.

BLOOD TRANSFUSION

The therapeutic replacement of blood or its components is indicated in many instances. However, appropriate **blood transfusion** is not a simple matter and requires several considerations. The reason for the transfusion must be carefully evaluated, and the potential benefit should outweigh any potential harm to the patient. Potential harm includes such considerations as the risk of transfusion-transmitted disease, and other possible transfusion reactions. The practice of blood banking is regulated by several different agencies in the United States. These include the National Center for Drugs and Biologics of the FDA, which requires compliance to regulations; the AABB, which has voluntary self-regulation of members; and the Joint Commission of Accreditation of Health Care Organizations (JCAHO).

Transfusion Reactions

Transfusion reactions can generally be characterized as hemolytic, febrile, allergic, or circulatory overload. Although the most life-threatening transfusion reaction is the hemolytic reaction that occurs with the destruction of incompatible red cells by antibodies in the patient's serum (usually ABO incompatibility), several other forms of transfusion reaction, with varying severity to the patient, also exist. These include immediate and delayed effects, both immunologic and nonimmunologic.

Immediate immunologic effects include febrile nonhemolytic reactions, usually to the donor's granulocytes. Anaphylaxis from antibody to IgA, urticaria (hives) from antibody to plasma proteins, and noncardiac pulmonary edema from antibody to leukocytes or complement activation are other immediate immunologic causes of transfusion reactions. Nonimmunologic immediate transfusion effects include marked fever with shock from bacterial contamination, congestive heart failure from increased blood volume, and hemolysis of infused red cells from the physical destruction of blood such as from freezing or overheating or mixing nonisotonic solutions with red blood cells.

In addition to the immediate causes of transfusion reactions, there are delayed adverse effects of transfusion. Delayed hemolysis may occur from prior sensitization to red cell antigens by antibodies which are not present or detectable in the blood immediately prior to transfusion. Graft-vs.-host disease may result from engraftment of transfused functional lymphocytes. Purpura (the presence of purple patches in the skin and mucous membranes) from bleeding as a result of the development of antiplatelet antibodies may occur. Or the patient may be sensitized and form antibodies to donor antigens on red cells, white cells, platelets, or plasma protein. Other delayed nonimmunologic adverse effects include iron overload from multiple (over 100) transfusions and the transmission of disease as a result of transfusion. These include hepatitis, acquired immunodeficiency syndrome (AIDS), and protozoan infections.

Benefits and Reasons for Transfusion

There are many indications for the transfusion of blood or blood components or derivatives. In general these may be divided into four major categories and the component to be transfused will depend on which of these categories applies.

First, transfusion may be used to restore or maintain *oxygen-carrying capacity* or hemoglobin. This is best done by the transfusion of red blood cells with plasma removed. The transfusion of whole blood is both unnecessary and contraindicated, as the inclusion of plasma will increase blood volume with possible circulatory overload.

The second basic indication of transfusion is to restore or maintain *blood volume*. This is necessary in cases of acute blood loss, as seen with massive bleeding, to prevent shock. Although whole blood may sometimes be indicated, as in actively bleeding patients who have lost over 25% to 30% of their blood volume, it is usually preferable to replace lost blood volume with crystalloid (electrolyte) solutions such as 0.9% sodium chloride (isotonic saline) or plasma substitutes. Lost hemoglobin can be replaced later with packed red cells although in most patients, about 20% of blood volume can be replaced with crystalloid solutions alone.

A third indicator of transfusion is to replace coagulation factors in order to maintain *hemostasis*. This is done with a variety of blood components and derivatives which vary with the particular situation in question. These include platelet concentrates, fresh frozen plasma, cryoprecipitate, and factor VIII, and factor IX concentrates.

Finally, transfusion may be indicated in order to restore or maintain *leukocyte function*. This is quite rare but may be necessary for severely granulocytopenic patients with infections that do not respond to antibiotics.

Donor Selection and Identification

The selection and proper identification of the potential blood donor is essential in assuring that the blood which is collected for transfusion is safe and will be of benefit to the recipient. Until about 15 years ago, much of the blood used for transfusion was obtained from donors who were paid for their blood donations. This practice has been almost completely replaced by voluntary donations which have significantly decreased the risk of hepatitis, as it has been demonstrated that paid donors are less likely to give a reliable history.

The selection of the blood donor involves a medical history and miniphysical examination. Two considerations must be kept in mind when the donor is to be selected. They are whether the procedure might be harmful to the donor, and whether the donor's blood might be harmful to the recipient. The actual selection process involves a series of questions to ensure safety to both the donor and recipient. Medical guidelines and requirements for the selection of donors have been developed by the FDA, AABB, American Red Cross, and College of American Pathologists (CAP). It is essential that guidelines and requirements be established for each blood bank and codified in its own standard operating procedures manual.

Collection of Blood

Blood for transfusion must be collected and handled under strictly sterile conditions to prevent contamination. According to the AABB it is collected only by trained personnel working under the direction of a qualified, licensed physician. The collection must be aseptic, must use a sterile closed collection system, and a single venipuncture. If more than one venipuncture is done, a new container and donor set must be used for each skin puncture. The AABB also requires that the phlebotomist sign or initial the donor record, whether or not a full unit is collected. The usual amount of blood drawn for 1 unit of whole blood is 450 mL. This is added to 63 mL of citrate phosphate dextrose (CPD) or CPD adenine (CPDA-1) anticoagulant solution which brings the total volume of a unit of blood to about 500 mL. When the proper amount of blood has been collected, pilot tubes and segments must be filled with up to 30 mL of blood for the various testing procedures that are required before the blood can be used.

Anticoagulants and Preservatives

Blood collected for transfusion must be treated with an anticoagulant. It must be collected into an FDA-approved container. These are usually plastic blood collection bags. They must be pyrogen-free, sterile, and contain anticoagulant sufficient for the amount of blood to be collected. The anticoagulant and preservative solution is generally a combination of citrate and dextrose. Citrate is used as an anticoagulant which binds calcium, thus preventing activation of the coagulation cascade. Dextrose is used to provide an energy source for the red blood cells. Inorganic phosphate buffer is added to increase adenosine triphosphate (ATP) production, which increases red cell viability. Adenine is another additive which is used to improve red cell survival and extend the storage period of blood. As mentioned, two commonly used anticoagulants are CPD and CPDA-1. CPD is approved by the FDA for 21-day storage of red cells at 1 to 6° C. CPDA-1 is approved for storage for up to 35 days at 1 to 6° C.

Labeling

Proper labeling of the collecting container is of the utmost importance. According to the AABB, each unit of blood or blood component must include the following information at a minimum. The name of the product (i.e., whole blood, red cells), the kind and amount of anticoagulant, the volume of the unit, the required storage temperature, the name and address of the collecting facility, the expiration date, and the unique donor identification number, together with an indication of whether the donor is a volunteer, autologous, or paid. The ABO blood group and Rh type are also shown on the label, once these tests are completed. The pilot tubes and segments for testing must also be properly labeled and a stoppered or sealed sample of donor blood retained and properly stored by the transfusion service for at least 7 days after transfusion.

Storage of Blood

Blood bank blood must be stored in a refrigerator with a constant temperature of 1 to 6° C. Some sort of alarm must be available that will go off whenever the temperature is not within these limits. A thermometer for recording the temperature should also be installed. Whole blood, collected with CPD can be stored for only 21 days; whole blood with CPDA-1 for 35 days. After 21 or 35 days, this blood is outdated and must be removed from the blood supply or treated with a rejuvenation solution and the time extended as described below.

Stored whole blood is inspected daily for color, turbidity, appearance of clots, and presence of hemolysis. Blood is removed when it does not meet the appearance criteria established by the laboratory.

Blood Processing Tests

The testing of each unit of donated blood is neither simple nor inexpensive. A series of tests must be performed in order to ensure that the blood will be as safe as possible so that it will truly benefit the patient. These tests include methods which ensure compatibility between donor and recipient (described previously) and tests to screen for transfusion-transmitted diseases. Tests to ensure compatibility include ABO and Rh typing and antibody screening. Screening for transfusion-transmitted disease includes tests for syphilis, hepatitis, and AIDS. Since one unit of blood is normally separated into several components which are transfused into several different recipients, the presence of viruses such as those causing hepatitis or AIDS would be truly disastrous.

Screening for Transfusion-Transmitted Disease

The most important factor in ensuring that blood is free of transmittable disease is the careful selection of the blood donor. The virtual elimination of commercial blood donation has significantly decreased the risk of hepatitis. This, together with procedures to allow for self-deferral of donors who have risk factors for human immunodeficiency virus (HIV), the causative agent of AIDS, has done much to ensure the safety of the blood supply. Nevertheless, blood is routinely screened for transmissible disease. The number of routine screening tests has increased dramatically in the past few years, from a single screening test for syphilis to a battery of tests for hepatitis and HIV.

Tests for Syphilis.—A screening test for syphilis continues to be required by the FDA; however, it is no longer required by the AABB.

Tests for Hepatitis.—At least four viruses have been associated with hepatitis after transfusion. The severity of disease varies, and the actual incidence of transfusion-transmitted hepatitis is not truly known. Nevertheless, transmission of hepatitis remains a risk in transfusion. For this reason, donated blood is screened with several tests for hepatitis virus. At present these include a test for hepatitis B surface antigen (HBsAg) by enzyme immunoassay or radioimmunoassay (RIA), and tests for non-A, non-B hepatitis by hepatitis B core antibody and ALT.

Tests for AIDS.—Because of the long incubation period of HIV, donor selection methods and self-deferral of donors is essential in the screening of blood for HIV. At present, all donated blood is screened with two different serologic tests for HIV. All units of blood must be tested with an FDA-licensed test for HIV-1 antibody and for human T-cell lymphotropic virus type 1 (HTLV-1) antibody.

Autologous Transfusions

A relatively new and now common practice in blood banking is the use of autologous transfusions. This is based on the knowledge that the safest blood a recipient can receive is his or her own blood. Not only does this prevent transfusion-transmitted infectious diseases, but it eliminates the formation of antibodies to antigens in the transfused blood, graft-vs.-host disease, and stimulates erythropoiesis by repeated preoperative phlebotomy. For these reasons, patients who meet certain criteria are encouraged to donate blood for themselves before anticipated surgery if they are likely to need blood transfusion.

Directed Transfusions

These are transfusions where the patient directly solicits blood for transfusion from family or friends. It is the public's response to concern about AIDS. However, it is based on a false assumption that blood donated by family or friends is safer than that from the regular volunteer donor population. This has not been found to be true as the directed donor is under significantly more pressure to donate than an anonymous donor. It is also felt that the extra paperwork and other logistics increase the probability of clerical errors.

Blood Components and Derivatives for Transfusion

From the preceding, it should be evident that whole blood is rarely used when transfusion is indicated. Rather, a variety of preparations including red cells, plasma, albumin, platelet concentrates, leukocytes, and other preparations and derivatives are used. These are summarized in Table 18–5 and in the material which follows. Materials prepared from blood by mechanical methods, especially by centrifugation, are called components, whereas those separated by more complex processes are called blood derivatives or *fractions*. Modern equipment, such as refrigerated centrifuges and plastic bags, has made blood component preparation within reach of most every blood bank laboratory. Blood fractionation is still a complex process and is done by the pharmaceutical industry from plasma pools of thousands of donor units.

The use of plastic bags for blood containers has been the most important advance for component blood therapy. By using plastic instead of glass, several containers can be interconnected in a sterile system. Blood drawn into the primary container bag can be easily separated into components, which are then transferred asepti-

cally into one or more of the satellite container bags. In this way, plasma and cells can be prepared, stored, and administered individually, without the potential for contamination that is always present when the blood container is "entered" for transfusion into the recipient or patient.

Whole Blood

Whole blood is made up of plasma and the formed elements (red cells, white cells, platelets). It is collected aseptically and must be free from transmissible diseases such as hepatitis and AIDS. Clotting is prevented by use of an anticoagulant solution such as CPD or CPDA-1. Whole blood can be stored for up to 21 days with CPD solution or 35 days with CPDA-1 if refrigerated at 1 to 6° C.

In cases of severe hemorrhage, whole blood may be used to replace red cells and plasma. However, whole blood is rarely transfused. It is generally separated into various components and derivatives both to ensure economic use of a valuable resource and for clinical appropriateness.

Red Blood Cells

Blood component preparation begins with the separation of plasma from whole blood, leaving the red cells. Red cells for transfusion can be prepared by sedimentation or centrifugation. The technique used must maintain the sterility of both the plasma and the red cells. If the container is not entered when the red cells are prepared, the expiration date for the red cells remains the same as for the original whole blood. If the container is entered, the red cells are considered usable for only 24 hours. Packed red cells are especially useful in treating certain anemic conditions.

Red cells have essentially replaced whole blood in transfusion except in the case of massive bleeding when over 25% to 30% of blood volume is lost. In most cases, even in massive bleeding, red cells, together with isotonic saline or plasma substitutes, are preferred.

Red cells may be further treated by removing leukocytes by centrifugation, washing, or filtration. Red cells may also be treated with additive solutions consisting of saline, adenine, glucose, and mannitol. In this case maximum amounts of plasma are removed shortly after phlebotomy and additive solutions are used to maintain red cell function. This process extends the shelf life of red cells to 42 days. Rejuvenation solutions have also been licensed to extend the life of stored blood for immediate use, or frozen for transfusion later. This is especially useful for rejuvenating outdated units of autologous donor blood.

Plasma

When the red cells are removed from whole blood, plasma remains. It is the liquid portion of blood that has been anticoagulated. Slightly more than half the volume of whole blood is plasma. Plasma should not be used to

TABLE 18-5.

Some Blood Components and Derivatives and Their Uses

Blood Component or Derivative	Use
Whole blood	Acute blood loss where both red cells and volume are desired; rarely indicated
Red blood cells	To increase red cell mass (e.g., therapy for anemia); use with colloids or crystalloids in active bleeding or massive transfusion
Red blood cells	
Additive solution added	Like red cells or whole blood
Leukocytes removed by centrifugation, washing, or filtration	To increase red cell mass and avoid febrile and allergic reactions from leukocytes or plasma proteins and to prevent anaphylactic reactions
Deglycerolized	To extend storage of red cells with rare blood types and autologous transfusion or to prevent HLA sensitization
Platelets (platelet concentrates, platelet-rich plasma, random or single donor by apheresis	Functional or quantitative platelet defects
Granulocytes, apheresis	Rare; for septic, severely granulocytopenic patients who do not respond to antibiotic therapy after 48 hrs of treatment
Fresh frozen plasma	In bleeding patients with multiple coagulation defects; also for treatment of factor V or XI deficiency
Cryoprecipitate	For treatment of von Willebrand's disease, factor XIII deficiency, or hypofibrinogenemia
Factor VII concentrate	For hemophilia A
Factor IX concentrate	For hereditary deficiency of factors II, VII, IX, or X
Albumin/plasma protein fraction (plasma substitutes)	For volume expansion and colloid replacement without risk of hepatitis or AIDS
Immune serum globulin	For treatment or prophylaxis of hypogammaglobulinemia and to prevent or modify hepatitis A and non-A, non-B hepatitis
Rh immune globulin	To prevent hemolytic disease of the newborn in Rh-negative women exposed to Rh-positive red cells

replace lost blood volume or protein, as much safer products exist. These include plasma substitutes such as albumin or plasma protein fractions, synthetic colloids, and balanced salt solutions. These have the advantage of not transmitting disease or causing allergic reactions. Plasma is appropriately used to replace coagulation factors.

Fresh Frozen Plasma.—When plasma is used it is often in the form of fresh frozen plasma. Fresh frozen plasma is a good source of labile clotting factors and can be used to replace all coagulation factors. It is especially useful in treating multiple coagulation deficiencies, as seen with liver failure, disseminated intravascular coagulation (DIC), vitamin K deficiency, warfarin toxicity, or with massive transfusions.

Cryoprecipitate.—Plasma is used to make other blood derivatives. One of these is cryoprecipitated antihemophilic factor (AHF). It is prepared by slowly thawing a unit of fresh frozen plasma at 1 to 6° C overnight. A small amount of white precipitate is formed. This is cryoprecipitate. The unit is centrifuged and all but 10 to 15 mL of the supernatant plasma is removed. The preparation contains AHF, also called factor VIII; fibrinogen; von Willebrand's factor; and factor XIII. Cryoprecipitate used to be the product of choice for severe hemophilic patients who were bleeding, but newer methods which inactivate viruses make pooled concentrates of factor VIII the product of choice. Cryoprecipitate is presently used in the treatment of severe von Willebrand's disease.

Plasma Substitutes.—These include albumin and plasma protein fractions which are prepared by the chemical fractionation of pooled plasma. The products are heat-treated to eliminate the risk of infectious disease such as hepatitis and AIDS. They are used to treat patients who need replacement of blood volume. Alternatively, crystalloid (either saline or electrolyte) solutions are used. The preferred product is debatable.

Platelets

Platelet concentrates are prepared from random donor whole blood units by differential centrifugation shortly after donation. They are used for patients who are bleeding due to low platelet counts or occasionally abnormally functioning platelets. Massive transfusions may also result in thrombocytopenia and require platelet concentrates. Occasionally, patients develop HLA antibodies that make transfused platelet concentrates ineffective. In such cases it may be necessary to select HLA-matched donors and prepare platelets by apheresis.

CONCLUSION

This chapter has been only a brief introduction to the complex field of immunohematology and blood banking, also known as transfusion medicine. Specific blood-grouping and crossmatching methods have been omitted. The current edition of the *Technical Manual of the American Association of Blood Banks* is useful for these procedures. Also, it is extremely important to *always* follow the manufacturer's instructions when using any specific blood-grouping or blood-typing antisera. Complete instructions are always included with the reputable commercial products. Other topics that have not been covered completely in this chapter but which must be understood before the student can work in the blood bank include causes of error, cleaning of glassware, organization of the blood bank, selection of blood donors, labeling of blood, and record-keeping protocols. Excellent discussions of these subjects have been published in standard blood bank texts. In addition, knowledge may be gained from firsthand experience in a licensed blood bank. Areas that have not been covered in this discussion include bone marrow transplants, organ transplants, and HLA typing and matching.

In the field of blood banking there are numerous situations that may result in error. In general, these may be organizational, clerical, or technical errors. Organizational and clerical errors may be made by the blood bank staff or by personnel in other services involved in the transfusion of blood. These errors often involve incorrect identification of the patient or of the blood removed from the patient and sent to the laboratory for testing.

Transfusion involves a series of tests that are performed by several persons. Included are clerical manipulations where even a mistake on the part of a typist in transcribing a laboratory report could result in fatal errors if adequate checks did not exist. Because of the number of persons and tests involved in blood transfusion, a blood bank has elaborate organizational procedures that must be followed exactly to ensure that the correct blood is transfused into the correct patient. The AABB and the FDA have definite requirements and recommendations. Organizational systems involve such items and procedures as request forms, methods of labeling tubes of blood from the patient, manner of recording results in the laboratory, labeling and numbering of donor blood, selection of blood donors, and storage of blood.

Technical errors are the direct responsibility of the blood banking laboratory and its staff. They may be personal errors, where the laboratorian is directly responsible, or impersonal errors resulting from various factors that enter into the laboratory technique. In any blood-grouping or compatibility testing method, impersonal technical factors can produce false-positive or false-negative results. Some may happen in all tests, and some are peculiar to a specific method. These sources of error are beyond the scope of this discussion but they must be understood by blood bank personnel if the results are to be reliable and accurate.

It is hoped that this brief outline of blood banking will serve as a useful introduction to the student. Work in this area will require much additional knowledge and study.

BIBLIOGRAPHY

Blood Group Antigens and Antibodies as Applied to Hemolytic Disease of the Newborn. Raritan, NJ, Ortho Diagnostics, 1968.

Bryant NJ: *An Introduction to Immunohematology,* ed 2. Philadelphia, WB Saunders Co, 1982.

Erskine AG, Socha WW: *Principles and Practices of Blood Grouping,* ed 2. St Louis, Mosby–Year Book, Inc, 1978.

Harmening D: *Modern Blood Banking and Transfusion Practices,* ed 2. Philadelphia, FA Davis Co, 1989.

Henry JB: *Clinical Diagnosis and Management by Laboratory Methods,* ed 18. Philadelphia, WB Saunders Co, 1991.

Huestis DW, Bove JR, Busch S: *Practical Blood Transfusion,* ed 3. Boston, Little, Brown & Co, 1981.

Issitt PD: *Applied Blood Group Serology,* ed 3. Miami, Montgomery Scientific Publications, 1985.

Mollison PL: *Blood Transfusion in Clinical Medicine,* ed 7. Oxford, Blackwell Scientific Publications, 1983.

Race RR, Sanger R: *Blood Groups in Man,* ed 6. Oxford, Blackwell Scientific Publications, 1975.

Walker RH (ed): *Technical Manual of the American Association of Blood Banks,* ed 10. Arlington, VA, American Association of Blood Banks, 1990.

Appendix A

Prefixes and Suffixes/Stem Words

Every specialty has a vocabulary of its own. The clinical laboratory is no different. Progress in learning the vocabulary of the laboratory and of medicine in general will come with experience, but some introductory information is important for anyone coming into the laboratory for the first time.

Most modern medical words are made up of parts derived from Greek or Latin, some with changes that have gradually been made over the years as the ancient words were adopted into English. All but the simplest medical terms are made up of two or three parts. For example, *pathology* is the study of disease. The root word is *pathos-,* from the Greek, meaning disease. The suffix *-logy* is also from the Greek word, *-logia,* from *logos,* meaning the study of. By examining the root or stem word along with the prefix or suffix, the meaning of most medical words can be understood.

Many of the common prefixes, suffixes, and stem words are listed below.

PREFIX/STEM WORD	MEANING
a-, an-	lack, not
ab-, a-	away from, outside of
ad-	to, toward
ambi-, ambo-	both
amyl-, amylo-	starch
angi-, angio-	vessel, vascular
ante-	before, preceding, in front of
arteri-, arterio-	artery, arterial
arthr-, arthro-	joint
aur-, auri-, auro-	ear
bi-	two, twice, double
bi-, bio-	life
brachi-, brachio-	arm, brachial
brady-	slow
bronch-, broncho-	bronchus, bronchial

PREFIX/STEM WORD	MEANING
cardi-, cardia-, cardio-	heart, cardiac
cephal-, cephalo-	head
cerebr-, cerebri, cerebro-	cerebrum, cerebral, brain
cervic-, cervico-	neck, cervix, cervical
chol-, chole-, cholo-	bile, gall
circum-	around, about
co-, com-, con-, cor-	with, together
col-, coli-, colo-	colon
contra-, counter-	against, opposite
crani-, cranio-	cranium, cranial
cyan-, cyano-	dark blue, presence of the cyanogen group
cyst-, cysti-, cysto-	gallbladder, urinary bladder, pouch, cyst
de-	undoing, reversal
dec-, deca-	ten, multiplied by ten
deci-	tenth, one-tenth of
derm-, derma-, dermo-	dermis, dermal, skin
dextr-, dextro-	toward, of, or pertaining to the right
di-, dis-	two, twice, double
dipl-, diplo-	twofold, double, twin
dis-, di-	separation, reversal, apart from
dys-	abnormal, diseased, difficult, painful, unlike
en-, em-	in, inside, into
end-, endo-	within, inner, internal
enter-, entero-	intestine, intestinal
ep-, epi-	upon, beside, among, above
erythr-, erythro-	red
eu-	good, well, normal, true
ex-, e-, ef-	out, away, without
extra-	outside of, beyond the scope of
ferri-	ferric, containing iron (III)
ferro-	ferrous, containing iron (II)
fibr-, fibro-	fiber, fibrous

PREFIX/STEM WORD	MEANING
gastr-, gastro-	stomach, gastric
gluc-, gluco-	glucose
glyc-, glyco-	sweet, sugar, glucose, glycine
gyne-	female, woman
hem-, hema-, hemo-	blood
hemi-	half, partial
hepat-, hepato-	liver, hepatic
heter-, hetero-	other, another, different
hex-, hexa-	six
hom-, homo-	common, like, same
hydr-, hydro-	water, hydrogen
hyp-, hypo-	deficiency, lack, below
hyper-	excessive, above normal
hyster-, hystero-	uterus, uterine, hysteria
icter-, ictero-	icterus, jaundice
immuno-	immune, immunity
in-, im-	not, in, into
inter-	between, among
intra-	within, inside
is, iso-	equality, similarity, uniformity
juxta-	near, next to
kerat-, kerato-	horn, horny, cornea
ket-, keto-	presence of the ketone group
kilo-	thousand
lact-, lacti-, lacto-	milk, lactic
lapar-, laparo-	flank, abdomen
laryng-, laryngo-	larynx, laryngeal
latero-	lateral, to the side
leuk-, leuc-, leuko-, leuco-	white, colorless, leukocyte
levo-	left, on the left
lith-, litho-	stone
lymph-, lympho-	lymph, lymphatic
macr-, macro-	large, great, long
mal-	wrong, abnormal, bad
mamm-, mammo-	breast
medi-, medio-	middle, medial, median
meg-, mega-, megal-	large, extended, enlarged, one million times as large as
micr-, micro-	small, minute, one-millionth
mon-, mono-	single, one, alone
morph-, morpho-	form, structure
multi-	many, much, affecting many parts
my-, myo-	muscle
myel-, myelo-	marrow
nas-, naso-	nose, nasal
ne-, neo-	new, recent
necr-, necro-	death

PREFIX/STEM WORD	MEANING
nephr-, nephro-	kidney
neur-, neuro-	neural, nervous, nerve
nitr-, nitro-	nitrogen
non-	not, ninth, nine
normo-	normal
nucle-, nucleo-	nucleus, nuclear
oo-	egg, ovum
orth-, ortho-	straight, direct, normal
ost-, oste-, osteo-	bone
ot-, oto-	ear
oxy-	oxygen
par-, para-	near, beside, adjacent to
path-, patho-	pathologic
peri-	about, beyond, around
phag-, phago-	eating, feeding
pharyng-, pharyngo-	pharynx, pharyngeal
phleb-, phlebo-	vein, venous
phon-, phono-	sound, speech, voice
phot-, photo-	light
physi-, physio-	natural, physical, physiologic
phyt-, phyto-	plant, vegetable
plasm-, plasmo-	plasma, protoplasm, cytoplasm
pneum-, pneumo-	air, gas, lung, respiratory
poly-	multiple, compound, complex
post-	after, behind
pre-	before
pro-	front, forward, before
proct-, procto-	rectum, anus
prot-, proto-	first, primitive, early
pseud-, pseudo-	false, deceptively resembling
psych-, psycho	psyche, psychic, psychology
pulmo-	lung, pulmonary
py-, pyo-	pus
pyel-, pyelo-	renal, pelvic
pykn-, pykno-, pycn- pycno-	compact, dense
pyr-, pyro-	fire, heat
radio-	radiation, radioactivity
re-	again, back
ren-, reni-, reno-	kidney, renal
retro-	back, backward, behind
rhin-, rhino-	nose, nasal
rubr-, rubri-, rubro-	red
sarc-, sarco-	flesh, fleshlike, muscle
semi-	half
ser-, seri,- sero-	serum, serous
sub-	under, less than
super-	above, upon, extreme
supra-	upon, above, beyond, exceeding

PREFIX/STEM WORD	MEANING
syn-, sym-	together, with
tachy-	rapid, quick, accelerated
thorac-, thoraci-, thoracio-, thoraco-	thorax, thoracic
thromb-, thrombo-	clotting, coagulation, blood platelets
thyr-, thyreo-, thyro-	thyroid
tox-, toxi-, toxo-	toxic, poisonous
trache-, tracheo-	trachea, tracheal
trans-	through, across
trich-, tricho-	hair, filament
un-	not, without
uni-	one
ur-, uro-	urine, urinary
uter-, utero-	uterus, uterine
vas-, vasi-, vaso-	vessel, vascular
ven-, vene-, veni-, veno-	vein, venous

SUFFIX/STEM WORD	MEANING
-algia	a painful condition
-ase	enzyme
-ation	action, process
-blast	sprout, shoot, germ, formative cell
-cele	tumor, hernia, pathologic swelling
-cyte	cell

SUFFIX/STEM WORD	MEANING
-desis	binding, fusing
-ectomy	surgical removal
-emia	blood
-ethesia	feeling, sensation
-gram	drawing, record
-graph	something written, recorded
-itis	inflammation
-logy	field of study
-lysis	dissolving, loosening, dissolution
-megaly	abnormal enlargement
-oma	tumor, neoplasm
-opia, -opy	defect of the eye
-osis	process, state, diseased condition
-pathy	disease, therapy
-penia	deficiency
-phil, -phile	having an affinity for
-plasty	plastic surgery
-rrhage, -rrhagia	abnormal or excessive discharge
-scope	viewing instrument
-scopy	inspection, examination
-stoma	mouth, opening
-stomy	operation establishing an opening into a part
-tomy	cutting, incision, section
-uria	of or in the urine

Appendix B

Abbreviations

AHG	antihuman globulin
AIDS	acquired immune deficiency syndrome
ANA	antinuclear antibody
APTT	activated partial thromboplastin time
ASCP	American Society of Clinical Pathologists
ASMT	American Society for Medical Technology
ASO	antistreptolysin O
BAP	blood agar (plate)
BT	bleeding time
CAP	College of American Pathologists
CBC	complete blood count
CDC	Centers for Disease Control
CFU	colony-forming unit
CLIA 88	Clinical Laboratory Improvement Amendments of 1988
CPD	citrate phosphate dextrose
CPDA-1	citrate-phosphate-dextrose with adenine
CPU	central processing unit
CRP	C-reactive protein
CRT	cathode ray tube
DAT	direct antiglobulin test
DIC	disseminated intravascular coagulation
DNA	deoxyribonucleic acid
EA	early antigen
EBV	Epstein-Barr virus
EDTA	ethylenediamine tetraacetic acid
EIA	enzyme immunoassay
ELISA	enzyme-linked immunosorbent assay; enzyme-labeled immunosorbent assay
EMB	eosin methylene blue agar
ESR	erythrocyte sedimentation rate
FIA	fluorescence immunoassay

Hb	hemoglobin
HBV	hepatitis B virus
HCV	hepatitis C virus; also called non-A, non-B hepatitis virus
HCFA	Health Care Financing Administration
Hct (or Ht)	hematocrit
HDN	hemolytic disease of newborn **Hgb** hemoglobin
HHS	Department of Health and Human Services
HIS	hospital information system
HIV	human immunodeficiency virus
HLA	human leukocyte antigen
HMWK	high molecular weight kininogen
IAT	indirect antiglobulin test
IDDM	insulin-dependent diabetes mellitus
IF	intrinsic factor
Ig	immunoglobulin
IM	infectious mononucleosis
IV	intravenous
IU	international unit
JCAHO	Joint Commission on Accreditation of Healthcare Organizations
L	liter
LAP	leukocyte alkaline phosphatase
LIS	laboratory information system
LISS	low ionic strength saline solution
M	meter
Mac	MacConkey (agar)
MCH	mean cell hemoglobin
MCHC	mean cell hemoglobin concentration
MCV	mean cell volume
MIC	minimal inhibitory concentration

MKC	megakaryocyte
mol	mole
MPV	mean platelet volume
MSDS	material safety data sheets
NAD$^+$	nicotinamide adenine dinucleotide, oxidized form
NADH	nicotinamide adenine dinucleotide, reduced form
NBS	National Bureau of Standards
NCCLS	National Committee for Clinical Laboratory Standards
NIDDM	non-insulin-dependent diabetes mellitus
OGTT	oral glucose tolerance test
OSHA	Occupational Safety and Health Administration
PCT	prothrombin consumption time
PCV	packed cell volume
PKK	plasma prekallikrein
PMN	polymorphonuclear neutrophil
PRP	platelet-rich plasma
PT	prothrombin time
PTT	partial thromboplastin time
QA	quality assurance
QC	quality control

RAM	random access memory
RBC	red blood cell
RCF	relative centrifugal force
RDW	red cell distribution width
RES	reticuloendothelial system
RF	rheumatoid factor
RhIG	Rh immune globulin
RIA	radioimmunoassay
SB	sheep blood (agar)
SI	International System of Units (le Système International d'Unités)
SLE	systemic lupus erythematosus
SPIA	solid-phase immunosorbent assay
TDM	therapeutic drug monitoring
TLC	thin-layer chromatography
VAD	vascular access device
VDRL	Venereal Disease Research Laboratory (test for syphilis)
vWD	vonWillebrand's disease
vWF	vonWillebrand's factor
WBC	white blood cell

Glossary

A

absolute cell count Concentration of a cell type expressed as a number per volume of whole blood, usually per liter; obtained by multiplying the relative percentage value by the total leukocyte count per liter.

absorbance spectrophotometry Utilizes Beer's law where the amount of light absorbed by a solution is directly proportional to the concentration of the solution; this measurement can be made only by mathematical calculation from the transmission data obtained by use of a quantitative analytical method, such as spectrophotometry.

absorbed light Light that is not transmitted.

accuracy Correctness of a result, freedom from error, or how close the answer is to the "true" value.

acholic stool Absence of bile; results in formation of colorless, chalky appearing fecal specimens.

acid-base balance Maintenance of a constant balance between acids and bases; maintenance of constant pH.

acid-fast stain Used to detect organisms that are difficult to decolorize, even with acid-alcohol solutions; typical organisms are those that cause tuberculosis or leprosy.

acute-phase reactants Group of glycoproteins associated with nonspecific inflammatory conditions.

acute-phase serum Serum collected early in the course of an illness, when little or no antibody has had time to develop.

additives, anticoagulants Additives usually are anticoagulants that prevent coagulation of the blood specimen. Several different anticoagulants are available for different testing purposes. Some laboratory tests require the use of plasma or whole blood for the assay, and these must be anticoagulated during the collection process.

aerobe Microbe that requires oxygen for growth.

aerosols Infectious particles that are airborne; fine mist in which particles are dispersed.

agglutination Visible clumping or aggregation of red cells or any particles, used as an indication of a specific antigen-antibody reaction.

albuminuria Presence of albumin in urine.

alignment Microscope adjustment that ensures that the light path from the light source throughout the microscope and ocular is physically correct.

alleles Variants of a gene for a particular trait.

amorphous material Crystaline material seen in the urine sediment as granules without shape or form.

anaerobe Microbe that cannot grow in an atmosphere of oxygen; special steps must be taken to provide an oxygen-free atmosphere for incubation and growth of these organisms.

analog computation Measurement derived directly from an instrument signal.

analytical balance Instrument used to weigh substances to a high degree of accuracy (e.g., chemicals used in the preparation of standard solutions.)

anemia Decrease in number of erythrocytes resulting in decreased delivery of oxygen to tissues (decreased red cell mass; decreased hemoglobin concentration or abnormal hemoglobin).

anion gap Concentration of undetermined anions; calculated as the difference between measured cations and measured anions.

antibody Protein substance found in the plasma or other body fluids that is formed as the result of antigenic stimulation and is specific for the antigen against which it is formed. In blood banking, antibodies are present in commercially prepared serum, called antiserum.

antibody titer Amount of antibody present or required to produce a reaction with a particular amount of another substance.

antigen Foreign (different from "self") substance that when introduced into the body of a person lacking the antigen results in an immune response and formation of its corresponding antibody. In blood banking, antigens are generally, but not always, found on the red cell membrane.

antihuman globulin (AHG) test (AGT) or reaction Method of detecting the presence of all human isoantibodies by using a specially prepared antiserum to human immunoglobulin and/or complement. May be a direct (DAT) or indirect (IAT) test. Also known as the Coombs' reaction or test.

antiserum Serum containing antibodies. In blood banking, a special highly purified preparation of antibodies used as a reagent to show the presence of antigen on red blood cells.

Apt test Test for maternal hemoglobin ingestion in newborn infants.

autoclave Apparatus for effecting sterilization using steam under pressure; when used with an automatic regulating pressure gauge, the degree of heat to which the contents are subjected is automatically regulated also.

automated differential counter Instrument designed to repeatedly and automatically determine the types and percentages of leukocytes present in a blood specimen.

automatic cell counter Instrument designed to repeatedly and automatically count the numbers of formed cellular elements present in a blood specimen, usually the erythrocytes, leukocytes, and platelets.

automatic pipette Device used to repeatedly and accurately measure volume of standard solutions, reagents, specimens, or other liquid substances.

B

B lymphocyte Blood cell that matures in the bone marrow; functions in antibody production or formation of immunoglobulin.

bacteriuria Bacteria in the urine.

bar code reader Optical reading device that converts a series of black lines into a sequence of numbers or letters for entry into a computer (e.g., names of patients, identification numbers, tests requested).

barrier precautions Personal protective devices (e.g., gloves, gowns) placed between blood or other body fluid specimen and the person handling it, to prevent transmission of infectious agents borne by specimens.

basic first aid Immediate care given after an injury before treatment is started by trained medical personnel.

batch analyzer Instrument that can analyze a batch of samples simultaneously for one particular analyte at a time.

bedside testing Capillary blood samples can be used to perform rapid testing procedures (many are utilizing commercial products) at the bedside; a common test is the glucose blood test done for management of diabetes mellitus patients.

Beer's law, Beer-Lambert law In a solution, color intensity at a constant depth is directly proportional to concentration.

bilirubin Vivid yellow pigment, major byproduct of normal red blood cell destruction.

biochemical properties and reactions Properties are characteristics (e.g., molecular weight, melting point) present in various types of chemicals; reactions involve the conversion of one chemical species, the reactant, to another chemical species, the product.

biohazard Symbol or term denoting any infectious material or agent that presents a possible health risk.

biohazard container All infectious materials are handled as potential biohazards. These special containers should be used for all blood, other body fluids, and tissues, and disposable materials contaminated with them; they should be tagged "Biohazard" or bear the universal biohazard symbol.

birefringence Ability of an object or crystal to rotate or polarize light.

blank solution Solution containing all the components, including solvents and solutes, except the compound to be measured.

blood transfusion Technique of replacing whole blood and/or its components.

bloodborne pathogens Infectious agents or pathogens carried by the blood.

body cavity fluid Fluid normally found in small amounts in various cavities or body spaces (e.g., cerebrospinal, pleural, abdominal, pericardial, peritoneal, and synovial fluid). In certain conditions, such fluid is aspirated and assayed.

brightfield microscope Illumination system used in the common clinical microscope.

buret Long cylindrical graduated tube with a stopcock delivery closing on one end used to control the delivery of the flow of liquid from the device; used to deliver measured quantities of fluid or solutions.

C

calibration Means by which glassware or other laboratory apparatus is checked to determine the exact units it will measure or deliver by relating them to a known concentration of an analyte.

capillary blood (peripheral blood) collection Blood drawn from the capillary bed by means of puncturing the skin.

capillary pipette Small glass or plastic tube used to collect small amounts of capillary blood, usually directly from a capillary puncture.

carcinogen Substance that can cause the development of cancerous growths in living tissues.

casts Structures that result from solidification of Tamm-Horsfall mucoprotein in the lumen of the kidney tubules; they form a mold, or cast, of the tubule and trap other material that may be present when formed. Several types exist. They represent a biopsy of the kidney and are clinically significant.

cathode ray tube, terminal, video display unit Television-like screen device used to monitor input, output, and general status of a computer system.

central memory Provides storage and rapid access for information (data).

central processing unit Part of the computer that controls and performs the execution of programs or instructions.

centrifugation Separation of a solid material from a liquid by application of increased gravitational force by rapid rotating or spinning.

cerebrospinal fluid (CSF) Formed by the choroid plexus in the ventricles of the brain and found within the subarachnoid space, the central canal of the spinal cord, and the four ventricles of the brain.

chromatography Method of analysis in which the solutes, dissolved in a common solvent, are separated from one another by differential distribution of the solutes between two phases (a mobile phase and a stationary phase).

chromosome Threadlike structure within the nucleus of each cell, made up of genes. Chromosomes exist in pairs in all cells except sex cells. Each species has a specific number of paired chromosomes.

Clinical Laboratory Improvement Amendments of 1988 (CLIA 88) Standards set for all laboratories to ensure quality patient care; provisions include requirements for quality control and assurance, for the use of proficiency tests, and for certain levels of personnel to perform and supervise work done in the clinical laboratory.

coagulation cascade Process of coagulation in which a series of biochemical reactions occur, converting inactive substances to active forms that in turn activate other substances; carefully controlled process responding to injury while maintaining normal blood circulation.

coagulation factor I, fibrinogen Synthesized in the liver; not dependent on vitamin K for production.

coagulation factor II, prothrombin, prethrombin Synthesized in the liver; dependent on vitamin K for production.

coagulation factor III, tissue thromboplastin, tissue factor Lipoprotein found in many body tissues; converts prothrombin to thrombin.

coagulation factor IV Calcium when it participates in the coagulation process. (Calcium is essential for coagulation.)

coagulation factor V, proaccelerin, labile factor, accelerator globulin (AcG) Necessary for conversion of prothrombin to thrombin; synthesized in the liver.

coagulation factor VII, proconvertin, stable factor, serum prothrombin conversion accelerator (SPCA), autoprothrombin I   Synthesized in the liver; dependent on vitamin K for production.

coagulation factor VIII, antihemophilic factor (AHF), antihemophilic globulin (AHG), antihemophilic factor A, platelet cofactor 1.   Production site unclear; factor deficient in the blood of persons with classical hemophilia (hemophilia A), and vonWillebrand's disease; necessary for normal platelet function.

coagulation factor IX, plasma thromboplastin component (PTC), antihemophilic factor B (AHB), Christmas factor, autoprothrombin II, platelet cofactor 2   Synthesized in the liver; is dependent on vitamin K for production. Deficiency results in hemophilia B or Christmas disease.

coagulation factor X, Stuart-Prower factor, Stuart factor, autoprothrombin III   Synthesized in the liver; is dependent on vitamin K for production.

coagulation factor XI, plasma thromboplastin antecedent (PTA), antihemophilic factor C   Synthesized in the liver; is not dependent on vitamin K for production.

coagulation factor XII, Hageman factor, glass or contact factor   Synthesized in the liver; is not dependent on vitamin K for production.

coagulation factor XIII, fibrinase, fibrin-stabilizing factor (FSF), Laki-Lorand factor.   May be synthesized in the liver; assists in formation of fibrin clot.

colony forming unit (CFU)   In microbiology, colony count; in hematology, a pluripotential, undifferentiated stem cell that is stimulated to proliferate and differentiate into colonies of a specific cell type.

common pathway   Final stages of the coagulation cascade, beginning with the convergence of the extrinsic and intrinsic pathways (factor X) and ending with formation of the fibrin clot.

compatibility testing   All of the tests performed before a transfusion to ensure that the transfused blood or component will benefit and not harm the recipient. These include tests on both recipient and donor blood, including a cross match between patient serum and donor red blood cells.

compensated polarized light   Modification of the normal brightfield microscope in which two crossed polarizing filters plus a first-order red compensator or filter are inserted to observe the presence or absence and type of birefringence. In the clinical laboratory, especially useful in examination of synovial fluid.

complement   Group of serum proteins that can produce inflammatory effects and lysis of cells when activated.

complement fixation   When complement is tied up or bound (fixed) to an antigen-antibody complex, it is no longer available to be activated.

complete blood count (CBC)   Generally includes hemoglobin, hematocrit, leukocyte count, and leukocyte differential; specific tests vary with the facility.

components   Portions of whole blood prepared for transfusion by physical means, especially centrifugation.

condenser   Part of the microscope that directs and focuses the beam of light from the light source onto the material under examination; positioned just under the stage, and can be raised or lowered by means of an adjustment knob.

conjugated bilirubin, direct bilirubin   Bilirubin that has been conjugated with glucuronate in the liver, exists in plasma unbound to any protein, as contrasted with unconjugated bilirubin; is water soluble, and high blood levels are excreted in the urine.

continous-flow analyzer   Instrument that constantly pumps reagent and sample through tubing and coil, forming a continuous stream.

control specimen   Material or solution with a known concentration of the analytes being measured; used for quality control where the test result for the control specimen must be with certain limits in order for the unknown values run in the same "batch" to be considered reportable.

coulometry   Technique in which the charge required to completely electrolyze a sample is measured.

Coulter principle   Means of counting particles and measuring their size or volume by impedence change caused by the particle in a current-conducting fluid (electrolyte); this principle is applied in many of the blood cell counters used in hematology laboratories (Coulter Counter).

creatinine clearance Estimate of the function of the glomerular filtration rate; obtained by measuring the amount of creatinine in plasma and its rate of excretion in the urine.

crystals, abnormal Urinary crystals of metabolic or iatrogenic origin that are generally of pathologic significance and require chemical confirmation.

crystals, normal Urinary crystals that may be found in normal urine specimens of an acid or alkaline pH; generally are not pathologic, and can be reported on the basis of morphologic appearance.

culture Growing of microorganisms or living tissue cells in special media.

cuvette Tube or receptacle used in a photometer for holding the sample to be measured.

cytocentrifugation Special slow centrifugation method used to prepare permanent microscope slides of fluids (e.g., urine, other body fluids), resulting in better morphologic preservation than by other centrifugation or preparation methods.

D

data base Systemic storage of information (data) that can be accessed by the operator or user of the computer system.

decontamination Process of eliminating something that has become contaminated or mixed with something that makes it impure.

deionization of water Process of removing ionized substances from water.

density Amount of matter per unit volume of a substance.

Department of Health and Human Services (HHS) Department of the U.S. government under which the Health Care Financing Administration (HCFA) is managed. Responsible for implementation of laws; writing of regulations that provide details of how various laws are to be carried out; publishes details of proposed regulations in the *Federal Register,* an official government document.

derivatives Blood products prepared from whole blood by more complex methods than components are. Also referred to as fractions.

diabetes mellitus Chronic metabolic syndrome of impaired carbohydrate, fat, and protein metabolism that is secondary to insufficiency of insulin secretion or to the inhibition of the activity of insulin; characterized by increased concentration of glucose in the blood and urine.

diazo reaction Coupling of a diazonium salt with another aromatic ring to give an azo dye.

differential stain Stain used to differentiate specific cellular details in a microorganism; more than one stain is used to produce the end result. Gram stain is an example of a differential stain.

digital computation Calculations that involve data available in the form of discrete units or numbers.

dilution Weaker solution made from a stronger solution. Describes the relative concentrations of the components of a mixture; the preferred method is to refer to the number of parts of the material being diluted in the total number of parts of the final product.

dilution factor Reciprocal of the dilution made; multiply the result by the reciprocal of the dilution to correct for the dilution used.

discrete sample analyzer Instrument that compartmentalizes each sample reaction.

distilled water As water is boiled, the steam is cooled and condensed, and collected as distilled water.

dry film reagent technology Instruments or tests that use a dry film layered device that supplies the necessary reagents for the reaction to take place when the serum sample is added to it; the specimen (serum) provides the solvent (water) necessary to rehydrate the dry reagents on the film.

E

effusion Abnormal accumulation of any of the extracellular fluids. Fluid escapes from the blood or lymphatic vessels into the tissues or body cavities (e.g., serous cavities: pericardium, peritoneum, or pleural) or the joints.

Ehrlich's aldehyde reaction Reaction of urobilinogen, porphobilinogen, and other Ehrlich-reactive compounds with *p*-dimethylaminobenzaldehyde in concentrated hydrochloric acid to form a colored aldehyde.

electrolyte battery Collection of tests for common electrolytes: chloride, bicarbonate, sodium, and potassium. These four electrolytes often are measured at the same time, because changes in the concentration of one almost always is accompanied by changes in one or more of the others.

electronic cell counting device Automatic instrument that counts cellular elements in the blood (usually erythrocytes, leukocytes, and platelets) repeatedly and accurately.

electrophoresis Movement of charged particles in an electrical field; technique used to separate mixtures of ionic solutes by the differences in their rates of migration in an electric field.

enumeration of formed elements Counting of cellular elements of the blood (usually erythrocytes, leukocytes, and platelets).

enzyme immunoassay (EIA) Uses enzymes as immunochemical labels in detection of antigen-antibody reactions.

enzyme-linked (or labeled) immunosorbent assay (ELISA) Immunoassay or test that uses an enzyme conjugated to antibodies or antigens to produce a visible end point; diagnostic test used to detect antigens or antibodies in a patient's specimen.

enzymology Study of the various biologic materials (proteins) that have catalytic activity; study of enzymes present in the blood.

epithelial cells Cells that make up the covering of the various internal and external organs of the body, including the lining of the blood vessels.

equivalent weight Mass in grams that will liberate, combine with, or replace 1 gm of hydrogen ion; generally is the molecular weight divided by the valence.

erythrocyte Red blood cell, one of the formed elements of the peripheral blood; chief role is to transport oxygen to the tissues.

erythrocyte sedimentation rate (ESR) Rate in millimeters at which the red blood cells fall or sediment in a given unit of time (usually 1 hour).

etiologic agent Agent causing a disease.

exponent Number used to indicate how many times a number must be multiplied by itself.

extravascular fluid Body fluid other than blood or urine.

extrinsic system of coagulation Coagulation pathway that is activated by tissue thromboplastin; necessary components are factor VII and calcium.

exudate Effusion that results from inflammatory conditions, such as infections and malignancies, that directly affect the membranes lining a cavity.

eyepiece (ocular) Microscope lens that magnifies the image formed by the objective.

F

fasting blood Blood collected after an 8- to 12-hour fast from food and liquids other than water. For some tests, additional patient restrictions are necessary, such as no smoking or administration of certain drugs during the fasting period.

fibrin End product of coagulation. Forms a visible clot, a fibrin mesh to entrap the blood cells. Is derived from fibrinogen, a plasma protein, by the action of thrombin.

fibrinogen, coagulation factor I Plasma protein that is the substrate for thrombin action in the formation of fibrin. Manufactured by the liver; is not vitamin K-dependent.

fibrinolysis Destruction of the fibrin clot by plasmin activity to keep the vascular system free from clots; under normal conditions, coagulation and fibrinolysis are kept in balance.

first morning urine specimen First urine voided in the morning. It is generally the most concentrated specimen of the day because less fluid or water is excreted during the night, yet the kidney has maintained excretion of a constant concentration of solid or dissolved substances.

flame emission photometry Atoms of certain elements, when sprayed into a hot flame, become excited and remit energy at wavelengths characteristic for that element. Utilizes a device (flame photometer) to measure the intensity of the colored flame. Solution containing metal ions is sprayed into a flame and the intensity and color of the flame is proportional to the amount of substance present in the solution.

flocculation Clumping of particles to form visible masses.

flow cytometry Enumeration and differentiation of blood cells by passing them through a focused beam of a laser.

fluorescent antibody technique Assay that uses antibodies that cause fluorescence as an indication of a reaction.

G

galvanometer Measures and records the amount of current (in the form of electrons) reaching it.

gaussian curve Particular symmetric statistical distribution; also known as "normal" distribution.

genitourinary tract specimen Specimen collected from the genital or urinary tract (e.g., vaginal cervix and perineal area in women, anterior urethra in men).

genotype Actual total genetic makeup. Often impossible to determine by laboratory testing, but requires additional family studies.

gestational diabetes Glucose intolerance that occurs during some pregnancies.

glomerular filtrate Ultrafiltrate of blood formed as blood is filtered through the glomerular capillaries of the glomerulus into Bowman's capsule. First step in urine formation, basically blood plasma without protein or fat.

glucose tolerance test Measures the response of the body to a challenge load of glucose; used to aid in the diagnosis of diabetes mellitus.

glucosuria, glycosuria Presence of glucose in urine.

grade of chemicals Varying quality of production criteria are placed on manufacture of chemicals for laboratory use, depending on the use to which the chemical is put; the grade indicates the level of quality.

graduated pipette, measuring pipette Cylindrical tube used to deliver a measured volume of liquid between two calibration (or graduation) marks on the tube; has several graduation or calibration marks on the tube, allowing a variety of measurements with the same device.

Gram's staining reaction Using the Gram's staining method, microorganisms retaining the violet (purple) color of the primary stain (crystal violet–iodine complex) are considered Gram "positive"; microorganisms having the red-pink color of the counterstain (safranin) are considered Gram "negative." Use of these properties serves to classify or differentiate organisms in microbiology. Differential stain.

granulocyte Leukocyte that contains prominent cytoplasmic granules; neutrophils, eosinophils, and basophils.

gravimetric analysis Analysis by measurement of mass.

group A β-hemolytic Streptococcus Microorganism that accounts for most infectious "strep throat." Organism is isolated from throat swabs by one of several methods (e.g., culture plates, rapid slide agglutination procedures).

gum guaiac Phenolic compound that turns blue when oxidized. Commonly used as the chromogen in tests for the detection of occult blood in feces.

Hansel's stain Stain containing eosin and methylene blue; used to stain for the presence of eosinophils.

hardware Physical elements of a computer system (e.g., central processing unit, printer, terminal).

hazard identification system Provides in words, symbols, and pictures information on presence of potential laboratory materials considered hazardous (e.g., flammable, health risk, chemical reactivity).

Health Care Financing Administration (HCFA) Agency of the U.S. Department of Health and Human Services; regulates and administers funding under the Health Insurance for the Aged Act of 1965 (Medicare); regulates reimbursement for Medicare-related activities. Medicare and Medicaid amendments to the Social Security Act authorize the regulation of specific laboratory services if the government is authorized to pay for these services to the aging and needy population of the U.S.; HCFA coordinates its regulatory functions with the Centers for Disease Control (CDC).

hematocrit Ratio of packed red blood cell volume to whole blood volume, expressed as a percent or ratio unit.

hematopoiesis Blood cell production.

hematuria Presence of red blood cells in urine.

hemocytometer Counting chamber used to perform manual cell counts.

hemoglobin   Iron-containing protein portion of the red blood cells that carries oxygen to the tissues; four globin chains, each containing a heme moiety.

hemolysis   Rupture of the red cell membrane and release of hemoglobin into the suspending medium or plasma; the plasma or serum appears reddish. In blood banking, hemolysis is used as an indicator of an antigen-antibody reaction.

hemolysis, alpha   In microbiology, partial destruction (lysis) of red blood cells in a blood agar plate; greenish color appears around the bacterial colony producing the alpha hemolysin.

hemolysis, beta   In microbiology, complete destruction (lysis) of red blood cells around a colony on a blood agar plate; leads to a completely clear zone surrounding the colony producing the beta hemolysin.

hemophilia   Hereditary deficiency of plasma coagulation proteins; results in a varying degree of bleeding disorders, mild to severe, depending on the specific deficiency.

hemophilia A   Classic bleeder's disease; sex-linked deficiency of the coagulant component of factor VIII (antihemophilic factor); *see* Hemophilia.

hemophilia B, Christmas disease   Sex-linked deficiency of factor IX; *see* Hemophilia.

hemosiderin   Iron-containing granules that may occur in urine after a hemolytic episode. Stain blue with Prussian blue stain for iron.

hemostasis   Cessation of blood flow from an injured blood vessel, with final intent to stop the bleeding.

hepatitis B virus (HBV)   Virus that can be directly transmitted by the blood, causing hepatitis, an acute viral illness. Hepatitis is an inflammation of the liver that is endemic worldwide. Complete recovery is usual; some patients, however, remain carriers or can develop chronic hepatitis.

hepatitis C virus (HCV), also known as non-A, non-B hepatitis virus   Can be transmitted directly by the blood, causing acute viral hepatitis. This infection does not show the serologic markers of hepatitis A or hepatitis B.

heterophil antibodies   Antibodies stimulated by one antigen that react with entirely unrelated antigens on the red cells from different mammalian species.

high-power objective   Usually a ×40 magnification objective used for more detailed examination of wet preparations.

hospital information system (HIS)   Main hospital data base; contains the base of information about the patient established when the patient was first admitted or registered by the hospital or clinic. This data base can be accessed by the laboratory information system (LIS) as necessary.

human chorionic gonadotropin (hCG)   Hormone produced by the placenta during pregnancy; used as a base for most rapid pregnancy tests.

human immunodeficiency virus (HIV)   Virus that can be transmitted by the blood and some body fluids; can cause HIV infection or acquired immune deficiency syndrome (AIDS).

hyaluronate (hyaluronic acid)   High molecular weight mucopolysaccharide found in synovial fluid, responsible for its normal viscosity. Secreted by the synovial fluid cells that line the joint cavity.

hyperglycemia   High concentration of blood glucose.

I

immune response   Any reaction demonstrating specific antibody response to antigenic stimulus.

immunoassay   Assay utilizing antigen-antibody reactions to detect the presence of a specific analyte.

indwelling line   Device used to administer therapeutic products (e.g., fluids, medications, blood products) to patients over long periods. With careful training, it is also possible to collect blood samples from these lines. Also called vascular access devices (VAD).

in vitro antigen-antibody reactions   Reactions between antigens and antibodies in a test tube or on a slide (outside the living body; *in vitro* is a Latin term meaning "in glass").

infection control   Set policy or program within a health care institution to prevent exposure to biologic hazards.

infusion set   Allows collection of blood from patients with small, fragile, or rolling veins.

inoculating loop or needle   Metal loop or needle attached to a long handle, used to inoculate culture media with specimens or to transfer colonies for subculture. Metal loops must be flamed between uses. Disposable varieties of these loops are available.

input device   Any device allowing data or instructions to be placed into a computer system.

interfacing data   Communications link that allows the transfer of data between the user and the computer system or between another processor and the computer system.

internal standard   Chemical compound of known amount added to a specimen and carried through all steps of an analytical procedure to provide a basis for accurate quantitation, despite variations in the procedural steps; is similar chemically and structurally to the substance being assayed; frequently used in gas chromatography and high-pressure liquid chromatography assays.

International System of Units   (SI units, from Système International d'Unités); standard international language of measurement.

interpretive report   Reporting of laboratory results in a usable format, including information about reference ranges or flagging of abnormal values, so the physician can find the results for the requested analyses in an efficient, clear manner.

intrinsic system of coagulation   Utilization of plasma contact factors to initiate coagulation, beginning with the activation of factor XII; all necessary factors required are contained in the circulating blood.

ion-selective electrode   Indicator electrode used in potentiometry devices to respond to specific ions in the solution.

iris diaphragm   Part of the microscope located at the bottom of the Abbe condenser, under the lens but within the condenser body; controls the amount of light passing through the material under observation; can be opened or closed to adjust contrast by means of a lever.

J

jaundice   Increased concentration of bilirubin in the blood (serum) and accumulation of bilirubin pigment in the tissues.

Joint Commission on Accreditation of Healthcare Organizations (JCAHO)   Voluntary organization, not governmental, made up of representatives from various health care associations (e.g., hospital, physician, dentist). Mission of JCAHO is to enhance the quality of health care provided to the public, and the organization is dedicated to improving the process to carry out this mission. One important function of JCAHO is accreditation of U.S. hospitals. Standards and guidelines are set for hospitals, and accreditation is carried out and monitored through a continual process of site visits, surveys, and reports. The organization also monitors other health care facilities (e.g., mental health facilities, nursing homes, home health agencies, hospices, managed care, and ambulatory care organizations).

K

ketoacidosis   Acidosis resulting from the presence of increased ketone bodies.

ketosis   Increased concentration of ketones in blood and urine.

L

laboratory information system (LIS)   Computer system designed for use by the clinical laboratory; includes collection of patient information, generation of test results, assembly of data output, production of ancillary reports, and storage of data.

laboratory procedure manual   Collection of information about the specific procedures for all analytical assays performed by the laboratory; includes information about specimen requirements and special collection or processing details, test request information, procedural information (how to perform the test, reagents used for the assay, control specimens used), calibration of instruments, quality control data, details about reference values and reporting of results, and any information about bibliographic resources.

laboratory report   Information about results of various assays performed by the laboratory; should be presented in a usable format; *see* Interpretive report.

latex agglutination procedures   Particles of latex are used to visualize an antigen-antibody agglutination reaction; test latex particles are coated with a specific antibody and clump together (agglutinate) when the specific antigen is present in the specimen being assayed.

leukemia Progressive malignant disease of the blood-forming organs characterized by abnormal proliferation of leukocytes and their precursors in body tissues. Peripheral blood cells and bone marrow cells are changed quantitatively and qualitatively.

leukocyte White blood cell; one of formed elements found in peripheral blood.

leukocyte differential Classification and recorded percentage of various types of leukocytes as seen on a stained blood film or as obtained from an electronic counting device.

leukocyte esterase Enzyme present in the azurophilic or primary granules of the granulocytic leukocytes; presence of this enzyme in urine indicates urinary tract infection.

light-emitting diode (LED) Readout device found in digital computerized equipment; a semiconductor device visualized as a glowing readout.

linkage (linked genes) Genes for different traits located on the same chromosome, positioned so closely they are inherited as a unit.

lithiasis Kidney stone formation.

low-power objective Usually a ×10 magnification objective used for the initial scanning and observation in most microscopic work.

M

malabsorption Inadequate, incomplete, or impaired absorption from the gastrointestinal tract; may be associated with presence of increased fat in the feces.

material safety data sheet (MSDS) Information about the hazards of each chemical are provided by the supplier or manufacturer of the chemical; any hazardous chemicals used in a laboratory should be accompanied by this information.

measurement of mass Gravimetric analysis; commonly, measurement of weight using various types of balances for preparation of laboratory reagents and standard solutions.

meconium Viscid, elastic, greenish black material composed of amniotic fluid, biliary and intestinal secretions, and epithelial cells passed from the intestine by newborn infants within the first 24 hours after delivery.

melena Black or tarry fecal specimens; dark color is due to the presence of blood, which is changed to a black substance as it passes through the gastrointestinal tract.

metric system Traditional system of weights and measures based on a decimal system using divisions and multiples of tens; based on a standard unit of length, the meter.

microorganisms Microscopic organisms; organisms seen only with the use of a microscope (e.g., bacteria, viruses, fungi, protozoa).

microsampling Obtaining very small amounts of blood or other body specimens (e.g., capillary blood, cerebrospinal fluid); usually requires micromethods for assay.

minimal inhibitory concentration (MIC) Minimum concentration of antimicrobial agent needed to prevent visually discernible growth of a bacterial or fungal suspension.

molarity Gram molecular mass or weight of a compound per liter of solution.

monoclonal antibody Highly specified antibody derived entirely from a single ancestral antibody-forming parent cell. Produced by hybridization; used in diagnostic testing.

mycology Study or science of fungi.

N

National Bureau of Standards (NBS) Department of the U.S. government. Maintains and supplies standard reference materials needed for the preparation of primary standard solutions; develops reference methods and reference materials.

National Committee for Clinical Laboratory Standards (NCCLS) Nonprofit educational organization that sets voluntary consensus standards for all areas of clinical laboratories.

nephron Working unit of the kidney, where urine is formed; includes the glomerulus, Bowman's capsule, proximal and distal convoluted tubules, and loop of Henle.

95% confidence interval Numerical limits within which a sample must fall to be part of the normal distribution of values; determined statistically, and is the basis for quality control "rules" for the acceptance or rejection of certain results; based on a gaussian curve where 95% of the population have observations within ± 2 standard deviations.

nomenclature of blood clotting factors International Committee on Nomenclature of Blood Clotting Factors ascertains consistency in terminology used; standardizes the complex nomenclature for the various clotting factors.

nonglucose reducing substances (NGRS) Substances other than glucose (including several sugars) that may be present in the urine and which have the ability to reduce heavy metal from a higher to a lower oxidation state. NGRS are not detected by the reagent strip tests specific for glucose.

normality Number of equivalent weights per liter of solution.

numerical aperture Index or measurement of the resolving power of a microscope. Also an index of the light-gathering power of a lens that describes the amount of light entering the objective. As the numerical aperture increases, resolution decreases.

O

objective Major part of the magnification system of the microscope. Most commonly used microscopes have three objectives: low power, high power, and oil immersion. Usually mounted in a rotating nosepiece that enables a quick change of objectives.

occult blood Blood not observable by the naked eye, but requires use of a chemical test to be detected.

Occupational Health and Safety Act of 1970 (OSHA) Created the Occupational Health and Safety Administration within the U.S. Department of Labor to set levels of safety and health for all workers in the United States. A federal agency.

oil-immersion objective Generally a $\times 100$ magnification lens with a relatively short working distance of 1.8 mm. Requires the addition of a special immersion oil placed between the objective and the slide or cover glass. Cannot be used with wet preparations.

optical density Term used to express the amount of light being absorbed when being passed through a solution; *see* Absorbed light.

osmolarity Number of osmoles of solute per liter of solution.

osmotic fragility Test to determine the ability of the red blood cells to withstand hypotonic or hypo-osmotic solutions. Measure of the resistance of the red cell membrane to rupture; cells with membrane defects (hereditary spherocytosis) have increased fragility.

output device Any device that allows information generated by a computer system to be used (e.g., results of calculations for a laboratory assay). Information output can be printed, displayed, or transferred to another processor.

oval fat body (OFB), renal tubular fat (RTF) bodies Renal epithelial cell (and possibly macrophage) filled with fat droplets.

P

parasitology Study or science of parasites.

Patient's Bill of Rights Document drawn up by health care institutions that declares certain rights for all patients being cared for in that facility. Being considerate of these rights constitutes good patient care. In the laboratory context, the Patient's Bill of Rights must be considered when collecting the various patient specimens needed for testing.

percent solution Somewhat outdated expression of concentration based on parts per hundred parts (e.g., 10% sodium chloride, which is 10 gm NaCl diluted to 100 mL with deionized water; currently expressed as 10 gm/dL).

percent transmittance Amount of light that passes through a colored solution compared with the amount of light that passes through a blank solution.

pericardial fluid Extravascular fluid that surrounds the heart.

peripheral blood film Blood smear prepared on a glass microscope slide using circulating peripheral, blood. Blood usually obtained by venipuncture or finger puncture.

peritoneal fluid Extravascular fluid that surrounds the abdominal and pelvic cavities.

peroxidase Enzyme that catalyzes release of free oxygen from hydrogen peroxide. Peroxidase activity of the heme portion of the hemoglobin molecule is the basis of the reagent strip tests for blood.

Petri dish or plate Shallow, flat glass or plastic plate with a loose-fitting deep cover, used to hold culture media.

pH Unit that describes the acidity or alkalinity of a solution.

phase contrast microscope Microscope illumination system that uses a special condenser with an annular diaphragm with a matched absorption ring in the corresponding objective. Used to give additional contrast in wet preparations; especially useful for counting platelets and observing urinary sediment.

phenotype Observable genetic makeup that can be determined by direct testing (i.e., blood type).

phlebotomist Person trained in drawing blood. Primarily trained to draw blood by venipuncture, but also trained to perform capillary collections and to do skin punctures of various types. Drawing blood specimens from indwelling lines is an additional technique performed by a trained phlebotomist.

photoelectric cell, photodetector Electronic device that measures the amount of light intensity being transmitted by a solution; produces electrons in proportion to the amount of light reaching it.

photometry Process of measuring the amount of light intensity using a specific device such as a spectrophotometer or colorimeter.

physical properties In urinalysis, color, transparency, odor, foam, and specific gravity of a urine specimen.

plasma Liquid portion of blood after it has been anticoagulated and centrifuged or otherwise allowed to settle.

plasma cell, plasmacyte Derivative of the B lymphocyte. Large, with a round or oval eccentric nucleus. Specialized for production of antibodies; rarely is seen in the peripheral blood.

plasmin Proteolytic enzyme that breaks down fibrin; is generated by the activation of a plasma precursor, plasminogen.

platelet adhesiveness, platelet retention Test that measures the ability of platelets to adhere to glass surfaces.

platelet aggregation Massing or clumping of platelets; test for platelet function.

platelet plug Formation of an aggregate or mass of platelets that physically plug or slow down the flow of blood at the site of an injury to a blood vessel.

pleural fluid Extravascular fluid that surrounds the lungs.

pluripotential stem cell (PSC) Stem cell that is uncommitted to any specific cell line; stimulation results in differentiation and maturation.

polarizing microscope Microscope illumination system that employs two crossed polarizing lenses, extinguishing the passage of light through the microscope. Used to detect objects or crystals that bend or polarize light, making them visible when viewed with crossed polarizing filters.

porphobilinogen An unstable intermediary product in the synthesis of heme; a significant increase in the urine can be seen in acute intermittent hepatic porphyria.

potentiometry Technique in which the potential difference between two electrodes is measured under equilibrium.

precipitation Visible result of an antigen-antibody reaction between a soluble antigen and its specific antibody.

precision, reproducibility Measure of the closeness of the results obtained when repeating the analysis on the same sample; agreement between replicate measurements.

proficiency testing Program under which samples are sent to a group of laboratories for analysis; results are compared with those of other laboratories participating in the program. Included as a component of quality assurance programs.

program Set of commands or steps that instruct the computer to perform a certain task.

proportion Two or more ratios having the same relative meaning but with different numbers.

protective isolation Measures used to protect the patient from infectious agents.

protein error of pH indicators Color change of a pH indicator due to the presence of protein rather than hydrogen ion concentration.

proteinuria Presence of protein, usually albumin, in urine.

prothrombin, coagulation factor II, prethrombin
Produced by the liver; is vitamin K–dependent.

pure culture Culture in which each colony is from a single isolated originating bacterial cell.

pyuria Presence of pus (leukocytes) in the urine; indicates a possible urinary tract infection.

Q

quality assurance "Comprehensive set of policies, procedures, and practices necessary to make sure that the laboratory's results are reliable. QA includes record keeping, calibration and maintenance of equipment, quality control, proficiency testing, and training."*

quality assurance program Plan to carry out policies and practices necessary to comply with quality assurance standards set by accreditation agencies to make certain that the laboratory's results are reliable and that these results are used in the best interest of the patient.

quality control "Set of laboratory procedures designed to ensure that the test method is working properly and that the results meet the diagnostic needs of the physician. QC includes testing control samples, charting the results, and analyzing them statistically."*

quality control chart Visual documentation of information derived from using control specimens; values for control specimen assays used for a particular substance are plotted on the chart on a regular basis and are statistically analyzed for trends of change.

quality control program Plan to carry out procedures established to make certain that laboratory assay methods are working properly and that the assay results meet the diagnostic needs of the physician; makes use of control specimens and standard solutions.

quantitative transfer Process of transferring the entire amount of a weighed or measured substance from one vessel to another; usually used in the process of reagent preparation where the weighed substance (chemical) must be transferred in its entirety

*NCCLS: *Tentative Guidelines: Physician's Office Laboratory Procedure Manual,* Glossary of Common Laboratory Terms, POL2-T, 9:5, Villanova, PA, National Committee for Clinical Laboratory Standards, 1989.

to a volumetric flask for dilution with deionized water.

quantitative urine culture method Traditional method of detecting urinary tract infection in which urine is cultured on an appropriate media and identified.

R

random access analyzer Instrument that does all the selected determinations on one sample before going on to the next sample.

random access memory (RAM) Central memory in the central processing unit (CPU) of a computer; commonly used as a means of storage of information that is frequently altered, changed, or updated.

rapid streptococcal antigen detection Basis for rapid tests in the presence of the specific streptococcal antigen, present in the causative organism for "strep throat," group A β-hemolytic streptococci.

ratio Amount of something in proportion to an amount of something else; always describes a relative amount.

reagin antibodies Antibody-like proteins that react in some serologic tests for syphilis.

red blood cell indices In hematology, the calculated values for red cell measurements, such as mean cell volume (MCV), mean cell hemoglobin (MCH), and mean cell hemoglobin concentration (MCHC).

reference range, normal range, normal values, reference values Range of values that includes 95% of the test results for a healthy reference population.

refractometer Temperature-compensated instrument used to measure refractive index.

relative centrifugal force (RCF) Expression of the number of revolutions per minute and the centrifugal force generated; method of comparing the forces generated by various centrifuges, taking into account the speed of rotation and the radius from the center of rotation.

reliability Ability of a laboratory assay to produce consistent results when testing is repeated successively.

renal threshold Level above which the substance cannot be reabsorbed by the renal tubules and is thus excreted into the urine.

resolution   Limit of usable magnification; tells how small and how close individual objects can be and still be recognized.

reticulocyte   Young red blood cell that has just extruded its nucleus. Characterized by the presence of RNA; becomes a normal, mature red cell when all the RNA is lost; stains with a supravital stain.

Rh immune globulin (RhIG)   Concentrated and purified form of anti-D antibody, used to immunosupress Rh negative women who deliver Rh positive babies, to prevent sensitization of the mother by her child's red blood cells.

Rh negative   Red blood cells lacking the D antigen (d/d).

Rh positive   Red blood cells containing the D antigen (D/D or D/d).

rheostat   Control used to adjust the amount of light entering the microscope.

rheumatoid factor (RF)   Autoantibodies present in the serum of patients with clinical features of rheumatoid arthritis; circulating complexes of immunoglobulins, known collectively as rheumatoid factor.

round off   Bring the digit (number) to the chosen number of significant figures.

S

safety manual   Current compilation of all safety practices and procedures, kept in a readily available format for the use by all persons in the specific laboratory setting; anything that could pose a potential safety hazard for persons in the laboratory must be described in this manual.

sediment   Solid material that has settled out of suspension (e.g., urinary sediment).

sensitivity to antimicrobial agents   Ability of certain antibiotics (antimicrobial agent) to inhibit the growth of an organism.

sensitization   Process in which an individual is made sensitive to a foreign antigen through exposure. Once sensitization has occurred, the individual responds to a repeated exposure with an accentuated immune response.

serial dilution   Progressive dilution of a substance in a series of tubes in predetermined ratios to give concentrations of a specific amount.

serous fluid   Fluid within the closed cavities of the body (e.g., pleural, pericardial, peritoneal).

serum   Liquid portion of plasma that remains after the clot is removed. Preferable to plasma when typing or otherwise testing blood for compatibility.

serum separator gel   Additive used to assist in obtaining serum after centrifuging a whole blood specimen. A special silicon gel layer is added to the collection tubes that moves to form a barrier between the cells and serum during centrifugation; the gel hardens to form an inert barrier, allowing easy serum separation or removal after the centrifugation process.

sharps container   Used disposable needles and other sharp objects must be safely discarded in these containers, which are made of rigid plastic, metal, or stiff paperboard. The containers must be conveniently located, easily recognizable, and marked as a biohazard. All skin lancets, needles, scalpel blades, and bleeding time devices must be discarded properly in a sharps container, with extreme caution.

significant figure   Digits of whole numbers or in decimal form, beginning with the leftmost nonzero digit and extending to the right; numbers should contain only digits necessary for the precision of the determination or measurement; the digits of a number that are known to be reliable.

simple stain   One stain that colors everything in the cell the same color.

software   Series of instructions or commands that direct the operation of the computer system.

specific gravity   Ratio of the density of a solution compared with the density of an equal volume of water at a constant temperature; depends on the weight and number of particles in a solution.

spectrophotometer   Device that quantitatively provides the relationship between the intensity of the colors of an unknown solution and that of the standard solution.

spectrophotometry   Quantitative measuring technique in which the color of a solution of an unknown concentration is compared with the color of a similar substance of known concentration.

standard curve   Plotting of percent transmission or absorbance readings on graph paper for several known standard solutions of varying concentrations will enable construction of a "standard curve" for a particular assay.

standard deviation (SD) Statistical measurement of the degree of variation from the mean of a series of measurements; measure of the precision or reproducibility.

standard solution Reference material that is of fixed and known chemical composition of the substance being assayed and can be prepared in a pure form for use in the laboratory; certified reference material that is generally accepted or officially recognized as the unique standard for the assay regardless of the purity of the analyte content.

steatorrhea Presence or increased quantities of fat in the feces.

stercobilin Pigment derived from bilirubin; responsible for normal color of the feces.

streak plate Culture plate prepared by inoculating so as to spread out colonies as much as possible, so that single, isolated colonies may be observed after incubation.

synovial fluid Extravascular fluid that surrounds the joints of the body.

syringe and needle collection system Separate syringes and needles of appropriate size and gauge are used to collect some blood specimens. Blood in the syringe is carefully added to the appropriate collection tube containing the necessary additive.

T

T lymphocyte Blood cell that matures in the thymus; functions in cell-mediated responses; makes up the majority of the lymphocytes in the peripheral blood.

Tamm-Horsfall protein Mucoprotein secreted by the renal tubular cells and not derived from the blood plasma. This protein forms the matrix of urinary casts.

therapeutic drug monitoring Testing of blood level of a drug to monitor or keep track of its medical effectiveness in treatment of a disease.

thin-layer chromatography Method of chromatography often used to do therapeutic drug monitoring tests; stationary phase is a thin layer of an adsorbent coated on a glass plate or sheet of plastic, the mobile phase is a solvent or a solvent mixture.

throat swab Sterile fibrous material (commonly dacron or rayon) fixed to a stick; used to collect material from the back of the throat for culture or rapid detection tests for diagnosis of "strep throat."

thrombin Activated form of factor II that acts as a serine proteolytic enzyme to cleave fibrinogen and form fibrin; is a reagent to test platelet aggregation.

thrombocyte, platelet One of the formed elements in the peripheral blood; chief function is its role in coagulation of blood.

thromboplastin Substance with ability to convert prothrombin to thrombin.

timed urine collection Urine collected over time (e.g., 2, 12, or 24 hours). Collection commonly is preserved by refrigeration between voidings, and is used when a quantitative assay is needed. It is important to adhere to specific time requirements and be certain that the collection time is noted on the container. Entire timed collection must be sent to the laboratory in the container.

titration Quantitative volumetric technique of measuring the concentration of an unknown solution by comparing it with a measured volume of a solution of known concentration.

to-contain pipette Pipette calibrated to contain a specific amount of liquid; to assure that all the liquid is emptied from the pipette, it must be rinsed well with a diluting solution.

to-deliver pipette Pipette calibrated to deliver a specified volume when filled properly and the liquid is allowed to drain completely into a receiving vessel.

tolerance Form of resistance to an antimicrobial agent.

torsion balance Laboratory balance commonly used to weigh chemicals; is assembled as a single flexible structure by means of highly tensed torsion bands of watch-spring alloy; has no knife edges to dull, or other loose parts.

tourniquet Elastic strip or cuff that can be tightened when applied around the arm, usually just above the elbow; allows the vein to become more prominent so that venipuncture can be more easily done.

toxicology Study of the origin, nature, and effects of poison. Toxicologic analyses are used to detect the amounts of substances that could be poisonous or toxic at certain concentrations.

transfusion reaction Any adverse effect of transfusion; generally characterized as hemolytic, febrile, allergic, or circulatory overload.

transmitted light Light that is not absorbed.

transudate Formation of an effusion as the result of filtration through a membrane.

triple-beam balance, "trip" balance Three-beamed balance. Each beam provides a different weighing scale; scales are provided with movable weights. Used commonly in preparation of laboratory reagents.

typing Testing of suspensions of red cells with known antibody solutions (antisera) to determine the identity of antigens, known as the blood type.

U

ultrafiltrate of plasma Filtrate of plasma over a membrane, where extremely small particles such as proteins are restricted, or not filtered.

unconjugated bilirubin, indirect bilirubin, free bilirubin Water-insoluble form of bilirubin that is formed as a breakdown product from heme by the reticuloendothelial system and carried in the bloodstream bound to albumin. Due to its insolubility, this form cannot be excreted by the kidney or found in the urine.

unexpected antibody Antibody that results from specific antigenic stimulus. In blood banking, the result of stimulation from pregnancy, transfusion, or injection of red cells. Also referred to as an immune antibody.

universal precautions Recommended safety policies used for handling *all* biologic (patient) specimens. Potential infectivity of any patient's blood or body fluids is unknown; therefore all blood and body substances (fluids) are considered equally infectious.

Unopette system Commercially available disposable self-filling pipette and diluent-reservoir system used to measure and dilute blood for testing purposes.

urinary system Consists of two kidneys and two ureters plus the bladder and urethra.

urine Fluid composed of the waste materials of blood; formed in the kidney and excreted from the body by way of the urinary system.

urobilinogen Group of colorless chromogens formed in the intestine by the reduction of bilirubin by bacteria present in the normal bacterial flora; normal product of bilirubin metabolism.

V

vacuum tube and needle collection system Blood collection system consisting of evacuated collection tubes with appropriate additives, double-ended needles, and needle holders; allows blood collection directly from the vein into the tube.

vascular access device (VAD) Device or indwelling line used to administer therapeutic products over a long period; *see* Indwelling line.

venipuncture Process of collecting blood from a vein.

virology Study or science of viruses; in the context of this textbook, the study of viruses that cause human disease.

visual colorimetry Determination or comparison of color intensity of a solution by use of the human eye; has all but been replaced by photoelectric colorimetry and spectrophotometry instrumentation.

voided midstream urine specimen Noncatheterized urine specimen collected after the first few milliliters have been deposited in the urinal or toilet; the urine is free-flowing, and the midportion of the collection is saved in a specimen container.

volume per unit volume Measured volume of a liquid added to a specific volume of another liquid.

volumetric glassware Glassware that has been manufactured of good-quality glass and calibrated under strict conditions to hold, contain, or deliver a specific volume of liquid (e.g., volumetric pipette, flask, buret).

volumetric pipette Extremely accurate, single-line pipette used to measure specimens, controls, and standard solutions, or anything requiring precise measurement.

W

wavelength of light Linear distance traveled by one complete wave cycle of a particular beam of radiant energy.

wet reagent chemistry Assay utilizing wet reagents. Traditional manual chemistry assays use wet reagent chemistry. Compare with dry reagent technology.

Wright's stain A mixture of eosin and methylene blue used to observe cellular morphology of blood cells when examining blood films; a polychromatic Romanovsky-type stain.

Wright-Giemsa stain Variation of Wright's stain. See Wright's stain.

X

xanthochromia Yellowish discoloration used to describe the supernatant spinal or other serous fluid, indicating the presence of previous hemorrhage. Strictly speaking, xanthochromia produces a yellow color; however, the term is applied to pale pink to orange or yellow when describing fluids.

Index